Procedures and Protocols
in the Neurocritical Care Unit

Niraj Arora
Editor

Procedures and Protocols in the Neurocritical Care Unit

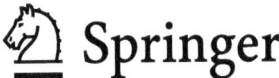

Editor
Niraj Arora
Department of Neurology
University of Missouri School of Medicine
Columbia, MO, USA

ISBN 978-3-030-90224-7   ISBN 978-3-030-90225-4 (eBook)
https://doi.org/10.1007/978-3-030-90225-4

© The Editor(s) (if applicable) and The Author(s), under exclusive license to Springer Nature Switzerland AG 2022
This work is subject to copyright. All rights are solely and exclusively licensed by the Publisher, whether the whole or part of the material is concerned, specifically the rights of translation, reprinting, reuse of illustrations, recitation, broadcasting, reproduction on microfilms or in any other physical way, and transmission or information storage and retrieval, electronic adaptation, computer software, or by similar or dissimilar methodology now known or hereafter developed.
The use of general descriptive names, registered names, trademarks, service marks, etc. in this publication does not imply, even in the absence of a specific statement, that such names are exempt from the relevant protective laws and regulations and therefore free for general use.
The publisher, the authors and the editors are safe to assume that the advice and information in this book are believed to be true and accurate at the date of publication. Neither the publisher nor the authors or the editors give a warranty, expressed or implied, with respect to the material contained herein or for any errors or omissions that may have been made. The publisher remains neutral with regard to jurisdictional claims in published maps and institutional affiliations.

This Springer imprint is published by the registered company Springer Nature Switzerland AG
The registered company address is: Gewerbestrasse 11, 6330 Cham, Switzerland

This book is dedicated to

Patients, who trust me to help them get better during difficult times,

Students, residents and fellows who inspired me to write this book,

My parents, who made me capable for my endeavours,

My wife and kids, for their unconditional love and support, without which this project would not have been complete!

Foreword

Dr. Arora has edited a practical, daily use excellent text on neurocritical care. I am delighted to review and provide an overview of this book. The state-of-the-art text is dedicated to current status of knowledge and management in neuroscience ICUs. The book includes coverage of both procedures and protocols being carried out in neuroscience ICU.

Each chapter focuses on one particular procedure or protocol and provides up-to-date knowledge about that topic. Dedicated chapters on the procedures both invasive and noninvasive for the care of the critically sick and protocols for important pathologies that one deals practically – to have all this in one place is a boon in itself during the crucial time of patient management.

This methodological approach with due consideration and review of each procedure and protocols related to the daily functioning and management in a neurocritical care ICU is a significant plus. I'm delighted with the format of this book. The breadth of the field of neurocritical care is wide, and with the developing new technological advancement, it is essential to know the basics as well as be up to date with the recent updates. The time available to the physician in training or service is limited, and the book covers all the important topics which a physician in training would deal in day-to-day practice and could serve as the best aid. Furthermore, the knowledge of the authors is clearly displayed by the quality of the content and undoubtedly will be picked up by the readers too.

I feel this will be very useful for day-to-day management in neuroscience ICUs by physicians, residents and fellows, nurse practitioners, and all others involved in care of patients with neurocritical issues anywhere. Whether at bedside or reading for reference, this book would be useful. It is rare to find such a book which could cover this wide range of topics and still keep focus on what it is important to the intensivist. This book will serve as a handy reference.

I commend Dr Niraj Arora and other contributors to this text for writing a hands-on manual for daily neuroscience ICU working!

Pradeep Sahota, MD, FAAN, FANA, FAASM
Professor & Chairman, Department of Neurology
University of Missouri – School of Medicine, University of Missouri Health Care
Columbia, MO, USA

Preface

Practice of Neurocritical care is an art and science. The sooner you realise, the better you become at it!

The field of Neurocritical Care is expanding leaps and bounds. With the abundance of knowledge about this exciting field, one is faced with a constant challenge to keep up with the pace of learning new things and keeping the basics of the understanding of disease pathology. As a resident, I struggled to procure a resource which could provide me with the knowledge of all essential materials which I will be dealing with during rotations of critical care, especially neurocritical care. There are a number of books in the market available which could provide you with the knowledge about the pathophysiology, diagnosis, and management of neurocritical care conditions. However, when it comes to the mind of a resident, they need some resources which could cover all the important procedures as well as the protocols which one could be potentially using during their rotation while taking care of the critically ill patient. This book has come as a dream project when I got the opportunity to work at the University of Missouri, Columbia. No work is accomplished without hard work and perseverance. This holds true for writing a book for sure. From the original thought to the writing of this preface has been a journey for me. Trying to catch up with the management of critically ill patients in neuroscience ICU and finishing up the write up of the chapters, working with residents and fellows, and coordinating with the publication staff, these all have been a wonderful experience.

The purpose of this book is to guide the physician about the procedures that are worth learning for the neurocritical care unit as a neurointensivist. Some of the procedures have been written by the experts in their own fields; however, the procedures could and should be learnt and performed in the neurosciences ICU. The neurocritical care curriculum mentions all these procedures which are included in this book. As the field expands and with technological advancements, certain procedures like tracheostomy and gastrostomy might be performed at the bedside by the intensivist. This might be an added advantage to the patient as well as hospital as significant resources and time are spent during the patient transport and those resources could be allocated for other reasons. The book will not only help the students, residents, or fellows but also anyone including nurse practitioners, advanced practice providers, and any interested person who wants to learn the principles of the critical care procedures and have an understanding of the management of diversified pathologies in neurosciences ICU.

The protocols mentioned in this book are being constantly used practically for the decision management of the patients. Since there is a significant practice variability based on the level of experience of the treating intensivist, the protocols serve as a basic structure which can guide the treatment. We are still not at the level where personalised treatment approaches could be provided, even though a lot of efforts are being made to tailor the treatment based on underlying genetic makeup of a patient and the use of artificial intelligence. Nevertheless, none of the advancements can replace a good bedside neurological exam, and the protocols mentioned in this book are based on the day-to-day experience and practice. The evidence for the protocols has been included in the references, and interested readers should practice the protocols in patient management and get additional help by using the references provided.

The goal of the book is to generate interest for the budding independent providers for the procedures in critical care practice as well as to make the management of critically ill patients less daunting when sometimes a single provider needs to take care of multiple patients at night (a common practice at some academic centres). "A life saved is a life gifted" – with the correct timely, vigilant management decisions and proper judicious monitoring, one could save someone's loved one. The tremendous joy that as a provider one might experience is when you manage the patient who otherwise would not have been salvaged without your due diligence.

With a strong belief that the first edition of this book will serve as the basis for the upcoming editions, I consider this as my small effort to educate. I hope that the book can become an essential guide during the rotations in the neurosciences ICU.

Columbia, MO, USA   Niraj Arora, MD

Acknowledgements

The book is a tireless effort on the part of many students, residents, fellows, and colleagues who have taken time from their schedules not just to shape this work but also making sure that the work is up to the mark. Special thanks to Dr. Pradeep Sahota for his constant encouragement and support.

Word of special thanks to the Springer Project coordinators, Abha Krishnan and Marie Felina Francois, who have been patiently working with me throughout the production of the book.

Contents

Part I Procedures

Vascular Access.   3
Niraj Arora and Shivangi Singh

Pulmonary Artery Catheters. 27
Taishi Hirai, John E. A. Blair, and Arun Kumar

Arterial Catheters. 39
Taishi Hirai, John E. A. Blair, and Arun Kumar

Airway Access. 43
Mohammed Alnijoumi

Thoracocentesis 103
Salman Ahmad

Chest Tube Thoracostomy. 113
Salman Ahmad

Pericardiocentesis. 125
Taishi Hirai, Bhradeev Sivasambu, and John E. A. Blair

Paracentesis. 137
Naren Nallapeta, Harleen Chela, and Yezaz A. Ghouri

**Lumbar Puncture and Intrathecal
Drug Administration** 157
Clayton Reece Burgoon, Will Bryan,
and Ambarish P. Bhat

Intracranial Access 173
Michael Ortiz Torres and Steven B. Carr

Point of Care Ultrasound 195
Armin Krvavac, Ramya Gorthi, Jennifer Minoff,
and Rajamurugan Subramaniyam

Transcranial Doppler Ultrasound. 241
Nanda Thimmappa

Cervical Traction. 265
Michael Ortiz Torres and Steven B. Carr

Part II Protocols

Sedation and Analgesia Management 277
Kathryn E. Qualls and Francisco E. Gomez

Intracranial Hypertension in Intensive Care Unit 289
Niraj Arora and Chandra Shekar Pingili

**Sepsis and Fever in the Neuro-Critical Care
Unit (NCCU)** 317
Chandra Shekar Pingili and Niraj Arora

Status Epilepticus 365
Kunal Bhatia and Komal Ashraf

Targeted Temperature Management 395
Francisco E. Gomez, Jesyree Veitia,
and David Convissar

Mechanical Ventilation and Weaning In ICU 411
Tijo Thomas, Ephrem Teklemariam,
and Chitra Sivasankar

Tracheostomy Care. 427
Mohammed Alnijoumi and Troy Whitacre

Hemodynamic Monitoring 445
Kia Ghiassi, Premkumar Nattanmai, and Niraj Arora

Endotracheal Intubation via Direct Laryngoscopy 497
Jonathan F. Ang and Blaine Michael Winterton

Vasospasm 509
Chandra Shekar Pingili and Niraj Arora

Phenobarbital for Alcohol Withdrawal Syndrome 535
Carly M. Guay and Kathryn E. Qualls

Diabetic Ketoacidosis and Hyperglycemia 549
Muhammad Waqar Salam and John Liu

Electrolyte Management 565
Kathryn E. Qualls and Niraj Arora

Plasmapheresis 579
Zeeshan Azeem, Angela Emanuel, and Kunal Malhotra

Intravenous Immunoglobulin 601
Biswajit Banik and Niraj Arora

Brain Death..617
Kunal Bhatia and Niraj Arora

Continuous Renal Replacement Therapy 649
Zeeshan Azeem, Angela Emanuel, and Kunal Malhotra

Delirium..679
Arpit Aggarwal and Oluwole Popoola

Index...695

Contributors

Arpit Aggarwal, MD Clinical Psychiatry, University of Missouri, Columbia, MO, USA

Salman Ahmad, MD, FACS, FCCM Division of Acute Care Surgery, University of Missouri Health, Columbia, MO, USA

Mohammed Alnijoumi, MD, FCCP Department of Medicine, University of Missouri, Columbia, MO, USA

Jonathan F. Ang, MD Division of Pulmonary, Critical Care and Environmental Medicine, University of Missouri, Columbia, MO, USA

Niraj Arora, MD Department of Neurology- Neurocriticalcare unit, University of Missouri, Columbia, MO, USA

Komal Ashraf, DO Department of Neurology, University of Missouri, Columbia, MO, USA

Zeeshan Azeem, MD Karl D Nolph Division of Nephrology, University of Missouri, School of Medicine, Columbia, MO, USA

Biswajit Banik, MD Department of Neurology, University of Missouri, Columbia, MO, USA

Ambarish P. Bhat, MD Department of Radiology, University of Missouri, Columbia, MO, USA

Kunal Bhatia, MD Department of Neurology, Division of Neurocritical Care, Washington University School of Medicine, St. Louis, MO, USA

John E. A. Blair, MD Department of Medicine, Division of Cardiology, University of Chicago, Chicago, IL, USA

Will Bryan, RRA Department of Radiology, University of Missouri, Columbia, MO, USA

Clayton Reece Burgoon, MSRS, RRA, RT(R) Department of Radiology, University of Missouri, Columbia, MO, USA

Steven B. Carr, MD Division of Neurosurgery, University of Missouri School of Medicine, Columbia, MO, USA

Harleen Chela, MD Department of Medicine, Division of Gastroenterology & Hepatology, University of Missouri School of Medicine, Columbia, MO, USA

David Convissar, MD Harvard University, Boston, MA, USA

Angela Emanuel, MBBS, FCPS Karl D Nolph Division of Nephrology, University of Missouri, School of Medicine, Columbia, MO, USA

Kia Ghiassi, DO Department of Neurology, University of Missouri, Columbia, MO, USA

Yezaz A. Ghouri, MD Department of Medicine, Division of Gastroenterology & Hepatology, University of Missouri School of Medicine, Columbia, MO, USA

Francisco E. Gomez, MD Pharmacy Department, University of Missouri Health Care, Columbia, MO, USA

Department of Neurology, University of Missouri Health Care, Columbia, MO, USA

Ramya Gorthi, MD Department of Internal Medicine, Saint Louis University School of Medicine, St. Louis, MO, USA

Carly M. Guay, PharmD Pharmacy Department, University of Missouri Health Care, Columbia, MO, USA

Contributors xxi

Taishi Hirai, MD Department of Medicine, Division of Cardiology, University of Missouri, Columbia, MO, USA

Armin Krvavac, MD Department of Internal Medicine, Saint Louis University School of Medicine, St. Louis, MO, USA

Arun Kumar, MD Department of Medicine, Division of Cardiology, University of Missouri, Columbia, MO, USA

John Liu, MD Division of Endocrinology, Diabetes and Metabolism, Department of Internal Medicine, University of Missouri, Columbia, MO, USA

Kunal Malhotra, MD Karl D Nolph Division of Nephrology, University of Missouri, School of Medicine, Columbia, MO, USA

Jennifer Minoff, MD Department of Internal Medicine, Saint Louis University School of Medicine, St. Louis, MO, USA

Naren Nallapeta, MD State University of New York, Buffalo, NY, USA

Premkumar Nattanmai, MD Department of Neurology, University of Missouri, Columbia, MO, USA

Chandra Shekar Pingili, MD Dayton Lung and Sleep Medicine, Inc, Dayton, OH, USA

Department of Neurocritical Care, University of Missouri, Columbia, MO, USA

Oluwole Popoola, MD, MPH Clinical Psychiatry, University of Missouri, Columbia, MO, USA

Kathryn E. Qualls, PharmD, BCPS, BCCCP Pharmacy Department, University of Missouri Health Care, Columbia, MO, USA

Muhammad Waqar Salam, MD Division of Endocrinology, Diabetes and Metabolism, Department of Internal Medicine, University of Missouri, Columbia, MO, USA

Shivangi Singh, MD Department of Neurology, University of Missouri School of Medicine, Columbia, MO, USA

Bhradeev Sivasambu, MD Department of Medicine, Division of Cardiology, University of Missouri, Columbia, MO, USA

Chitra Sivasankar, MD Division of Anesthesiology/Neurosurgery, Thomas Jefferson University, Philadelphia, PA, USA

Rajamurugan Subramaniyam, MD Department of Internal Medicine, Saint Louis University School of Medicine, St. Louis, MO, USA

Ephrem Teklemariam, MD Thomas Jefferson University, Philadelphia, PA, USA

Nanda Thimmappa, MD University of Missouri, Columbia, MO, USA

Tijo Thomas, MD Thomas Jefferson University, Philadelphia, PA, USA

Michael Ortiz Torres, MD Division of Neurosurgery, University of Missouri School of Medicine, Columbia, MO, USA

Jesyree Veitia, MD Yale University, New Haven, CT, USA

Troy Whitacre, RRT, RRT-ACCS Respiratory Care Services, MU Health Care, Columbia, MO, USA

Blaine Michael Winterton, DO Department of Medicine, University of Missouri, Columbia, MO, USA

Part I
Procedures

Vascular Access

Niraj Arora and Shivangi Singh

1 Peripheral Vascular Catheters

1.1 Introduction

Peripheral access is achieved with peripheral intravenous catheters (PIVCs), midline catheters and peripherally inserted central lines (PICCs). Choosing among them depends on the specific indications, anticipated length of insertion and patient comorbidities.

Catheters are typically either derived from silicone or polyurethane with similar overall rates of complications for both in peripheral lines. The major difference noted between the two catheters is increased incidence of mechanical phlebitis in polyurethane catheters, given stiffer material [1]. These catheters come in different sizes depending on the outer diameter and the flow rate. The gauge system developed in Birmingham

---

N. Arora (✉)
Department of Neurology- Neurocriticalcare unit, University of Missouri, Columbia, MO, USA
e-mail: arorana@health.missouri.edu

S. Singh
Department of Neurology, University of Missouri School of Medicine, Columbia, MO, USA

© The Author(s), under exclusive license to Springer Nature Switzerland AG 2022
N. Arora (ed.), *Procedures and Protocols in the Neurocritical Care Unit*, https://doi.org/10.1007/978-3-030-90225-4_1

which was originally used for sizing the iron wires and later adapted for hollow needles and catheters is widely prevalent. Even though it does not correlate well with the outer diameter this system is commonly used in the peripheral vascular catheters. French system of catheter sizing is more systematic and simple. With the increase of one French unit, there is an increase of 0.33 mm in outer diameter. Most common vascular catheters range between 4 to 10 French in size. This system is commonly used for multi lumen catheters or speciality catheters (Table 1).

TABLE I Vascular catheters

Peripheral vascular catheters

Gauge size	Outside Diameters (mm)	
12	2.64	
14	2.03	
16	1.62	
19	1.22	
18	1.02	
20	0.91	Length varies from 3 to 5 cm
21	0.81	
22	0.71	
23	0.61	
24	0.56	
25	0.5	
26	0.45	

TABLE 1 (continued)

Midline catheters

Size (French)	Length (cm)	Number of lumens
4	8–20 cm	1–2
5	8–20 cm	1–2

PICC catheters

Size (French)	Length (cm)	Number of lumens	Gauge size	Flow rate (L/h)
5	50	Single	16	1.75
5	70	Single	16	1.3
5	50	Distal	18	0.58
		Proximal	20	0.16
5	70	Distal	18	0.44
		Proximal	20	0.12

Central venous catheters

Size (French)	Length (cm)	Number of lumens	Lumen size (Gauge)	Flow rate (L/h)
7	16	Distal	16	3.4
		Middle	18	1.8
		Proximal	18	1.9
7	20	Distal	16	3.1
		Middle	18	1.5
		Proximal	18	1.6
7	30	Distal	16	2.3
		Middle	18	1
		Proximal	18	1.1

(continued)

TABLE 1 (continued)

Hemodialysis catheters

Size (French)	Length (cm)	Number of Lumens	Lumen size	Flow rate (L/h)
12	16	Proximal	12	23.7
		Distal	12	17.4
12	20	Proximal	16	19.8
		Distal	12	15.5

It is essential to know that flow (Q) through a hollow rigid tube is directly proportional to the pressure gradient (ΔP) and inversely proportional to resistance. ($Q = \Delta P \times 1/R$). Also according to the Hagen-Poiseuille equation, flow (Q) is directly proportional to the fourth power of the inner radius of the tube (r^4) and inversely proportional to the length of the tube (L).

$$\text{Hagen Poiseuille equation}: Q = P \times \left(\pi r^4 / 8\mu L\right)$$

This equation influences the flow rate of the catheters. With increase in the inner radius of the catheters, the flow rate would increase significantly. It should also be noted that the flow in the 30 cm catheters would be less than half the flow rate in the 5 cm catheter.

Peripheral access catheters can be inserted using a direct visual approach or via visualization devices such as infra-red or ultrasound technology. Details of insertion will be discussed in the text below.

A. Peripherally Inserted Venous Catheters (PIVC) (Figs. 1, 2) The majority of hospitalized patients have at least one peripheral intravenous catheter (PIVC), making PIVC one of the most common clinical procedures. In the United States, over 300 million PIVCs are used for hospitalized patients

Vascular Access 7

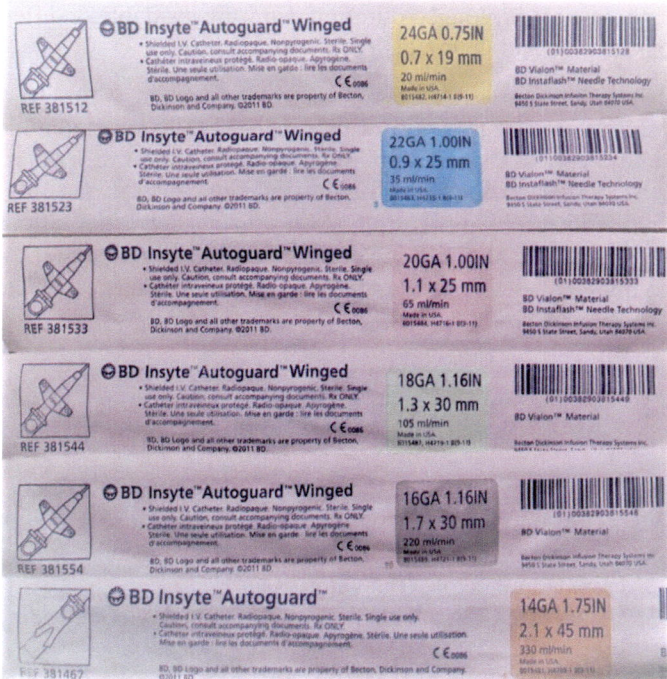

Figure 1 Peripheral vascular catheters

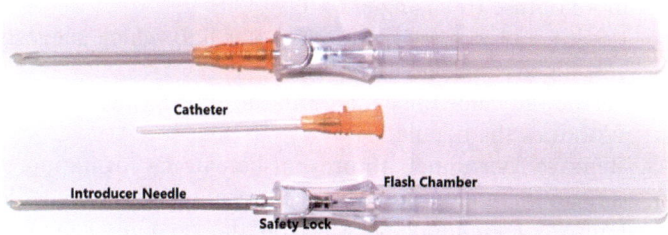

Figure 2 Peripheral catheters and its parts. Top: Catheter-over-needle device, Bottom: Parts of the peripheral vascular catheter

annually [2, 3]. These catheters are usually made up of polyethylene and provoke a strong inflammatory response on contact with blood vessels [1]. This limits the use of these catheters for prolonged duration. They are available in different lengths and diameters (Table 1).

Indications: Treatment with peripherally compatible solutions (less than 900 mOSm/liter, not vesicant or irritant) for less than 5 days [4, 5]. The larger bore catheters (14,16G) are used in rapid fluid resuscitation as in emergency situations like trauma or shock. Smaller bore catheters (20G) are most commonly used to cannulate the vein for most clinical conditions.

1.2 Method of Insertion [6]

1. Tourniquet should be applied in the arm to ensure adequate venous filling without causing patient discomfort or local ischemia.
2. Palpate and inspect the vein.
3. Clean area with alcohol swab or povidone-iodine solution.
4. Anchor the selected vein by applying gentle traction.
5. Insert catheter needle into the vessel at a 15-to-30° angle using the dominant hand. If using deeper veins, use a more obtuse (60°) angle.
6. Look for blood flash in the catheter hub, which suggests vessel penetration.
7. Further advance the catheter to the appropriate location. Withdraw the needle.
8. Remove tourniquet. To prevent hematoma formation, it is recommended to remove the tourniquet before needle removal and apply pressure on the area after needle removal.
9. Attach IV tube.
10. Secure catheter with tape and a sterile transparent dressing.
11. Assess catheter function and distal blood flow.

Advantages: Peripheral access is considered less invasive than central and has a lower risk of infection (0.5/1000 catheter days) [7, 8]. Cyclic or episodic chemotherapy management can also be considered when less than 3 months in duration with non-vesicant product infusion [9]. These catheters can be inserted in different locations like the neck (e.g., external jugular vein) or lower extremity (e.g., foot veins) in emergency situations [9].

Disadvantages: Access could be difficult in obese patients, patients without adequate veins, increased risk of infection and phlebitis in high risk patients (e.g., diabetics).

If repeated insertion attempts fail, it's appropriate to consider the designation of difficult intravenous access and explore the access site with ultrasound or other visualization technologies like using infrared rays [5]. Access through the distal portions of the upper extremity are preferred in patients with chronic kidney disease in order to preserve peripheral and central veins for hemodialysis, fistulas or grafts [10].

B. Midline Catheters (Fig. 3)

These catheters are inserted just like peripheral catheters, but they are of longer length (8–20 cm) compared to periph-

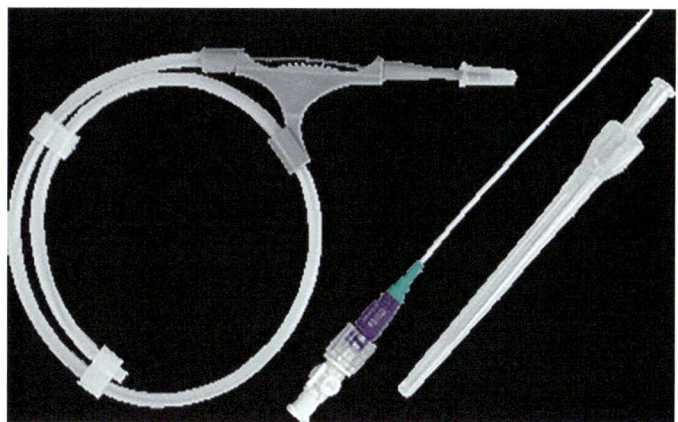

FIGURE 3 Bard Powerglide Midline Catheter 20G, 10 cm with guidewire

eral catheters (3–5 cm). These catheters can be single or dual lumen; however, a single-lumen catheter is typically preferred [9].

Indications:
When treatment is likely indicated for more than 6 days with up to 14 days being permissible. Patients with difficult intravenous access despite ultrasound-guided peripheral catheter attempts may also be considered for a midline catheter [9, 10].

Advantages:
Lower phlebitis rates than peripheral catheters and lower rates of infection compared to other central catheters [9].

Disadvantages:
Require more training and are more intensive than traditional PIVCs.

C. Peripherally Inserted Central Catheter (PICC) (Fig. 4)
PICC lines compromise more than half of all devices used to obtain central access [11]. These are long catheters inserted into the basilic or cephalic arm veins (above the antecubital fossa) and advanced into the superior vena cava. Because the basilic vein has a larger diameter compared to the cephalic vein and a straighter course in the arm, it is the preferred

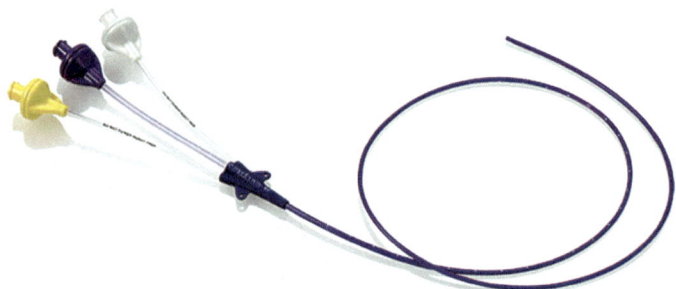

Figure 4 Medcomp triple-lumen PICC catheter

route for PICCs. PICCs are indicated in patients requiring intravenous access for more than 14 days or those necessitating continuous infusions of vesicant, parenteral nutrition, chemically irritating or peripherally incompatible solutions of any duration [10]. Cyclic chemotherapy of more than 3 months is another indication. PICCs may also be used in patients requiring frequent phlebotomy (e.g. every 8 h for more than 6 days). Burn patients, patients requiring chronic or lifelong access (e.g. sickle cell disease, cystic fibrosis or short gut) or those requiring frequent hospitalizations should also be considered for PICC insertion. PICC lines may also be used for cardiac monitoring or vasopressor administration in hemodynamically unstable patients [9]. Finally, using antimicrobial-coated PICC lines may help reduce significant reduction in risk of infections [12].

1.3 Technique [6, 13]

PICC lines are inserted under ultrasound guidance. The procedure is performed under strict aseptic precautions and the length of the catheter to be used is predetermined by measuring the distance from the antecubital fossa to the shoulder and then from shoulder to the right sternoclavicular joint, then down to the right 3rd intercostal space. After the basilic vein is located and cannulated, the catheter is advanced in the vein upto the lower third of the superior vena cava, just above the right atrium. The chest X-ray is performed to confirm the location of the catheter tip.

1.4 Pitfalls

General:
1. If having difficulty locating a vein, you can tap on the vein, ask the patient to grip and relax his/her hands repeatedly or apply a warm compress for at least 2–3 min. If still unable to isolate a vein, can also use ultrasound guidance.

Avoid venous access near sites of infection or injury. Also avoid using extremities with previous arteriovenous fistulas or grafts or lymph node dissections [6, 14].
2. When advancing the catheter after getting a blood flash, make sure further entry is smooth. If you meet resistance, withdraw the catheter as you may have penetrated the posterior wall of a vessel.
3. If you suspect that you pierced an artery, apply pressure at site.
4. If having difficulty securing the catheter, use multiple transparent dressings.
5. If induration, erythema or significant pain is reported at the insertion site, there may be concern for phlebitis or infection. Remove the catheter if infection is suspected and monitor for ongoing signs of sepsis.
6. If concerned for extravasation of fluids, apply compresses (e.g. using sterile gauze) and elevate the extremity [6].
7. Deep vein thrombosis is a potential complication of venous access. If this is a concern, evaluate using ultrasound.

PICC Related:
1. Venous air embolism: When advancing a catheter into the thorax, the negative intrathoracic pressure in spontaneously breathing patients can allow for air to enter the venous system if the catheter is open to the atmosphere. Presentation can range from dyspnea to R heart failure, pulmonary edema and embolic stroke. Prevention in such patients is by ensuring the patient is in Trendelenburg position [15].
2. Malposition seen on Chest Radiograph: A properly placed PICC should be in the SVC, with the tip 1–2 cm above the R atrium (near the tracheal carina) [16]. If the tip is below the carina, there is a concern for Right atrial entry and potential perforation; thus, retraction is recommended.

2 Central Vascular Catheters

2.1 Introduction

First described in 1929, central venous catheters (CVCs) have become an important part of hospital care. More than seven million units per year of central venous access devices are used in the United States; per 2016 data, the number increases to ten million worldwide [11].

Canalization sites include internal jugular (IJ), femoral and subclavian veins with advancement into the vena cava. Per CDC recommendations, to minimize infection risk, subclavian is preferred over jugular and femoral locations in adult patients when using non-tunneled CVC. No recommendation regarding anatomic preference is indicated for tunneled CVCs. Subclavian CVCs, however, should be avoided in hemodialysis patients and patients with chronic kidney disease to prevent subclavian vein stenosis. Additionally, when using IJ for canalization, the right side of the neck is preferred due to a vessel course [13, 17].

If ultrasound is available, the CDC recommends its use in placing CVCs to limit cannulation attempts and mechanical complications [17]. Complication rates increase with each additional attempt or percutaneous puncture [6].

2.2 Indications

2.2.1 Non-tunneled CVCs (Fig. 5)

Non-tunneled CVCs are indicated in patients requiring emergent care (i.e. unstable, requiring hemodynamic monitoring or large fluid infusions). They can also be used for parenteral nutrition. Typically, they are used for short-term access and are preferred over PICCs in patients requiring 14-day access. Additionally, they can be used to deliver parenteral nutrition and chemotherapy lasting more than 3 months [9].

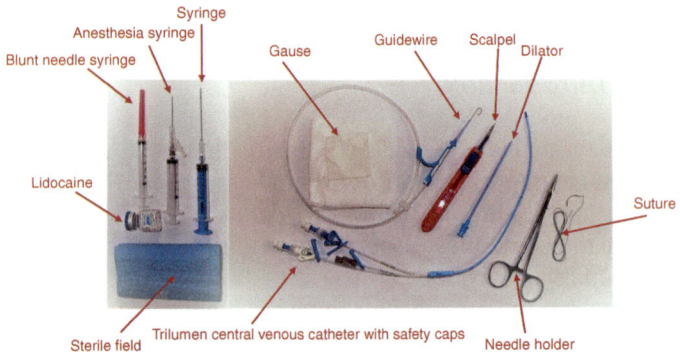

FIGURE 5 Central venous catheter kit

Their infection rate is similar to that of PICCS; antimicrobial coating agents are also used to reduce infection risk by 40% when access is required for more than 5 days [10]. Both chlorhexidine/silver sulfadiazine and minocycline/rifampin are available as antimicrobial coating agents [13, 18].

2.2.2 Tunneled CVCs

Tunneled CVCs are inserted using a subcutaneous tunnel in the mid-chest region. Such types of catheters are indicated in patients receiving treatment exceeding 31 days or those requiring multiple treatments over several months. They are used for delivery of vesicant, irritant, parenteral nutrition or chemotherapy medications (regardless of duration). Another consideration is for patients requiring more than 6 annual hospitalizations with each necessitating at least 15 days of therapy or those in whom a PICC is indicated but limited due to thrombosis risk [9].

2.3 Technique of Insertion for Non-tunneled Catheters [6, 13] (Fig. 6)

1. Maintain sterile precautions, including caps, masks, sterile gloves, sterile gowns and a sterile drape for the patient from head to toe [17].
2. Identify vessels using ultrasound. Hand hygiene before and after palpating the insertion site using an alcohol-based rub is recommended [17].

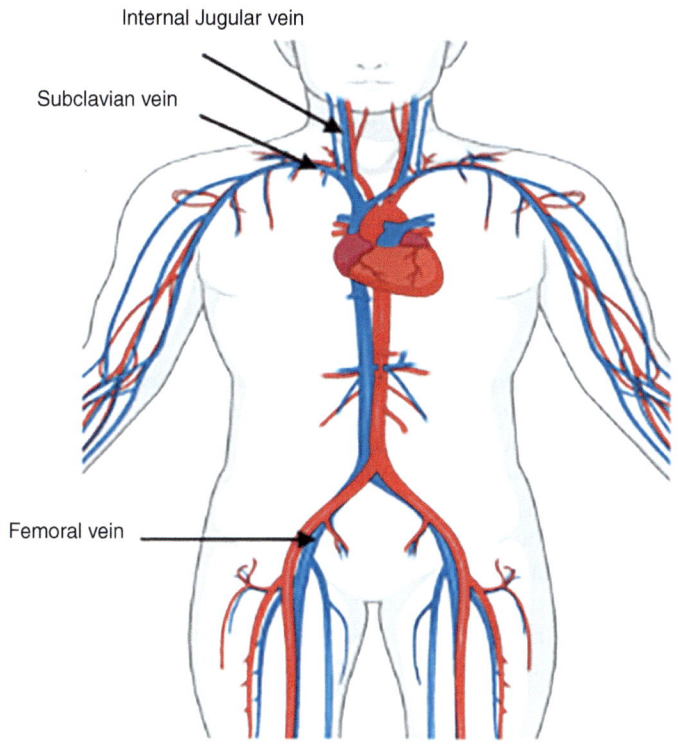

FIGURE 6 Sites of central venous access

A. Internal Jugular Vein (IJV): The IJV is located under the sternocleidomastoid (SCM) muscle and runs diagonally down the neck when a line is drawn from the pinna to the sternoclavicular joint. Insertion of the catheter can be done blindly by inserting the needle at the apex of the angle formed by the sternal and clavicular heads of the sternocleidomastoid muscle. Carotid artery is palpated on the lateral side of the sternal head of the sternocleidomastoid while the vein is superficial to it (about 1–2 cm depth from the skin usually). Care must be taken to point the needle to the ipsilateral nipple to avoid puncture of the carotid artery. Distance from the cannulation site to the right atrium is about 15 cm, so the shortest CVCs should be used. For left IJV, a 20 cm catheter may need to be considered. To identify the vessel, have the patient in Trendelenburg position and the head slightly turned to the opposite side to further straighten the venous course. Avoid turning the head beyond 30° because it can stretch the vessel and reduce diameter. Using US, place the probe at the triangle created by the two heads of the SCM. Right side IJV is preferred over left side due to the short and straight course to the heart.

B. Subclavian Approach: The subclavian courses underneath the clavicle and continues in the thoracic inlet. The vein is approached usually using landmarks with index finger at the sternal notch and thumb placed at the angle of the clavicle, two-thirds of the way lateral from the sternal notch.. The vessel may be difficult to identify using US because of the overlying clavicle; thus, surface landmarks are often used. To locate, identify the clavicular head of the SCM and the vein lies under the clavicle in this area. Cannulation can be done from above or below the clavicle.

C. Femoral Approach: The femoral vein is located in the femoral canal, along with its corresponding nerve and artery. At the level of the inguinal crease, the vein is medial to the artery and is easiest to cannulate with the hip abducted. The vein can be located by palpating the femoral artery pulse and US can be used to further locate the vein.

3. Apply chlorhexidine to the insertion site. Allot 2 min for it to dry.
4. Anesthetize insertion site by injecting 1–2% lidocaine in all conscious patients.
5. Using an 18-gauge introducer needle with an attached 10 ml syringe, introduce the needle into the skin and subcutaneous tissue until a flash of blood is seen in the hub. Perform this using your dominant hand.
6. Stabilize the needle with your nondominant hand.
7. Assure that the syringe has constant venous flow. If no flow is seen, withdraw the needle as you may have breached the posterior vessel wall.
8. Remove the attached syringe and occlude the catheter with your finger to prevent air entry.
9. Insert the guidewire through the needle, maintaining a firm grip on the guidewire.
10. Advance the guidewire. If you meet resistance, reposition the needle to assert proper needle position.
11. Remove the needle once the guidewire is inserted at least 10 cm into the vessel.
12. Make a small incision at the insertion site using a #11 scalpel blade to accommodate dilator/catheter. Do not cut the guidewire.
13. Advance the dilator/catheter over the guidewire with a gentle twisting motion.
14. Maintaining a grip on the guidewire, advance the catheter to its appropriate depth.
15. Remove the guidewire.
16. Aspirate and flush all ports to assert catheter function.
17. Secure the catheter with a suture and apply transparent dressing.
18. Obtain chest radiograph to confirm catheter placement in the superior vena cava.

2.4 Pitfalls

General
- If it is felt at any point that the sterile field is compromised, make sure to replace equipment.
- When preparing the insertion site, make sure to prep a wider region in case multiple cannulation attempts are required.
- Arterial puncture can occur in up to 15% of CVC placements, resulting in mediastinal hematoma, hemothorax, tracheal compression with possible asphyxiation and retroperitoneal hemorrhage [19–21]. A higher incidence is reported with internal jugular attempts [21–23] with carotid artery puncture being the most feared complication. Prevention includes using US guidance. If suspected, confirm with measurement of venous waveform; management includes either applying pressure at site to prevent further bleeding and removing the catheter slowly or leaving it in. Immediate removal may lead to more hemorrhage, pseudoaneurysm or fistula development, with a greater risk in patients on anticoagulant agents [24, 25].
- Make sure the guidewire passes easily when inserted. Do not force the guidewire. If it does not pass, then needle position may need to be adjusted.
- In the case of injury to the right atrium during canalization procedure (e.g. patient develops arrhythmias), Advanced Cardiac Life Support (ACLS) protocols should be followed. If perforation of the right atrium is suspected (e.g. potential cardiac tamponade), immediate assessment and pericardiocentesis may be indicated [24, 25].
- If the guidewire is lost at any point after insertion, make sure to obtain a chest radiograph to assess retention. Improper guidewire placement can lead to right atrial irritation and premature ventricular contractions or dysrhythmias.
- When advancing a catheter into the thorax, the negative intrathoracic pressure in spontaneously breathing patients

can allow for air to enter the venous system if the catheter is open to the atmosphere. Presentation can range from dyspnea to right heart failure, pulmonary edema and embolic stroke. Prevention in such patients is by ensuring the patient is in Trendelenburg position [15].
- Monitor patient for catheter-related infection (erythema at insertion site or fever, chills, hypotension without another confirmed source). Etiologies include skin flora, infection of catheter hub with repeated manipulation and hematogenous seeding from bacteremia. Prevention includes sterile technique, chlorhexidine application, avoidance of femoral line and removing unnecessary catheters [26, 27]. If a catheter-related infection is suspected, one should assess the need for continued catheter used and remove if possible. Blood cultures should be ordered with additional workup as indicated [28].
- If concerned for an occluded catheter (e.g. thrombosis, precipitation of medications), assess cause and consider re-insertion. Stenosis of subclavian veins is of greater concern than for other sites, which is the impetus for avoiding using this site in patients requiring an AV fistula for hemodialysis using the ipsilateral arm [29].
- If malposition of catheter is seen on chest radiograph, assess for pneumothorax and reposition catheter. Pneumothorax risk is minimal with IJ access because the veins are in the neck; however, risk increases with using surface landmarks as a guide [23].
- Lymphatic injuries (especially during internal jugular or subclavian vein canalization) can be seen. Treatment is with nitric oxide, thoracoscopic fibrin glue or percutaneous coiling [30].
- Tracheal injury due to accidental puncture is rarely reported; management is primarily surgical. Immediate consultation with an otorhinolaryngologist or a trauma surgeon is recommended [24].

3 Specialty Catheters

These catheters are used for a specific purpose only. Their long term use in hospital or intensive care settings is not indicated and alternative approaches should be performed if needed. They include hemodialysis catheters, introducer sheaths and pulmonary artery catheters. The Pulmonary artery Catheter is discussed in the next chapter while hemodialysis catheter and introducer sheath are discussed below.

3.1 Hemodialysis Catheters: (Fig. 7)

Hemodialysis requires direct access to the circulation, preferably via an atrioventricular fistula (AVF). In urgent cases or in patients with chronic renal failure requiring a bridge to AVF, atrioventricular graft or transplant therapy, dual-lumen dialysis catheters may be used. These catheters contain both an arterial and venous lumen that withdraws from and returns blood to the patient, respectively. They are placed into the internal jugular or femoral veins and may be tunneled or tunneled with subcutaneous cuffs. Typically, they are associated with a two- to three-fold increased risk of infection compared to AVF or AV grafts [31]. Flow rate is between 200 and 5000 mL/min [32].

Indicated in patients requiring urgent dialysis or in patients needing bridge therapy to an AVF, atrioventricular graft or transplantation.

3.2 Introducer Sheaths: (Fig. 8)

Catheter introducer sheaths facilitate percutaneous entry of intravascular devices, helping protect the vessel from injury as wires and catheters are introduced. Most have a 5- to 9-French inner diameter and vary in lengths depending on the intervention site. A one-way valve prevents bleeding through the sheath [33]. These catheters are indicated as part

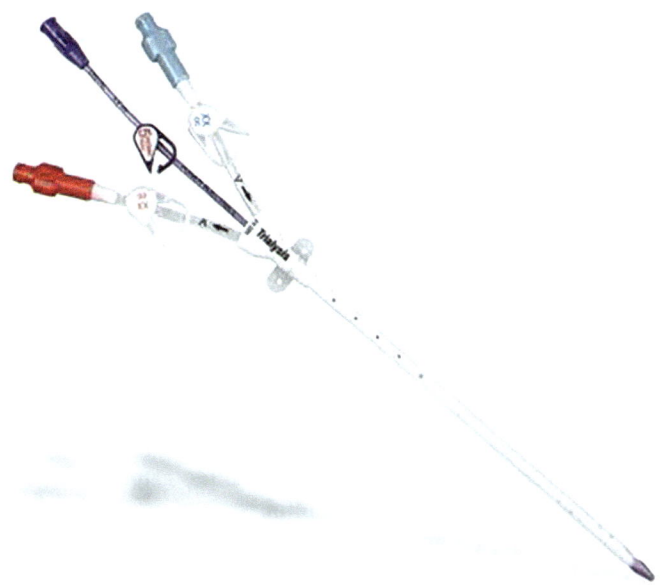

FIGURE 7 Bard power-triple lumen dialysis catheter 13 Fr × 20 cm

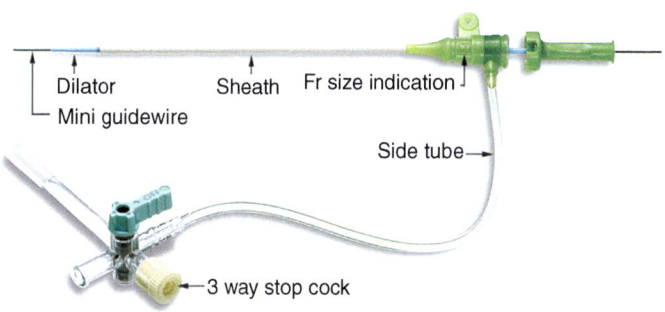

FIGURE 8 Radifocus introducer sheath

of endovascular catheterization devices to prevent blood vessel injury. Pulmonary artery catheters can also be introduced through the sheaths. They also can be used for rapid infusion of fluids or blood products during hemodynamic resuscitation. Along with the pressurized infusion system, the flow rates of 850 ml/min have been reported [34].

3.3 Technique

3.3.1 Hemodialysis Catheter

Insertion of hemodialysis catheter is similar to other forms of central venous access. The most important thing to consider during the procedure is to make a slightly bigger nick compared to the one for central line insertion. This helps as two dilation has to be done twice during this procedure. The smaller dilator primes the track for the bigger dilator. Dilator should be rotated clockwise holding it from the distal end (preferably with a gauze piece) for better grip. Each time, care should be taken to avoid pulling on the guidewire. Firm pressure should be applied with the gauze piece at the dilation site to avoid excess bleeding. The guidewire should always be moving freely within the dilator and the insertion should be smooth. If during the procedure significant resistance is felt, the position of the guidewire should be checked with should be placed at the site of the while introducing, summarized below. Further details as mentioned under "central venous access" [35].

3.3.2 Introducer Sheath [36]

The insertion requires identification of the target vessel, using ultrasound if necessary, introduction of micro-puncture needle into artery until a flash of blood appears, followed by guidewire insertion and introducer needle removal. The sheath with the accompanying dilator is threaded over the guidewire and eventually the dilator and guidewire is removed as a unit with the sheath left within the vessel.

References

1. Seckold T, Walker S, Dwyer T. A comparison of silicone and polyurethane PICC lines and postinsertion complication rates: a systematic review. J Vasc Access [Internet]. 2015 May 23 [cited 2020 Sep 30];16(3):167–77. Available from: http://journals.sagepub.com/doi/10.5301/jva.5000330.
2. Alexandrou E, Ray-Barruel G, Carr PJ, Frost S, Inwood S, Higgins N, et al. International prevalence of the use of peripheral intravenous catheters. J Hosp Med [Internet]. 2015 Aug 1 [cited 2020 Sep 15];10(8):530–3. Available from: https://pubmed.ncbi.nlm.nih.gov/26041384/.
3. Zingg W, Pittet D. Peripheral venous catheters: an under-evaluated problem. Int J Antimicrob Agents [Internet]. 2009 [cited 2020 Sep 15];34 Suppl 4. Available from: https://pubmed.ncbi.nlm.nih.gov/19931816/.
4. Periard D, Monney P, Waeber G, Zurkinden C, Mazzolai L, Hayoz D, et al. Randomized controlled trial of peripherally inserted central catheters vs. peripheral catheters for middle duration in-hospital intravenous therapy. J Thromb Haemost [Internet]. 2008 Aug [cited 2020 Sep 13];6(8):1281–8. Available from: https://pubmed.ncbi.nlm.nih.gov/18541001/.
5. Gorski LA. The 2016 infusion therapy standards of practice. Home Healthc Now [Internet]. 2017 Jan [cited 2020 Sep 13];35(1):10–8. Available from: http://journals.lww.com/01845097-201701000-00003.
6. Wyatt C. Vascular access. In: Tintinalli JE, Ma OJ, Yealy DM, Meckler GD, Stapczynski JS, Cline DM, et al., editors. Tintinalli's emergency medicine: a comprehensive study guide, 9e [Internet]. New York: McGraw-Hill Education; 2020. Available from: http://accessmedicine.mhmedical.com/content.aspx?aid=1166528709.
7. Maki DG, Kluger DM, Crnich CJ. The risk of bloodstream infection in adults with different intravascular devices: a systematic review of 200 published prospective studies. Mayo Clin Proc [Internet]. 2006 [cited 2020 Sep 13];81(9):1159–71. Available from: https://pubmed.ncbi.nlm.nih.gov/16970212/.
8. Hadaway L. Short peripheral intravenous catheters and infections. J Infus Nurs [Internet]. 2012 July [cited 2020 Sep 13];35(4):230–40. Available from: https://pubmed.ncbi.nlm.nih.gov/22759827/.

9. Moureau N, Chopra V. Indications for peripheral, midline and central catheters: summary of the MAGIC recommendations. Br J Nurs [Internet]. 2016 [cited 2020 Sep 15];25(8):S15–24. Available from: https://pubmed.ncbi.nlm.nih.gov/27126759/.
10. Chopra V, Flanders SA, Saint S, Woller SC, O'Grady NP, Safdar N, et al. The Michigan appropriateness guide for intravenous catheters (MAGIC): results from a multispecialty panel using the RAND/UCLA appropriateness method. Ann Intern Med [Internet]. 2015 Sep 15 [cited 2020 Sep 15];163(6):S1–39. Available from: https://pubmed.ncbi.nlm.nih.gov/26369828/.
11. Vascular access devices market analysis, size, trends | United States | 2020–2026 | MedSuite - iData Research [Internet]. [cited 2020 Sep 15]. Available from: https://idataresearch.com/product/vascular-access-devices-market-united-states/.
12. Rutkoff GS. The influence of an antimicrobial peripherally inserted central catheter on central line-associated bloodstream infections in a hospital environment. J Assoc Vasc Access. 2014;19(3):172–9.
13. Marino P. Marino's The Little ICU Book. 2016. 904 p.
14. Mbamalu D, Banerjee A. Methods of obtaining peripheral venous access in difficult situations. Postgrad Med J [Internet]. 1999 [cited 2020 Sep 15];75(886):459–62. Available from: https://www.ncbi.nlm.nih.gov/pmc/articles/PMC1741330/?report=abstract.
15. Vesely TM. Air embolism during insertion of central venous catheters. J Vasc Interv Radiol [Internet]. 2001 [cited 2020 Sep 15];12(11):1291–5. Available from: https://pubmed.ncbi.nlm.nih.gov/11698628/.
16. Stonelake PA, Bodenham AR. The carina as a radiological landmark for central venous catheter tip position. Br J Anaesth [Internet]. 2006 [cited 2020 Sep 15];96(3):335–40. Available from: https://pubmed.ncbi.nlm.nih.gov/16415318/.
17. O'Grady NP, Alexander M, Burns LA, Dellinger EP, Garland J, Heard SO, et al. Guidelines for the prevention of intravascular catheter-related infections. Clin Infect Dis [Internet]. 2011 May [cited 2020 Sep 15];52(9):e162. Available from: https://www.ncbi.nlm.nih.gov/pmc/articles/PMC3106269/.
18. Casey AL, Mermel LA, Nightingale P, Elliott TS. Antimicrobial central venous catheters in adults: a systematic review and meta-analysis [Internet]. Lancet Infect Dis. 2008 [cited 2020 Sep 15];8:763–76. Available from: https://pubmed.ncbi.nlm.nih.gov/19022192/.

19. Jobes DR, Schwartz AJ, Greenhow DE, Stephenson LW, Ellison N. Safer jugular vein cannulation: recognition of arterial puncture and preferential use of the external jugular route. Anesthesiology [Internet]. 1983 Oct 1 [cited 2020 Sep 15];59(4):353–5. Available from: http://pubs.asahq.org/anesthesiology/article-pdf/59/4/353/307685/0000542-198310000-00017.pdf.
20. Jobes DR, Ellison N, Troianos CA, Weber M, Huber C, Oates A, et al. Complications and failures of subclavian-vein catheterization [Internet]. N Engl J Med. Massachusetts Medical Society; 1995 [cited 2020 Sep 15];332:1579–81. Available from: http://www.nejm.org/doi/abs/10.1056/NEJM199506083322313.
21. Ruesch S, Walder B, Tramèr MR. Complications of central venous catheters: internal jugular versus subclavian access - a systematic review. Crit Care Med [Internet]. 2002 [cited 2020 Sep 15];30(2):454–60. Available from: https://www.ncbi.nlm.nih.gov/books/NBK69121/.
22. Feller-Kopman D. Ultrasound-guided internal jugular access: a proposed standardized approach and implications for training and practice. Chest [Internet]. 2007 [cited 2020 Sep 15];132(1):302–9. Available from: https://pubmed.ncbi.nlm.nih.gov/17625091/.
23. Hayashi H, Amano M. Does ultrasound imaging before puncture facilitate internal jugular vein cannulation? Prospective randomized comparison with landmark-guided puncture in ventilated patients. J Cardiothorac Vasc Anesth [Internet]. 2002 Oct 1 [cited 2020 Sep 15];16(5):572–5. Available from: http://www.jcvaonline.com/article/S1053077002000629/fulltext.
24. Kornbau C, Lee K, Hughes G, Firstenberg M. Central line complications. Int J Crit Illn Inj Sci [Internet]. 2015 [cited 2020 Sep 15];5(3):170. Available from: http://www.ijciis.org/text.asp?2015/5/3/170/164940.
25. Bowdle A. Vascular complications of central venous catheter placement: evidence-based methods for prevention and treatment [Internet]. J Cardiothoracic Vasc Anesth. W.B. Saunders; 2014 [cited 2020 Sep 15];28:358–68. Available from: https://pubmed.ncbi.nlm.nih.gov/24008166/.
26. Philip KNG, Ault MJ, Gray Ellrodt A, Maldonado L. Peripherally inserted central catheters in general medicine. Mayo Clin Proc [Internet]. 1997 [cited 2020 Sep 15];72(3):225–33. Available from: https://pubmed.ncbi.nlm.nih.gov/9070197/.
27. Sherertz RJ, Ely EW, Westbrook DM, Gledhill KS, Streed SA, Kiger B, et al. Education of physicians-in-training can

decrease the risk for vascular catheter infection. Ann Intern Med [Internet]. 2000 Apr 18 [cited 2020 Sep 15];132(8):641–8. Available from: https://pubmed.ncbi.nlm.nih.gov/10766683/.
28. McConville JF, Patel BK. Intravascular devices in the ICU. In: Hall JB, Schmidt GA, Kress JP, editors. Principles of critical care, 4e [Internet]. New York: McGraw-Hill Education; 2015. Available from: http://accessmedicine.mhmedical.com/content.aspx?aid=1126247143.
29. Hernández D, Díaz F, Rufino M, Lorenzo V, Pérez T, Rodríguez A, et al. Subclavian vascular access stenosis in dialysis patients: natural history and risk factors. J Am Soc Nephrol. 1998;9(8):1507–10.
30. Kusminsky RE. Complications of central venous catheterization [Internet]. J Am Coll Surg. Elsevier; 2007 [cited 2020 Sep 15];204:681–96. Available from: http://www.journalacs.org/article/S1072751507001305/fulltext.
31. Dhingra RK, Young EW, Hulbert-Shearon TE, Leavey SF, Port FK. Type of vascular access and mortality in U.S. hemodialysis patients. Kidney Int [Internet]. 2001 [cited 2020 Sep 15];60(4):1443–51. Available from: https://pubmed.ncbi.nlm.nih.gov/11576358/.
32. Anwer B. Interventional radiology. In: Elsayes KM, Oldham SAA, editors. Introduction to diagnostic radiology [Internet]. New York: McGraw-Hill Education; 2015. Available from: http://accessmedicine.mhmedical.com/content.aspx?aid=1115261680.
33. Lin PH, Bechara CF, Chen C, Veith FJ. Arterial disease. In: Brunicardi FC, Andersen DK, Billiar TR, Dunn DL, Kao LS, Hunter JG, et al., editors. Schwartz's principles of surgery, 11e [Internet]. New York: McGraw-Hill Education; 2019. Available from: http://accessmedicine.mhmedical.com/content.aspx?aid=1164312731.
34. Barcelona SL, Vilich F, Cote CJ. A comparison of flow rates and warming capabilities of the Level 1 and Rapid Infusion System with various-size intravenous catheters. Anesth Analg. 2003;97:358–63.
35. Ahmed HM, Aquina CT, Gracias VH, Provencio JJ, Pennisi MA, Bello G, et al. Dialysis catheter. In: Encyclopedia of intensive care medicine [Internet]. Berlin Heidelberg: Springer; 2012 [cited 2020 Sep 15]. p. 714. Available from: https://www.ncbi.nlm.nih.gov/books/NBK539856/.
36. Input® Introducer Sheaths [Internet]. [cited 2020 Sep 15]. Available from: https://www.medtronic.com/us-en/healthcare-professionals/products/cardiovascular/interventional-guidewires-accessories/input-introducer-sheaths.html.

Pulmonary Artery Catheters

Taishi Hirai, John E. A. Blair, and Arun Kumar

1 Introduction

The Swan-Ganz catheter was invented by Dr. Harold JC Swan and his colleague Dr. William Ganz at Cedar-Sinai Hospital in 1970s. The right heart catheterization performed using this catheter allows the operator to assess the hemodynamics and tailor the treatment for the patients.

2 Indications

Among number of indications to perform right heart catheterization, the two main indications for placement in the intensive care unit are for differentiation of shock and assessment of volume status.

T. Hirai (✉) · A. Kumar
Department of Medicine, Division of Cardiology, University of Missouri, Columbia, MO, USA
e-mail: hirait@health.missouri.edu; kumararun@health.missouri.edu

J. E. A. Blair
Department of Medicine, Division of Cardiology, University of Chicago, Chicago, IL, USA
e-mail: jblair2@bsd.uchicago.edu

© The Author(s), under exclusive license to Springer Nature Switzerland AG 2022
N. Arora (ed.), *Procedures and Protocols in the Neurocritical Care Unit*, https://doi.org/10.1007/978-3-030-90225-4_2

(a) Differentiation of shock.

Shock is clinically defined as systolic blood pressure (SBP) <90 mmHg for >30 min or requirement of vasopressor support to maintain SBP >90 mmHg and evidence of end organ hypoperfusion [1].

Right heart catheterization is useful in differentiating the cause of shock by assessing the three components: preload, cardiac output, and afterload. First, the preload of left ventricle: Left ventricular end-diastolic pressure (LVEDP) can be estimated by measuring the pulmonary capillary wedge pressure (PCWP), which is equal to left atrial pressure and LVEDP in the absence of valvular disease or precapillary pulmonary hypertension. Second, the cardiac index and cardiac output are obtained by applying the Fick method or using a thermodilution method. Finally, the systemic vascular resistance, considered afterload of the left ventricle is obtained using the mean arterial pressure, right atrial pressure, and the cardiac output (Fig. 1).

The cause of shock can be differentiated utilizing these three parameters assessed by the right heart catheterization (Table 1).

(b) Guidance of therapy for severe heart failure or cardiogenic shock.

Severe heart failure:

The assessment of volume status of patients with severe heart failure can be challenging. When the hemodynamics and volume status is clear to the treating physician, routine right heart catheterization is not necessary. On the other hand, right heart catheterization is useful when the patient's hemodynamic status is unclear, such as in patients with worsening kidney function despite diuresis, evidence of hypoperfusion concerning for low output state or clinical suspicion for right ventricular failure.

Cardiogenic shock:

Right heart catheterization should be utilized in patients with suspected cardiogenic shock to guide the timing and degree of hemodynamic support with inotropes such as

$$\text{Cardiac Output (CO) (L/min)} = \frac{\text{Oxygen Consumption}}{13.4 \times \text{Hgb (g/dl)} \times (\text{SaO2-SvO2})}$$

$$\text{Cardiac Index (CI) (L/min/m}^2) = \frac{\text{CO}}{\text{BSA}}$$

$$\text{Systemic Vascular Resistance (dyne} \cdot \text{sec} \cdot \text{cm}^{-5}) = \frac{\text{MAP} - \text{CVP}}{\text{CO}}$$

$$\text{Pulmonary Artery Pulsatility Index (PAPI)} = \frac{\text{sPAP} - \text{dPAP}}{\text{RA}}$$

$$\text{Cardiac Power Output (CPO)} = \frac{\text{MAP} \times \text{CO}}{451}$$

FIGURE 1 Cardiac output, cardiac index, systemic vascular resistance, cardiac power and pulmonary pulsatility index obtained from hemodynamic parameters. Hgb: hemoglobin, SaO2: arterial saturation, SvO2: mixed venous saturation, BSA: body surface area, MAP: mean arterial pressure, CVP: central venous pressure, sPAP: systolic pulmonary artery pressure, dPAP: diastolic pulmonary pressure, RA: right atrial pressure

TABLE 1 Differentiation of the three most common types of shock based on hemodynamics

	Blood Pressure	PCWP (Preload)	CO (Contractility)	SVR (Afterload)
Distributive	↓	↓	↑	↓
Cardiogenic	↓	↑	↓	↑
Hypovolemic	↓	↓	↓	↑

PCWP PULMONARY CAPILLARY WEDGE PRESSURE, *CO* CARDIAC OUTPUT, *SVR* SYSTEMIC VASCULAR RESISTANCE

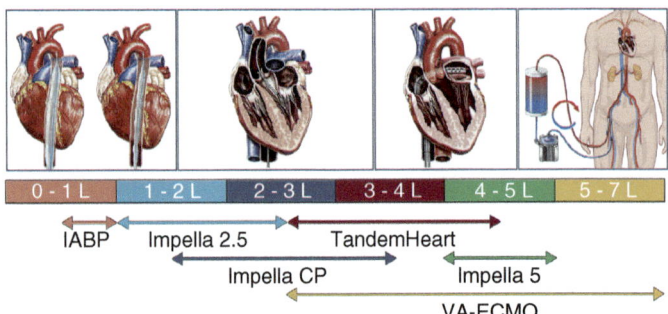

FIGURE 2 Types of percutaneous hemodynamic support devices and degree of hemodynamic support

dobutamine or milrinone, and/or mechanical circulatory support devices. There are four different types of percutaneous mechanical circulatory support devices that can be used in patients with cardiogenic shock: Intra-aortic balloon pump, Impella, Tandem heart and Extracorporeal Membrane Oxygenation (ECMO). Each device can provide different degree of hemodynamic support as summarized in Fig. 2 [2]. The escalation and de-escalation of inotropic therapy and mechanical circulatory support can be decided based on information obtained by right heart catheterization, such as cardiac power output (CPO) and pulmonary artery pulsatility index (PAPI) [3]. Therefore, continuous hemodynamic monitoring is routinely performed with "leave-in" Swan-Ganz catheter in patients with cardiogenic shock.

(c) Diagnosis of pulmonary hypertension:

Pulmonary hypertension can be diagnosed with mean pulmonary artery pressure (PAP) >20 mmHg and severe pulmonary hypertension is defined as mean PAP >40 mmHg [4]. Pulmonary vascular resistance (PVR) and PCWP are measured to differentiate the types of pulmonary hypertension: pre-capillary, post-capillary and combined pre and post capillary. If primary pulmonary hypertension is diagnosed with normal PCWP and elevated PVR, reversibility study can be performed with nitric oxide, nitroglycerin or nitroprusside to assess for the response to pharmacologic treatment.

(d) Assessment for intracardiac shunting:

When an intracardiac shunt is suspected, such as atrial septal defect, ventricular septal defect or anomalous pulmonary venous return, multiple samples of oxygen saturation can be measured at a variety of locations within the cardiac chambers. The shunt fraction can be measured by assessing the ratio of pulmonary arterial blood flow (Qp) and the systemic blood flow (Qs). This will aid the diagnosis in addition to the information obtained from the imaging studies, such as echocardiogram and cardiac magnetic resonance imaging.

(e) Hemodynamic assessment during high-risk percutaneous coronary intervention (PCI):

When performing a complex intervention to a patient with a higher risk for decompensation with reduced ejection fraction and/or high-risk anatomy, placement of percutaneous hemodynamic support devices can be considered during the PCI [5]. When percutaneous hemodynamic support devices are used, right heart catheterization is recommended to assess the hemodynamics to guide the escalation and de-escalation of support. There are variety of algorithms to decide which patient needs hemodynamic support, and the clinical practice still varies among the operators. In general, hemodynamic support is considered in patients with decreased cardiac output and increased PCWP.

3 Technique/Methods

Right heart catheterization can be performed either in the cardiac catheterization laboratory or at the bedside. Right heart catheterization at the bedside is performed via the internal jugular vein or subclavian vein, as it is challenging to position the catheter from the femoral vein without continuous fluoroscopic guidance.

In the cardiac catheterization laboratory, right heart catheterization can be performed from the internal jugular vein, subclavian vein, basilic vein or femoral vein. Among the access points, basilic vein is most comfortable for the patients, and therefore it is the first choice at the authors' institutions if the catheter does not need to be kept in for hemodynamic monitoring. Basilic access is not suitable for continuous hemodynamic monitoring as the patient cannot move the arm.

For internal jugular, subclavian or femoral vein:

(a) Obtain ultrasound-guided venous access with insertion of a 6–8 Fr sheath. A micro-puncture sheath and catheter, or 18-gauge needle can be used. Micropuncture needle is a 21-gauge needle, which could decrease the risk of bleeding and can be dilated with a dilator to accommodate 0.035-inch guidewire after confirming good entry-site (Fig. 3).
(b) After checking the balloon and flushing all ports, the catheter is inserted through the venous sheath.
(c) Once inserted the balloon tip is inflated for it to be inserted into the cardiac chambers by the flow of blood.
(d) Pressure of each chamber (right atrial, right ventricle, pulmonary artery) are measured (Fig. 4).
(e) For pulmonary capillary wedge pressure, the catheter is inserted until the pulmonary arterial tracing drops and the tracing appears atrial. To re-sample pulmonary

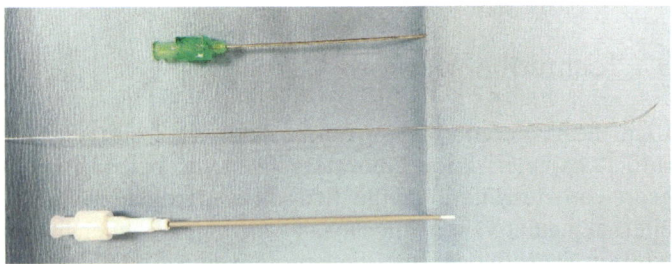

FIGURE 3 A micropuncture needle, guidewire, and dilator

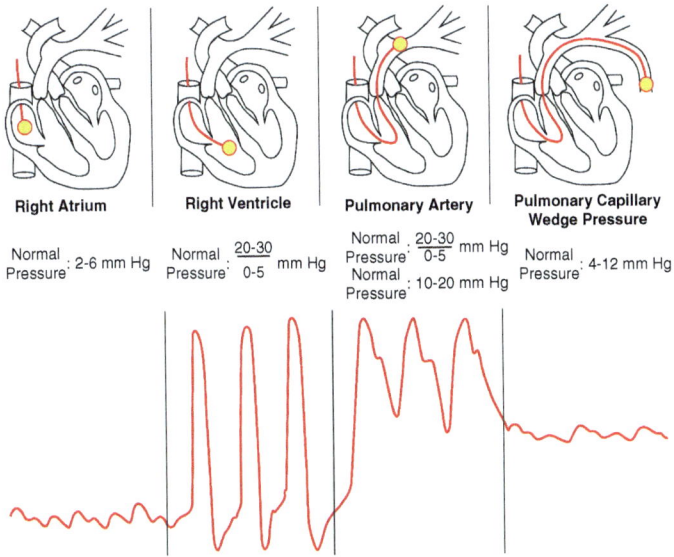

FIGURE 4 Normal pressure waveforms in each chamber

pressure or to obtain pulmonary arterial oxygen saturation, the balloon is deflated.
(f) Pulmonary arterial saturation and right atrial saturation are measured. If arterial access is available, arterial saturation is measured to evaluate the cardiac output using the Fick method. If not, the peripheral saturation of the pulse oximetry can be used to calculate cardiac output and cardiac index.
(g) Thermodilution technique can also be performed to measure the cardiac out put and cardiac index. Heparinized saline is injected from the proximal port for three to four times.
(h) The procedure may be performed using pressure waveforms alone, however fluoroscopy is useful in patients with intracardiac devices such as pacemakers, and in patients with complex anatomy such as congenital heart disease.
(i) If the catheter is left in, it is sutured in place and locked at the hub with a protective sleeve to maintain sterility.

From basilic vein:

(a) Intravenous access can be obtained at bedside or in the cardiac catheterization laboratory using 20–22-gauge peripheral intravenous catheters. The peripheral catheter is exchanged to a 6 Fr radial sheath over a guidewire (Fig. 5).

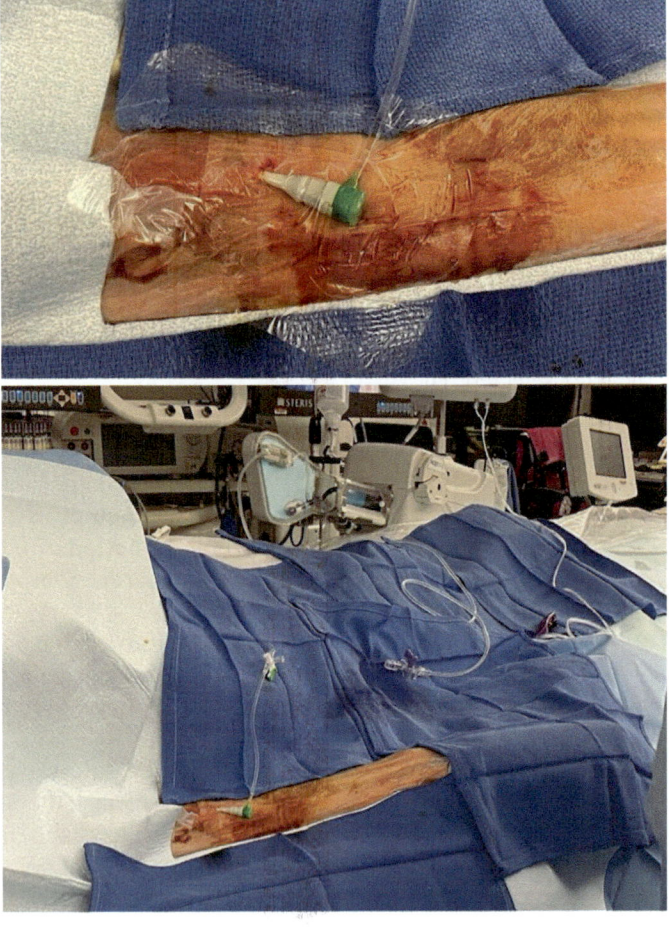

FIGURE 5 A 6 French sheath advanced into the basilic vein

(b) After checking the balloon and flushing all ports, Swan-Ganz catheter is inserted through the venous sheath. The catheter is advanced without balloon inflation until it reaches the axillary vein. The balloon is then inflated in the axillary vein and advanced into each chamber.

4 Types of Kits Available

Swan-Ganz catheter without thermodilution (Fig. 6):

This catheter comes in a variety of sizes from 4 Fr to 8 Fr. The 5 Fr or 6 Fr catheters are typically used when advancing from the basilic access. Although smaller catheters are easier to advance through smaller vessels, the tradeoff is accuracy of the measurement as the larger lumen size allows for more accurate and consistent waveforms.

Swan-Ganz catheter with thermodilution: (Fig. 7):

This catheter allows for continuous monitoring of cardiac output and mixed venous saturations at bedside. When the catheter is left in for continuous monitoring, this device is typically selected. The size of the catheter is 7.5 Fr or 8 Fr.

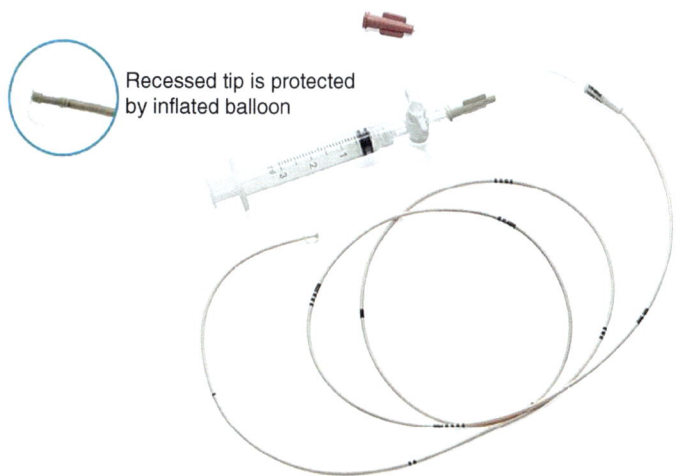

FIGURE 6 Swan-Ganz catheter without thermodilution capability

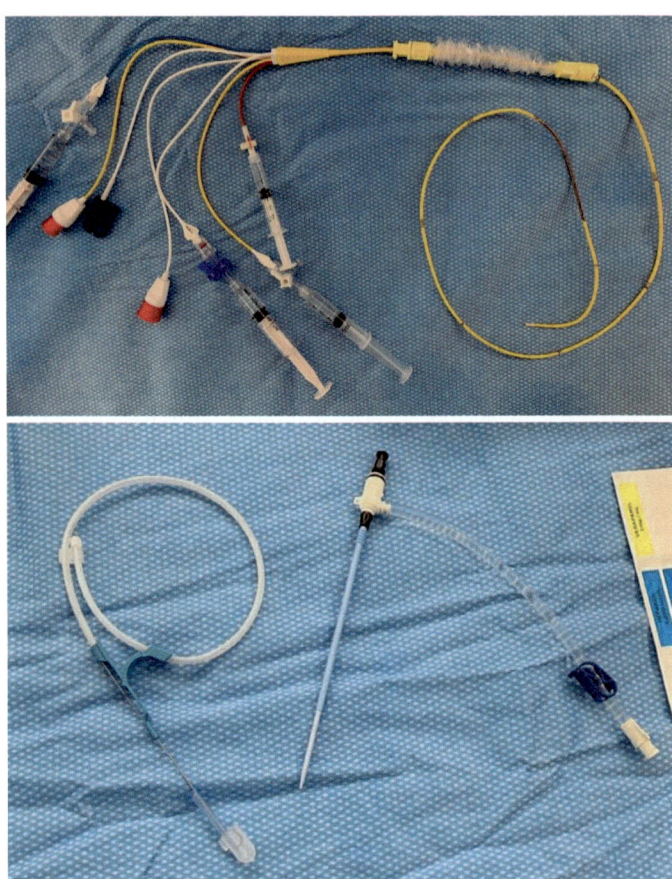

FIGURE 7 Swan-Ganz catheter with thermodilution capability

5 Pitfalls and Troubleshooting

(a) Cannot obtain accurate wedge pressure:

The position of the catheter is checked by fluoroscopy and the pressure waveform. If the pressure waveform is unclear, wedge saturation can be obtained to confirm catheter position. Especially in patients with severe pulmonary hypertension, it can be difficult to obtain accurate wedge pressure. Operators can deflate the balloon, advance the catheter, and slowly inflate the balloon until the balloon wedges. If accurate waveform cannot be obtained, advancing to a different branch of pulmonary artery can be considered. It is important for the operator to review the morphology of the waveform in the various chambers to be confident in the placement of the catheters.

(b) The waveform is not correct:

If the waveform is not correct in the ICU setting this is typically due to either air or clot in the catheter or the pressure line. Catheter is flushed after aspirating a small amount of blood. It is also important to check all the tubing and connections are tightly fastened as loose connection can be a cause of inaccurate waveform.

(c) Catheter in the right ventricle:

When the catheter is in the right ventricle, it can be typically detected at bedside by the change in the pressure waveform from a PA waveform to a RV waveform. The catheter will need repositioning as it can become a cause of arrhythmia. If this occurs, first confirm the position with a portable chest X-ray. If the access point is in the internal jugular vein or subclavian vein, the position can be adjusted at bedside. If the catheter is coiled in the right ventricle, the catheter is withdrawn to the superior vena cava before advancing again with balloon inflated. If the access point is the femoral vein, the position will need to be adjusted in the cardiac catheterization laboratory with continuous fluoroscopic guidance.

(d) Complete heart block:

In a patient with underlying left bundle branch block, complete heart block can occur with irritation of the right bundle with the catheter during the right heart catheterization. These are typically transient and improve with removal of the catheter.

(e) Catheter cannot be advanced to the pulmonary artery.

Especially in patients with right ventricular dilation and/or severe tricuspid regurgitation, advancing the catheter to the pulmonary artery can be challenging. If the catheter cannot be advanced to position at bedside, it can be performed in the cardiac catheterization laboratory under continuous fluoroscopic guidance. In addition, an 0.018–0.021-inch guidewire can be used to navigate the catheter.

(f) Improper zero:

Prior to recording measurements, the pressure transducer must be zeroed at the mid chest level of the patient. Improper zeroing of the pressure transducer will lead to inaccurate measurements, which can adversely impact clinical decisions.

Acknowledgement The authors acknowledge Jennifer Higgins RCIS for preparation of the photographs and Jose Aceituno for graphical design.

References

1. Hochman JS, Sleeper LA, Webb JG, et al. Early revascularization in acute myocardial infarction complicated by cardiogenic shock. SHOCK Investigators. Should We Emergently Revascularize Occluded Coronaries for Cardiogenic Shock. N Engl J Med. 1999;341:625–34.
2. Atkinson TM, Ohman EM, O'Neill WW, Rab T, Cigarroa JE, Interventional Scientific Council of the American College of C. A practical approach to mechanical circulatory support in patients undergoing percutaneous coronary intervention: an interventional perspective. JACC Cardiovasc Interv. 2016;9:871–83.
3. van Diepen S, Katz JN, Albert NM, et al. Contemporary management of cardiogenic shock: a scientific statement from the American Heart Association. Circulation. 2017;136:e232–68.
4. Maron BA, Kovacs G, Vaidya A, et al. Cardiopulmonary hemodynamics in pulmonary hypertension and heart failure: JACC review topic of the week. J Am Coll Cardiol. 2020;76:2671–81.
5. O'Neill WW, Kleiman NS, Moses J, et al. A prospective, randomized clinical trial of hemodynamic support with Impella 2.5 versus intra-aortic balloon pump in patients undergoing high-risk percutaneous coronary intervention: the PROTECT II study. Circulation. 2012;126:1717–27.

Arterial Catheters

Taishi Hirai, John E. A. Blair, and Arun Kumar

1 Introduction

Arterial catheters are essential for continuous hemodynamic monitoring when treating patients in the intensive care unit.

2 Indications

The two main reasons for placement of an arterial catheter in the intensive care unit are continuous hemodynamic monitoring and frequent arterial blood gas monitoring in patients with respiratory failure often managed by mechanical ventilation.

(a) Continuous hemodynamic monitoring

T. Hirai (✉) · A. Kumar
Department of Medicine, Division of Cardiology, University of Missouri, Columbia, MO, USA
e-mail: hirait@health.missouri.edu; kumararun@health.missouri.edu

J. E. A. Blair
Department of Medicine, Division of Cardiology, University of Chicago, Chicago, IL, USA
e-mail: jblair2@bsd.uchicago.edu

Patients in shock, which is clinically defined as systolic blood pressure (SBP) <90 mmHg for >30 min or requirement of vasopressor support to maintain SBP >90 mmHg require continuous hemodynamic monitoring Vasopressor and inotropic therapy are titrated based on the invasive blood pressure obtained by the arterial catheter. On the other hand, in patients with severe hypertension such as those presenting with hypertensive emergency, intravenous antihypertensive medications are titrated based on the invasive blood pressure.

(b) Frequent monitoring of arterial blood gas

Patients who require mechanical ventilation or non-invasive ventilation require frequent arterial blood sampling for blood gas analysis to monitor the response to treatment and for adjustment of ventilator settings. To avoid frequent arterial punctures for these samples, an arterial line is often placed as the blood sample can be easily drawn from the catheter.

3 Technique/Methods

The arterial catheter is placed using sterile technique and is commonly placed in the radial artery. If the pulse is not palpable or in a patient with a small radial artery, ultrasound guidance is useful to guide the direction of the needle.

Femoral arterial catheters can be placed when radial arterial access is not an option. Ultrasound guidance is recommended to confirm the entry location of the catheter is in the common femoral artery.

4 Types of Kits Available

(a) Radial arterial catheterization kit with guidewire integration (Fig. 1):

This catheter has a 20 gauge catheter which is loaded over a 22 gauge needle. Arterial puncture by the 22 gauge needle

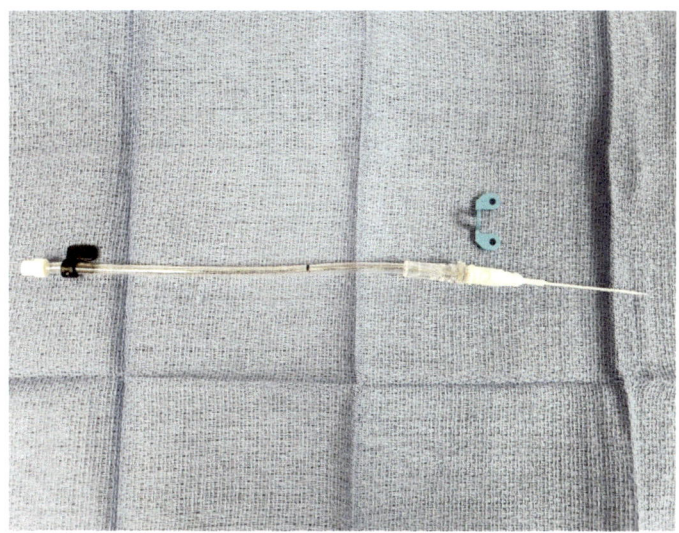

FIGURE 1 Radial arterial catheterization kit with needle and guidewire integration

is confirmed by a small flashback of blood. A 0.018 inch guidewire is advanced by advancing the black knob. Arterial catheter is advanced over this guidewire into the artery.

(b) Arterial catheter kit with separate needle and guidewire (Fig. 2):

After arterial puncture, the guidewire is advanced through the needle. The needle is then removed, and the arterial catheter is inserted over the guidewire. As there is a small size difference between the guidewire and the catheter, making a small skin nick with a scalpel will allow the catheter to advance smoothly into the vessel.

5 Pitfalls and Troubleshooting

(a) The guidewire cannot be advanced through the needle:

If the guidewire cannot be advanced into the arterial lumen, the needle tip could be touching the posterior wall of

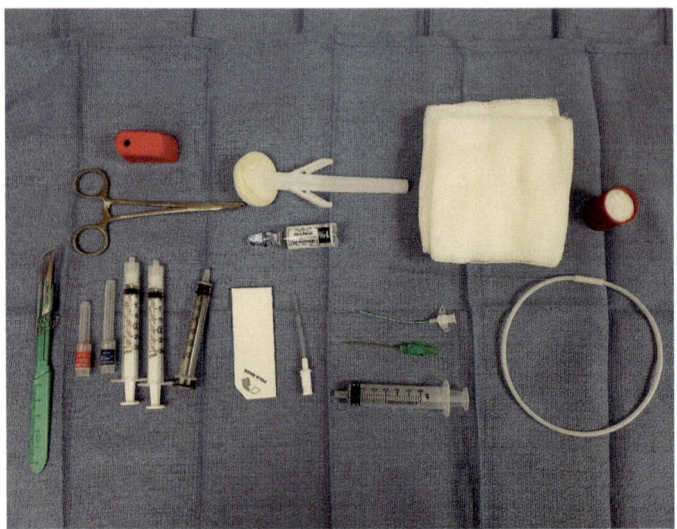

Figure 2 Arterial catheter kit with separate needle and guidewire

the vessel or a lesion. Angle down the needle and make small adjustments by withdrawing the needle slowly until the guidewire can be advanced without resistance. Hydrophilic guidewires that are used when inserting radial arterial sheaths can be considered. Hydrophilic guidewires should be used with caution, as they may cause dissection if advanced improperly.

(b) The waveform is not correct.

This typically occurs with either air or clot in the catheter or pressure line. Flushing of the catheter should be performed and if the waveform is still inaccurate, replacement of the arterial catheter is necessary.

(c) Proper zero

Prior to recording measurements, the pressure transducer must be zeroed at the mid chest level of the patient. Improper zeroing of the pressure transducer will lead to inaccurate measurements, which can adversely impact clinical decisions.

Airway Access

Mohammed Alnijoumi

Introduction

The patent airway is one of the mainstays of survival. It is protected by reflexes and muscular tone which maintains airway patency. Loss of such reflexes or tone could lead to airway obstruction, which in turn could be detrimental if swift decisions are not taken. Such decisions could be the difference between life and death.

The physician's job in those situations is to determine if proceeding with intubation is required or not. Such a decision is the catalyst of what happens next.

In this chapter, we discuss different methods to access the airway to maintain patency either electively or emergently. In addition, we discuss bronchoscopy as a specialized method to access the distal bronchial structures for diagnostic or therapeutic purposes.

M. Alnijoumi (✉)
Department of Medicine, University of Missouri,
Columbia, MO, USA
e-mail: alnijoumim@health.missouri.edu

© The Author(s), under exclusive license to Springer Nature Switzerland AG 2022
N. Arora (ed.), *Procedures and Protocols in the Neurocritical Care Unit*, https://doi.org/10.1007/978-3-030-90225-4_4

Airway Anatomy

A basic understanding of airway anatomy is important. It forms the foundation of airway management. This upcoming anatomy discussion is by no means meant to be exhaustive, but rather a basic review. Consulting with anatomy books is encouraged if further details are needed.

The mouth, or oral cavity, extends from the lips anteriorly to the pharynx posteriorly. It is bound by the hard palate superiorly and the mandible inferiorly. It contains the tongue, which is a muscular structure that is attached to the hyoid bone and the mandible. In an unconscious patient, the tongue would fall backward and potentially obstructs the airway. Hence, a jaw thrust especially after opening the mouth is very effective in opening the patient's airway.

The nose, or nasal cavity, is the space from the roof of the mouth to the cranial base. It extends from the nares anteriorly to the pharynx posteriorly. Each nostril has a highly vascularized network of capillaries on the nasal septum, known as Kiesselbach plexus or Little's area. Epistaxis mostly occurs from this area and caution is taken when a nasal airway is planned. It is for the vascularity of the nasal septum that the nasal mucosa is most sensitive to vasoconstricting agents. The widest opening in the nose is located between the inferior nasal turbinate and the nasal floor. This part of the airway tilts slightly downwards along its path. It forms the preferred space to use when nasopharyngeal airway or nasotracheal intubation is attempted. The paranasal sinuses drain into the nasal cavity and hence could be blocked with the prolonged presence of a nasal airway increasing the risk of paranasal sinus infection. Additionally, mucosal depression at the nasopharynx where the eustachian tube enters forms a potential weak space that could be injured by nasal airways.

The larynx is an air passage that extends from the tongue to the trachea. It is a mobile structure. It contains the epiglottis, vocal cords, arytenoid cartilages, and ends inferiorly at the cricoid cartilage. It is the most innervated structure in the body, and exciting it in the conscious patient would lead to significant vagal and sympathetic discharges. The epiglottis is the most important anatomical structure that must be identified during direct or video laryngoscopy. The intubating blade would have to be passed either anterior or posterior to it based on the type of blade used. The cricothyroid membrane extends from the inferior aspect of the thyroid cartilage cephalad to the superior border of the cricoid cartilage caudad. It is a thin membrane and is punctured during cricothyroidotomy. It is easily identified in a male compared to a female given the lower position of the larynx and the larger laryngeal prominence or Adam's apple. Given the proximity of the cricothyroid membrane to the vocal cords, large-size tubes should be avoided to reduce the risk of vocal cords injury or subglottic stenosis. Due to laryngeal mobility, stabilizing the larynx is helpful during laryngeal procedures.

The trachea extends from the cricoid cartilage to the main carina. It measures about 12–16 mm in diameter and extends about 12 cm in length. The size of the trachea depends on the gender and height of the individual. The tracheal lumen is bound anteriorly by C-shaped cartilaginous rings and posteriorly by a muscular wall that lies anterior to the esophagus. The posterior wall could be punctured forming a tracheo-esophageal fistula.

The main carina divides the bronchial tree into right and left. The right lung has three lobes, and the left has 2 anatomical lobes. Correct identification of those lobes is a prerequisite during flexible bronchoscopy.

1 Supraglottic Devices

The supraglottic device is a collective term describing airway access devices that, as the name implies, sits in the supraglottic space, i.e. the Larynx. The hallmark device is the Laryngeal Mask Airway, LMA. Additionally, oropharyngeal airways and nasopharyngeal airways play an important role in maintaining a patent airway. In this section, we will discuss those devices, their indications, techniques of inserting them, and any pitfalls that could arise with their use.

1.1 Oropharyngeal and Nasopharyngeal Airways

Introduction

The oropharyngeal airway (OPA) and Nasopharyngeal airway (NPA) (Fig. 1) are rounded tubes that extend across the oropharynx and nasopharynx respectively to maintain airway

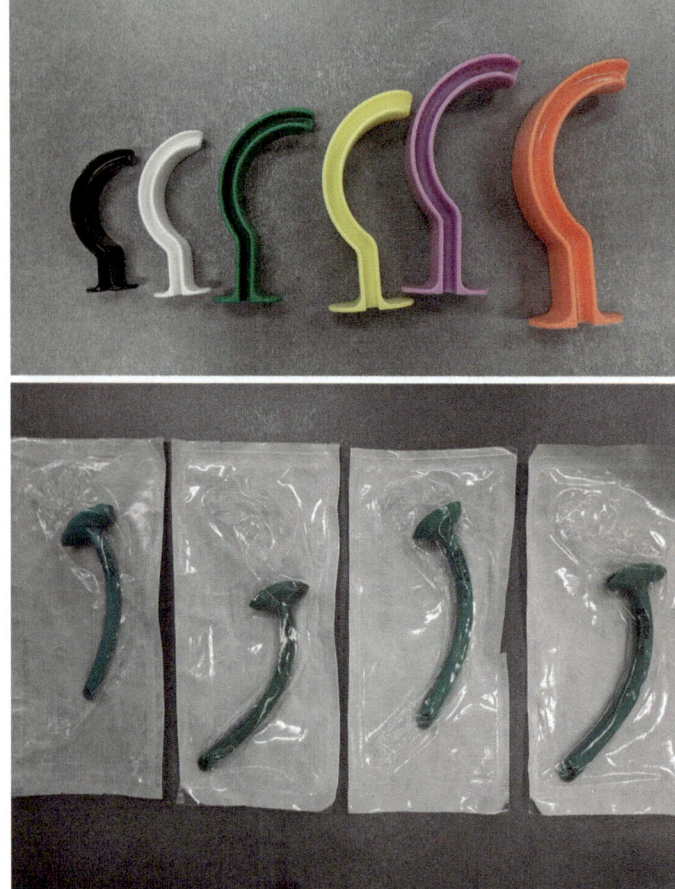

FIGURE 1 Top: Oropharyngeal airway (OPA); Bottom: Nasopharyngeal airway (NPA)

patency. In a sedated or unconscious patient, airway obstruction occurs if the tongue falls backward obstructing the oropharynx or if the epiglottis falls onto the Larynx. Relaxation of the jaw also leads to airway obstruction. It is known that head tilt and jaw thrust help to open the airway. However, this occupies both provider's hands and could be a daunting task when Bag-Mask ventilation (BMV) is underway. The OPA and NPA would work as an adjunct to help maintain airway patency during BMV or when delivering Oxygen via a facemask.

Indications and Contraindications

The main indication (Table 1) of an OPA or an NPA is to maintain airway patency and as an adjunct airway during bag-mask ventilation. This is more important in those patients who are unconscious or with a depressed level of consciousness. NPA has the advantage over OPA in patients who are semi-conscious or have an intact cough and gag reflexes, those with limited mouth opening, or the presence of macroglossia.

The biggest contraindication for OPA is a conscious patient as they are expected to have an intact gag reflex. The NPA should be avoided, if possible, in suspected cases of a base of skull fractures. Other general contraindications include the use of anticoagulation and patients with bleeding diatheses.

Complications vary and are usually limited when inserted attentively. For an OPA, complications arise mainly from injury to soft tissues, injury to dental structures, or inadvertent aspiration of the OPA. In the case of an NPA, the most feared complication is intracranial placement. Moreover, soft tissue injury and epistaxis could occur, and migration into the nasopharynx when the NPA flange is rather small.

Sizing

OPA comes in different sizes, 1 through 4. Those sizes refer to the length of the OPA, from its flange anteriorly to its distal end. The OPA is sized generally by measuring the distance from the angle of the mouth to the angle of the jaw at the auricle of the ear (Fig. 2a). This can be done quickly by plac-

TABLE 1 Indications, contraindications, & complications of oropharyngeal and nasopharyngeal airways

Oropharyngeal airway:	Nasopharyngeal airway:
Indication:	Indication:
Maintain airway patency in unconscious patients	Maintain an airway in unconscious or semiconscious patient.
Contraindications:	Contraindications:
Conscious or semiconscious patient	Suspected base of skull fracture
Intact gag reflex	Maxillofascial fractures
Use of anticoagulation (relative)	Use of anticoagulation
Small mouth opening	
Macroglossia or angioedema	
Complications:	Complications:
Injury to soft tissues or dental structures	Injury to soft tissues and mucosa
Migration	Submucosal passage
Aspiration	Intracranial insertion
	Migration.

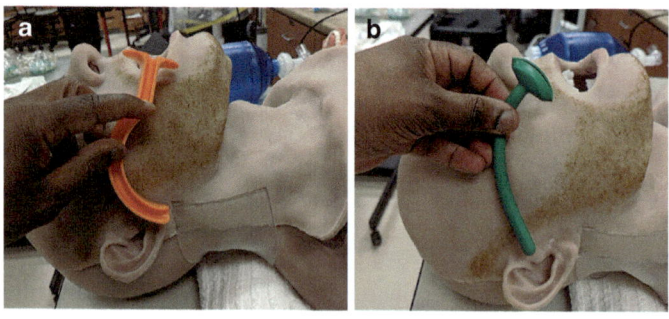

FIGURE 2 (**a**) Sizing the OPA. (**b**) Sizing the NPA

ing the chosen oral airway at the side of the face and measure as above. Generally, sizes 3 and 4 are used for most adults.

Similarly, NPA comes in different sizes, ranging from 5 to 9 mm (or 20F to 36F). In contrast to OPA, the size refers to the inner diameter of the NPA. Generally, sizes 6 and 7 are used in most adults. The traditional teaching of sizing the NPA is by using the diameter of the patient's smallest finger. However, this method has not been validated. The length of the NPA could be estimated similarly to the sizing of the OPA as above (Fig. 2b).

Techniques and Methods

OPA is inserted by two different methods:

1. The OPA is held upside down, with the curvature pointing upwards. It is inserted halfway through the oral cavity before it is rotated 180° and advanced further until the flange sits against the patient's lips.
2. The OPA is held in the correct position, with the curvature pointing downwards. The mouth is opened, and the tongue is advanced outwards either by a jaw thrust or pulled manually. The OPA is inserted and advanced until it seats in position as above.

NPA is inserted through the nares, using the inferior most aspect of the nares above the hard palate, i.e. parallel to the nasal floor. The NPA should be well lubricated with generous amounts of lubricants before insertion. The tip of the NPA is positioned laterally such as the opening is pointing medially. This avoids injury to Little's area or Kiesselbach Plexus and hence epistaxis. The NPA is advanced gently with slight rotational movement. If resistance is encountered, the NPA should not be forced into the nares any further and rather pulled back to avoid mucosal injury and submucosal insertion. The other nares could be tried or the NPA is switched to a smaller size. If time permits, using a 4% atomized lidocaine or 2% lidocaine jelly with or without a vasoconstricting agent is encouraged.

NPA is preferred when there are limitations with mouth opening or patients with large tongues as angioedema or macroglossia. However, OPA is preferred in cases of a suspected base of skull fractures.

1.2 Laryngeal Mask Airway (LMA)

Introduction

Dr. Archie Brain, a British anesthesiologist is known as the inventor of the Laryngeal Mask Airway. Despite being an anesthesiologist, he applied engineering practices to develop the LMA. He believed the best method to connect two tubes is to connect them "end-to-end". At that time, the year 1981, anesthesia was delivered via an endotracheal tube inserted into the anatomical airway, or a facemask with or without oral or nasal airway. He successfully published his initial experience with the laryngeal mask airway in the British Journal of Anesthesia in 1983. Since then, the uses of LMA and the studies to support its use were aplenty highlighting the clinical benefits of the LMA.

The LMA of Dr. Brain, or classical LMA, is the prototype and the proverbial parent of the other supraglottic devices that came afterward. Studies supporting other types of LMA demonstrate either equivalency or lack of inferiority comparing them to the classical LMA, while not demonstrating superiority over it.

Anatomy

The LMA is made primarily out of Polyvinyl Chloride (PVC). Other materials are used for non-disposable LMA. It has a curved tube (Fig. 3), with a connector at its proximal end. This connector allows means of artificial ventilation to be connected to the LMA. At the distal end of the LMA, a bowl is present that matches the shape of the larynx. This bowl is surrounded by a balloon cuff or mask that helps in sealing the larynx. The balloon cuff is inflated using the inflation balloon through the pilot balloon on the outside of the patient.

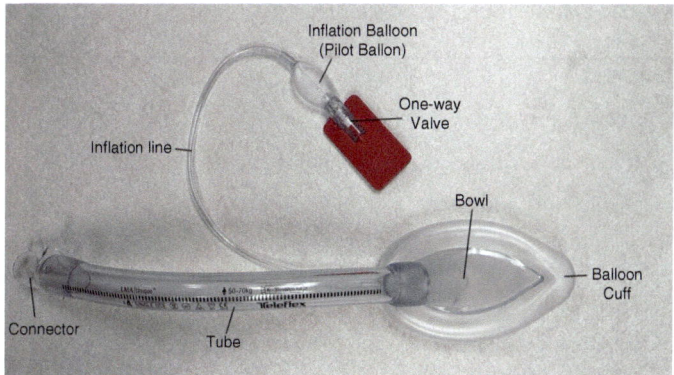

FIGURE 3 Components of the laryngeal mask airway

Indications and Contraindications

The main indication of supraglottic device use is to secure the airway in different clinical scenarios (Table 2). Those scenarios can be as follows:

- Elective general anesthesia cases, e.g., oral and maxillofacial surgeries
- Acute airway management as a rescue device in difficult airway intubation, i.e., in "cannot intubate, cannot oxygenate" situations.
- During Cardiopulmonary Resuscitation (CPR) and in prehospital care.
- In an unresponsive patient.

The LMA is adequately tolerated by patients with minimal side effects or complications. However, malposition could occur in up to 40% of cases. There is a real risk of aspirating gastric contents and secretions as it doesn't violate the airway to protect against aspiration. It is contraindicated in patients who are at increased risk of aspiration as those with a full stomach, increased intraabdominal pressure, or decreased gastric emptying. However, the use of second2generation LMA could help reduce the risk of aspiration. Since LMA insertion requires traversing the oral cavity, it is contraindi-

Table 2 Indications, contraindications, and complications of Laryngeal Mask Airway (LMA)

Indications:

   Elective Surgery

   Rescue device in acute airway management

   During CPR

   In the unresponsive patient

Contraindications:

   Emergency surgery where full stomach is expected

   Increased intrabdominal pressure, e.g. pregnancy, obesity, and decreased gastric emptying or gastroparesis.

   Small mouth opening.

Complications:

   Aspiration of gastric contents

   Malposition and loss of tidal volumes during artificial ventilation.

cated in patients with smallmouth opening or difficulty opening the oral cavity.

Techniques and Methods

The supraglottic device, as the name implies, would sit snuggly on the larynx. This allows for direct communication between the supraglottic device and the tracheobronchial tree. Those devices have to traverse the oropharynx to be effectively placed over the larynx.

(a) The LMA device is prepared. The cuff is inflated with 30-cc of air. Then, the balloon cuff is pressed gently against a flat service to partially deflate the cuff (Fig. 4). Alternatively, the cuff is only inflated with 10-cc of air. Partial inflation of the LMA balloon would provide it with enough rigidity needed at the time of insertion.

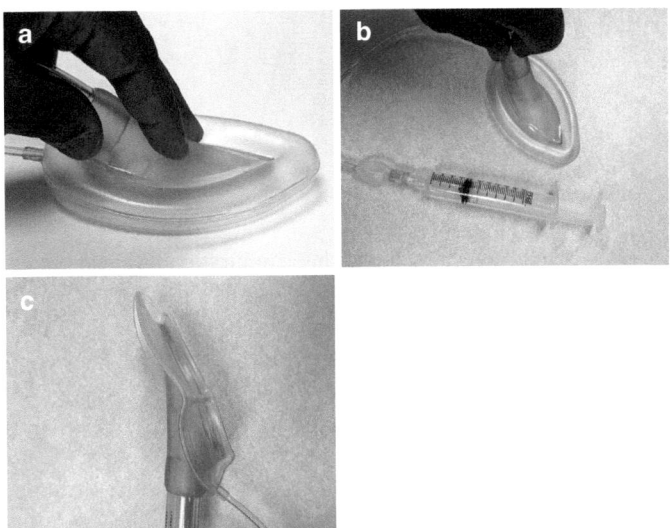

FIGURE 4 (**a**) Deflating the LMA to ensure enough inflation of the balloon to maintain the rigidity of its tip. (**b**) Attaching a syringe to the pilot balloon helps opening the one-way valve. (**c**) A fully deflated LMA balloon. Notice the lack of rigidity of the LMA tip

(b) The patient is positioned in a supine position, and the head is tilted slightly backward. The mouth is then opened.
(c) The LMA is held in the operator's dominant hand (Fig. 5). The distal end of the LMA is held between the index finger and the thumb at the junction of the cuff and the tube. Lubricating the LMA is optional.
(d) The LMA is advanced through the oral cavity with the tip following the hard and soft palate.
(e) The LMA is advanced further until it is seated well over the Larynx. As the LMA clears the soft palate and the oral cavity, a slight "give off" would be encountered before it seats on the larynx with a snug fit. This "give off" or release acts as feedback for adequate seating on the Larynx (Fig. 6). Such excellent seating or positioning is seen on

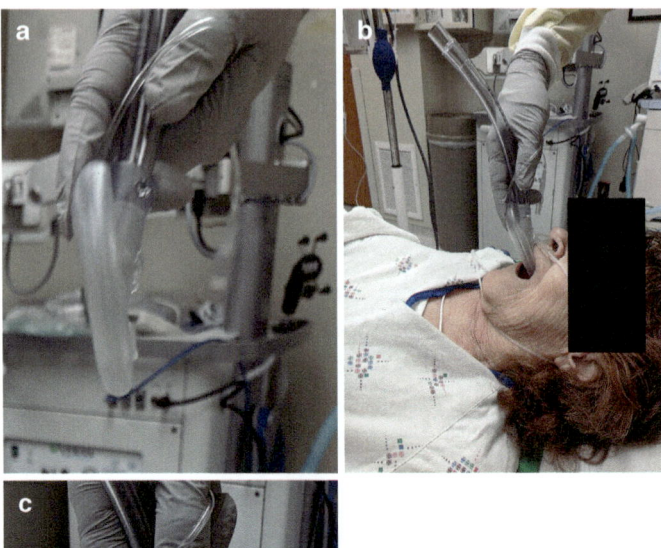

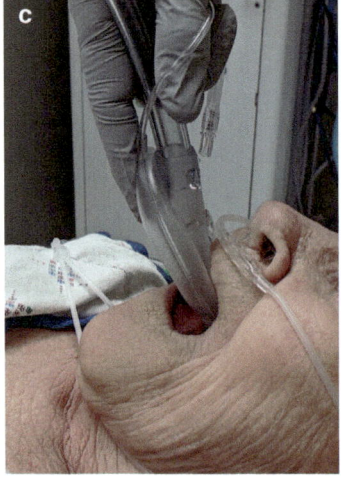

FIGURE 5 (**a**) Laryngeal Mask Airway is held in the dominant hand between the index finger and the thumb at the junction of the cuff and tube. (**b**) The LMA is advanced with the index finger against the roof of the mouth following its curvature. (**c**) Close up of LMA as it is advanced using the index finger into the oral cavity

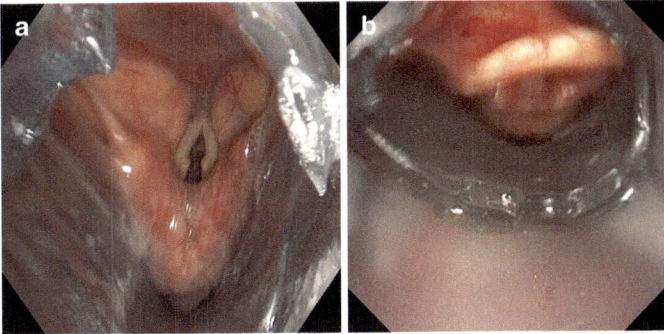

FIGURE 6 (**a**) Endoscopic view of a well seated Laryngeal Mask Airway. (**b**) Endoscopic view of a malpositioned Laryngeal Mask Airway

    flexible laryngoscopy with the tip of the LMA lies within the upper esophageal sphincter, its bowl hugs the larynx while keeping the epiglottis out of the bowl against the posterior oropharynx as it rests on the inflated cuff. This would provide uninterrupted access to the airway

(f) The LMA is then secured in place. Ventilation would ensue using either a bag-mask device or a mechanical ventilator. Connecting a colorimetric capnometer or waveform capnography and monitoring tidal volumes on the ventilator ensures adequate positioning and seating on the Larynx.

Other Types of Supraglottic Devices

The classic LMA was an excellent invention. It was manufactured by the Laryngeal Mask Airway Company before it was bought by Teleflex company. The classic LMA is backed up by millions of case use and thousands of peer-reviewed research papers. However, different types (Fig. 7) of the LMA made that company have been introduced since the classic LMA. Those include:

- LMA Unique
- LMA Flexible

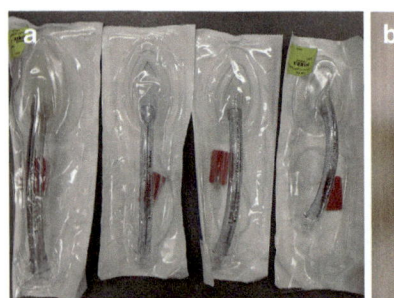
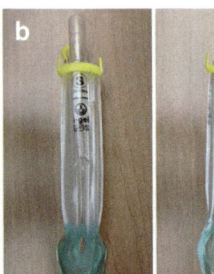
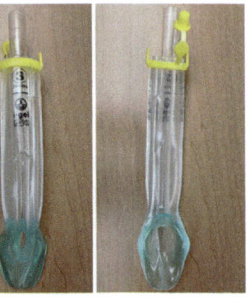

FIGURE 7 Different Laryngeal Mask Airways (LMA). (**a**): LMA unique. (**b**): iGel LMA

- LMA ProSeal
- LMA Supreme
- Intubating LMA or Fastrach

Other manufacturers of similar laryngeal mask airways include:

- Ambu
- Cookgas AirQ
- iGel

It is worth noting that supraglottic devices are divided into a first and second generation, by the presence of a gastric drainage tube in the second generation. This gastric drainage tube reduces the risk of aspiration as it vents out in addition to allowing insertion of an orogastric tube to decompress the stomach.

Pitfalls/Troubleshooting

1. Malposition: This a rather common occurrence, as much as 40% in one series. Radiologically, malposition has been detected in as much as 50–80%. Mispositioning of the LMA occurs from inadequate insufflation pressure (too high or too low), inadequate sizing (too large or too small), or level of insertion (too deep or too shallow). Malposition could occur ventrally or laterally. A malpositioned LMA would increase the risk of gastric insufflation, aspiration of

gastric contents, and air leak with loss of tidal volumes. Removing the LMA and correcting the above issues should improve its positioning and airway seal.
2. A fully deflated LMA (Fig. 4c) could be difficult to insert as it doesn't maintain its shape and can bend on insertion. Having the LMA balloon partially filled with air would mitigate this (see above discussion).
3. Difficulty in advancing the LMA through the oral cavity could be encountered. This usually happens if the mouth opening is small or inadequate. Advancing the jaw should help if this issue arises. If mouth opening is rather limited a different method of airway access should be attempted.

2 Infraglottic Devices

Introduction

The infraglottic devices are tubes that are inserted into the airway to allow for direct access to the airway. Those tubes could be inserted via the oropharynx or the nasopharynx. As their name implies, they are intended to be placed below the level of the glottis at their final position. The hallmark device of this group is the Endotracheal Tube (ETT). The ETT is inserted via direct laryngoscopy (DL) or video laryngoscopy (VL) for an orotracheal route. In the hands of a very experienced operator, blind nasotracheal intubation could be achieved when needed. Once inserted, those tubes allow for the delivery of artificial ventilation. The presence of a balloon cuff near its tip allows for adequate delivery of artificial breaths and reduces the risk of aspiration.

Indications and Contraindications

Endotracheal intubation is indicated (Table 3) in elective procedures requiring deep sedation or general anesthesia, in acute respiratory failure requiring mechanical ventilation, or for the unconscious patients. Inserting an ETT has become more common for bronchoscopy and endobronchial interventions. However, in cases of airway trauma or obstruction

TABLE 3 Indications, contraindications, & complications of Endotracheal intubation and Endotracheal (ET) tubes

Indications:

Elective procedure with deep sedation or general anesthesia.

Acute respiratory failure.

The Unconscious patient.

Acute respiratory failure.

Contraindications:

Trauma to the upper airway

Obstruction of the upper airway

Complications:

Tracheal stenosis

Infections and Ventilator-associated pneumonia

Bleeding

Soft tissue injury

of the upper airway, the ETT cannot be passed and hence contraindicated. The surgical airway should be considered. The extended presence of an ETT could cause tracheal stenosis, and increased risk of infection and ventilator-associated pneumonia. During its insertion, bleeding and injury to the oropharyngeal and upper airway can occur.

Anatomy

The endotracheal tube (Fig. 8) is a long cylindrical tube of about 30 cm in length. It is made of Polyvinyl Chloride (PVC). It comes in different sizes based on its inner diameter. The proximal end has a connector that allows the ETT to connect to a bag-mask device or a mechanical ventilator for ventilation. The distal end of the ETT, or the tip, is usually tapered to allow for easy insertion. The taper is to the left as this allows for good visualization at the time of insertion. It also has a side port, known as Murphy's eye. This allows for

Airway Access 59

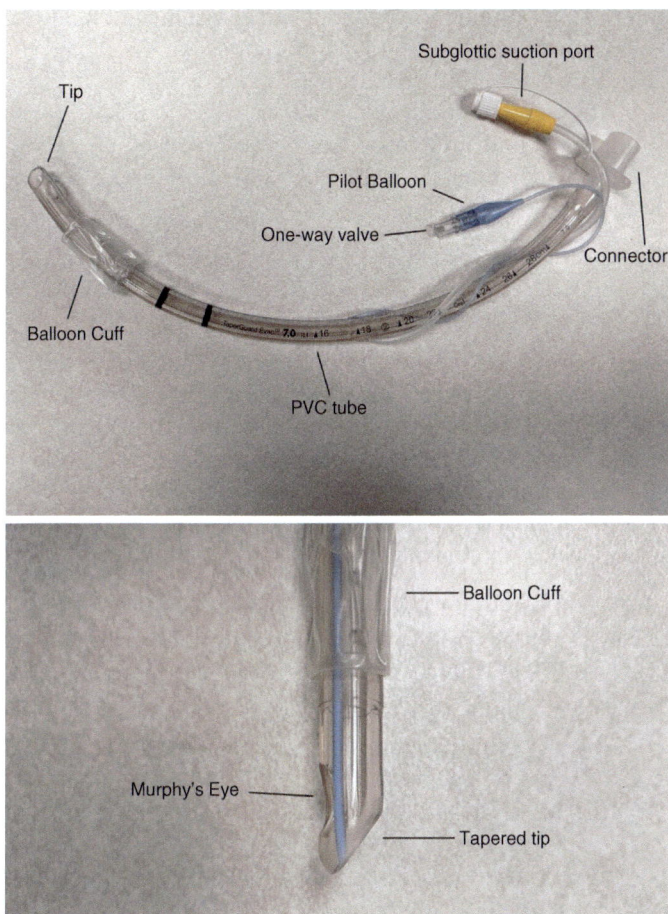

FIGURE 8 Top: Anatomy of the ETT. Bottom: Closeup of the ETT tip

the continued delivery of ventilation if the distal orifice is blocked by secretions or occluded by tracheobronchial wall tissue. It is worth noting that specialty endotracheal tubes are commercially available.

Insertion

Inserting the ETT requires traversing the oropharynx and larynx with the eventual passage of the ETT into the tracheal lumen. This is done mostly under direct visualization. Direct visualization constitutes the cornerstone of inserting the ETT. This can be either a Direct Laryngoscopy or a Video Laryngoscopy to obtain adequate visualization. It is worth noting that blind intubation can be achieved by an experienced provider. Such discussion of blind intubation is beyond the scope of this chapter.

2.1 Direct Laryngoscopy

Direct Laryngoscopy (DL) is a procedure that allows visualization of the Larynx. Once visualized, an ETT could be passed under direct visualization into the trachea. Direct laryngoscopy is an invasive procedure and hence sedation or paralysis is required. Occasionally, awake direct laryngoscopy could be achieved in the hands of an experienced operator in certain special circumstances.

(a) A preprocedural checklist should be completed before direct laryngoscopy and endotracheal intubation. This checklist, at a minimum, should include:
- (i) Universal time-out procedures.
- (ii) Good Intravenous access with at least two peripheral IV lines.
- (iii) Medications for sedation or rapid sequence intubation
- (iv) Preferred ETT size and a backup one of a smaller size.
- (v) An oral suction catheter or a Yankauer suction tip.
- (vi) Direct laryngoscope with handle and blade, including a light source.
- (vii) Intravenous fluids
- (viii) Bag-Mask device
- (ix) Supplemental Oxygen.
- (x) 10-cc syringe
- (xi) Colorimetric Capnometer (CO_2 detector)
- (xii) A stethoscope.

(b) The ETT should be checked and prepared first. This includes unpacking the ETT and inflating the balloon using the 10-cc syringe to ensure its intactness. The balloon is then deflated and retracted manually to form a slim profile at its tip. Lubricating the tip of the ETT is optional but encouraged.
(c) A malleable stylet is inserted into the lumen of the ETT which is shaped into a "hockey stick" by bending the distal few centimeters of the ETT to about 30° (Fig. 9).
(d) The direct laryngoscope is then checked, and a blade is chosen. It can not be stressed enough how important to check

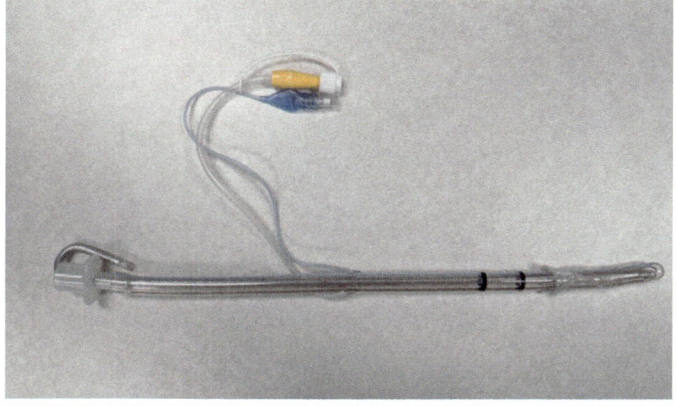

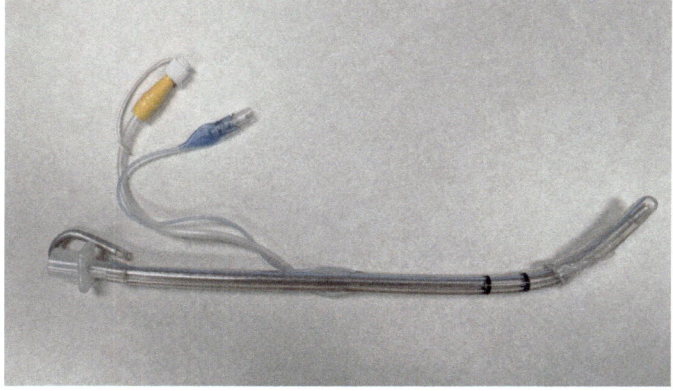

FIGURE 9 Top: ETT with Malleable style. Bottom: ETT with malleable stylet in "Hockey stick" shape

that the light source and the batteries are in a good functioning condition at this point, before proceeding any further.

Blades available for Direct Laryngoscopy are:

(i) A curved blade (Fig. 10), or Macintosh, with a left-facing shelf or flange, and a wide tip reinforced into a knob at its tip.

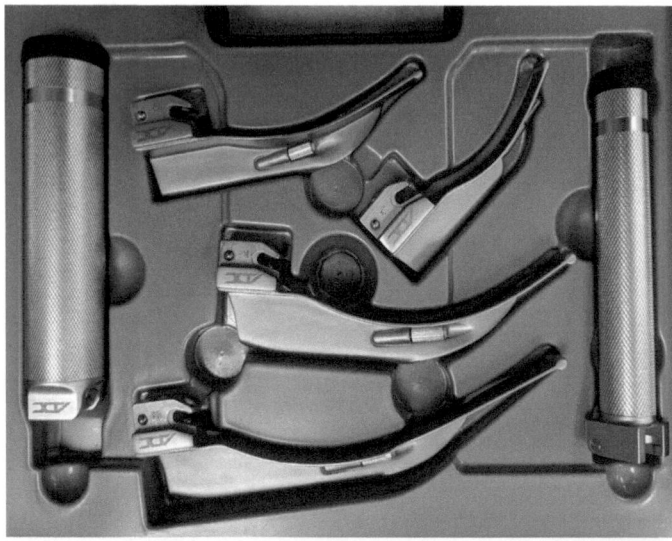

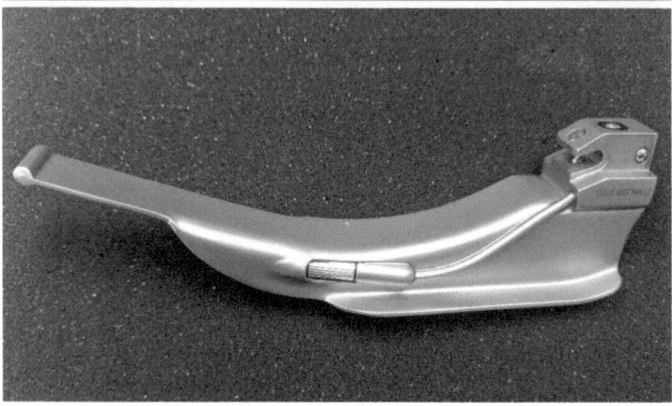

FIGURE 10 Macintosh blade

(b) The ETT should be checked and prepared first. This includes unpacking the ETT and inflating the balloon using the 10-cc syringe to ensure its intactness. The balloon is then deflated and retracted manually to form a slim profile at its tip. Lubricating the tip of the ETT is optional but encouraged.
(c) A malleable stylet is inserted into the lumen of the ETT which is shaped into a "hockey stick" by bending the distal few centimeters of the ETT to about 30° (Fig. 9).
(d) The direct laryngoscope is then checked, and a blade is chosen. It can not be stressed enough how important to check

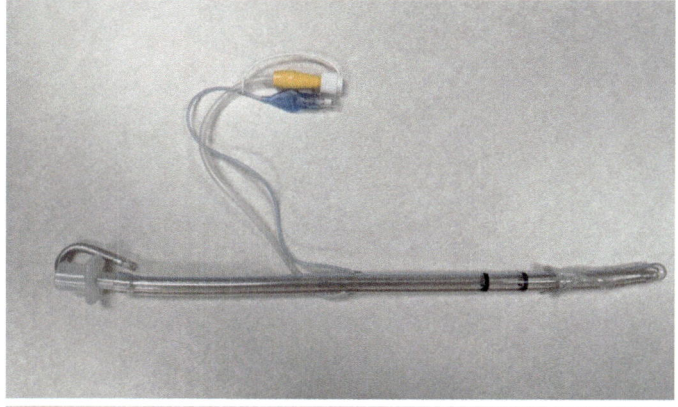

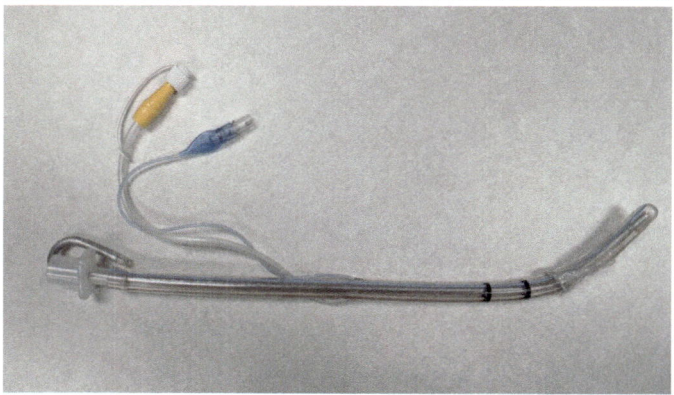

FIGURE 9 Top: ETT with Malleable style. Bottom: ETT with malleable stylet in "Hockey stick" shape

that the light source and the batteries are in a good functioning condition at this point, before proceeding any further.

Blades available for Direct Laryngoscopy are:

(i) A curved blade (Fig. 10), or Macintosh, with a left-facing shelf or flange, and a wide tip reinforced into a knob at its tip.

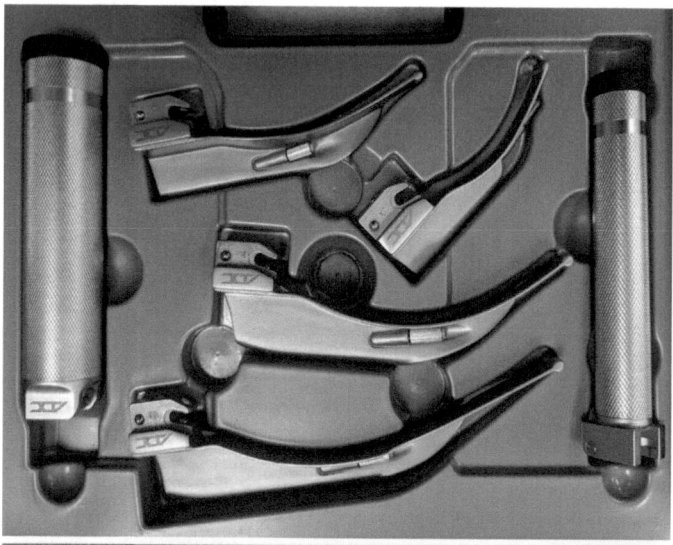

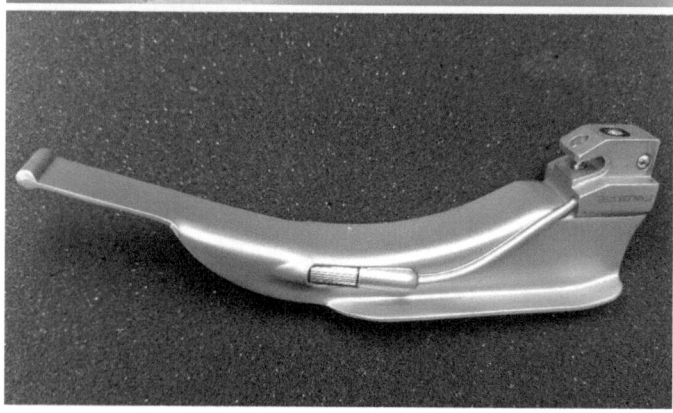

Figure 10 Macintosh blade

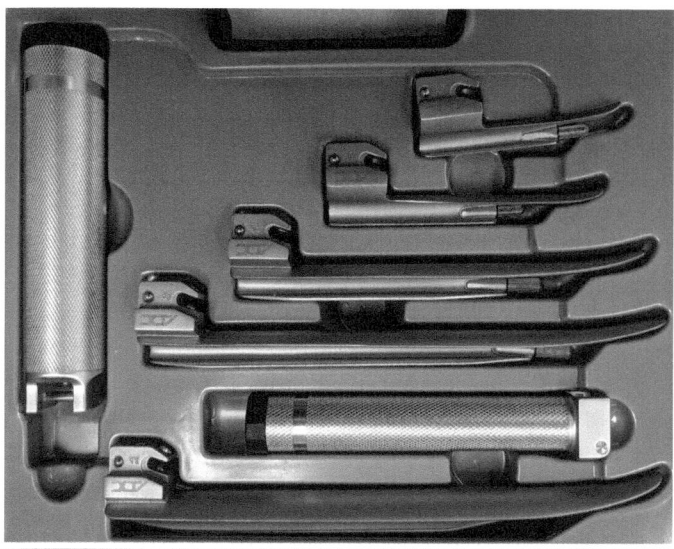
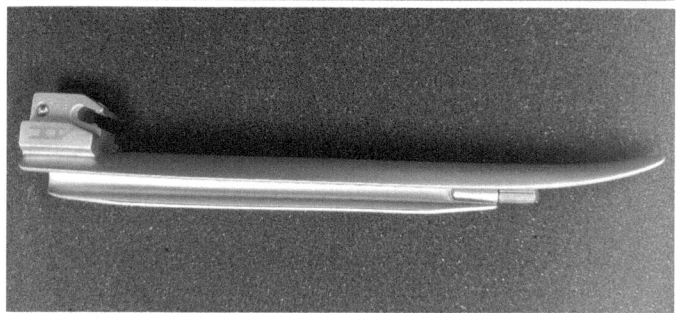

FIGURE 11 Miller blade

(ii) A straight blade (Fig. 11), or Miller, has a slimmer profile with a smaller left-facing flange and without a reinforced or thick tip.

(e) Patient weight is confirmed and intended sedation and paralytics are drawn up by nursing staff or a provider responsible for sedation.

(f) The bed is positioned in a way that would allow the intubating provider to be standing up with the arms and hands are at a comfortable level for intubation.

(g) The patient is positioned in a "sniff-position". At that position, the patient's oral axis, pharyngeal axis, and laryngeal axis are aligned allowing for optimum intubation condition.
(h) The blade is held in the left hand (Fig. 12), regardless of the operator's dominant hand. It is held firmly at the lower half of the handle.

The next steps would vary depending on the chosen blade

Curved Blade (Macintosh):

1. The blade is inserted from the right corner of the mouth and advanced slightly. The blade is quickly moved to the midline, "sweeping" the tongue to the left. The tongue is carried by the flange during this maneuver.
2. The blade is advanced further inwards. Intermittently, the handle is lifted at the operator's shoulder. This allows the operator to evaluate the anatomy before advancing the blade further. The lifting maneuver happens at the operator's shoulder, not the elbow.
3. The above step is repeated as the blade is advanced further inwards, until the epiglottis is identified. The epiglottis is the anatomical landmark that must be identified during direct laryngoscopy.
4. The blade is then advanced **anterior** to the epiglottis and into the hyo-epiglottic ligament. As the reinforced knob is advanced into the hyoepiglottic ligament, the epiglottis will lift. Further lifting occurs at the shoulder of the operator, not the elbow, to provide a good view of the larynx and vocal cords.
5. The ETT is advanced from the right corner of the mouth and directed towards the vocal cords. This would result in direct visualization of the intubation process as the tube is inserted endotracheally.

Straight Blade (Miller):

1. The blade is inserted through the midline. A sweeping action is not necessarily needed.

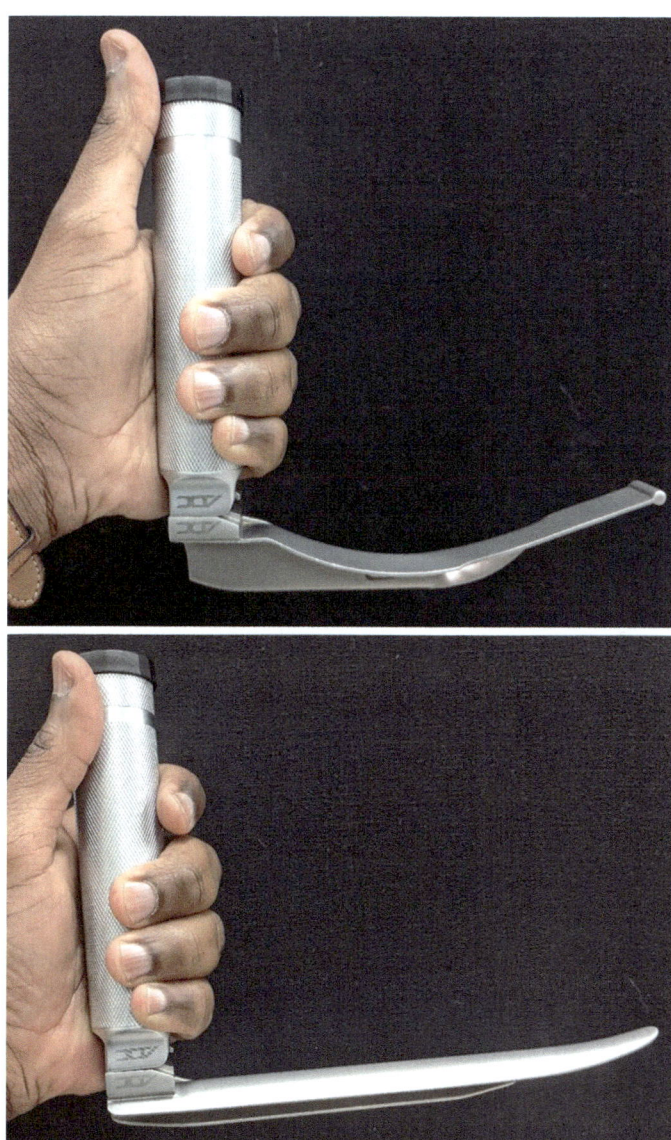

FIGURE 12 Holding the intubating blade

2. The blade is raised intermittently during advancement to view anatomical landmarks. Again, the epiglottis is the anatomical landmark to be visualized.
3. Once the epiglottis is identified, the miller blade is advanced **posterior** to it.
4. Lifting the handle at the shoulder would result in lifting the epiglottis and opening the airway to visualize the larynx and vocal cords.
5. The ETT is advanced from the right corner of the mouth and observed as it enters the trachea.

Once the ETT is inserted into the trachea, the following steps could be completed:

(i) The malleable stylet is removed partially. This will help straighten the distal end of the endotracheal tube, allowing it to be advanced into the airway easily.
(j) The balloon of the ETT is inflated using the 10-cc syringe.
(k) The tube position is checked. This can be done in different ways.

1. Waveform capnography or a color-changing CO_2 detector.
2. Auscultation over both bilateral lung fields and the stomach area.
3. A suction esophageal detection device.
4. Bronchoscopic view of the endotracheal lumen.

Pitfalls/Troubleshooting
1. Starting with smaller blade size. Size 4 blade (for both Macintosh and Miller blades) is a reasonable starting size as it allows access to the laryngeal structures. However, if a smaller size is chosen and later discovered not to be adequate to visualize the laryngeal structures, changing it to a larger size is appropriate and strongly encouraged.
2. Inability to visualize the vocal cords. This would lead to difficult intubation. There are different plausible explanations and solutions to this:

(a) Lifting the blade at the shoulder should help, as it would lift the head of the patient upwards and anteriorly lining the oral, pharyngeal, and laryngeal axes better.
(b) Adequate positioning of the patient to align the oral, pharyngeal, and laryngeal axes.
(c) While in between attempts, analyzing the steps are taken in the process and what could have gone wrong would allow for self-correction and improvement with the next attempt.
(d) Changing the type of blade could also help if the vocal cords are not well visualized.
(e) Occasionally, and in the hands of an experienced operator, visualizing the posterior arytenoid cartilages and advancing the ETT anterior to those structures would lead to successful intubation.
(f) Arm fatigue would lead to difficulty lifting the blade and visualizing the vocal cords.

3. Arm fatigue. Swapping operators would help if this happened. Novice operators would experience arm fatigue sooner than their experienced counterparts. Assigning BMV with jaw thrust and chin lift to a different provider minimizes the chances of the intubating provider's arm fatigue.

2.2 *Video Laryngoscopy*

The development and evolution of fiberoptic fibers and miniaturization of the video cameras have facilitated the development of video laryngoscopy. Contrary to conventional direct laryngoscopy, they mostly provide an indirect view of the laryngeal structures during intubation via an external monitor or attached screen. There are different manufacturers of video laryngoscopes (Fig. 13), with different types and angulation of the blades (Fig. 14). Some manufacturers have

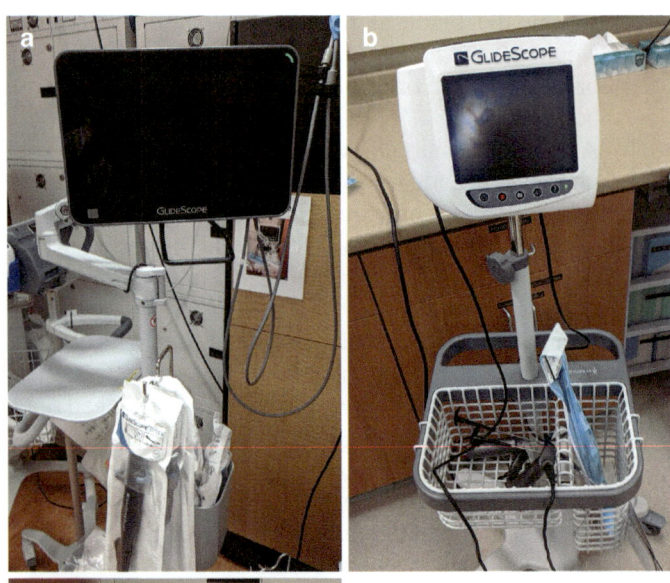
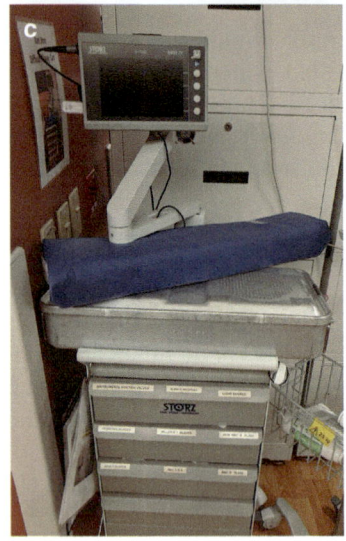

FIGURE 13 Video Laryngoscopes. (**a**) GlideScope. (**b**) GlideScope. (**c**) Karl Storz C-MAC

Airway Access 69

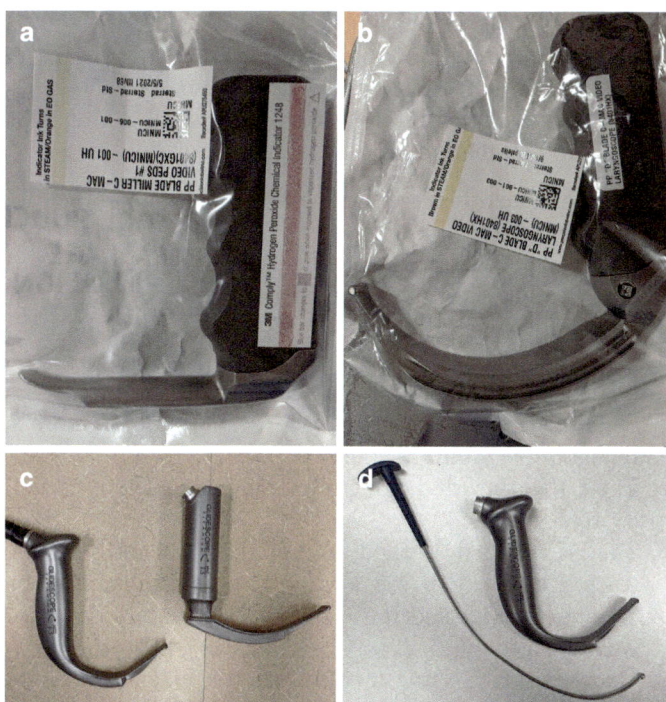

FIGURE 14 Video Laryngoscope Blades (**a**) Pediatric Miller Blade for Karl Storz C-MAC. (**b**) Adult Macintosh Blade for Karl Stroz C-MAC. (**c**) GlideScope LoPro T3 blade (left) and MAC T3 (right). (**d**) GlideScope T3 LoPro blade with proprietary angulated stylet. Notice the matching angulation to the blade

manufactured Mac & Miller blades to use with video laryngoscopy. Video laryngoscopy and the angulated blade allow to maneuver around the oropharyngeal and laryngeal structures, instead of compressing and mobilizing them as with direct laryngoscopy. Additionally, video laryngoscopy provides an improved angle of view.

Techniques

The steps required for intubation using a video laryngoscope are rather similar to direct laryngoscopy discussed above. The preparatory, and post-intubation steps are similar. The differences in the intubation process are as follow:

1. The angulated blade is inserted through the midline into the open mouth.
2. The blade is advanced following the curvature of the oropharynx and the anatomical structures until the epiglottis comes in view.
3. Once the Epiglottis is in view, the tip of the angulated blade is directed in the hyoepiglottic space, anterior to the epiglottis. This is achieved by a rocking motion, more so than a lifting motion.
4. The ETT is inserted along the midline and advanced until it comes in view.
5. The ETT is then directed through the vocal cords into the trachea until slight resistance is met. This happens as the angulated stylet and the ETT meet the anterior tracheal wall.
6. Once resistance is met, the stylet should be removed before further advancement of the ETT.
7. The ETT is then advanced further into the tracheal lumen.

Advantages

1. Video laryngoscopy allows the operator to maneuver around tissue instead of compressing it.
2. It facilitates the teaching of learners, either by demonstrating to them while they observe the anatomy or allowing their supervisor to observe and provide real-time feedback during intubation.
3. It increases the success rate of the first-time pass, although the studies yielded contradicting results.
4. Reduces arm fatigue, as less force is being used during the intubation process.
5. Allow for photographic and videographic documentation.

Pitfalls/Troubleshooting

1. Video laryngoscope requires the operator to look at the screen at all times as she or he is intubating the patient. However, the eyes of the operator should be directed to the patient's mouth when the ETT and stylet are introduced into the oral cavity. Otherwise, injury to the oral structures will ensue.
2. Some video laryngoscopy manufactures have proprietary angulated stylets that are used with their video laryngoscopes. If they are not available, a malleable stylet could be used. It is imperative to closely match the angulation of the angulated blade when this type of stylet is used.
3. Advancing the blade deeper into the hyoepiglottic space would lead to the further lifting of the epiglottis. Directing the ETT in those situations would prove difficult. Relaxing the rocking motion and hence the lifting action of the epiglottis would help mitigate this.
4. It is natural to feel rushed to intubate a patient, especially in urgent or emergent situations. However, video laryngoscopy will inherently take longer than direct laryngoscopy. It is advisable not to rush through the laryngoscopy or the intubation process to increase the chance of successful intubation.

3 Surgical Airway

Introduction

Surgical techniques to access the airway provide an excellent alternative to securing the airway in case of an emergency (cricothyroidotomy or surgical/open tracheostomy), or as a method of delivering prolonged mechanical ventilation when needed. Tracheotomy and Tracheostomy, although used interchangeably, have different meanings. The former indicates the incision into the trachea, while the latter is the formed stoma between the trachea and the skin.

Here, we will review the indications of surgical airway access, contraindications, and possible complications. Surgical airway access includes cricothyroidotomy and surgical tracheostomy creation. We will primarily discuss Cricothyroidotomy. We will briefly discuss the surgical creation of tracheostomy; however, a detailed discussion is beyond the scope of this chapter. In the next section, we will discuss percutaneous tracheostomy as a separate procedure.

Indications

Surgical airway access is employed when the translaryngeal approach is not accessible or the use of which is rather prolonged. Hence, indications for such procedures (cricothyroidotomy and tracheostomy) can be divided into three general groups (Table 4):

TABLE 4 Indications, contraindications, and complications of surgical airway

Indications:

   Prolonged mechanical ventilation

   Airway and laryngeal obstruction.

   Airway protection and secretion management.

Contraindications:

   Lack of procedural knowledge and operator's inexperience.

   Soft tissue infection

   Bleeding diathesis

   Recent sternotomy & history of head and neck surgery.

Complications:

   Bleeding

   Site infection

   Injury to soft tissue – larynx, vocal cord, trachea

   Pneumothorax & Pneumomediastinum.

1. Prolonged mechanical ventilation
2. Airway or laryngeal obstruction
3. Airway protection. It is worth noting that airway protection or secretions management could be achieved by different means as well.

It is imperative to understand that cricothyroidotomy is the preferred method of surgical airway access when an airway establishment is needed emergently. Tracheostomy, on the other hand, is preferred to maintain the airway in cases where prolonged mechanical ventilation is needed or expected. Such surgical techniques required a very good knowledge of airway anatomy.

Contraindications of surgical airway access include:

1. Overlaying soft tissue infection
2. Inability to palpate anatomy adequately.
3. Bleeding diathesis or uncorrectable coagulopathy or thrombocytopenia.
4. Operator inexperience
5. Recent sternotomy
6. History of head and neck surgery.

Technique/Methods

A. **Cricothyroidotomy:**

Cricothyroidotomy involves a puncture of the cricothyroid membrane to give access to the upper trachea. This opening can be created either surgically or percutaneously.

1. **Surgical Cricothyroidotomy:**

    (a) Standard preprocedural steps should be performed before the start of the procedure if possible. This includes standard timeout protocol and aseptic techniques and precautions.
    (b) The operator stands on the side of his dominant hand, mostly the right side of the patient.
    (c) Palpate neck anatomy. Identify the thyroid cartilage, which is the prominent protrusion in the

neck. The prominence of the thyroid cartilage is more noticeable in males.
(d) Slide the finger down the Thyroid cartilage to the cricothyroid membrane. This membrane extends from the Thyroid cartilage superiorly to the cricoid cartilage inferiorly. Identifying the cricoid cartilage before sliding the palpating finger cephalad into the cricothyroid membrane is an acceptable alternative.
(e) Pin the Larynx in position by the thumb and the long finger of the non-dominant hand. This would leave the index finger free to palpate the anatomy and the cricothyroid membrane.
(f) Using a #15 scalpel on the dominant hand, make a vertical 1.5–2.0 cm incision.
(g) A horizontal incision is made at the caudal end of the cricothyroid membrane.
(h) A tracheal hook is inserted into the airway in the horizontal orientation with the opening towards the operator.
(i) The tracheal hook is then rotated 90° clockwise before it is pulled cephalad to hook the thyroid cartilage. Others have recommended hooking the cricoid cartilage by rotating the tracheal hook 90° counterclockwise. This would decrease the risk of injury to the vocal cords, given their proximity to this location.
(j) A Trousseau dilator or a Kelly clamp is then inserted into the tracheal incision from the side and opened to dilate the incision.
(k) The cricothyroidotomy tube with the introducer is inserted into the trachea going caudad. At the same time, the Trousseau dilator or the Kelly clamp is rotated 90° counterclockwise to facilitate the entry of the cricothyroidotomy tube into the airway.
(l) The introducer is then removed entirely leaving the cricothyroidotomy tube in the airway.

(m) The balloon cuff is inflated and the patient is connected to a Bag-Mask or a mechanical ventilator for assisted ventilation.
(n) The new cricothyroidotomy tube is then secured in position with soft ties.
(o) Post tracheostomy/cricothyroidotomy care ensues.
(p) The cricothyroidotomy is eventually converted to a tracheostomy as soon as the patient's condition stabilizes or within 24–48 h.

2. **Percutaneous Cricothyroidotomy – Seldinger Technique:**

   There are similarities between the two approaches, but the percutaneous cricothyroidotomy might be easier to learn by non-surgeons given the use of the Seldinger technique and the similarities with the central venous access method.

   Steps (**a**) to (**f**) and steps (**m**) to (**p**) are like the surgical technique.

   (g) A 16- to 18-gauge catheter over the needle is connected to a saline-filled syringe and inserted at 45° caudally at the lower end of the cricothyroid membrane. Successful puncture of the airway is confirmed by aspirating air (bubbles in the saline-filled syringe).
   (h) The needle and syringe are removed, leaving the 6F catheter in place
   (i) A guidewire is then inserted through the catheter a few centimeters into the airway.
   (j) The 6F catheter is removed while leaving the guidewire in place.
   (k) The cricothyroidotomy tube loaded onto a dilator is inserted over the guidewire and into the airway caudally.
   (l) The dilator and guidewire are then removed completely leaving the newly placed cricothyroidotomy tube in place.

3. **Rapid 4-step Technique:**
   This method was described by Brofedl in 1996. It involves 4 steps that are easy to recall. It also requires no specialized equipment. A clinician will need a scalpel, a tracheal hook, and a tracheostomy tube or an endotracheal tube.

   (a) Palpation:
   The clinician stands on the left side of the patient, palpate anatomy using the left index finger while fixing the larynx between the thumb and the long finger. Identification of the cricothyroid membrane is essential. Occasionally, a skin incision might be required to facilitate palpation of anatomy.
   (b) Stab incision:
   This is completed by inserting a #20 surgical scalpel held in the right hand at the inferior aspect of the cricothyroid membrane. Once the membrane is stabbed, the scalpel position is maintained.
   (c) Inferior traction:
   A tracheal hook held in the left hand is inserted caudad to the scalpel. Once into the tracheal lumen, it is rotated 90° clockwise and caudal traction is applied to the superior border of the cricoid cartilage. Traction is maintained and the scalpel is removed.
   (d) Tube insertion:
   Using a cricothyroid tube, a size 6.0 tracheostomy tube, or a small endotracheal tube held in the right hand is then inserted into the newly created stoma and directed caudad into the airway. This is now secured in place and connected for artificial ventilation.

B. **Surgical Tracheostomy:**
Surgical tracheostomy is an ancient procedure performed in extremis to open the airway. With the advancement in anesthesia, it became a common procedure for

those who need an established airway. Chevalier Jackson has described the procedure in the early twentieth century which remained similar to the present day.

(a) A preprocedural checklist is followed, adhering to Time-out protocols and aseptic techniques as per local practices.

(b) The patient is positioned in a supine position. Neck hyperextension is achieved by placing a pillow or a shoulder strap behind the shoulders. This helps to expose the neck and the laryngeal/tracheal anatomical landmarks.

(c) The skin is marked identifying the anatomical landmarks (Thyroid cartilage, Cricoid Cartilage, and sternal notch). The location of the planned surgical incision is marked as well at this time.

(d) The skin at the intended surgical incision is infiltrated with 1% lidocaine with epinephrine. Lidocaine would provide the local anesthesia and, more importantly, the epinephrine will provide adequate vasoconstriction to the area.

(e) The skin incision is made, soft tissue is divided down to the strap muscles. The skin incision is usually made horizontally; however, a vertical incision could be made.

(f) The strap muscles are separated laterally at the midline. This helps in identifying the thyroid isthmus. They are held in place using surgical retractors.

(g) The thyroid isthmus is clamped, then divided between the clamps and oversewn.

(h) The cricoid cartilage and tracheal rings are identified. The preferred entry point between tracheal rings is chosen. It is imperative to avoid a sub-cricoid insertion.

(i) At this point, different approaches could be taken:

  (i) Silk stay-sutures are inserted in the paramedian area to allow holding the trachea open as

a vertical midline incision is made. Additionally, the stay sutures help to pull the trachea up to the skin. The tracheostomy tube could be inserted through that incision.
  (ii) A window of cartilage could be removed to create the tracheostomy; however, this risks the development of tracheal stenosis and tracheomalacia.
  (iii) A Bjork flap could be formed by an inverted U-shaped incision to create the tracheotomy. However, the flap could obstruct the tracheal opening if it comes undone.
 (j) The tracheostomy tube is secured with sutures and soft trach ties applied.
 (k) Post-tracheostomy care.

Pitfalls and Troubleshooting

- Making the horizontal incision in the cricothyroid membrane at its superior end. This could injure the vocal cords, and more importantly the cricothyroid vasculature leading to bleeding. Using an ultrasound before the procedure, when time permits, would help with the correct placement of the horizontal incision.
- Forgetting to insert the Trousseau dilator into the vertical incision. This helps with vertical dilation of the entry point to the tracheal lumen.
- Attempting to control bleeding before establishing the airway. As the cricothyroidotomy is THE final step in the "cannot intubate, cannot ventilate" emergency airway algorithm, time is of the essence and should not be wasted controlling bleeding. This could be achieved after the airway is secured.
- A clinical fixation on a cricothyroidotomy tube. Similar to the point above, an appropriate airway must be placed if a cricothyroidotomy tube is not available. Common alternatives would be a cuffed Shiley 6.0 tracheostomy tube or a cuffed endotracheal tube of a small outer diameter.

- Inserting a large diameter tube should be avoided when possible, to reduce the risk of vocal cord injury and subglottic stenosis.

4 Percutaneous Dilatation Tracheostomy (PDT)

Introduction

Performing a tracheostomy for the airway can either be an open tracheostomy (i.e., surgical approach) or a percutaneous dilatation tracheostomy (PDT). Percutaneous dilatational tracheostomy involves creating a tracheal stoma percutaneously before dilating it for the eventual placement of a tracheostomy tube. Studies have demonstrated no differences between the two techniques, although PDT has the slight advantage of less stomal infection. Another advantage is the ability to perform percutaneous dilatational tracheostomy at the bedside, minimizing the need for patient transportation or using Operating Room time. Most of the time, PDT is performed with moderate or deep sedation, and infrequently a neuromuscular blockade is needed. General Anesthesia is rarely if ever used. The indications for percutaneous tracheostomy are similar to those for surgical airway access. Tracheotomy and Tracheostomy are used interchangeably although they carry some differences.

Technique

Like any other invasive procedure, a preprocedural checklist is completed confirming informed consent, coagulation status, review of bloodwork, history, physical examination, and current or recent medications. Additional equipment that is preferred to be available, electrocautery machine, open tracheostomy kit, an airway box for emergent re-intubation in the event of inadvertent extubation (Fig. 15). There are different commercially available kits to complete the PDT procedure. E.g. Portex ULTRAperc Single Dilator kit (Smiths

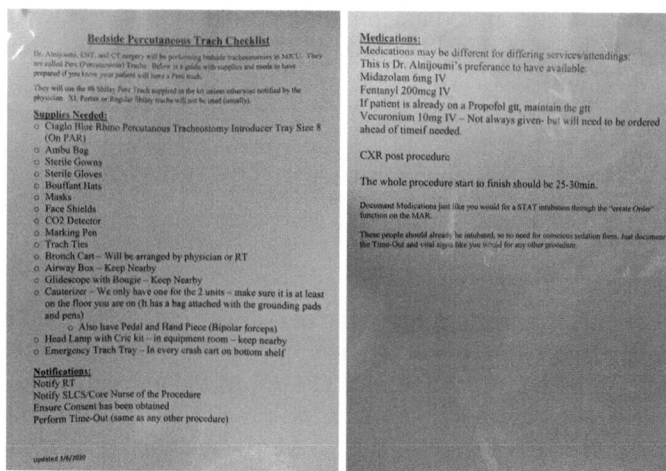

FIGURE 15 A checklist for equipment and medications for bedside percutaneous dilatational tracheostomy

Medical), Ciaglia Blue Dolphin kit using balloon dilation (Cook Medical), & Ciaglia Blue Rhino Percutaneous tracheostomy kit (Cook Medical). We commonly use the Ciaglia Blue Rhino percutaneous kit (Fig. 16), and the following steps apply to that kit specifically. The principle is similar, to dilate a tracheostomy tract percutaneously.

1. The patient is positioned in the supine position with a hyperextended neck. Neck hyperextension is achieved by placing a shoulder roll behind the patient.
2. Neck anatomy is palpated, and landmarks are marked using a skin marker. Those landmarks are thyroid cartilage, cricoid cartilage, and the suprasternal notch.
3. Using an ultrasound to examine this space is rather optional. However, it helps in identifying those structures adequately, namely thyroid cartilage, cricoid cartilage, and tracheal rings. Additionally, ultrasonography helps in selecting the entry site and identifying vascular structures around it. Hence, the use of ultrasonography is strongly encouraged if pulsation is palpated around the entry site or the suprasternal notch.

Airway Access 81

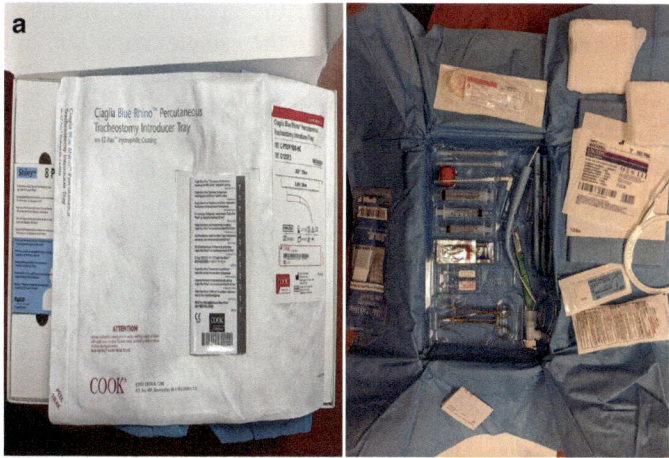

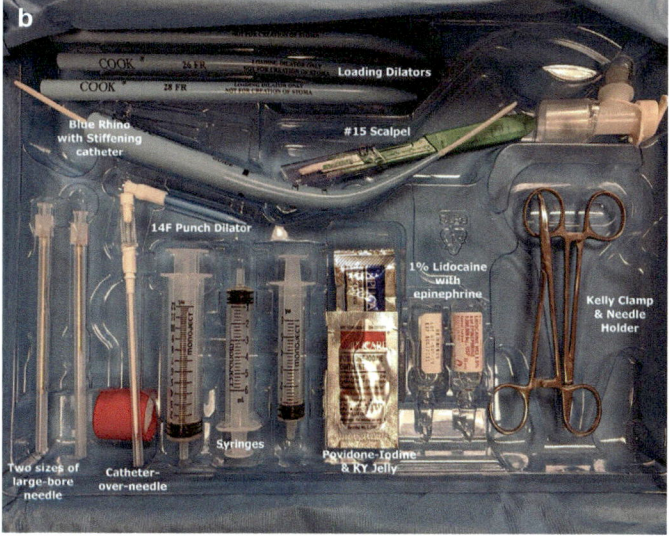

Figure 16 (**a**) Ciaglia Blue Rhino Percutaneous Tracheostomy Kit.
(**b**) Contents of the Blue Rhino Tray Kit

4. The kit is opened and prepped, including checking the balloon of the tracheostomy tube. While deflating the balloon, it is encouraged to pull back on the balloon as much as to shrink the outer profile of the tube. The tracheos-

tomy tube is then loaded on the appropriate tracheostomy loader, by matching the single digit of the tracheostomy loader to the size of the trach – e.g., 28F dilator for the 8.0 tracheostomy tube.
5. The operator should stand at the side of the patient that corresponds to the operator's dominant hand.
6. The neck is cleaned with povidone-iodine or 2% Chlorhexidine sticks, following the manufacturer recommended instructions.
7. A fenestrated drape is applied, exposing the surgical site.
8. A topical anesthetic, 1% Lidocaine with epinephrine, is injected at the incision site and allowed adequate time. The epinephrine helps achieve vasoconstriction and minimize site bleeding.
9. The non-dominant hand of the operator is used to hold the skin taught before a surgical incision, about 2 cm in length, is made at the insertion site. Although a horizontal incision can be used, we prefer to use a vertical incision starting just below the cricoid cartilage. Such a vertical incision helps avoid the laterally located thyroid arteries and the external jugular veins. It also allows for repositioning of the insertion needle if need be. The incision can also be extended if the need arises.
10. Blunt dissection of the subcutaneous fat to the pretracheal fascia is carried out with the operator's dominant index finger or a hemostat clamp.
11. Optimally, reexamination and palpation of the cricoid cartilage and the tracheal rings after blunt dissection is performed.
12. The bronchoscopist, at the head of the bed, would have already inserted a flexible bronchoscope through the endotracheal tube into the tracheobronchial tree. The airway is suctioned as needed.
13. The flexible bronchoscope is retracted slowly within the lumen of the endotracheal tube while observing for transillumination. This allows for confirming the entry position.

14. The bronchoscope is advanced to the tip of the endotracheal tube until only a rim of the ETT is within view.
15. The ETT is loosened, and the bronchoscope with the ETT is slowly retracted as one unit while observing for transillumination. Experienced bronchoscopists could observe for the bronchoscopic view of the cricoid cartilage and the subglottic shelf to avoid inadvertent extubation.
16. Maintaining the bronchoscope within the ETT would help minimize any inadvertent needle injury and damage to the flexible bronchoscope. However, the use of disposable bronchoscopes makes this step insignificant.
17. The introducer needle with or without a saline-filled syringe is bounced off the wall of the trachea to ensure the intended puncture site is on an intercartilagenous membrane and not on tracheal cartilage. If it was felt to be on a tracheal ring, the needle tip is tilted slightly caudad or cephalad to guide the needle's tip on the intercartilagenous membrane to avoid any tracheal ring fracture. Tracheal ring fracture could lead to future tracheal or subglottic stenosis. Moreover, bouncing the needle off the tracheal wall would ensure an adequate central position. It is worth noting that there are two insertion needles in the kit. One with a catheter-over-needle allowing the guidewire to be inserted through the catheter after removal of the needle. The other is a larger-gauge needle allowing direct insertion of the guidewire into the airway through the needle's lumen.
18. The entry point should be between first & second, or second & third tracheal rings, at a location between 10 O'clock and 2 O'clock. It is preferred to be as close to noon position as possible.
19. The needle is inserted into the trachea under direct bronchoscopic visualization and positioned caudad. It is important to ensure that the tip of the needle remains within the lumen of the airway and not advanced any further to risk puncture to the posterior wall.
20. The guidewire is inserted through the catheter or the lumen of the larger-gauge needle into the airway towards

the carina under direct bronchoscopic visualization. The needle or the catheter is then removed leaving the guidewire in place.
21. The 14F punch dilator is inserted over the guidewire into the airway with or without twisting motion under direct bronchoscopic visualization. Focused attention is on protecting and avoiding any injury to the posterior wall. The punch dilator is then removed, leaving the guidewire in place.
22. The one-step dilator, The Blue Rhino, with the white stiffening catheter is held in a pincer position and inserted over the guidewire into the airway in a motion that follows the airway. This is done under direct bronchoscopic visualization while ensuring that the posterior wall is not in its path. The Blue Rhino is advanced up to the "skin-level" mark. It could be left in place for few seconds or removed immediately after reaching that mark. This motion could be repeated once if needed to ensure adequate dilation.
23. The Blue Rhino is then removed leaving the stiffening catheter and the guidewire in place.
24. The appropriate size tracheostomy tube loaded on its dilator is inserted over the guidewire and the stiffening catheter into the airway under direct bronchoscopic visualization. Adequate airway insertion is indicated by a two-step release felt as the balloon clears the stoma into the tracheal lumen. This is a personal observation, not documented by peer-reviewed sources. The author describes this as the "two-pop" feedback.
25. The white stiffening catheter and the guidewire are then removed.
26. The bronchoscope is then taken out of the ETT and inserted into the newly placed tracheostomy tube. Bronchoscopic visualization of the distal tracheal rings and the main carina confirms adequate placement of the tracheostomy tube within the tracheal lumen. The bronchoscope is removed promptly.

27. The inner cannula of the tracheostomy tube is inserted, the balloon inflated, and the tracheostomy tube is connected to the mechanical ventilator circuit. Ventilator graphics is monitored to ensure adequate ventilation with the return of delivered tidal volumes. The use of colorimetric capnometry or end-tidal CO_2 capnography is an additional optional step confirming correct positioning.
28. The tracheostomy tube is either sutured to the skin or not. Clinical evidence is lacking to prefer one approach over the other. Published guidelines encourage using sutures. It is in the author's opinion to avoid suturing the tracheostomy tube as the presence of sutures conveys a false sense of security if trach issues arise. If sutures are placed, they should be removed within few days.
29. Tracheostomy ties are then placed around the patient neck, allowing enough space for two fingers to fit in snuggly. Avoid overtightening the tracheostomy ties as they could prevent blood supply and drainage when the neck muscles are contracted with neck movement or coughing.
30. Post-tracheostomy care.

Pitfalls and Troubleshooting

- Bleeding:
  Most of the bleeding that occurs during percutaneous tracheostomy is venous. Such venous bleeding usually stops with the insertion of the tracheostomy tube as it tamponades such bleeding. In the event of arterial bleeding, electrocautery could be used with special attention to the delivered FiO_2 to avoid airway fire. More preferably, a hemostat could be applied to the bleeding vessel before it is ligated.
- Difficulty puncturing into the trachea:
  Such difficulty in puncturing into the trachea could be encountered in the younger population. Further blunt dissection into the pre-tracheal fascia could help with this issue.

- Mobile Trachea:

   The larynx is a mobile structure, and hence pinning it down between the thumb and long finger of the non-dominant hand would help when this is encountered. The free index finger of the non-dominant hand could be used to direct the insertion needle. More commonly, the index finger could be fixed onto the cricoid cartilage to guard against a sub-cricoid entry.
- Pliable Trachea:

   The trachea could be pliable and would bow as the pressure exerted on the insertion needle is transferred to the anterior tracheal wall. Exerting less pressure on the needle before its entry into the tracheal lumen might mitigate this.
- Difficulty inserting the single dilator or the tracheostomy tube into the trachea:

   If this happens, then repeating the preceding step is essential and cannot be stressed enough. This ensures adequate opening of the puncture site or its adequate dilation before re-entering the trachea
- Inadequate site:

   If the needle puncture into the trachea was in a less than optimal location, then removing the large-bore needle or the catheter-over-needle and attempting again at a different location is reasonable. This is essentially important before the punch dilator is inserted. Once used to open the entry point further indicates a commitment to the entry site.
- It is important to adequately choose the appropriate tracheostomy tube size for the patient before the procedure. This minimizes any complications related to the procedure or the post-placement care of a tracheostomy tube.

5 Bronchoscopy

Introduction

Gustav Killian is considered the father of bronchoscopy. He was a German otolaryngologist in Heidelberg Germany. He described the use of a laryngoscope to examine and remove a pork bone from the airways of 3 patients. He was credited with coining the term "Direct Bronckoscopie". Bronchoscopy in its early days, the 1870s, was a rigid steel pipe inserted into the airways for the examination and removal of various foreign bodies. The development of fiberoptic imaging helped in the development of the Flexible Bronchoscope, which became commercially available in 1968. In the decades to follow, the use of flexible bronchoscopes surpassed the number of rigid bronchoscopes performed. Further advancement in the video image processing units led to further advancement in the design and reach of the flexible bronchoscope (Fig. 17). Single-use disposable bronchoscopes, developed by different manufacturers, are commercially available.

For this section, bronchoscopy will be referring to Flexible Bronchoscopy. The use of rigid bronchoscopes is limited to specially trained physicians.

Anatomy

The bronchoscopist must become familiar with the anatomy of the bronchoscope as it would allow for adequate use of the equipment. There is the actual bronchoscope and then there is the video processing unit along with a light source. The video processing unit is what allows for the projection of the bronchoscopic view onto a monitor. Thus, helping the bronchoscopist and potentially learners to observe the inside of the airway during the diagnostic and therapeutic portions of the procedure. Although the video processing unit is usually operated by a bronchoscopy technician, this should not deter the clinician from having at minimum a basic understanding of its operation. The bronchoscope could be divided into (1) handle, (2) fiberoptic and light bundle, (3) tip. The handle (Fig. 18a) houses the angulating lever that controls the tip of the bronchoscope in a single plane of directions, a suction controller, several buttons for different functions, and a working channel that allows the insertion of instruments into the bronchial tree. It is worth remembering that the working channel and the suction channel are shared along the shaft of

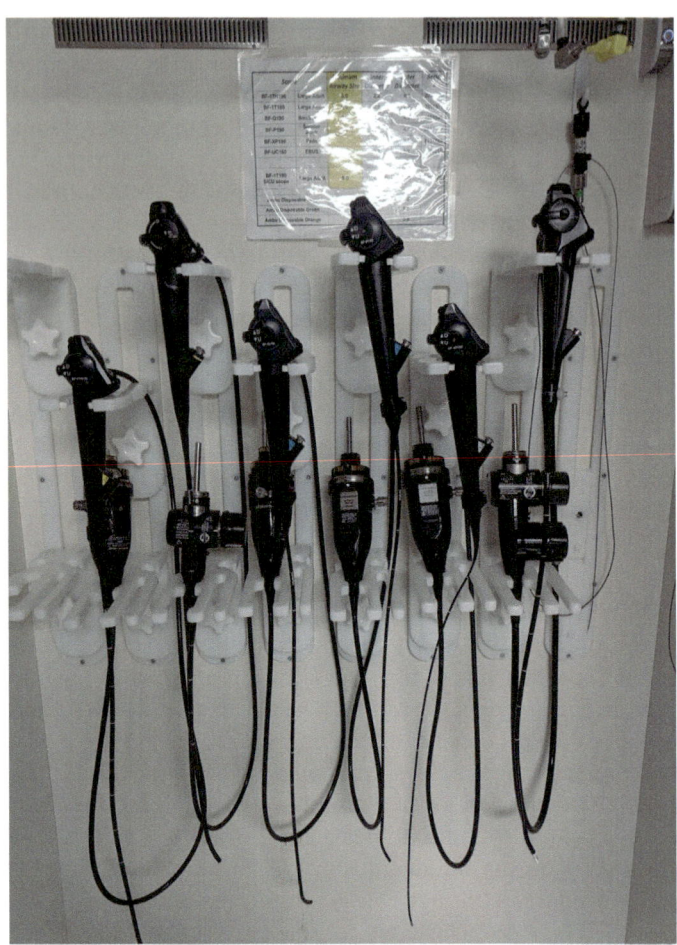

Figure 17 The Flexible Bronchoscope

the bronchoscope. At the left side of the handle, the fiberoptic and light cables emerge and are carried in a protected bundle to the image processing unit and transmission of the image. The tip of the bronchoscope, (Fig. 18b), has the working/suction channel, two light sources, and the miniaturized camera.

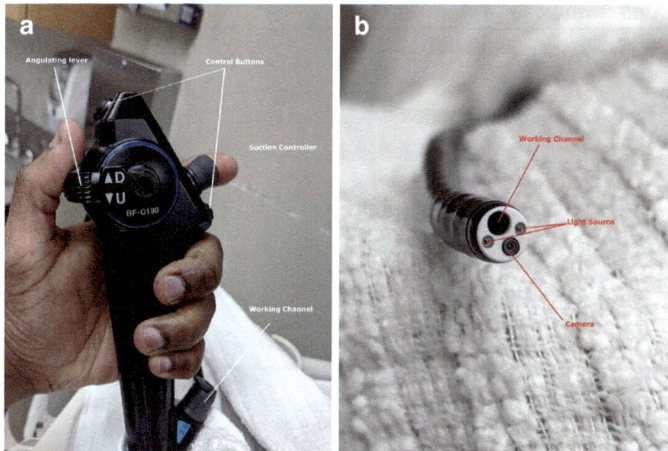

FIGURE 18 (**a**) The handle of the bronchoscope. (**b**) The tip of the bronchoscope

Indications

The indications (Table 5) of bronchoscopy could be divided into diagnostic and therapeutic indications. Those could range from a simple inspection bronchoscopy, up to airway debridement and reestablishment of airway patency.

(a) Diagnostic Bronchoscopy:

  (i) Mucus Plug removal.
  (ii) Foreign body retrieval.
  (iii) Symptoms and signs of respiratory diseases.
  (iv) Hemoptysis.
  (v) Lung transplant donors.
  (vi) Diagnosis of lung cancer.
  (vii) Diagnosis of thoracic lymphadenopathy.

(b) Diagnostic and Therapeutic:

  (i) Hemoptysis.
  (ii) Airway obstruction.
  (iii) Lung cancer treatment.

TABLE 5 Indications for bronchoscopy

Diagnostic Bronchoscopy:	Diagnostic & Therapeutic:
Mucus plug removal	Hemoptysis
Foreign body retrieval	Airway obstruction
Symptoms & Signs of respiratory diseases	Lung cancer treatment
Hemoptysis	
Diagnosis of lung cancer and thoracic lymphadenopathy	

Technique and Methods

As bronchoscopy allows access to the lower tracheobronchial tree, it must traverse the upper airway (pharynx and larynx) through either the nose or the mouth. Such trip to the lower airways could be through the natural orifices or bypassed with an artificial airway, e.g. Laryngeal mask airway (LMA) or an endotracheal (ET) tube. The first few steps will differ slightly based on the route of entry and whether an artificial airway is present or not.

(a) Basic and Standard Pre-procedure Steps:

 (i) Standard Time-out protocol:
 This step is important in any procedure performed. It allows the healthcare team to "pause" from what each team member is doing and focus on the procedure. During this step, a checklist is completed before the procedure. The components of this checklist can vary among different institutions (Fig. 19). However, the correct patient, medical record number, date of birth, patient's allergies, N.P.O status, planned procedure(s), and dispositions of the patient are reviewed. Any concerns from any member of the healthcare team are brought up and resolved at this critical step before the procedure. The importance of this step cannot be emphasized enough.

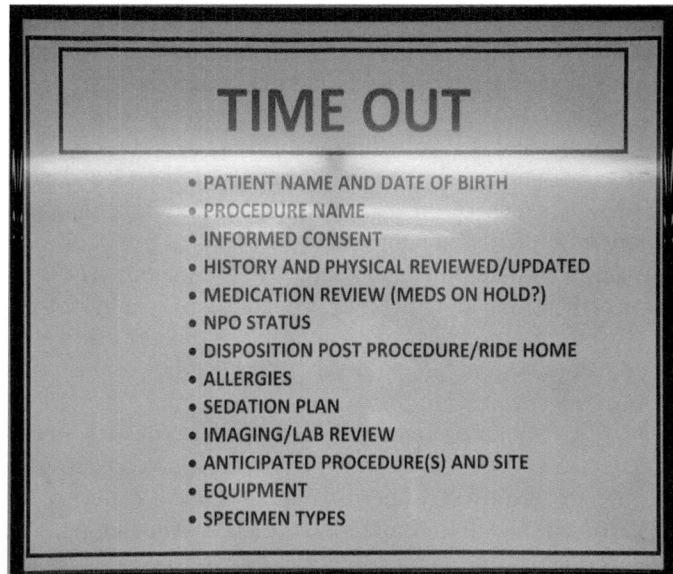

FIGURE 19 Example of Time-Out protocol

(b) Airway Preparation:

This step is usually conducted by the bronchoscopy technician or the respiratory therapist. Depending on the route of entry, the airway is anesthetized with topical lidocaine. Topical lidocaine can be 1%, 2%, or 4%. Such application could be as viscous jell, liquid form, or nebulized. Nebulization of lidocaine would allow the lidocaine to reach further down to the lower airways. This step is important as it allows for patient comfort and to conduct the procedure safely. This step could be minimized or skipped if the patient is deeply sedated with the presence of an artificial airway. However, if the LMA is the artificial airway, the application of topical anesthesia directly to the vocal cords via the bronchoscope is encouraged.

(c) Patient Sedation:

Sedating a patient for bronchoscopy is important. It helps with patient comfort and allows the proceduralist to complete the procedure with competency to achieve the intended results of the procedure. Based on local practices, this step is usually done by a healthcare team member with skills in sedation management or by the bronchoscopist. Sedation can be moderate or deep. Occasionally, general anesthesia might be needed with the presence of an anesthesiologist. Sedation management is discussed somewhere else in this textbook (see chapter "Sedation and Analgesia Management"). It is worth noting that flexible bronchoscopy could be performed in an awake patient in the hands of an experienced operator.

(d) Airway Evaluation:

This step represents the bulk of the procedure. In this step, the bronchoscopist steers the bronchoscopy through the upper airway, either through a natural orifice or an artificial airway, into the lower tracheobronchial tree.

The flexible bronchoscope is usually held in the left hand of the bronchoscopist (Fig. 20). Using the left hand would free up the right hand for handling any instruments inserted through the working channel. The left hand should wrap around the bronchoscope handle comfortably. The thumb would be on the angulating lever, the index finger is used to press the suction valve and to operate the control buttons on the bronchoscope, while the remainder of the fingers would wrap around the handle of the bronchoscope.

There are three basic movements of the bronchoscope. The combination of which would lead to the smooth steering of the bronchoscope through the tracheobronchial tree. Those three basic movements are used to break down the procedure for the aspiring bronchoscopist. With time they would "muscle memory" leading to the seamless steering of the bronchoscope.

Those movements are (1) rotation, which occurs at the wrist of the operator and allow the tip of the bronchoscope to look either right or left and if needed can look posteriorly if twisted far enough. (2) flexion and exten-

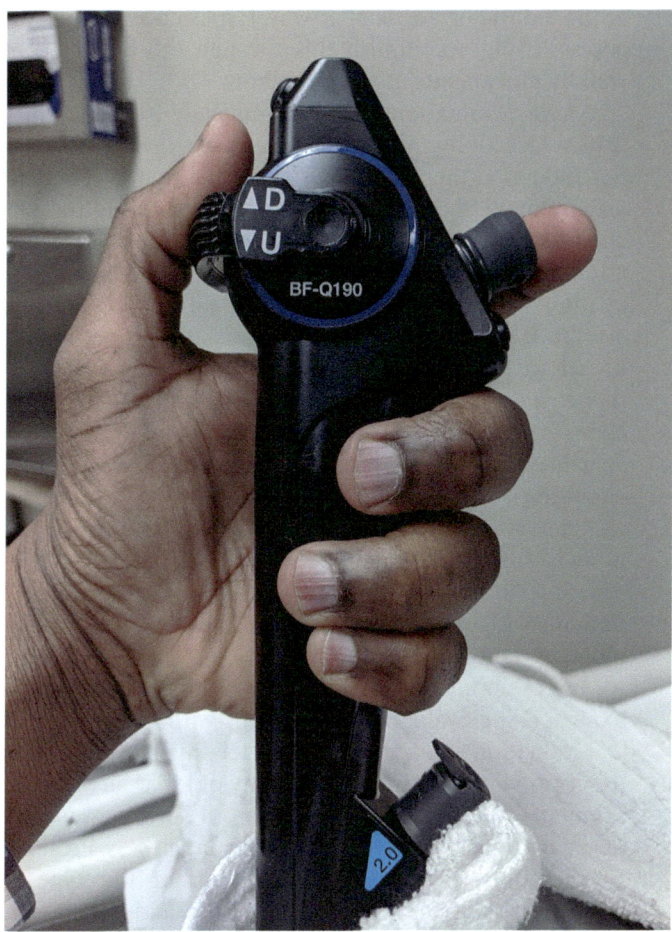

Figure 20 Holding the Bronchoscope

sion, which occur at the lever controlled by the operator's thump. Flexion will lead the tip of the camera to look upwards while extension would direct the camera downwards. (3) advancement and retraction of the bronchoscope in and out of the airway, which is usually handled by the right hand of the operator closer to the entry point at the natural or artificial airway. Experienced bronchoscopists could accomplish this through the left hand as well by movements at the left elbow.

Airway evaluation starts anatomically from the entry orifice describing the nasal cavity or the oral cavity, depending on the route of entry. Evaluation of the pharynx is completed at this point. Before entering the tracheobronchial tree, the larynx is evaluated with special attention to the vocal cords. Lidocaine should be instilled at the level of the vocal cords. Thereafter, patients who are moderately sedated would be asked to take a deep breath to allow for the abduction of the vocal cords, and thence easy transition of the bronchoscope into the trachea. Upon entering the trachea, the subglottic space is visualized, followed by the upper trachea. As the bronchoscope is advanced further distally, the lower trachea is evaluated until the main carina comes into view. The main carina divides the right from the left bronchial tree. The side to be examined first is the "normal side" for patients with expected anatomical or radiological pathology based on the indication, leaving the "abnormal side" to be examined last. However, if no pathology was expected, the evaluation would start with the right side.

Evaluation of each bronchial tree involves a detailed description of the mucosa, anatomy of lobar airways and segments, any anatomical variation of such, presence or absence of secretions, or endobronchial masses. Presence of secretions warrants a description of the type of secretions, their amount, viscosity, color, and if they were obstructing the airways or not.

This usually concludes the airway examination. However, if further diagnostic or therapeutic interventions were carried out during the procedure, those deserve detailed descriptions.

It is worth noting that the presence of an artificial airway would limit the description of the oropharynx or

nasopharynx (for both LMA and ETT), and larynx and upper trachea including the subglottic space (for ETT).
(e) Post-procedural Care:

Documentation is preferred to be immediate or soon after, describing the above findings. Documentation should include the indication for the procedure, diagnosis, sedation used if not documented by a separate provider who managed sedation, route of bronchoscope entry, bronchoscopic findings, endobronchial interventions if any, condition of the patient post-procedure, and any complications that might have occurred. When sedation is provided by the bronchoscopist, the medications used and their total doses should be documented. The type or model of the bronchoscope and its number should be noted. Such a numbering system is locally developed and adopted for tracking and infection control.

Since almost all bronchoscopies are performed with sedation, the patient should be monitored for at least 2 h to ensure the adequate return of vital signs to their pre-procedure baseline before the resumption of usual nursing care or discharge. Patients who are expected to take enteral nutrition are preferred to be NPO for 2 h post-procedure, as topical anesthesia of the upper airway increases the risk of aspiration. NPO status is not lifted unless the patient has an intact gag reflex, or as directed by the bronchoscopist or treating physician.

Pitfalls

Like all other procedures, some pitfalls should be kept in mind:

- Always maintain the bronchoscope in the center of the airway during the examination of the airway to minimize mucosal injury.
- Always maintain the shaft of the bronchoscope in a straight position. This would allow for proper transfer of the hand/wrist motion to the tip of the bronchoscope.

- Maintain adequate orientation during tracheobronchial airway evaluation. Whenever in doubt, retract to the previously known landmark. It is not uncommon to return to the main carina to gain adequate orientation.
- Labelling landmark structures and segmental airway orifices during bronchoscopic inspection would help with keeping track of your location while you are working your way through the tracheobronchial tree. This is important in solidifying segmental bronchial anatomy for the novices as they are learning the procedure.
- It is easy to delay documentation, however, the sooner you document, the more comprehensive and accurate your documentation would be.

6 Summary

Airway access is an important subject for the practicing clinician. It is conducive to the preservation of life when those skills are needed. Besides the technical aspects, factual knowledge is equally important for the clinical decision. This chapter has covered different aspects of airway access, procedures and methods involved. Continued practice and review are imperative to increase oneself preparedness.

Bibliography

1. Brown CA, Sakles JC, Mick NW. The Walls manual of emergency airway management. Philadelphia: Wolters Kluwer; 2018.
2. Tseng WC, Lin WL, Cherng CH. Estimation of nares-to-epiglottis distance for selecting an appropriate nasopharyngeal airway. Medicine (Baltimore). 2019;98(10):e14832.
3. Bullard D, Brothers K, Davis C, Kingsley E, Waters J 3rd. Contraindications to nasopharyngeal airway insertion. Nursing. 2012;42(10):66–7.
4. Roberts K, Whalley H, Bleetman A. The nasopharyngeal airway: dispelling myths and establishing the facts. Emerg Med J. 2005;22(6):394–6.

5. Baskett TF. Arthur Guedel and the oropharyngeal airway. Resuscitation. 2004;63(1):3–5.
6. Roberts K, Porter K. How do you size a nasopharyngeal airway. Resuscitation. 2003;56(1):19–23.
7. Lee CM, Song KS, Morgan BR, Smith DC, Smithson JB, Sloane RW, et al. Aspiration of an oropharyngeal airway during nasotracheal intubation. J Trauma. 2001;50(5):937–8.
8. Kok PH, Kwan KM, Koay CK. A case report of a fractured healthytooth during use of Guedel oropharyngeal airway. Singap Med J. 2001;42(7):322–4.
9. Stoneham MD. The nasopharyngeal airway. Assessment of position by fibreoptic laryngoscopy. Anaesthesia. 1993;48(7):575–80.
10. Gordon J, Cooper RM, Parotto M. Supraglottic airway devices: indications, contraindications and management. Minerva Anestesiol. 2018;84(3):389–97.
11. Jannu A, Shekar A, Balakrishna R, Sudarshan H, Veena GC, Bhuvaneshwari S. Advantages, disadvantages, indications, contraindications and surgical technique of laryngeal airway mask. Arch Craniofac Surg. 2017;18(4):223–9.
12. Timmermann A, Bergner UA, Russo SG. Laryngeal mask airway indications: new frontiers for second-generation supraglottic airways. Curr Opin Anaesthesiol. 2015;28(6):717–26.
13. Ramaiah R, Das D, Bhananker SM, Joffe AM. Extraglottic airway devices: a review. Int J Crit Illn Inj Sci. 2014;4(1):77–87.
14. Ingrande J, Lemmens HJ. Medical devices for the anesthetist: current perspectives. Med Devices (Auckl). 2014;7:45–53.
15. Brain AI, Verghese C, Strube PJ. The LMA 'ProSeal'--a laryngeal mask with an oesophageal vent. Br J Anaesth. 2000;84(5):650–4.
16. Kapila A, Addy EV, Verghese C, Brain AI. The intubating laryngeal mask airway: an initial assessment of performance. Br J Anaesth. 1997;79(6):710–3.
17. Brain AI, Verghese C, Addy EV, Kapila A, Brimacombe J. The intubating laryngeal mask. II: a preliminary clinical report of a new means of intubating the trachea. Br J Anaesth. 1997;79(6):704–9.
18. Brain AI, Verghese C, Addy EV, Kapila A. The intubating laryngeal mask. I: Development of a new device for intubation of the trachea. Br J Anaesth. 1997;79(6):699–703.
19. Asai T, Morris S. The laryngeal mask airway: its features, effects and role. Can J Anaesth. 1994;41(10):930–60.
20. Janssens M, Lamy M. Laryngeal mask. Intensive Care World. 1993;10(2):99–102.

21. Brain AI. The laryngeal mask--a new concept in airway management. Br J Anaesth. 1983;55(8):801–5.
22. Van Zundert AA, Kumar CM, Van Zundert TC. Malpositioning of supraglottic airway devices: preventive and corrective strategies. Br J Anaesth. 2016;116(5):579–82.
23. Latorre F, Eberle B, Weiler N, Mienert R, Stanek A, Goedecke R, et al. Laryngeal mask airway position and the risk of gastric insufflation. Anesth Analg. 1998;86(4):867–71.
24. Gao YX, Song YB, Gu ZJ, Zhang JS, Chen XF, Sun H, et al. Video versus direct laryngoscopy on successful first-pass endotracheal intubation in ICU patients. World J Emerg Med. 2018;9(2):99–104.
25. Bhattacharjee S, Maitra S, Baidya DK. A comparison between video laryngoscopy and direct laryngoscopy for endotracheal intubation in the emergency department: a meta-analysis of randomized controlled trials. J Clin Anesth. 2018;47:21–6.
26. Lascarrou JB, Boisrame-Helms J, Bailly A, Le Thuaut A, Kamel T, Mercier E, et al. Video laryngoscopy vs direct laryngoscopy on successful first-pass orotracheal intubation among ICU patients: a randomized clinical trial. JAMA. 2017;317(5):483–93.
27. Hypes C, Sakles J, Joshi R, Greenberg J, Natt B, Malo J, et al. Failure to achieve first attempt success at intubation using video laryngoscopy is associated with increased complications. Intern Emerg Med. 2017;12(8):1235–43.
28. Buis ML, Maissan IM, Hoeks SE, Klimek M, Stolker RJ. Defining the learning curve for endotracheal intubation using direct laryngoscopy: a systematic review. Resuscitation. 2016;99:63–71.
29. Silverberg MJ, Li N, Acquah SO, Kory PD. Comparison of video laryngoscopy versus direct laryngoscopy during urgent endotracheal intubation: a randomized controlled trial. Crit Care Med. 2015;43(3):636–41.
30. Lakticova V, Koenig SJ, Narasimhan M, Mayo PH. Video laryngoscopy is associated with increased first pass success and decreased rate of esophageal intubations during urgent endotracheal intubation in a medical intensive care unit when compared to direct laryngoscopy. J Intensive Care Med. 2015;30(1):44–8.
31. Haas CF, Eakin RM, Konkle MA, Blank R. Endotracheal tubes: old and new. Respir Care. 2014;59(6):933–52; discussion 52-5.
32. Durbin CG Jr, Bell CT, Shilling AM. Elective intubation. Respir Care. 2014;59(6):825–46; discussion 47-9.

33. Griesdale DE, Liu D, McKinney J, Choi PT. Glidescope(R) video-laryngoscopy versus direct laryngoscopy for endotracheal intubation: a systematic review and meta-analysis. Can J Anaesth. 2012;59(1):41–52.
34. Hurford WE. Techniques for endotracheal intubation. Int Anesthesiol Clin. 2000;38(3):1–28.
35. Poole O, Vargo M, Zhang J, Hung O. A comparison of three techniques for cricothyrotomy on a manikin. Can J Respir Ther. 2017;53(2):29–32.
36. Siddiqui N, Arzola C, Friedman Z, Guerina L, You-Ten KE. Ultrasound improves cricothyrotomy success in cadavers with poorly defined neck anatomy: a randomized control trial. Anesthesiology. 2015;123(5):1033–41.
37. Rowshan HH, Baur DA. Surgical tracheotomy. Atlas Oral Maxillofac Surg Clin North Am. 2010;18(1):39–50.
38. Hart KL, Thompson SH. Emergency cricothyrotomy. Atlas Oral Maxillofac Surg Clin North Am. 2010;18(1):29–38.
39. Elliott DS, Baker PA, Scott MR, Birch CW, Thompson JM. Accuracy of surface landmark identification for cannula cricothyroidotomy. Anaesthesia. 2010;65(9):889–94.
40. Mace SE, Khan N. Needle cricothyrotomy. Emerg Med Clin North Am. 2008;26(4):1085–101, xi.
41. Pracy JP, Watkinson JC. Surgical tracheostomy--how I do it. Ann R Coll Surg Engl. 2005;87(4):285–7.
42. Fikkers BG, van Vugt S, van der Hoeven JG, van den Hoogen FJ, Marres HA. Emergency cricothyrotomy: a randomised crossover trial comparing the wire-guided and catheter-over-needle techniques. Anaesthesia. 2004;59(10):1008–11.
43. DiGiacomo C, Neshat KK, Angus LD, Penna K, Sadoff RS, Shaftan GW. Emergency cricothyrotomy. Mil Med. 2003;168(7):541–4.
44. Eisenburger P, Laczika K, List M, Wilfing A, Losert H, Hofbauer R, et al. Comparison of conventional surgical versus Seldinger technique emergency cricothyrotomy performed by inexperienced clinicians. Anesthesiology. 2000;92(3):687–90.
45. Brofeldt BT, Panacek EA, Richards JR. An easy cricothyrotomy approach: the rapid four-step technique. Acad Emerg Med. 1996;3(11):1060–3.
46. Buchanan G. Successful case of tracheotomy in croup, and other surgical cases in private and hospital practice. Glasgow Med J. 1862;9(36):396–403.
47. Madsen KR, Guldager H, Rewers M, Weber SO, Kobke-Jacobsen K, White J, et al. Danish Guidelines 2015 for percuta-

neous dilatational tracheostomy in the intensive care unit. Dan Med J. 2015;62(3):C5042.
48. Lukas J, Duskova J, Lukas D, Paska J, Stritesky M, Haas T. Standard surgical versus percutaneous dilatational tracheostomy in intensive care patients. Saudi Med J. 2007;28(10):1529–33.
49. Flaatten H, Gjerde S, Heimdal JH, Aardal S. The effect of tracheostomy on outcome in intensive care unit patients. Acta Anaesthesiol Scand. 2006;50(1):92–8.
50. Mittendorf EA, McHenry CR, Smith CM, Yowler CJ, Peerless JR. Early and late outcome of bedside percutaneous tracheostomy in the intensive care unit. Am Surg. 2002;68(4):342–6. discussion 6-7
51. Ciaglia P. Differences in percutaneous dilational tracheostomy kits. Chest. 2000;117(6):1823.
52. Trottier SJ, Hazard PB, Sakabu SA, Levine JH, Troop BR, Thompson JA, et al. Posterior tracheal wall perforation during percutaneous dilational tracheostomy: an investigation into its mechanism and prevention. Chest. 1999;115(5):1383–9.
53. Ciaglia P. Percutaneous tracheostomy is really better-if done correctly. Chest. 1999;116(4):1138–9.
54. Ciaglia P. Improving percutaneous dilatational tracheostomy. Chest. 1997;112(1):295.
55. Marx WH, Ciaglia P, Graniero KD. Some important details in the technique of percutaneous dilatational tracheostomy via the modified Seldinger technique. Chest. 1996;110(3):762–6.
56. Ciaglia P, Graniero KD. Percutaneous dilatational tracheostomy. Results and long-term follow-up. Chest. 1992;101(2):464–7.
57. Ciaglia P, Graniero KD. Percutaneous tracheostomy. Chest. 1991;100(4):1178–9.
58. Ciaglia P, Firsching R, Syniec C. Elective percutaneous dilatational tracheostomy. A new simple bedside procedure; preliminary report. Chest. 1985;87(6):715–9.
59. Miller RJ, Casal RF, Lazarus DR, Ost DE, Eapen GA. Flexible bronchoscopy. Clin Chest Med. 2018;39(1):1–16.
60. Panchabhai TS, Mehta AC. Historical perspectives of bronchoscopy. Connecting the dots. Ann Am Thorac Soc. 2015;12(5):631–41.
61. Du Rand IA, Blaikley J, Booton R, Chaudhuri N, Gupta V, Khalid S, et al. British Thoracic Society guideline for diagnostic flexible bronchoscopy in adults: accredited by NICE. Thorax. 2013;68(Suppl 1):i1–i44.
62. Becker HD. Bronchoscopy: the past, the present, and the future. Clin Chest Med. 2010;31(1):1–18, Table of Contents.

63. Ernst A, Silvestri GA, Johnstone D. American College of Chest P. Interventional pulmonary procedures: guidelines from the American College of Chest Physicians. Chest. 2003;123(5):1693–717.
64. Pue CA, Pacht ER. Complications of fiberoptic bronchoscopy at a university hospital. Chest. 1995;107(2):430–2.
65. Simpson FG, Arnold AG, Purvis A, Belfield PW, Muers MF, Cooke NJ. Postal survey of bronchoscopic practice by physicians in the United Kingdom. Thorax. 1986;41(4):311–7.
66. Zavala DC. Complications following fiberoptic bronchoscopy. The "good news" and the "bad news". Chest. 1978;73(6):783–5.
67. Pereira W Jr, Kovnat DM, Snider GL. A prospective cooperative study of complications following flexible fiberoptic bronchoscopy. Chest. 1978;73(6):813–6.
68. Dreisin RB, Albert RK, Talley PA, Kryger MH, Scoggin CH, Zwillich CW. Flexible fiberoptic bronchoscopy in the teaching hospital. Yield and complications. Chest. 1978;74(2):144–9.

Thoracocentesis

Salman Ahmad

1 Introduction

This section will review the procedure of inserting a needle and catheter into the thoracic cavity to sample or drain fluid. Thoracentesis is reserved for elective indications rather than emergencies which are more readily treated with a chest tube thoracostomy or thoracotomy. Fluid can be aspirated for culture and cytology and a small diameter catheter can be placed for continuous drainage. As with any procedure, appropriate indications and contraindications must be considered and procedural consent must be obtained.

2 Indications

Indications for thoracentesis include the diagnosis and/or treatment of pleural effusion, empyema and retained hemothorax requiring thrombolytic therapy [4]. One could also electively evacuate a pneumothorax using a thoracentesis catheter in lieu of a chest tube thoracostomy. A properly

---

S. Ahmad (✉)
Division of Acute Care Surgery, University of Missouri Health, Columbia, MO, USA
e-mail: ahmadsa@missouri.edu

placed catheter can differentiate the contents of pleural fluid and guide your management. While the evacuation of pus or blood from a chest tube is diagnostic of an empyema or retained hemothorax, respectively; it can also be therapeutic by allowing clinicians to infuse thrombolytic medications into the pleural cavity through the tube to facilitate evacuation and obviate the need for more invasive procedures such as a thoracotomy or video-assisted thoracoscopic surgery (VATS) [2, 6]. Antibiotics are no longer routinely recommended for either emergent or elective chest tube thoracostomy [1]. While not included in this discussion, ultrasound can be a very useful adjunct in correct thoracentesis insertion and catheter placement [3, 5].

3 Technique/Methods

3.1 Prepare the Patient

(a) Perform a Time-Out to confirm the correct patient, procedure, side, medications/allergies and other concerns.
(b) Direct assistants appropriately; i.e. nursing, residents, students. Include respiratory therapy if the patient is on the ventilator or will need supplemental oxygen during conscious sedation.
(c) Prepare any necessary medications; sedation (conscious or deep), analgesia (IV and local). Antibiotics are no longer recommended.
(d) Position the patient in their hospital bed. If the patient can cooperate, sit them upright on the side of their bed with a table or Mayo stand and pillow to lean on. If not, roll them into a lateral decubitus position with the procedure side up, all while maintaining necessary spinal precautions. Both positions may require sliding the patient closer to the provider's side of the bed to minimize back strain. Likewise, raise or lower their bed to the most comfortable height for the provider.

(e) Use sterile, Chlorhexidine-based skin prep to create the sterile field around the ipsilateral procedure landmarks (Fig. 1).

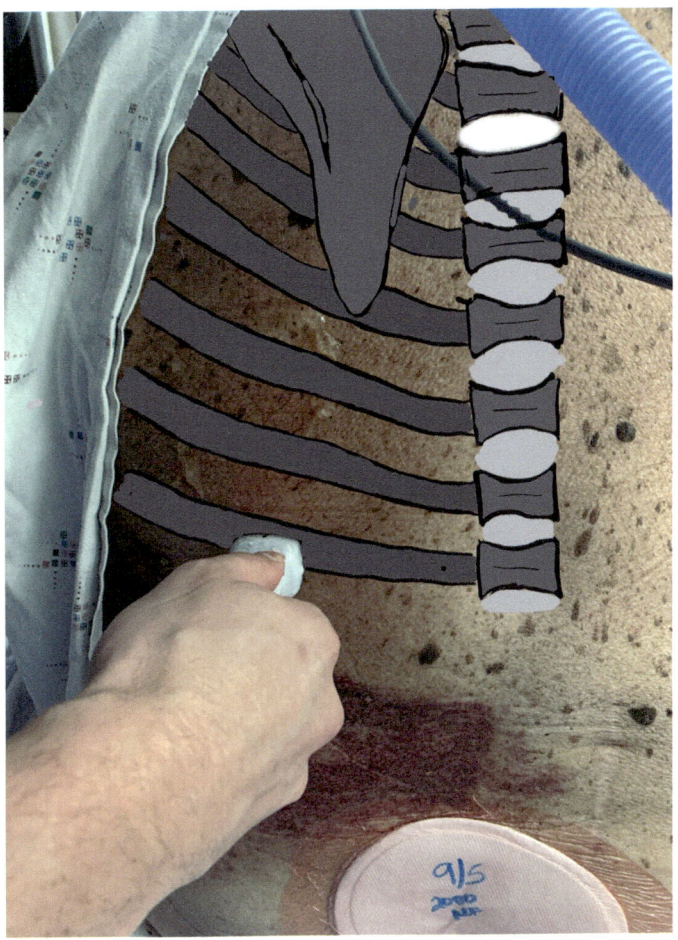

FIGURE 1 Thoracentesis anatomic landmarks (Ahmad, S)

3.2 Prepare Equipment and Yourself

(a) Open your sterile equipment on a rolling bedside table (Fig. 2).
(b) Open and prepare a pleural fluid collection bag, which will need to be connected to the catheter.
(c) Don cap, mask, gown and glove yourself (or with the aid of your assistant).
(d) Position equipment in the order you will need it (will make sense during procedure walkthrough, confirm w/ Fig. 2)

   1. Towels or surgical field drape
   2. Local anesthetic
   3. Scalpel #11 or #15 blade
   4. Gauze

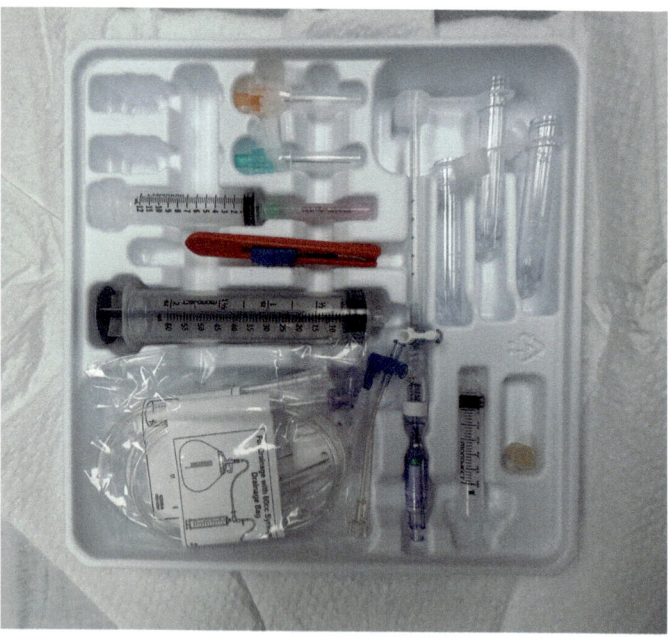

FIGURE 2 Thoracentesis collection bag and tubing (Ahmad, S)

5. Introducer or spinal needle and sheath with aspiration syringe
   6. Collection vials
   7. Drainage or pigtail catheter
   8. Wound dressing or bandage

3.3 Procedure Walkthrough

   1. Lay towels or field sterile drape around your anatomic boundaries. The visible field should include the ipsilateral scapula, midline spine and enough clearance inferiorly over the diaphragm. Include extra towels on the bed to lay the equipment and catheters on the field without contaminating them.
   2. Use the marking pen to demarcate the anatomic landmarks of your incision. In either upright or decubitus position, this will be along the mid-scapular line two finger breadths inferior to the scapular tip (Fig. 1). While not described here, ultrasound can be used to identify the fluid as well as follow diaphragm movement.
   3. With local anesthetic loaded in your syringe, infiltrate a skin wheal at your incision site (Fig. 3). You may also perform an optional intercostal block by palpating for the rib above, below and under your skin incision. Insert the local needle inferior to the ribs while aspirating. Infiltrate local anesthetic in these locations as long as you're not within an intercostal artery. This will temporarily anesthetize the pleural lining which can be the most painful part of the catheter insertion for awake patients.
   4. Insert your introducer or spinal needle connected to a syringe into the skin incision above the rib while aspirating gently. Stay parallel to the floor and continue advancing until you aspirate fluid or blood (Fig. 4).
   5. If you wish to extract a sample of pleural fluid for laboratory studies, aspirate here and remove the syringe. Inject the fluid into your specimen vials (usually 2 or 3 are included in the kit).

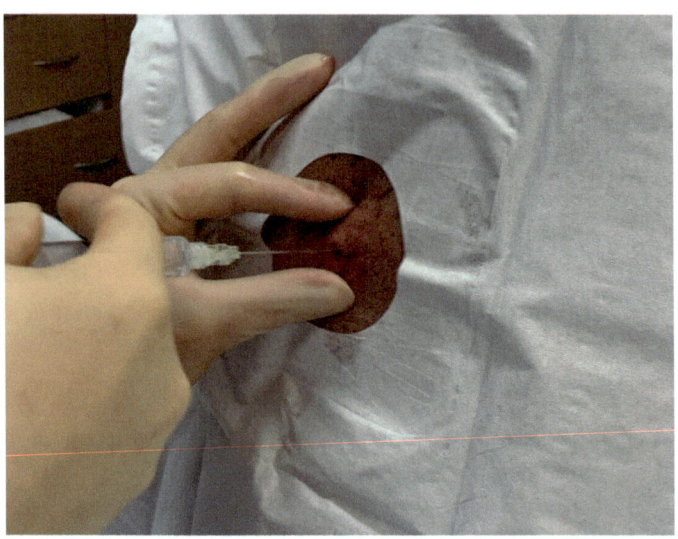

Figure 3 Prepped skin local anesthetic infiltration (Ahmad, S)

6. Make a longitudinal incision or nick in the skin less than 0.5 cm in length at your needle insertion site to accommodate the drainage catheter (Fig. 5). Use the gauze sponges to control bleeding.
7. After confirming the correct location of your pleural fluid, withdraw the needle and syringe and insert the drainage catheter or pigtail into the same incision while aspirating gently (Fig. 6). Keep in mind, most pleural drainage catheters only allow you to connect to a collection bag or chamber once the introducer needle inside it is completely removed. Once this is removed it cannot be reinserted as the valve shuts permanently.
8. Connect the tubing to the side valve and your collection chamber/syringe/bag of choice and turn the three-way stopcock to open allowing the fluid to drain through your catheter (Fig. 7). The drainage catheter or sheath is not usually left within the pleural cavity and is removed after drainage.

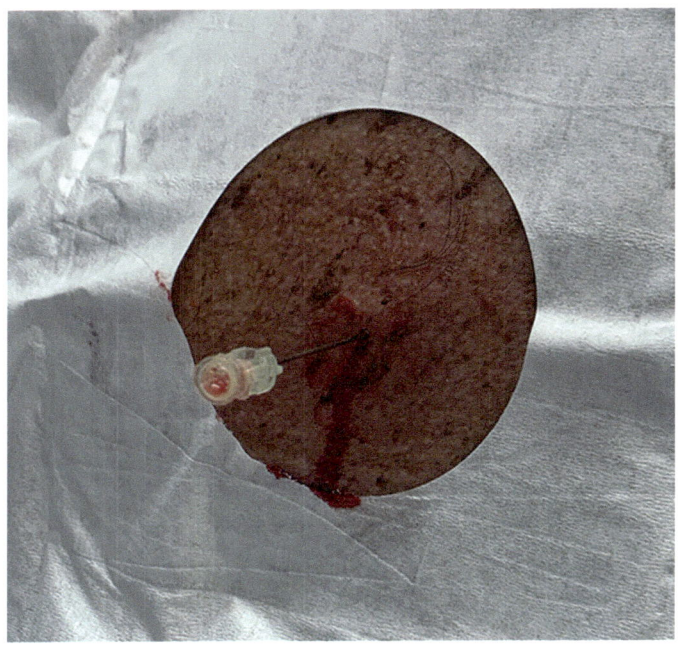

FIGURE 4 Introducer needle with fluid aspirate. (Ahmad, S)

9. If you have inserted a pigtail catheter, advance the catheter to insure most of the curved distal tail of the catheter resides within the pleural cavity and remove the wire. Then follow step #8 and secure your pigtail catheter to the skin using an adhesive clasp provided.
10. Apply a gauze or small bandage to your insertion site or a dressing if your catheter will remain in the pleural cavity.
11. Obtain a chest radiograph to confirm position of catheter and success of your drainage procedure as well as to rule out a pneumothorax which can occur with sudden drainage of a significant amount of fluid.

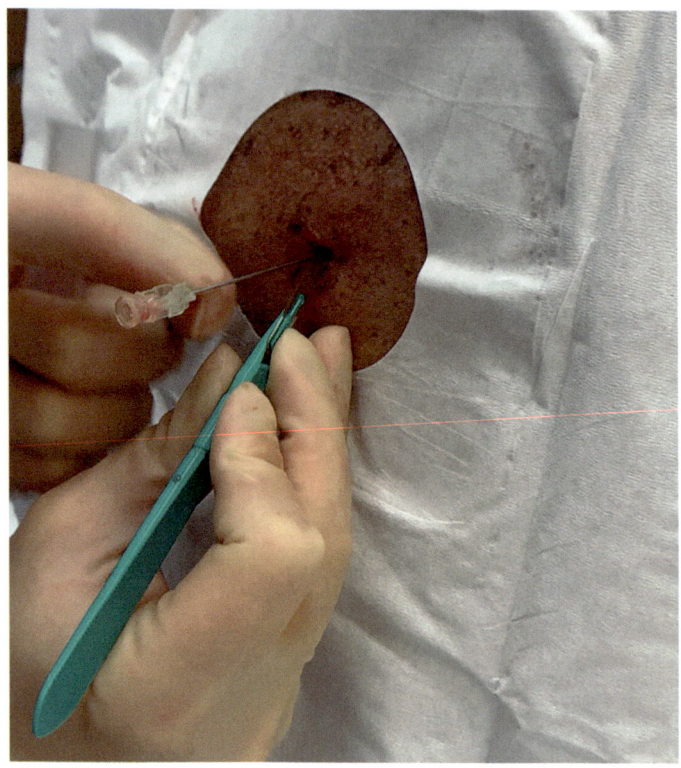

Figure 5 Scalpel incision around introducer needle (Ahmad, S)

4 Pitfalls/Troubleshooting

1. Pneumothorax & Re-expansion Pulmonary Edema

   Lung collapse may occur from inadvertent needle puncture or drainage of a significant amount of fluid which may result in disruption of the lung-pleural interface or cause rapid lung expansion. A pneumothorax should be suspected with the sudden onset of dyspnea or hypoxia. This can be confirmed by an immediate chest radiograph and

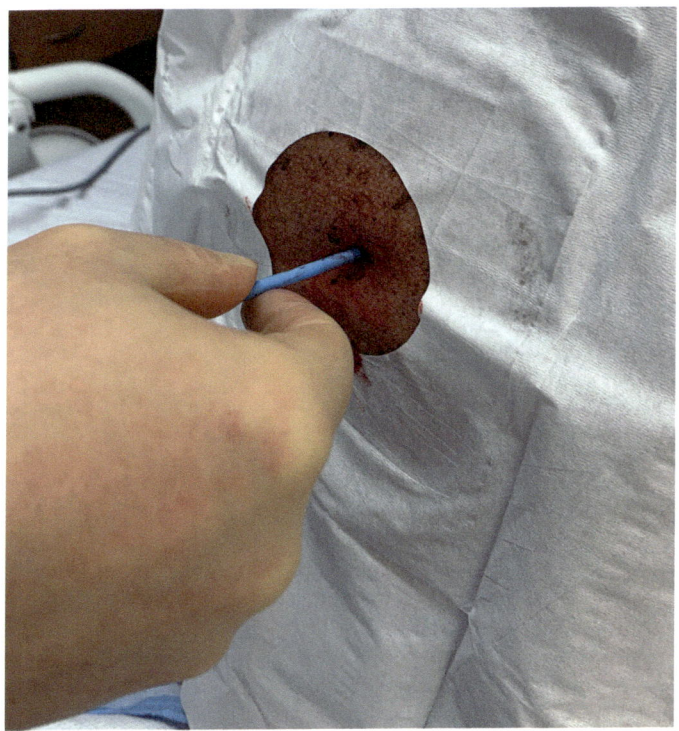

FIGURE 6 Pigtail insertion (Ahmad, S)

treated with a tube thoracostomy. Pulmonary edema can also be suspected by chest radiograph and treated with diuresis if tolerated.

2. Cannot identify fluid collection

    This possibility can be avoided by using ultrasound (if available) to isolate the collection or a thorough physical exam to percuss the thoracic cavity. This will help to demarcate the different densities of air (lungs), liquid (effusion) and solid (diaphragm). It is important to position the patient either upright or in the lateral decubitus position so that their fluid collection lies in a dependent position.

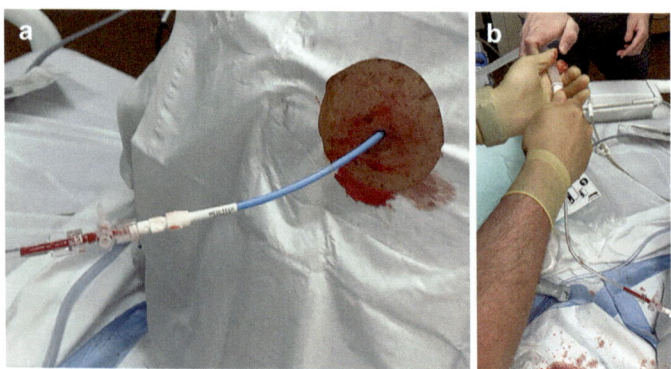

Figure 7 (a) Pigtail connected to drainage tubing. (b) Drainage catheter connected to pleural collection chamber (Ahmad, S)

References

1. Cook A, Hu C, Ward J, Schultz S, Moore FOD, Funk G, Juern J, Turay D, Ahmad S, Pieri P, Allen S, Berne J. Presumptive antibiotics in tube thoracostomy for traumatic hemopneumothorax: a prospective, Multicenter American Association for the Surgery of Trauma Study. Trauma Surg Acute Care Open. 2019;4(1):e000356.
2. DuBose J, Inaba K, Demetriades D, Scalea T, O'Connor J, Menaker J, Morales C, Konstantinidis A, Shiflett A, Copwood B. Management of post-traumatic retained hemothorax: a prospective, observational, multicenter AAST study. J Trauma Acute Care Surg. 2012;72:11–24.
3. Feller-Kopman D. Ultrasound-guided thoracentesis. Chest. 2006;129(6):1709–14. https://doi.org/10.1378/chest.129.6.1709
4. Hendriksen B, Kuroki M, Armen S, Reed M, Taylor M, Hollenbeak C. Lytic therapy for retained traumatic hemothorax: a systematic review and meta-analysis. Chest. 2019;155(4):805–15.
5. Krackov R, Rizzolo D. Real-time ultrasound-guided thoracentesis. JAAPA. 2017;30(4):32–7.
6. Redden MD, Chin TY, van Driel ML. Surgical versus non-surgical management for pleural empyema. Cochrane Database Syst Rev. 2017;3(3):CD010651.

Chest Tube Thoracostomy

Salman Ahmad

1 Introduction

This section will review the procedure of inserting a tube into a patient's chest, or a chest tube thoracostomy. A thoracotomy, on the other hand, is the procedure of opening the pleural cavity for exploration much like a laparotomy is the procedure of opening the abdominal cavity. A thoracostomy can be performed emergently or electively; however, it should follow the same principles outlined below to ensure a good outcome and minimize the risk of complications. There are elective conditions which can also be remedied with the placement of a thoracentesis catheter instead of a chest tube thoracostomy; i.e. pleural effusion, empyema, or retained hemothorax requiring thrombolytic therapy [3]. As with any procedure, appropriate indications and contraindications must be considered and informed procedural consent must be obtained.

S. Ahmad (✉)
Division of Acute Care Surgery, University of Missouri Health, Columbia, MO, USA
e-mail: ahmadsa@missouri.edu

2 Indications

Emergent indications for a chest tube thoracostomy include life-threatening thoracic compartment syndrome from tension pneumothorax or massive hemothorax. Increased intrathoracic pressures can substantially compromise superior and inferior vena caval blood return to the heart which results in obstructive shock and must be relieved quickly to avoid cardiac arrest. Elective indications for a chest tube thoracostomy also include a pneumothorax or hemothorax but without the presence of immediate life-threatening obstructive shock. One can clearly recognize how this procedure can be therapeutic, but a thoracostomy can also be diagnostic. A pleural effusion on an upright chest x-ray may consist of blood, serous fluid, chyle, pus or any combination thereof. A properly placed tube can differentiate the contents of pleural fluid and guide your management. In a trauma scenario, drainage of a hemothorax can be therapeutic not only for relieving intrathoracic pressures, but also for the auto-transfusion of evacuated blood using special equipment in the correct clinical scenario; i.e. without contamination. While the evacuation of pus or blood from a chest tube is diagnostic of an empyema or retained hemothorax, respectively; it can also be therapeutic by allowing clinicians to infuse thrombolytic medications into the pleural cavity through the tube to facilitate breakdown and clearance of the fluid collections and obviate the need for more invasive procedures such as a thoracotomy or video-assisted thoracoscopic surgery (VATS) [2, 5]. More recent data suggests that bigger is not better, and most hemothoraces are more readily drained with smaller bore chest tubes; i.e. less than 28 Fr [4]. For reference, the French designation refers to the approximate tube circumference in millimeters. Elective thoracostomy tubes can be placed in patients with coagulopathy or clotting disorders, but bedside clinical judgment must be used to assess the benefits of the procedure over risks of secondary hemorrhage and determine if the dyscrasia needs to be corrected chemically prior to the procedure. Antibiotics are no longer routinely recommended for either emergent or elective chest tube thoracostomy [1].

3 Technique/Methods

3.1 Prepare the Patient

(a) Perform a Time-Out to confirm the correct patient, procedure, side, medications/allergies and other concerns.
(b) Direct assistants appropriately; i.e. nursing, residents, students. Include respiratory therapy if the patient is on the ventilator or will need supplemental oxygen during conscious sedation.
(c) Prepare any necessary medications; sedation (conscious or deep), analgesia (IV and local). Antibiotics are no longer recommended.
(d) Position the patient in their hospital bed. This includes elevating or extending the ipsilateral upper extremity out of the surgical field. With the patient supine, raise or lower their bed to the most comfortable height for the provider.
(e) Use sterile, Chlorhexidine-based skin prep to create the sterile field around the ipsilateral procedure landmarks (Fig. 1).

3.2 Prepare Equipment and Yourself

(a) Open your sterile equipment on a rolling bedside table (Fig. 2).
(b) Open and prepare pleural fluid collection chamber (Fig. 3). Keep sterile white cap on the end until just before you need to connect it to your chest tube. Fill the water seal chamber, connect to continuous wall suction and set pressure regulator to 30 cm H20. This will ensure a steady pressure through the system regardless of what the wall suction regulator is set to.

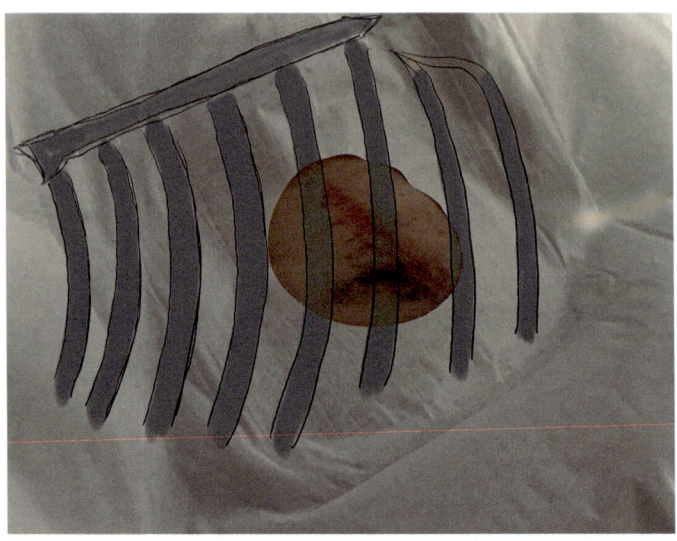

FIGURE 1 Prepped chest tube landmarks (Ahmad, S)

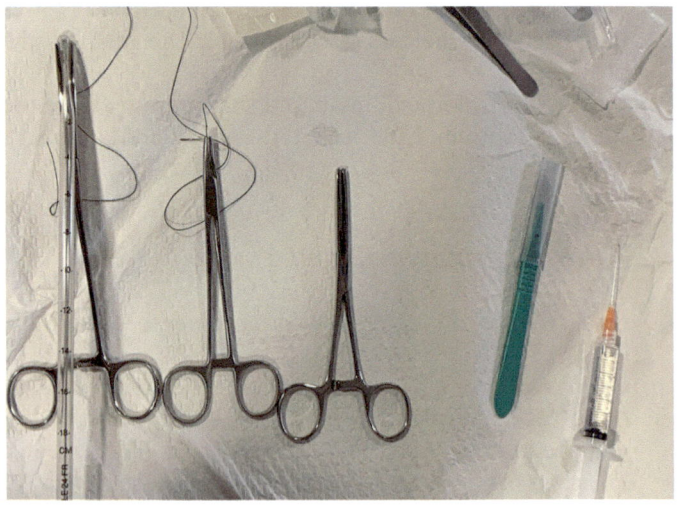

FIGURE 2 Equipment layout (Ahmad, S)

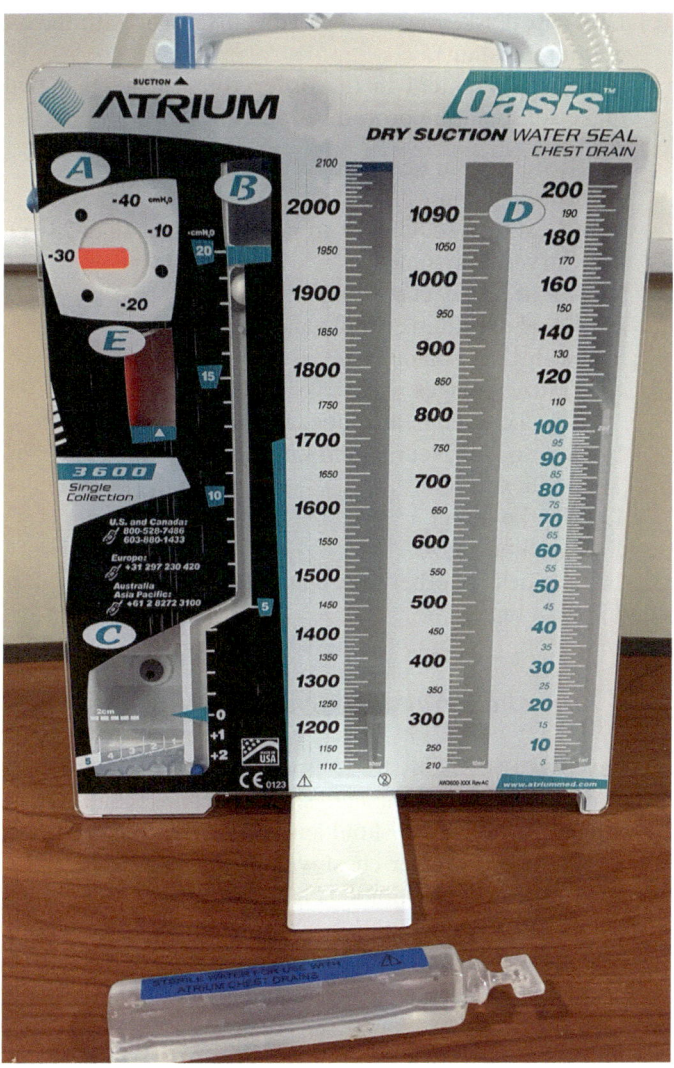

FIGURE 3 Pleural evacuation 3-chamber system (Ahmad, S)

(c) Don cap, mask, gown and glove yourself (or with the aid of your assistant).
(d) Position equipment in the order you will need it (will make sense during procedure walkthrough):

   1. Towels or surgical field drape
   2. Marking pen
   3. Chest tube (curved or straight, no larger than 28 Fr)
   4. Curved Mayo scissors
   5. Large Kelley clamps ×2
   6. Local anesthetic needle and syringe
   7. Scalpel #15 blade
   8. Gauze sponges
   9. Small curved hemostatic clamp
   10. Syringe for pleural fluid sample collection
   11. 0-Silk suture
   12. Needle driver
   13. Vaseline gauze
   14. Zip ties (or other tube clamping ties)
   15. Skin tape

3.3 Procedure Walkthrough

1. Lay towels or field sterile drape around your anatomic boundaries. The visible field should include the ipsilateral nipple, clavicle and shoulder head, lateral flank costal margin and posterior chest wall down to the bed. If you must use a smaller drape (Fig. 1) you should attempt to palpate those landmarks when identifying your tube insertion point. Include extra towels on the bed to lay the chest tube down on the field without contamination.
2. Use the marking pen to demarcate the anatomic landmarks of your incision. This should be just anterior to the mid-axillary line, at the 5 or 6th intercostal space which also correlates with the inframammary fold in men and women.
3. Prepare your chest tube by first cutting off the pointed distal end to a flat edge. This point exists to facilitate retrograde insertion of the tube through a thoracotomy inci-

sion from the inside out where it can be clamped and withdrawn out of the chest wall and skin. A flat edge is easier to attach over the pleural drainage system's adapter and secure with Zip ties.

4. You have the option of cutting extra wedge-shaped drainage holes in your chest tube to facilitate evacuation of larger pleural fluid collections. However, these should only be cut along the radiopaque white line running the length of the tube. This allows them to be easily identified on a chest x-ray.

5. Apply one Kelley clamp to the distal tip of the tube as shown in (Fig. 4). Measure the approximate intrathoracic length of your tube from the tip near the sternal notch to the skin exit incision with a slight bend to it. Place your second Kelley clamp at this part of the tube to guide your insertion depth.

6. With local anesthetic loaded in your syringe, infiltrate a skin wheal at your incision site. Then perform an intercostal block by palpating for the rib above, below and under your skin incision. Insert the local needle inferior to the ribs while aspirating. Infiltrate local anesthetic in these locations as long as you're not within an intercostal artery.

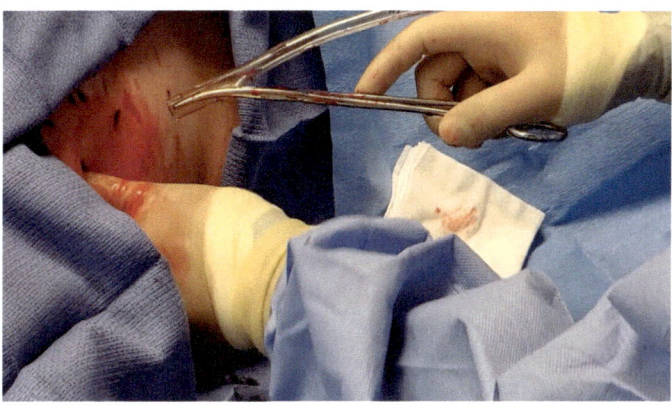

FIGURE 4 Clamp on chest tube (Ahmad, S)

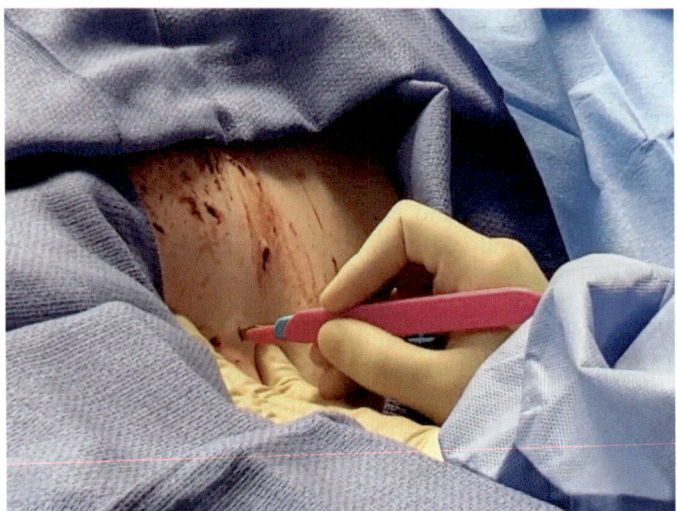

FIGURE 5 Skin incision with #11 Scalpel (Ahmad, S)

This will temporarily anesthetize the pleural lining which can be the most painful part of the tube insertion for awake patients.

7. Make a vertical 1–2 cm incision using the #11 or #15 scalpel blade (Fig. 5). This should go through skin and subcutaneous fat. Use the gauze sponges to control bleeding.
8. Use the small hemostatic clamp to bluntly dissect the subcutaneous space to the thoracic wall including the intercostal muscles (Fig. 6). More important, aim your dissection superiorly and slightly posteriorly as this will be the ideal path of your chest tube to insure it tracks superior and posterior in the thoracic cavity and minimize the chances of an intraparenchymal lung injury or fissured placement. Dissect down to the *superior* margin of the rib above your skin incision site.
9. With a good stable foot stance and using both hands, gently push the closed clamp through the intercostal muscles *above* the rib and into the thoracic cavity through the pleural lining. You will feel resistance followed by a quick

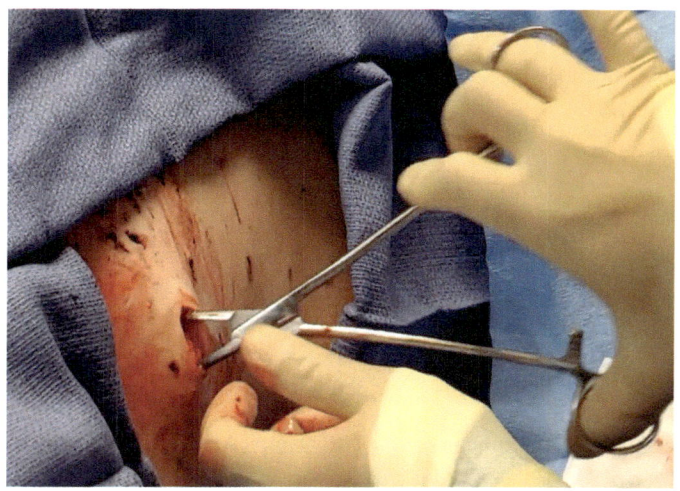

FIGURE 6 Clamp skin dissection (Ahmad, S)

pop when you penetrate the cavity and may also release air and blood. Keep your clamp in place and open it as you withdraw to widen the hole in the pleural lining. It will always be smaller than you think and difficult to find once the clamp is removed.

10. Once the insertion clamp is removed, use a single finger to bluntly enter the thoracic cavity through this same pleural defect and feel for the lung and diaphragm if possible. This serves to reassure yourself that you are in the thoracic and not abdominal cavity as well as allows you to sweep away any adhesions trapping the lung against the chest wall. Failure to perform this latter step increases the risk of lung injury from an intraparenchymal tube placement.
11. With the Kelley clamps in proper position on your chest tube, insert the tube through the chest wall defect using the distal clamp as a handle (Figs. 4 and 7). Aim the tip posteriorly and superiorly and hub to the distal Kelley clamp position only if you meet minimal resistance. The distal clamp should remain on the tip of the chest tube as

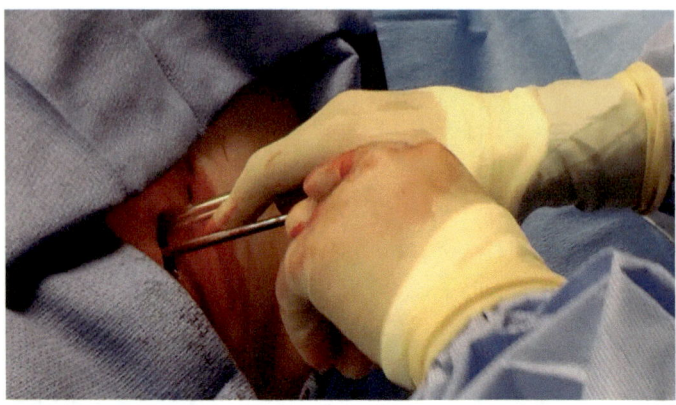

Figure 7 Chest tube insertion with clamp (Ahmad, S)

far as possible to insure adequate trajectory of the chest tube. Rotating the chest tube 360° after the distal clamp has been removed can sometimes confirm adequate placement without intraparenchymal or fissured trajectory. Note the depth of chest tube insertion here with the centimeter hash markings on the tube at the level of the distal Kelley clamp.

12. If you wish to extract a sample of pleural fluid for laboratory studies, attach your syringe at the distal cut-off end of the tube and remove your Kelley clamp.
13. Remove the white cap from the pleural evacuation collection chamber tubing and firmly connect to the cut-off distal end of your chest tube. Now remove your distal Kelley clamp if not already done. Be sure to hold your chest tube in position as the heavier collection tubing may exert traction and withdraw it.
14. Suture your tube in place by running through your skin incision then wrapping around the tube. Leave enough of a tail to use to close the skin once the tube is removed.
15. Apply the Vaseline gauze around the tube at the skin incision to limit air leaks.
16. Place additional padded gauze sponges between the tube and the chest wall to gently direct it away from the patient

in a anterior/lateral fashion. Apply skin tape to secure the tube to the chest wall leaving a portion of mesentery that helps offset the tube from the wall. Avoid the flexible foam-type tape as it does not withstand tension off the skin very well.
17. Apply the Zip ties or similar tube securing devices both proximal and distal to the plastic tree connector between the chest tube and the pleural fluid evacuation tubing.
18. Obtain a chest radiograph to verify the correct position of your tube and successful drainage of air and/or fluid.

4 Pitfalls/Troubleshooting

(a) Incorrect insertion site
 If your skin incision and subsequent chest wall insertion site are too low, you could inadvertently pass the chest tube into the abdominal cavity through the diaphragm. This reinforces the need for proper anatomic landmarks prior to any incisions or thoracic cavity penetration. It is imperative that your chest wall insertion defect is large enough to accommodate your finger which sweeps within the pleural cavity ensuring that you are in the chest and that the lung is not scarred and adhered to the chest wall. The latter may allow you to penetrate the lung parenchyma with your chest tube which could result in significant hemorrhage from laceration of a pulmonary arterial branch or in a significant air leak from a distal bronchial injury.
(b) Chest tube is in the chest wall but outside of the pleural cavity
 This is most likely to occur within morbidly obese patients with significant soft tissue between your skin incision and their chest wall. One can avoid this mistake by enlarging your skin incision enough to accommodate enough fingers and your chest tube and allow more definitive access to the chest wall defect. Once this is identified you are more likely to insert the chest tube and clamp into the pleural cavity through the defect rather than tunnel within the subcutaneous extra-thoracic space.

(c) Chest tube will not advance; i.e. sentinel hole not inside pleural cavity

This often occurs because the chest tube trajectory is into the lung parenchyma or a lobar fissure, producing resistance to further advancement. Do not force the tube into position. If you have properly estimated the depth of insertion prior to place your tube as suggested, you will know how deep the tube should lie. By placing the clamp at the appropriate position and angle on the tip of your tube, you can facilitate passage along the posterior-lateral chest wall and align the tube's trajectory towards the apex. A larger skin incision may also allow you to pass your finger alongside the chest tube within the pleural cavity for additional guidance. Some providers will roll the chest tube along its long axis after the clamp is removed to ensure it is not lodged within a fissure as they advance it.

References

1. Cook A, Hu C, Ward J, Schultz S, Dell FO, Iii M, Funk G, Juern J, Turay D, Ahmad S, Pieri P, Allen S, Berne J, Antibiotics A, Dell FO, Iii M. Presumptive antibiotics in tube thoracostomy for traumatic hemopneumothorax: a prospective, Multicenter American Association for the Surgery of Trauma Study. Trauma Surg Acute Care Open. 2019;4:1–6.
2. DuBose J, Inaba K, Demetriades D, Scalea T, O'Connor J, Menaker J, Morales C, Konstantinidis A, Shiflett A, Copwood B. Management of post-traumatic retained hemothorax: a prospective, observational, multicenter AAST study. J Trauma Acute Care Surg. 2012;72:11–24.
3. Hendriksen B, Kuroki M, Armen S, Reed M, Taylor M, Hollenbeak C. Lytic therapy for retained traumatic hemothorax: a systematic review and meta-analysis. Chest. 2019;155(4):805–15.
4. Inaba K, Lustenberger T, Recinos G, Georgiou C, Velmahos GC, Brown C, Salim A, Demetriades D, Rhee P. Does size matter? A prospective analysis of 28-32 versus 36-40 French chest tube size in trauma. J Trauma Acute Care Surg. 2012;72(2):422–7.
5. Redden MD, Chin TY, van Driel ML. Surgical versus non-surgical management for pleural empyema. Cochrane Database Syst Rev. 2017;3(3):CD010651.

Pericardiocentesis

Taishi Hirai, Bhradeev Sivasambu, and John E. A. Blair

1 Introduction

The heart is surrounded by visceral and parietal pericardium, normally <1 mm thick, and a small amount of fluid between the two layers of pericardium (15–30 cc). Cardiac tamponade is a life-threatening condition when excess fluid accumulation compresses the cardiac chambers leading to impaired diastolic filling and hemodynamic compromise [1]. Rapid percutaneous fluid removal and decompression of the pericardial space can be life-saving. In this chapter, we discuss a practical approach of pericardiocentesis.

T. Hirai (✉) · B. Sivasambu
Department of Medicine, Division of Cardiology, University of Missouri, Columbia, MO, USA
e-mail: hirait@health.missouri.edu;
sivasambub@health.missouri.edu

J. E. A. Blair
Department of Medicine, Division of Cardiology, University of Chicago, Chicago, IL, USA
e-mail: jblair2@bsd.uchicago.edu

© The Author(s), under exclusive license to Springer Nature Switzerland AG 2022
N. Arora (ed.), *Procedures and Protocols in the Neurocritical Care Unit*, https://doi.org/10.1007/978-3-030-90225-4_7

2 Indications

The two main indications for pericardiocentesis is for treatment of cardiac tamponade, and evaluation of the etiology of pericardial fluid.

(a) Cardiac tamponade

Cardiac tamponade is a clinical diagnosis defined by hemodynamic instability in patients with pericardial effusion. There are also specific echocardiographic criteria to assess cardiac tamponade such as diastolic collapse of the right ventricle, respiratory variation of mitral and tricuspid inflow and dilation of inferior vena cava. Patients with hemodynamic instability or echocardiographic evidence of cardiac tamponade should undergo an urgent drainage of the pericardial effusion to improve the cardiac filling and hemodynamic status. The threshold amount of pericardial effusion that causes tamponade physiology will depend on the acuity of the pericardial fluid accumulation and stiffness of the pericardium. In patients with slow accumulation of pericardial fluid, the pericardial sac can stretch and accommodate large amounts of fluid (2 liters or more) before developing tamponade physiology [2]. On the other hand, in patients with rapid accumulation of pericardial fluid such as bleeding due to coronary perforation, a small amount of effusion can cause tamponade physiology as there is little compensatory stretching of the pericardium.

(b) Diagnostic pericardial fluid sampling

Although the etiology of pericardial effusion can be diagnosed without pericardial fluid analysis in some instances, patients with suspected bacterial, tuberculous, or malignant pericardial effusion require pericardiocentesis to make the diagnosis and to better tailor the treatment.

3 Equipment

A pericardiocentesis kit typically includes the following (Fig. 1)

(a) 18-gauge needle
(b) 0.035 inch guidewire
(c) Dilator
(d) 6 or 8 French pigtail catheters
(e) Plastic drainage bag
(f) Local anesthetic
(g) Three-way stopcock

In addition to the kit above, we often utilize the micropuncture needle and the guidewire (Cook Medical, Bloomington, IN) (arrow). Micro-puncture needle is a 21-gauge needle that allows for smaller puncture. A standard 7 cm micro-puncture needle will often suffice for apical approach. For subxiphoid approach, 12 cm needle may be necessary depending on the patient's body habitus. After

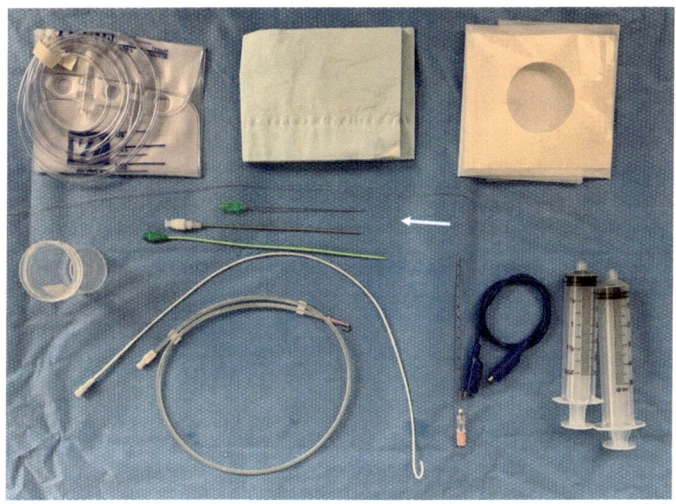

Figure 1 Equipment required for pericardiocentesis

inserting the micro-puncture sheath over a 0.018-inch guidewire, an 0.035-inch standard guidewire is advanced, and the pericardial drain is placed over this guidewire.

4 Technique/Methods

Pericardiocentesis is typically performed under fluoroscopic and echocardiographic guidance at cardiac catheterization laboratory or in a hybrid operating room [3]. While a pericardiocentesis at bedside using only anatomic landmarks can be performed, it is not performed unless it is an emergent situation, with a critically ill patient rapidly deteriorating from the effusion that cannot be safely transported to the cardiac catheterization laboratory [4].

There are three approaches that can be utilized. Although the subxiphoid approach has been the standard method, the apical approach has increasingly been used with echocardiographic guidance. Parasternal approach can be used in patients who are not suitable for subxiphoid or apical approach, however, it is considered a third option for most operators.

Pre-procedural assessment with the echocardiogram is essential to locate the size and distribution of the pericardial effusion. The subcostal/subxiphoid view can identify the amount of effusion accessible by the subxiphoid approach, located anterior to the right ventricle. Whereas the apical four chamber view is often used to assess the depth and size of the effusion that is approachable from transapical approach.

Although most pericardial effusions can be treated with percutaneous drainage, surgical approach may be necessary in patients with posterior effusion, loculated effusions, recurrent effusion, or pericardial hematoma with clot formation.

(a) Subxiphoid approach

The patient is positioned either in a wedge position at 30–45° angle or supine position depending on the operator's preference. The needle is inserted 1 cm below and 1 cm left to

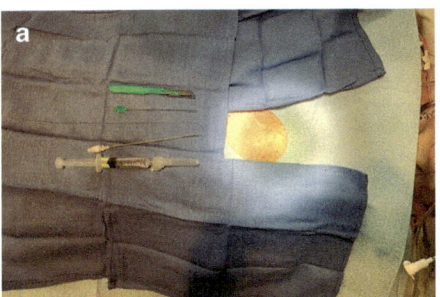 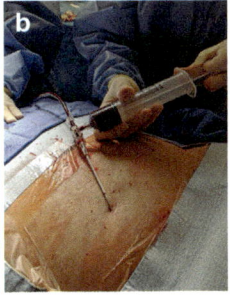

FIGURE 2 (**a**) Draping and preparation when performing subxiphoid approach. (**b**) Pericardial fluid is removed from the drain using a larger syringe

the xiphoid process (Fig. 2), however this may be adjusted to be more inferior in patients with larger body habitus to ensure a 30–45° angle results in the needle passing immediately beneath the costal margin. The needle is typically directed toward the left mid-clavicular line at 30–45° angle to the skin. The needle is advanced with continuous aspiration and directed immediately to the inferior costal margin until the pericardium is pierced and fluid is aspirated [2]. To ensure that no debris in the needle prevents aspiration of fluid and to anesthetize the sensitive peri-costal space, we recommend intermittent aspiration and injection of 1% lidocaine. In addition, we recommend advancement of the needle at a fixed trajectory until the costal margin is felt, then the needle tip may be directed under the costal margin to ensure the needle does not puncture abdominal or thoracic structures. If no fluid is aspirated, the needle should be withdrawn and redirected rather than redirected in the body where cardiac structures may be inadvertently lacerated. The direction of the needle can be assessed under fluoroscopic guidance using the heart border or using the ultrasound.

(b) Apical approach

The patient is positioned either in a wedge position at 30–45° angle or supine position depending on the location of

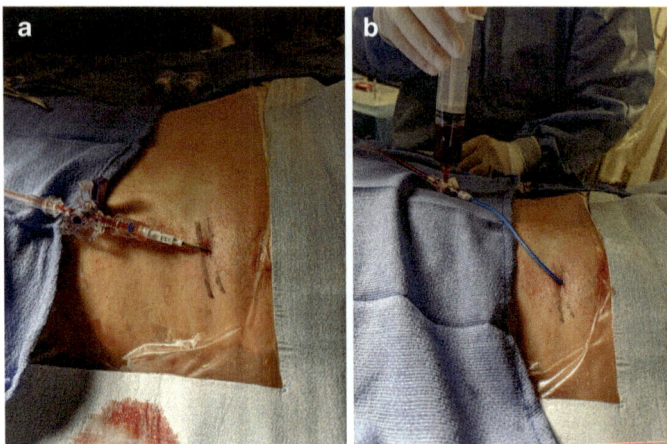

FIGURE 3 (**a**) The location of needle entrance in transapical approach. The upper and lower border of the rib is marked to avoid injury to the neurovascular bundle. The micro-puncture dilator is connected to pressure transducer prior to dilation, to confirm the catheter position. (**b**) Pericardial fluid is removed

fluid and operator's preference. The cardiac apex is identified using the ultrasound. The apex typically is free of overlying lung tissue. In addition, as the cardiac apex lacks major coronaries, this approach has the lowest risk of damaging the coronary arteries. The needle is inserted at the cephalic border of the rib to avoid injury to the neurovascular bundle running along the lower border of the ribs (Fig. 3). This approach is ideally performed ensuring the ideal trajectory using ultrasound guidance. We recommend the same intermittent aspiration technique as described above.

(c) Parasternal approach

Parasternal approach is used within 1 cm lateral to the left sternal border with the needle entry angle of 90° over the cephalic border of the fifth or sixth intercostal space. To prevent injury of the left internal mammary artery, lateral puncture (greater than 1 cm) should be avoided. In selected situations, right parasternal puncture can be performed if the fluid is more accessible from the right side.

5 Management After Pericardiocentesis

The specimen is typically sent for cell count, gram stain, bacterial and fungal culture and cytology. Other tests such as AFB stain, mycobacterial culture, adenosine deaminase, PCR study for viral infections can be considered depending on the clinical context. However, it should be noted that Light's criteria that is typically applied for assessment of pleural fluid is not reliable in discerning exudative and transudative pericardial fluid.

The drain is sutured in position (Fig. 4) and can be intermittently aspirated or continuously drained to gravity. At our institution, the drain is left to gravity and kept in place until the drain output is less than 50 cc over 24-h period. After the

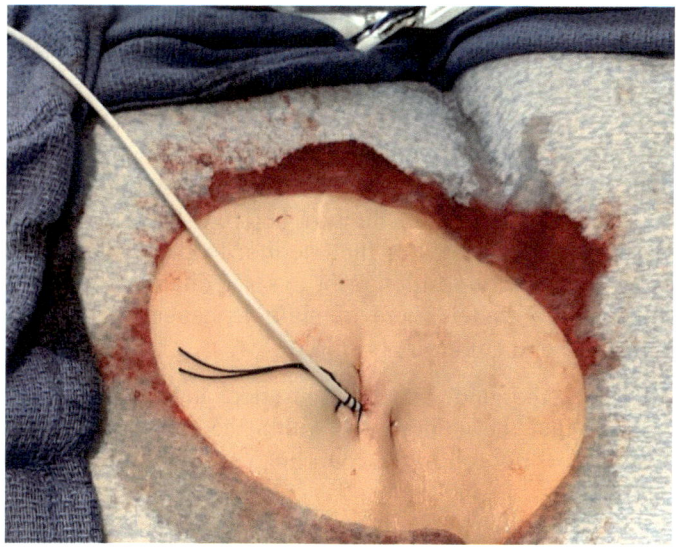

FIGURE 4 The drain is secured in place using a "purse string suture"

drain output has decreased, a limited echocardiogram is performed to confirm the resolution of the pericardial effusion. If there is significant residual pericardial effusion, patient motion can be encouraged and drain position can be adjusted for better drainage unless the effusion is loculated.

6 Complications

With the use of fluoroscopic and echocardiographic guidance, the complication rate is 1–2% in experienced operators' hands [3]. The operator should discuss the possible complications with the patient prior to the procedure.

The most serious and immediate complications of pericardiocentesis are myocardial puncture or laceration, vascular injury (coronary, intercostal, internal mammary or intra abdominal), pneumothorax, air embolism and arrhythmia [5]. Other complications include pneumomediastinum, pneumopericardium, liver laceration and bowel injury in patients with hiatal hernia.

7 Tips to Avoid Complications

Laceration usually occurs when the angle of the needle is changed within the tissue. Therefore, it is important to withdraw the needle close to the skin before the needle is redirected. It is important for the operator to check the needle and the guidewire position prior to serial dilation and placement of the catheter. There are multiple maneuvers to check the needle and guidewire position.

(a) Check the guidewire position under fluoroscopy. Make sure that the guidewire is within the cardiac silhouette but does not follow the course of a specific cardiac chamber (Fig. 5).
(b) Connect the needle or micropuncture dilator to a pressure line and measure the pressure. This will confirm the

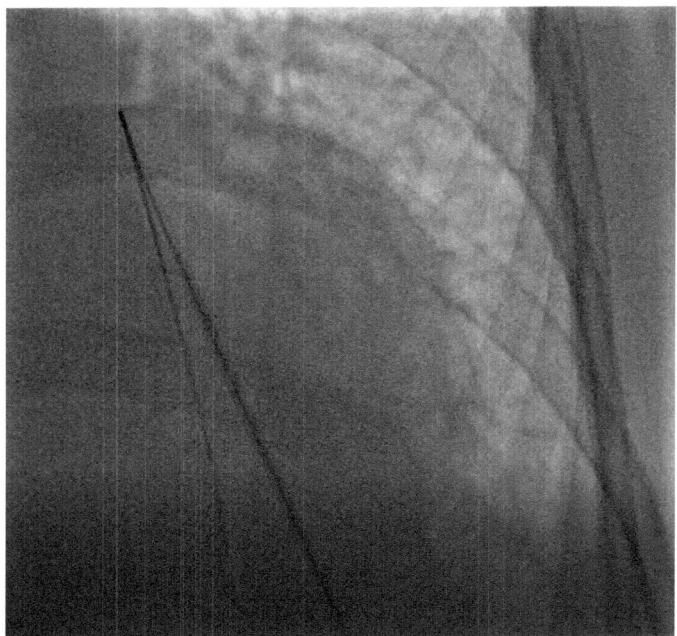

FIGURE 5 Guidewire position is within the cardiac silhouette but is not within any cardiac chamber

pericardial waveform and rule out the right ventricular waveform (Fig. 6).
(c) Small gentle contrast injection under fluoroscopy.
(d) Visualization of guidewire using ultrasound (Fig. 7).
(e) Injection of agitated saline through the needle under ultrasound visualization.
(f) Soak a gauge with a small amount of pericardial fluid. If the fluid is non-hemorrhagic, "halo-sign" will be seen. On the other hand, there will be no "halo-sign" if it is bloody effusion or if the fluid was aspirated from a cardiac chamber (Fig. 8).
(g) Connect the needle to the telemetry leads. Monitor for ST elevation which suggests the needle is touching the myocardium.

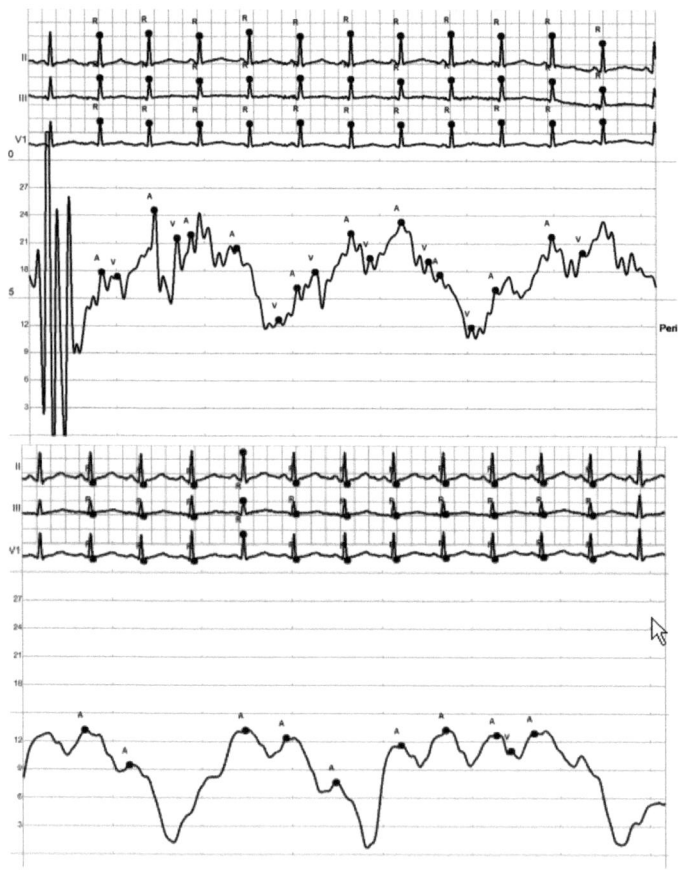

FIGURE 6 Pericardial pressure tracing pre and post pericardiocentesis

It is recommended for the operator to confirm the needle and guidewire position with at least two different methods before committing to dilation of the tract. Usually, even if the needle and/or wire is in a cardiac chamber and not in the pericardial space, bleeding and perforations rarely occur if you simply remove the needle and/or wire and re-attempt placement in the pericardial space. At our institution, the

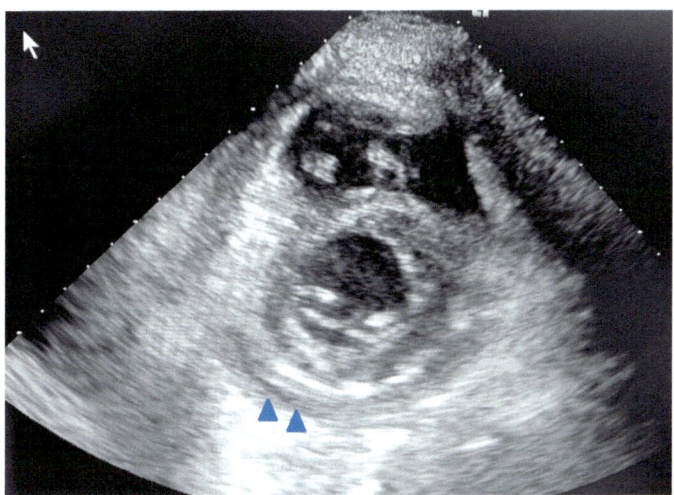

FIGURE 7 Guidewire position (arrows) confirmed by the echocardiogram

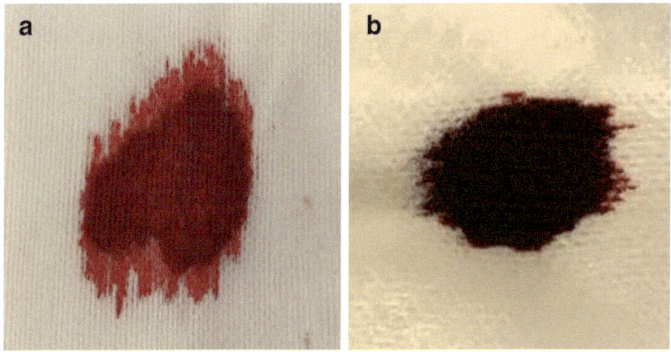

FIGURE 8 (**a**) "halo sign" seen in patients with non-hemorrhagic pericardial effusion. (**b**) Hemorrhagic pericardial effusion without a "halo sign"

position is typically confirmed using fluoroscopy and by obtaining the pressure waveform. If despite the above precautions are taken, the dilator or pigtail is inserted into a cardiac chamber (typically right ventricle, rarely the right atrium or left ventricle), it is important not to remove the catheter to prevent further bleeding. The catheter should be kept inside and percutaneous closure using a ductal occluder device or surgical repair should be considered.

Acknowledgement The authors acknowledge Jennifer Higgins RCIS for preparation of the photographs.

References

1. Little WC, Freeman GL. Pericardial disease. Circulation. 2006;113:1622–32.
2. Spodick DH. Acute cardiac tamponade. N Engl J Med. 2003;349:684–90.
3. Tsang TSM, Freeman WK, Sinak LJ, Seward JB. Echocardiographically guided pericardiocentesis: evolution and state-of-the-art technique. Mayo Clin Proc. 1998;73:647–52.
4. Ragosta M. Textbook of clinical hemodynamics. 1st ed. Elsevier; 2008.
5. Heffner AC. Emergency pericardiocentesis. UpToDate. 2019.

Paracentesis

Naren Nallapeta, Harleen Chela, and Yezaz A. Ghouri

1 Introduction

Abdominal paracentesis, synonymous with peritoneal tap or ascitic tap, is a routinely performed bedside procedure involving removal of peritoneal fluid from the peritoneal cavity using a needle for diagnostic and/or therapeutic purposes [1]. Normally the peritoneal cavity contains about 20 mL of fluid which is primarily secreted by the cells lining the visceral layer of the peritoneum. It helps in achieving frictionless motility of the bowels during peristalsis. Excess accumulation of this fluid is known as ascites [2]. Abdominal paracentesis is usually a safe and effective way to determine the cause of ascites and is performed by the physician at the bedside or by a radiologist in a radiology suite with ultrasound guidance [3].

N. Nallapeta
State University of New York, Buffalo, NY, USA
e-mail: narennal@buffalo.edu

H. Chela · Y. A. Ghouri (✉)
Department of Medicine, Division of Gastroenterology & Hepatology, University of Missouri School of Medicine, Columbia, MO, USA
e-mail: chelah@health.missouri.edu; ghouriy@health.missouri.edu;
https://muhealth.org/doctors/Yezaz-ghouri-md

© The Author(s), under exclusive license to Springer Nature Switzerland AG 2022
N. Arora (ed.), *Procedures and Protocols in the Neurocritical Care Unit*, https://doi.org/10.1007/978-3-030-90225-4_8

Physical exam-based detection of ascites followed by insertion of a needle to drain the fluid can also be performed without using ultrasound assistance.

The collected ascitic fluid is evaluated for biochemical analysis, cytological contents, and microbiological organisms. These include cell counts with differential, gram stain and culture, albumin level, total protein level, lactate dehydrogenase level, glucose level, amylase level, flow cytometric analysis and various other tests [4, 5]. Serum-to-ascites albumin gradient (SAAG) obtained by the subtraction of ascites albumin concentration from serum albumin concentration helps to determine if ascites is driven by portal hypertension or not. When the SAAG is ≥1.1 g/dL it is suggestive of portal hypertension [6]. The result of this analysis helps in diagnosing various conditions and illnesses.

2 Indications for Abdominal Paracentesis

The American association for the study of liver diseases (AASLD) is a leading organization of scientists and health care professionals working towards preventing and curing various liver diseases. AASLD provides practice guidelines which are evidence based and updated regularly by a panel of experts in hepatology. This includes recommendations regarding preferred approaches in diagnostic, therapeutic, and preventive aspects of medical care for individuals with liver diseases. The European association for the study of the liver (EASL) is also a key facilitator of excellence in liver research and liver-related clinical care. They assist physicians and healthcare providers with a range of state-of-the-art approaches for the diagnosis and treatment of liver diseases (Fig. 1).

Based on the current guidelines and recommendations provided by AASLD and EASL, the following are the common indications for paracentesis [4, 7].

1. Evaluation of new onset ascites: AASLD recommends diagnostic abdominal paracentesis for all patients with new-onset ascites. This should help with providing information regarding the etiology and guide further manage-

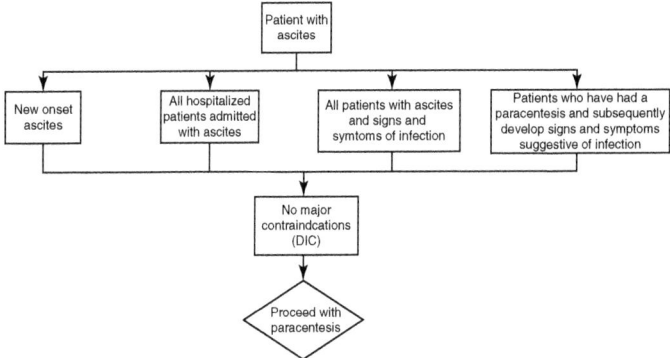

FIGURE 1 Decision making tree to determine the need for paracentesis among patients who present with ascites

ment of these patients by calculating the SAAG. Fluid accumulation due to portal hypertension can be readily differentiated from fluid accumulation due to other causes.
2. Hospitalized patients with ascites: Initial assessment must be made for all patients admitted to the hospital with cirrhosis associated ascites or new onset ascites. The rationale behind performing a paracentesis procedure in cirrhotic patients admitted to the hospital is mainly to assess spontaneous bacterial peritonitis (SBP). SBP is thought to be a leading cause of death in patients with chronic liver disease who have developed ascites. It is advisable to obtain an ascitic fluid sample for fluid analysis and culture before administration of antibiotics.
3. Patients with ascites and signs and symptoms of infection: The ascitic fluid must be assessed for cell counts and sent for culture and sensitivity testing, since appropriate antibiotic treatment is necessary for treating patients with peritonitis. A clinical diagnosis of peritonitis or the absence of it should be confirmed with fluid analysis.
4. Patients who have had a paracentesis and subsequently develop signs and symptoms suggestive of infection, such as:

- Fever
- Leukocytosis

- Abdominal pain or tenderness
- Findings on physical examination suggestive of peritonitis: Inspection showing reduced movement of abdominal muscles (silent abdomen), diffuse abdominal tenderness with voluntary or involuntary guarding and rigidity.
- Increased volume of ascites (on physical exam or radiologic studies)
- Unexplained encephalopathy
- Deteriorating liver function
- Acute kidney injury

5. Therapeutic relief of symptoms in patients with refractory ascites, ascites causing respiratory distress or abdominal discomfort from ascites [8, 9].

   Paracentesis is generally considered to be a safe procedure, but it is recommended for the provider to discuss its risks and benefits with the patient, in order for the patient to make an informed decision and give consent for the procedure [5, 10].

3 Contraindications

1. Absolute contraindications

   (a) Disseminated Intravascular Coagulation (DIC)
   (b) Acute abdomen requiring immediate intervention

2. Relative contraindications:

   (a) Uncooperative patient
   (b) Cellulitis of the abdominal wall
   (c) Distended bowel
   (d) Distended bladder
   (e) Pregnancy
   (f) Abdominal surgeries on the abdomen with intra-abdominal adhesions [11]

Individuals with acute liver failure or cirrhosis, tend to develop thrombocytopenia and coagulopathy which increases the risk of bleeding secondary to procedures. Studies have shown that major bleeding after paracentesis is quite rare despite thrombocytopenia or elevation in the international normalized ratio (INR). One such study included 612 patients who underwent large volume paracentesis having a platelet count of less than 50,000/μL but showed no major bleeding complications. There is no indication for routine use of blood products such as platelet concentrates or fresh frozen plasma in patients with such liver diseases [12].

4 Steps Involved in Performing Abdominal Paracentesis

The steps involved in performing bed-side paracentesis using ultrasound guidance have been detailed below.

1. Preparation:

    (a) Informed written consent: The consent should be obtained after a detailed discussion with the patient about potential risks and benefits of the procedure, including alternative techniques for performing paracentesis. The written consent should include the indication, benefits and potential risks associated with the procedure.
    (b) Patients should be asked to urinate if necessary, in order to empty the urinary bladder prior to procedure.
    (c) An additional assistant must be present to assist with the procedure once the individual performing the procedure has worn sterile gloves [13].

2. Patient positioning and identifying the site of needle puncture:

    (a) The patient is asked to lie down in a supine position.
    (b) The head-end of the bed is elevated to 30–45°.
    (c) To determine the site of paracentesis, percussion of the abdominal wall is performed to find the point of maxi-

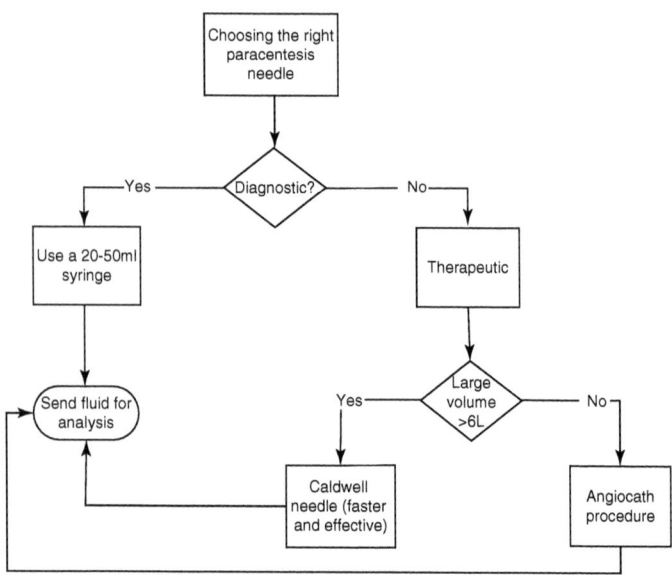

FIGURE 2 Algorithm to help choose the correct needle for paracentesis

mal dullness, usually sites of paracentesis include over the midline about 2 cm inferior to the umbilicus, right or left lower quadrant 2–3 cm lateral to the anterior rectus muscle avoiding the collateral vessels which run bilaterally close to the midline. One can also use the anatomical landmark by marking a site that is 3 cm medial and 3 cm cephalad to the anterior superior iliac spine as a point of reference. A bedside ultrasound machine, if available, is used to accurately identify prominent fluid pockets (Fig. 2).

(d) Once the site is chosen, a skin marker is used to mark the point of entry, usually with an 'X' mark. While identifying the site of puncture, abdominal wall vessels and previous surgical scars should be avoided.

3. Skin preparation:

Universal precautions are to be followed while performing the procedure. Initially the needle entry point on

the skin is sterilized using iodine, chlorhexidine, or ethanol. A drape is then used to form a sterile field around the marked site on the abdominal wall.
4. Equipment selection:

    (a) Paracentesis kit (commercially available kits)
    (b) Iodine, chlorhexidine, or ethanol wipes
    (c) Skin marker
    (d) Sterile gloves
    (e) Sterile gauze (4×4 inches size)
    (f) Sterile drape with a central clearing
    (g) Sterile syringes (5 mL syringe for local anesthesia, 20 mL syringe for diagnostic paracentesis)
    (h) Needles

    - 18 gauge needle to draw the anesthetic solution
    - 25 or 27 gauge and 1.5 inch long needle for administering local anesthetic
    - 18 gauge and 1.5–3.5 inch long needle for paracentesis

    (i) 1% or 2% lidocaine 10 mL solution, with or without epinephrine
    (j) #11 blade scalpel
    (k) Face mask
    (l) Two blood culture bottles (one for aerobic and the other for anaerobic culture)
    (m) Red-top tube and purple-top EDTA tube (for lab work)
    (n) Multiple 1–2 L vacuum bottles, if therapeutic paracentesis is performed
    (o) 3-way stopcock
    (p) Non-collapsible tubing for therapeutic paracentesis

5. Choosing the paracentesis needle: (Fig. 3)

    (a) Diagnostic paracentesis: Use a 20 to 50 mL syringe with an 18 gauge needle. A 1.5 to 3-inch long needle can be utilized to perform the paracentesis.
    (b) Therapeutic paracentesis: The two commonly used needles include the Caldwell needle and angiocath

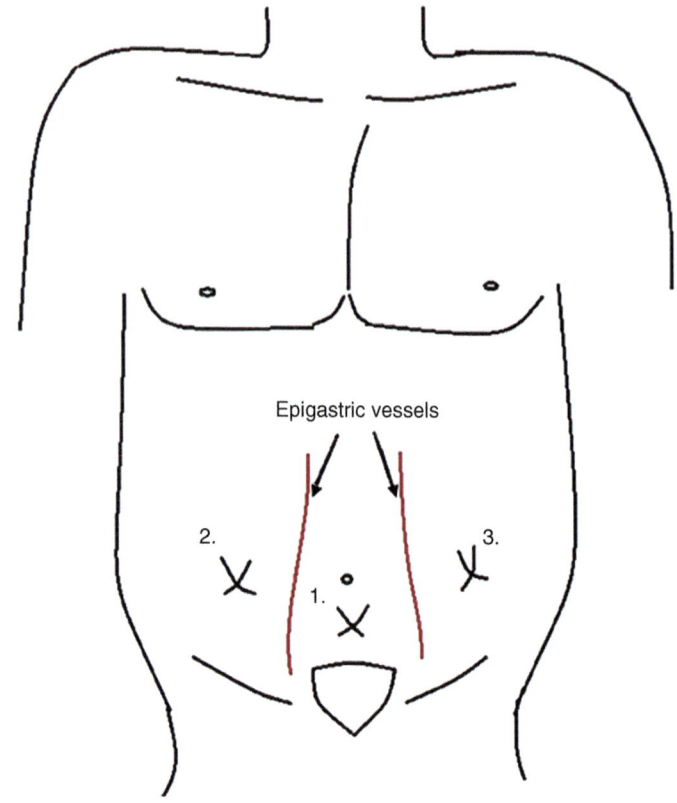

FIGURE 3 Surface anatomical landmarks over the abdomen and sites of needle entry during paracentesis. Site 1 represents the location for needle entry in the midline over the linea alba, Sites 2 & 3 represent the locations for needle entry in the traditional lateral approach technique

needle. The Caldwell needle is preferred for large volume paracentesis due to its larger bore size which facilitates faster drainage of ascitic fluid [14].

6. Anesthetizing the entry site:
   After reconfirming the point of entry using the bedside ultrasound, the skin around the marked area 'X' is anesthe-

tized using lidocaine solution, a 5 mL syringe, and a 1.5-inch-long needle; to infiltrate the skin and subcutaneous tissue. The needle is inserted into the skin using small increments of 3 to 4 mm. The plunger must be withdrawn before advancement to ensure the needle hasn't traversed a blood vessel or a superficial vein. Then the skin and subcutaneous tissue is carefully infiltrated with the local anesthetic while ensuring there is no active bleeding [15].

7. Paracentesis needle insertion:

   (a) A scalpel blade is used to create a small nick of 0.5 cm depth over the anesthetized skin and subcutaneous tissue, to ensure adequate space for the larger bore paracentesis needle to enter the peritoneal cavity. Avoid making larger nicks to minimize leakage of ascitic fluid post-procedure.

   (b) The paracentesis needle should be inserted into the previously anesthetized skin using the Z-track technique. This technique ensures minimal leakage of ascitic fluid after the procedure is completed.

   (c) The Z-track technique is performed as follows: (Fig. 4)

      (i) The first step involves applying superficial traction on the skin using a gloved hand while avoiding displacement of deeper abdominal tissues. Gauze pads can be used to create this traction and usually 1.5–2 cm traction of the skin is adequate.

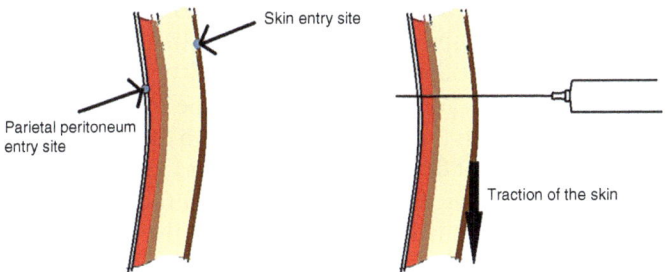

FIGURE 4 Anatomical description of layers of abdominal wall and needle insertion during paracentesis

(ii) Using the other gloved hand, insert the 3.5 inch needle through the abdominal wall while continuing to apply traction to the skin. The dominant hand is preferably used to insert the needle to apply graded and appropriate amount of pressure.
(iii) Gently advance the needle while constantly aspirating to look for any ascitic fluid return during the process. Generally, the proceduralist will experience a letting go sensation or a 'pop' as the needle penetrates the parietal peritoneum and enters the abdominal cavity. At this point the skin traction can be released, which allows the skin to slip back into its original position, this provides a seal to reduce the likelihood of post-procedure fluid leak.

Alternatively, to the Z-track technique, an angular mode of entry can be used to enter the peritoneal cavity. This involves entering the abdominal wall by inserting the needle at an angle rather than perpendicular to the skin to prevent leakage of fluid after procedure.

(d) Advance the needle slowly, while gently aspirating the syringe with every advancement to look for fluid return into the syringe. The ultrasound probe can be used to direct the needle towards the pocket of fluid.
(e) Once the needle has entered the peritoneal cavity, the bedside ultrasound can be used to confirm the location of needle. If the plan is to proceed with a large volume paracentesis, 25 to 50 mL of fluid should be initially obtained for fluid analysis at this time by withdrawing the fluid into the syringe connected to the needle.
(f) If the flow of fluid gets interrupted or there is difficulty in withdrawing fluid, it is possible that the omentum or bowel wall has been suctioned into the bevel of the needle. At this point, the needle must be slightly withdrawn, twisted, and reinserted at small increments to advance into a pocket of free fluid.

(g) For large volume paracentesis, the catheter that is over the needle is held in place while the needle is withdrawn.
(h) The catheter is then connected to the vacuum bottle with the tubing and placed at a level lower than the patient's abdomen to facilitate fluid drainage with gravity.
(i) During large volume paracentesis, it is advised to monitor the vitals of the patient at regular intervals. If more than 5 liters of fluid is removed, then it is recommended to infuse 10 g of albumin per liter of aspirated fluid. This is critical especially in case of cirrhotics who can develop hepato-renal syndrome following large volume paracentesis.
(j) Once the required amount of fluid has been aspirated, the needle must be withdrawn from the abdominal cavity in a rapid swift motion, while holding a 4×4 gauze piece at the site of needle entry. The gauze piece should be is held in place with constant pressure for 2 to 3 min.
(k) A pressure dressing with tape is then applied over the puncture site.
(l) Monitor for any further bleeding or fluid leak at the site for the next few minutes [16–18].

5   Analyzing Peritoneal Fluid

The peritoneal fluid obtained during the paracentesis is sent for the following analysis:

- Gram stain and culture
- Cell count with differential
- Fluid albumin
- Glucose level
- Lactate dehydrogenase (LDH) level
- Amylase level (if indicated)
- Bilirubin level (if indicated)
- Triglyceride level (if indicated)
- Cell cytology for ruling out malignancy (if indicated)

- Acid-fast bacilli (AFB) stain (if indicated)

Concomitantly, blood is drawn to obtain the following parameters:

- Serum chemistry
- Serum albumin
- Serum LDH

The results from fluid analysis can help in diagnosing various conditions, some of these interpretations have been listed below.

- Ascitic neutrophil count of >250 cells/µL is diagnostic of SBP. (Remember to subtract 1 neutrophil for every 250 red blood cells counted in the ascitic fluid)
- A SAAG of ≥1.1 is suggestive of portal hypertension, which usually occurs secondary to liver cirrhosis.
- When the fluid has a high amylase level of >200 IU/L, it suggests pancreatic inflammation causing leakage of pancreatic enzymes into the peritoneal space.
- Triglycerides of >200 mg/dL is suggestive of chylous ascites, which can occur due to injury to major lymphatic ducts.
- Often bloody ascitic fluid tap is thought to be secondary to malignancy, sometimes malignant cells maybe identified on flow cytometry.
- AFB positive bacilli seen on fluid microscopy is pathognomonic of Mycobacterium tuberculosis associated ascites [19].

6 Complications

Paracentesis is generally considered to be a safe procedure but just like any invasive medical procedure it can be associated with complications.

1. Bleeding: Insertion of needle or angiocath can cause injury to a blood vessel, leading to hemoperitoneum. Depending on the severity of bleed it can be managed with watchful waiting, angiographic embolization, or laparotomy. Packed red blood cells can be transfused if hemoglobin level sig-

nificantly decreases. In cases where platelet counts are low or if the patient is coagulopathic; platelet concentrates or fresh frozen plasma can be transfused, respectively. Case reports have been described in patients with acute on chronic liver disease or in patients with cirrhosis where splenic injury and subsequent splenic hematoma was noted. Rarely abdominal wall hematomas resulting in shock has been reported.

2. Ascitic fluid leakage: This is the most common complication associated with paracentesis and can take up to a few hours or sometimes few days to resolve by spontaneous healing of the needle tract created during the procedure. A colostomy bag is sometimes placed at the site to quantify the amount of fluid collected. The skin around the leak should be kept clean and dry to prevent skin irritation.

3. Bowel perforation: It is a rare complication and usually seals by itself without any active intervention. Monitor the patient closely and watch for any signs of peritonitis such as fever, chills, leukocytosis, and abdominal pain or tenderness. Broad spectrum antibiotics are generally administered for a period of 1 to 2 weeks.

4. Hypotension: This may develop during or soon after the procedure, but it tends to be transient and occurs due to shifting of fluids from vascular space as result of loss of fluid from the third space. Albumin infusion is recommended for large volume paracentesis.

5. Infection: This is a rare complication noted in a minute number of patients who undergo paracentesis. Intra-abdominal infection is extremely rare while skin infections and cellulitis may be seen in cases where sterile techniques are not adopted. This can be minimized by following universal precautions and using sterile equipment during the procedure.

6. Acute kidney injury: With large volume paracentesis when >10 liters of fluid is removed, it has been shown to cause hypotension especially when albumin is not infused. Hepatorenal syndrome is another possible complication noted in case reports as a result of large volume paracentesis due to splanchnic vasoconstriction.

7 Types of Kits Available

There are various commercially available paracentesis kits that contain the required equipment for paracentesis. If a large volume paracentesis is being planned, then a pre-assembled paracentesis kit is convenient instead of gathering individual equipment. In case a diagnostic tap is being performed and the aim is to obtain a small volume of ascitic fluid, then individual items can be gathered for cost-effectiveness.

The paracentesis kits that are widely used are the 'safety paracentesis kits' without much difference between various commercial brands. The availability of kits may vary depending on cost and facility of medical practice. Kits may not contain items such as sterile gloves, gown, bouffant, face masks or shield and these may need to be collected separately. Blood culture bottles should be arranged for if ascitic fluid is to be collected and sent for culture and sensitivity testing. The culture bottles are inoculated first when ascitic fluid is initially collected during the procedure, this decreases the risk of iatrogenic contamination by commensal organisms.

If performing a diagnostic tap when a small volume of fluid is collected, then only the following pieces of equipment are required [20].

- Drape
- Sterile gauze
- Betadine or alcohol based sterilizing agent/swab
- 10 mL syringe
- 18 gauge needle
- 1% lidocaine
- Tape

Some examples of commercially available kits include the Avanos, Arrow (Figs. 5 and 6), Haylard, GI supply, and Renova RP system. An advantage of the Renova RP system is that it contains a portable device into which the ascitic fluid

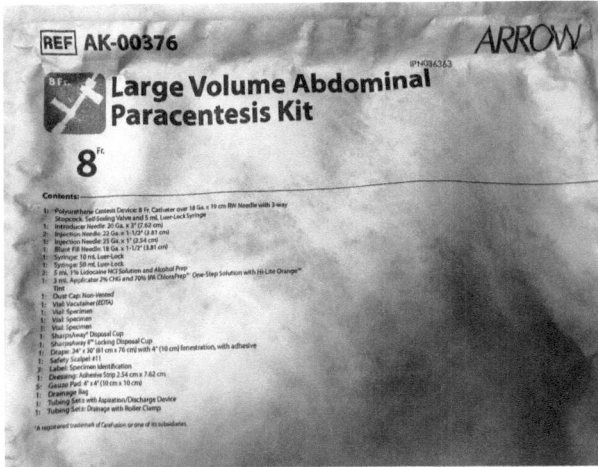

FIGURE 5 The Arrow large volume safety paracentesis kit. This is a pre-assembled kit that contains all the necessary equipment to perform a paracentesis other than the protective wear for the operator

drains and it abates the need for bottles [21]. The portable system contains two bags into which the fluid drains and it prevents interruption that occurs when a bottle is at capacity and needs to be exchanged for a new one. The system allows for controlled rate of fluid removal which may improve tolerability for the patients [22].

8 Pitfalls of Paracentesis

Paracentesis is a bedside procedure and is generally considered to be safe. But there are potential challenges that may arise while performing the procedure.

1. Difficulty in localizing the fluid pocket: In obese patients, the percussion method may not provide the most accurate localization of a fluid pocket. Physical examination may be hindered by body habitus or overlying bowel loops or

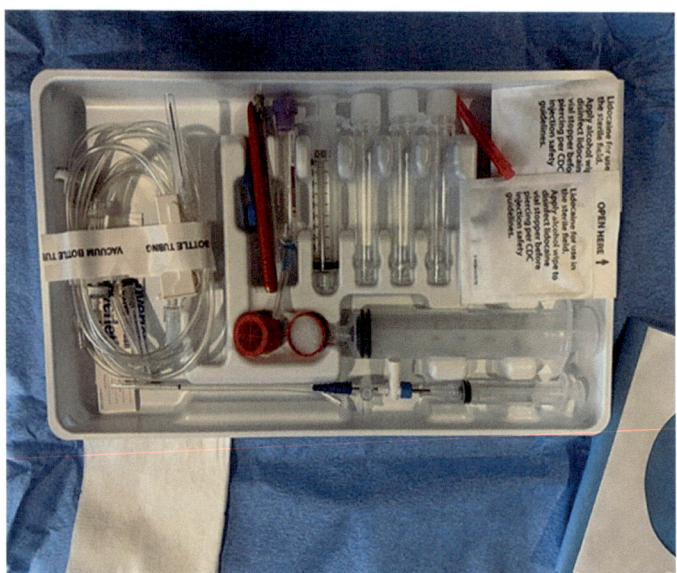

FIGURE 6 Sample cover of the Arrow paracentesis kit with its listed contents

organs. In general, an ultrasound should be used in order to identify the maximal sized fluid pocket for the safe aspiration of ascitic fluid.
2. Injecting local anesthetic: A skin wheal should be created at a planned skin entry site by injecting the local anesthetic solution using a narrow-gauge needle. The needle should be parallel to the skin instead of being perpendicular or at a large angle to help create the wheal. Once the wheal is created the needle is pulled out then reinserted in a perpendicular fashion to inject the solution along the proposed tract of paracentesis needle insertion. If the local anesthetic solution is not injected appropriately then the patient will experience pain during the procedure and lead to poor tolerance and early termination of procedure.
3. Lack of aspiration of fluid: When the paracentesis needle is being inserted, a constant suction on the syringe is maintained to detect the ascitic fluid as soon as the abdominal

cavity is entered. Sometimes even after complete insertion of the needle there may not be any fluid aspirated into the syringe. This usually occurs due to angle of insertion of the needle, incorrect localization of fluid pocket or bowel loops obstructing the flow. Repositioning the needle and withdrawing slightly can help overcome this challenge. Ideally ultrasound can be used to accurately advance the needle tip into the peritoneal cavity.

4. Cessation of flow of ascitic fluid: The ascitic fluid flow rate may sometimes spontaneously decrease or completely subside, in such cases, try to reposition the catheter by withdrawing slightly and/or reposition the patient so that the fluid shifts into the area where the tip of the catheter is located. As the fluid pocket decreases in size, the rate of fluid collected will decrease. The flow may stop if the fluid pocket is drained completely, loops of bowel have obstructed fluid flow, premature removal of the catheter or kinking of the tubing. At times, the catheter tip can be blocked by formation of a blood clot from the blood that enters the catheter when the needle/catheter is initially inserted. At that point, one has no choice but to remove the catheter and use a new needle/catheter to be re-inserted into the existing tract. Prior to insertion, use an ultrasound to confirm that there is still an adequate amount of fluid remaining. Avoid inserting in a different site if possible. Less commonly, the stopcock may not be turned in the proper direction and this will prevent flow of ascitic fluid. Be mindful of this occurring when a new bottle is being exchanged for one that is full, during which the stopcock is operated to stop or direct the flow of fluid.

5. Post-procedural ascitic fluid leak: This most commonly occurs due to insertion of a needle using improper Z-track technique or not using the technique at all. It can also occur when there is tense ascites and a small volume of ascitic fluid is collected for diagnostic purposes. Applying pressure dressing can prevent leakage but, in some cases when the leakage continues, a colostomy bag is applied at the site to measure the collected fluid and to protect the

surrounding skin. The fluid eventually stops leaking in most cases in hours to a few days. If the leakage is constant and prominent then a surgical suture can be applied at the site of leakage.

References

1. Babb RR. Diagnosing ascites: the value of abdominal paracentesis. Postgrad Med. 1978;63(5):219–23.
2. Rudralingam V, Footitt C, Layton B. Ascites matters. Ultrasound. 2017;25(2):69–79.
3. Cho J, Jensen TP, Reierson K, Mathews BK, Bhagra A, Franco-Sadud R, et al. Recommendations on the use of ultrasound guidance for adult abdominal paracentesis: a position statement of the Society of Hospital Medicine. J Hosp Med. 2019;14:E7–E15.
4. Runyon BA. Management of adult patients with ascites due to cirrhosis: an update. Hepatology. 2009;49(6):2087–107.
5. McGibbon A, Chen GI, Peltekian KM, van Zanten SV. An evidence-based manual for abdominal paracentesis. Dig Dis Sci. 2007;52(12):3307–15.
6. Shahed FHM, Mamun Al M, Rahman S. The evaluation of serum ascites albumin gradient and portal hypertensive changes in cirrhotic patients with ascites. Euroasian J Hepatogastroenterol. 2016;6(1):8–9.
7. EASL clinical practice guidelines on the management of ascites, spontaneous bacterial peritonitis, and hepatorenal syndrome in cirrhosis. J Hepatol. 2010;53(3):397–417.
8. Al Knawy B, Shiffman M. Percutaneous liver biopsy in clinical practice. Liver Int. 2007;27(9):1166–73.
9. Skye E. Abdominal paracentesis. 4th ed. 2020. p. 1461–5.
10. Hall DE, Prochazka AV, Fink AS. Informed consent for clinical treatment. CMAJ. 2012;184(5):533–40.
11. De Gottardi A, Thevenot T, Spahr L, Morard I, Bresson-Hadni S, Torres F, et al. Risk of complications after abdominal paracentesis in cirrhotic patients: a prospective study. Clin Gastroenterol Hepatol. 2009;7(8):906–9.
12. Mannucci PM, Tripodi A. Liver disease, coagulopathies and transfusion therapy. Blood Transfus. 2013;11(1):32–6.
13. Fyson J, Chapman L, Tatton M, Raos Z. Abdominal paracentesis: use of a standardised procedure checklist and equipment kit

improves procedural quality and reduces complications. Intern Med J. 2018;48(5):572–9.
14. Grabau CM, Crago SF, Hoff LK, Simon JA, Melton CA, Ott BJ, et al. Performance standards for therapeutic abdominal paracentesis. Hepatology. 2004;40(2):484–8.
15. Dancygier H. Ascites. Oxford: John Wiley & Sons, Ltd; 2014. p. 209–26.
16. De Gottardi A, Yeo CM, Garcia-Tsao G. Paracentesis. Oxford: Wiley-Blackwell; 2012. p. 1158–62.
17. Tuggy MMD, Garcia JMD. Paracentesis. 2011. p. 168–70.
18. Whiffen JD. The diagnostic abdominal paracentesis. Clin Med (Northfield). 1964;71:39–41.
19. Lemos J. Abdominal procedures. 1st ed. CRC Press; 2015. p. 95–100.
20. Jandrey KE. Abdominocentesis. Hoboken: John Wiley & Sons, Inc; 2018. p. 1206–9.
21. Paracentesis – Stanford University. Available from: http://dx.stanford.edu/procedures/Procedures_Paracentesis.pdf.
22. RenovaRP® Paracentesis Management System. Available from: https://www.gi-supply.com/product/paracentesis-pump/.

Lumbar Puncture and Intrathecal Drug Administration

Indications, Techniques, Variants, and Complications

Clayton Reece Burgoon, Will Bryan, and Ambarish P. Bhat

1 Introduction

Lumbar puncture is a routine procedure performed as a diagnostic tool and/or as a therapeutic application for certain treatment protocols. Understanding the various approaches and techniques increases the likelihood of a successful lumbar puncture. This review discusses the origin of the lumbar puncture, approaches to patient positioning, differences in needle variants, use of imaging guidance, and complications related to the procedure. Lumbar puncture was first performed in 1890 by Heinrich Ireneo Quincke when he inserted a needle between the third and fourth lumbar vertebra to collect the cerebrospinal fluid (CSF) from a 21-month-old child in a coma from suspected tuberculous meningitis [1]. This concept, with procedural improvements, continues to be the method of choice for collecting CSF samples, as well as obtaining measurements of intrathecal pressure, intrathecal drug administration, myelography, and spinal anesthesia [2].

C. R. Burgoon · W. Bryan · A. P. Bhat (✉)
Department of Radiology, University of Missouri,
Columbia, MO, USA
e-mail: bhatap@health.missouri.edu

© The Author(s), under exclusive license to Springer Nature Switzerland AG 2022
N. Arora (ed.), *Procedures and Protocols in the Neurocritical Care Unit*, https://doi.org/10.1007/978-3-030-90225-4_9

While many experienced practitioners can perform lumbar punctures at the patient's bedside, not all patients are candidates. Traditionally, locating both of the patient's iliac crests by palpation and drawing an imaginary line, called Tuffier's line, which crosses the L4-L5 joint space, can be used when attempting a blind puncture [3]. When patient body habitus prevents clinicians from palpating bony landmarks, an image-guided approach to view spinal anatomy can be used [4]. The path of the needle can be visualized and controlled with fluoroscopy, computed tomography, or ultrasound. This decreases puncture attempts and redirection of the needle, as well as the number of traumatic or failed attempts, especially in patients with a larger body mass index [5]. In fact these patients should be directly referred to diagnostic imaging for fluoroscopy guidance to ensure a successful attempt [4].

2 Indications

- Diagnostic lumbar punctures were traditionally performed to obtain CSF for laboratory testing and analysis in patients suspected to have meningitis, however in recent years lumbar punctures are performed to diagnose a wide range of autoimmune, degenerative, and neoplastic diseases [6]. A lumbar puncture is often ordered when patients present with vision changes, papillary edema, headache, altered mental status etc.
- A therapeutic lumbar puncture is performed in patients suspected to have an overproduction of spinal fluid resulting in intracranial hypertension, to accurately measure the CSF pressure, and subsequently drain fluid to relieve symptoms [7].
- A lumbar puncture is also used to administer medications within the intrathecal space.
  - Certain radiopaque contrast media can be injected, usually under image guidance, in order to better visualize the spinal cord and spinal nerves for any signs of nerve impingement but can also be used to evaluate for CSF leak if there is cause for perforation or rupture in the dura mater.

- Chemotherapy agents, such as Methotrexate or Cytarabine, can also be injected into the intrathecal space for treatment of Acute Lymphoblastic Leukemia, Burkitt Lymphoma/Leukemia, or Lymphoblastic Lymphoma [8].
- A test bolus of Baclofen is injected into the intrathecal space in patients with spinal spasticity or patients with spinal cord injury to assess for symptom improvement. Depending on the results, the patient may be a candidate for an intrathecal baclofen pump [9].
- Spinraza is an FDA approved treatment in patients with Spinal Muscle Atrophy and is injected into the intrathecal space with 4 loading doses over the course of 2 months and maintenance doses every 4 months thereafter [10].

3 Contraindications

Lumbar punctures are contraindicated in patients with increased intracranial pressure at the risk of cerebellar tonsillar herniation, in patients with a platelet count below 50×10^9/L, skin infection/rash in the area of needle placement [7, 11]. Image guided lumbar punctures involving ionizing radiation, such as fluoroscopy or computed tomography (CT), are contraindicated in women who are pregnant [4].

4 Anatomy, Positioning, and Needle Location

4.1 Anatomy

From superficial to deep the needle traverses the following layers prior to entry into the thecal space.

- Skin.
- Subcutaneous tissue- made up of adipose, connective tissue, and blood vessels.
- Ligamentum Flavum- band of tissue connecting the anterior aspects of adjacent lamina and helps to maintain

upright posture [12]. This is the site where the performing practitioner may feel a "pop" as the needle passes through the ligament and into the epidural space. This sensation is appreciated at a higher rate when an atraumatic needle is used, whereas the traumatic needle cuts through the tissue and the sensation is appreciated at a lesser rate.
- Epidural Space- the area superficial to the dura, contains fat and small blood vessels. This area is accessed for epidural anesthesia and epidural blood patches [12].
- Dura Mater- the outer tough layer that covers the arachnoid membrane, below which is the subarachnoid space containing CSF [12].

4.2 Position Techniques

When performing a lumbar puncture, the patient can be sitting, prone, or in the lateral decubitus position, depending on the patient's ability and cooperation. When measuring cerebrospinal fluid pressure, the lateral decubitus position is the most accurate [1, 2]. When positioning for an image-guided approach with fluoroscopy or computed tomography, the patient is prone when possible [5].

4.3 Spine Level Location

The L3–L4 and L4–L5 interspinous spaces, below the level of the conus medullaris are the usual locations chosen for needle puncture [3, 13, 14]. For individuals receiving multiple lumbar punctures (e.g., patients receiving scheduled intrathecal injections), alternating the level of injections is considered good practice to allow for tissue healing.

Lumbar puncture kit (Fig. 1): Basic lumbar puncture kit should include all the things as mentioned in the kit.

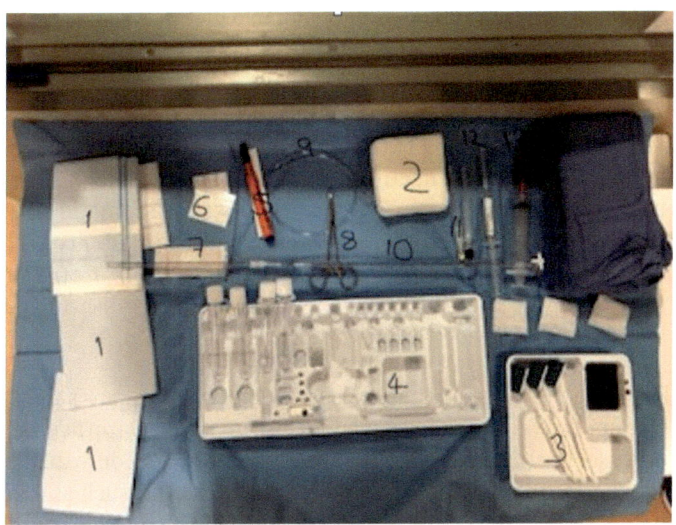

FIGURE 1 LP/Myelogram Sterile Tray: 1. Sterile Drapes/Towels, 2. Sterile 4″ by 4″ or 2″ by 2″ gauze, 3. Betadine prep solution with prep sponges, 4. Lumbar puncture kit with sterile test tubes, 5. Sterile marking pen, 6. Sterile labels, 7. Sterile bandage, 8. Radiopaque marking device, 9. Sterile drainage tubing, 10. Sterile manometer, 11. Spinal needle with size as needed for procedure, 12. 1% lidocaine for local anesthesia, 13. Empty syringe with blunt fill needle if performing myelography

5 Needle Variants

5.1 Needle Type

Two types of needles could be employed- traumatic and atraumatic [15]. The Quincke needle is a traumatic needle because of the sharp cutting tip. This allows for easier needle direction when advancing through the tissue, but increases the risk of developing a post lumbar puncture headache [16]. The Whittacre needle is an atraumatic needle and has a pencil-point or cone-shaped tip. These needles have a hole located near the distal tip on the side of the shaft, and are more difficult to advance through tissue [15]. The benefit of using an atraumatic needle is decreasing the risk of the patient developing a post procedure headache [1]. Most standard pre-packaged lumbar puncture kits come with a cutting needle to be exchanged for an atraumatic needle if the clinician chooses to do so [1]. Despite data to suggest benefit to the use of atraumatic needles when performing lumbar punctures, very few physicians regularly choose atraumatic needles likely due to lack of training and needle availability [17].

5.2 Needle Gauge

The general recommendation is to use needles that are at least 22-gauge. Available data suggests use of larger size needles increase the chances of developing a post-procedure headache [2, 15, 18]. The use of a smaller gauge needle, such as a 22 or 25-gauge, albeit safer, will decrease the rate at which fluid is collected, and thereby increase the total procedure time.

6 Imaging Guided

6.1 Ultrasound Guidance

Ultrasound guidance and mapping of anatomical landmarks can be used to assist lumbar puncture [18]. This is currently the only alternative to image assisted lumbar punctures for patients with contraindications for ionizing radiation (e.g., pregnancy). Ultrasound has demonstrated the ability to produce reliable and accurate depictions of the lumbar spine anatomy, especially deep within subcutaneous tissues [19]. Although there are some studies supporting the use of ultrasound guidance in the clinic or emergency room, it is still not very widely used to guide a lumbar puncture [3].

6.2 Fluoroscopy Guidance (Fig. 2)

Direct visualization of the needle with intermittent fluoroscopy during lumbar puncture, ensures a high level of success.

Lumbar Puncture and Intrathecal Drug Administration 163

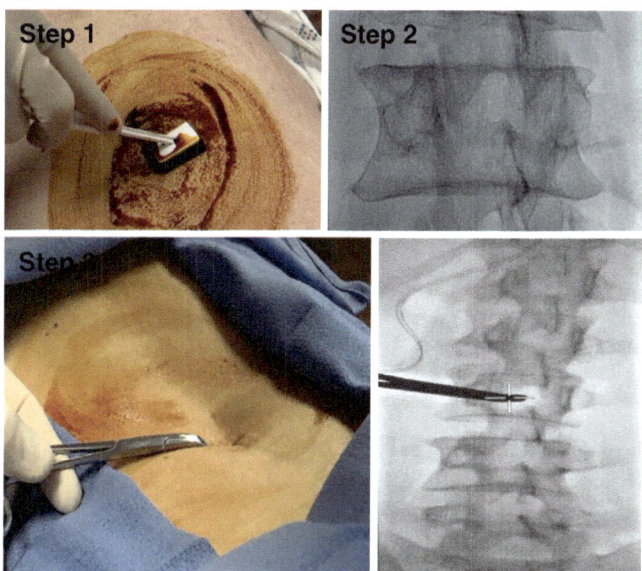

FIGURE 2 Technique for lumbar puncture

Step 1: The posterior lumbar spine region is prepped with betadine solution and draped with sterile drapes or towels

Step 2: Spot fluoroscopic image of interlaminar space (white arrowhead) as target for lumbar puncture. The black arrows show the lamina. The white arrows correspond to pedicles

Step 3: Under fluoroscopic guidance, the interlaminar space (+) is identified with a radio-opaque marker

Step 4: 1% lidocaine is administered in the skin and subcutaneous structure for local anesthesia

Step 5: Initial Needle Placement: Fluoroscopy is used to localize skin entry point

Step 6: Once skin entry point has been localized, puncture the skin and position the needle so it is parallel with the fluoroscopy beam. Advance the needle into the thecal sac

Step 7: Once in the thecal sac, remove the stylette and free flow of CSF should be seen

Step 8: Once intrathecal access has been obtained, connection tubing can be attached to the needle for CSF drainage. Mediations can be injected with via tubing or injecting straight into the needle. Replace stylette and remove needle when completed

Step 9: Once complete, clean skin prep solution from patient's back and place sterile bandage over puncture site

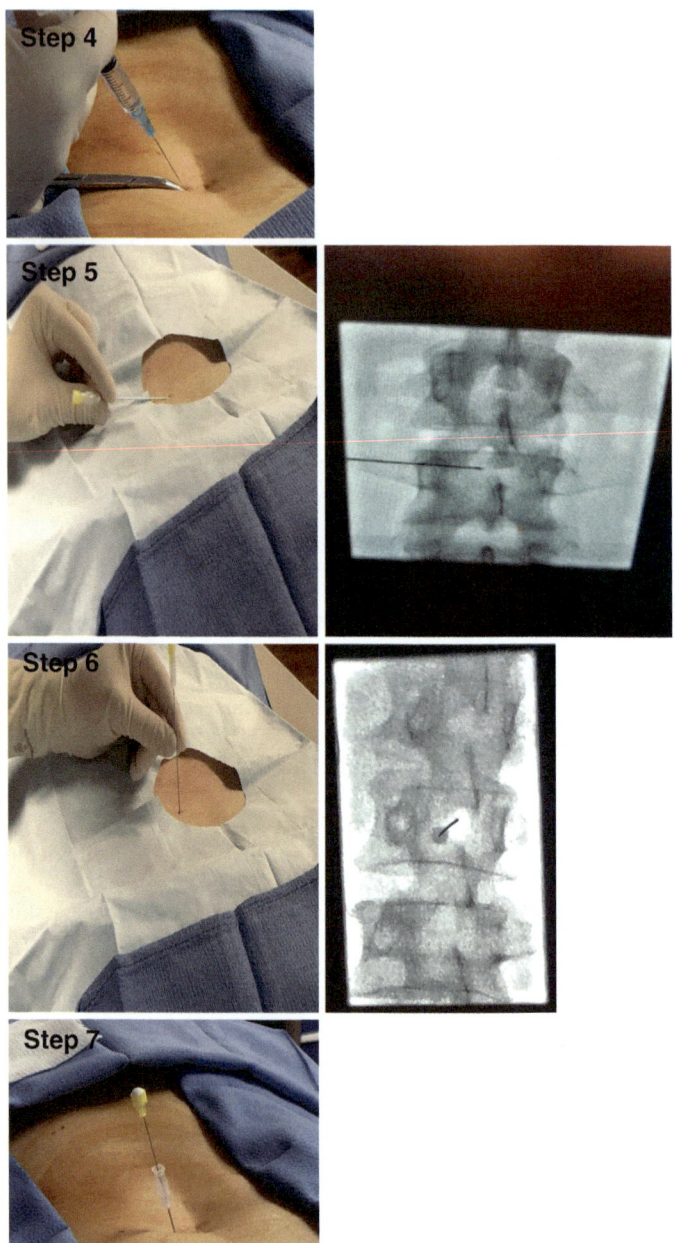

FIGURE 2 (continued)

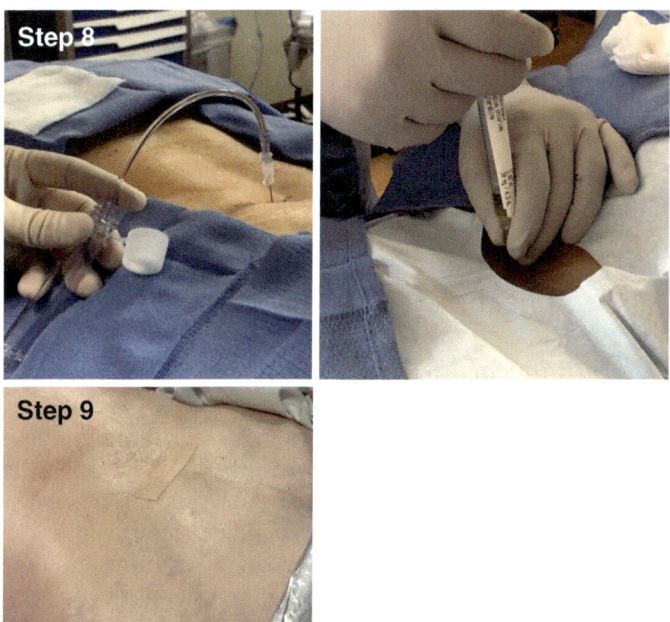

FIGURE 2 (continued)

It is the most commonly used method for guidance after a failed blind attempt [4]. Despite using ionizing radiation, fluoroscopic-guided technique to access the thecal sac is safer and more successful than blind attempts [5]. An attempt should be made to reduce patient dose with protective shielding unless the anatomy of interest would be obscured. Likewise, any staff in the room during a radiographic guided attempt should also use personal protective shielding to reduce occupational radiation exposure.

6.3 CT Guidance

The use of CT for guided lumbar puncture offers the benefit of an anatomical map with complete visualization of the thecal sac, layers of soft tissue, and nearby bony structures to assist the clinician advance the needle tip with millimeter accuracy directly into the sac [5]. The downside to using CT for guidance is the increased cost involved and the lack of ability to obtain various angulations (that could be performed by fluoroscopic guidance), especially in elderly people to move the hypertrophic spinous processes and lamina off the needle trajectory.

7 Complications

7.1 Intrathecal Lidocaine

During the initial lidocaine injection, the performing practitioner must be constantly aware of the depth at which the subcutaneous lidocaine is being injected. While it is necessary to adequately anesthetize the surrounding superficial tissue, there is a risk of inadvertently injecting lidocaine into the intrathecal space which could result in transient loss of sensation and power in the lower extremities.

7.2 Epidural Hematoma

Patients with underlying coagulopathy or on anticoagulation that has not been adequately reversed, are at an increased risk of developing an epidural/subarachnoid hematoma after a lumbar puncture procedure. The hematoma could create mass effect and impinge on the spinal cord or spinal nerves, possibly warranting urgent decompressive surgery [20].

7.3 Infection

Inadequate skin preparation or inadvertently contaminating the sterile field could result in infection. Special consideration is needed when selecting an antiseptic for lumbar puncture procedure. Chlorhexidine is contraindicated for lumbar punctures and neurosurgical procedures, as it is neurotoxic and should not be introduced into the cerebrospinal fluid. Ideally, utilizing a povidone-iodine solution is recommended, unless contraindicated (due to allergy or adverse reaction). Iopropyl alcohol (60–90% concentration) is recommended if the patient is unable to tolerate an iodine-based solution, however alcohol is flammable and extra precautions must be taken to prevent injury [21]. Introducing a contaminate directly into the cerebrospinal fluid could cause meningitis. Be sure to check the sterile supplies or signs of compromise and immediately change sterile gloves if there is a question of contamination are good methods to implement in everyday practice to keep this risk to a minimum.

7.4 Post Lumbar Puncture Headache

A post lumbar puncture headache is the most common complication caused by a persistent leak of CSF from the thecal sac into the surrounding tissues after needle penetration [14, 15]. In the study conducted by Özdemir et al., headaches were reported in 41% of cases performed [2]. These type of headaches typically occur in the occipital and/or frontal areas within 5 days after a lumbar puncture and the symptoms are exacerbated within minutes of sitting or standing upright and improve with lying down [14, 16]. Instructing the patient to remain supine for 4 to 6 h after the procedure will reduce the risk of developing a post lumbar puncture headache [16]. Additionally, instructing the patient to stay hydrated and increase the amount of caffeine intake over the first few days can further reduce this risk. If after a few days the patient is still experiencing symptoms associated with an orthostatic headache, the next usual step is to perform an epidural blood patch. This is when an average of 20 to 30 mL of the patient's own fresh, venous blood is injected into the epidural space. The normal clotting factors within the blood serve to "patch" the defect made in the thecal sac by the spinal needle and halting the leak of cerebrospinal fluid. Blood patches are contraindicated in patients who have a fever, local infection at the needle access site, or have known bleeding disorders [22]. Different institutions will utilize various post procedure protocols for patients who recently received a lumbar puncture as well as how to handle post procedure complications.

7.5 Needle Deformation

As the needle is advanced through the tissue, a number of situations can alter the physical shape of the shaft and bevel tip. If an aggressive technique is taken when trying to direct the needle tip instead of backing the needle out and redirecting, the needle can become permanently deflected off the original axis, adding additional complications to any further attempts with the same needle [2]. Thin-walled atraumatic needles have the tendency to deflect off axis frequently and with more severity than the traumatic cutting needles because they are more flexible [15]. If the needle's shaft or tip become compromised during an unsuccessful attempt, a new needle should be introduced before a second attempt to improve the chance of success.

8 Conclusion

The lumbar puncture is a common procedure performed to collect cerebrospinal fluid samples for evaluation, measure intracranial pressure and administer intrathecal medications. Currently many of these procedures are performed with imaging guidance, to increase the accuracy and make them safer. Hopefully the review of indications, contraindications, complications, types of needles used, implications of imaging guided approaches, associated radiation risks that have been discussed helps imaging departments, radiology employees, clinicians, and students to increase personal understanding of the procedure and overall patient care.

References

1. Butson B, Kwa P. Lumbar puncture. Emerg Med Australas. 2014;26(5):500–1. Available from: http://doi.wiley.com/10.1111/1742-6723.12290.
2. Özdemir HH, Demir C, Varol S, Arslan D, Yildiz M, Akil E. The effects of needle deformation during lumbar puncture. J Neurosci Rural Pract. 2015;6(2):198–201. Available from: https://www.ncbi.nlm.nih.gov/pmc/articles/PMC4387811/.
3. Mofidi M, Mohammadi M, Saidi H, Kianmehr N, Ghasemi A, Hafezimoghadam P, et al. Ultrasound guided lumbar puncture in emergency department: time saving and less complications. J Res Med Sci. 2013;18(4):303–7. Available from: https://www.ncbi.nlm.nih.gov/pmc/articles/PMC3793375/.
4. Edwards C, Leira EC, Gonzalez-Alegre P. Residency training: a failed lumbar puncture is more about obesity than lack of ability. Neurol Int. 2015;84(10):e69–72. Available from: https://pubmed.ncbi.nlm.nih.gov/25754807/.
5. Brook AD, Burns J, Dauer E, Schoendfeld AH, Miller TS. Comparison of CT and fluoroscopic guidance for lumbar puncture in an obese population with prior failed unguided attempt. J Neurointerv Surg. 2014;6(4):324–8. Available from: https://miami.pure.elsevier.com/en/publications/comparison-of-ct-and-fluoroscopic-guidance-for-lumbar-puncture-in.
6. Zambito Marsala S, Gioulis M, Pistacchi M. Cerebrospinal fluid and lumbar puncture: the story of a necessary procedure in the history of medicine. Neurol Sci. 2015;36(6):1011–5. Available from: https://link-springer-com.proxy.mul.missouri.edu/article/10.1007/s10072-015-2104-6.
7. Hoffman KR, Chan SW, Hughes AR, Halcrow SJ. Management of cerebellar tonsillar herniation following lumbar puncture in idiopathic intracranial hypertension. Case Rep Crit Care. 2015;2015:1–4.
8. Kwong YL, Yeung DYM, Chan JCW. Intrathecal chemotherapy for hematologic malignancies: drugs and toxicities. Ann Hematol. 2009;88:193–201.
9. McIntyre A, Mays R, Mehta S, Janzen S, Townson A, Hsieh J, et al. Examining the effectiveness of intrathecal baclofen on spasticity in individuals with chronic spinal cord injury: a systematic review [Internet]. J Spinal Cord Med. 2014;37:11–8. Available from: https://pubmed.ncbi.nlm.nih.gov/24089997/.

10. Pearson SD, Thokala P, Stevenson M, Rind D. The effectiveness and value of treatments for spinal muscular atrophy: a summary from the institute for clinical and economic review's new England comparative effectiveness public advisory council [Internet]. J Manag Care Spec Pharm. Academy of Managed Care Pharmacy (AMCP). 2019;25:1300–6. Available from: https://pubmed.ncbi.nlm.nih.gov/31778620/.
11. Kaufman RM, Djulbegovic B, Gernsheimer T, Kleinman S, Tinmouth AT, Capocelli KE, et al. Platelet transfusion: a clinical practice guideline from the AABB [Internet]. Ann Intern Med. American College of Physicians. 2015;162:205–13. Available from: https://pubmed.ncbi.nlm.nih.gov/25383671/.
12. Leffert LR, Schwamm LH. Neuraxial anesthesia in parturients with intracranial pathology: a comprehensive review and reassessment of risk [Internet]. Anesthesiology. 2013;119:703–18. Available from: https://pubmed.ncbi.nlm.nih.gov/23584382/.
13. Burns J, Scheinfeld MH. Back to the scanner: expected and unexpected imaging findings following spinal puncture and access. Emerg Radiol. 2013;20:291–7.
14. Kim M, Yoon H. Comparison of post-dural puncture headache and low back pain between 23 and 25 gauge Quincke spinal needles in patients over 60 years: randomized, double-blind controlled trial. Int J Nurs Stud. 2011;48(11):1315–22.
15. Pelzer N, Vandersteene J, Bekooij TJS, Schoonman GG, Wirtz PW, Vanopdenbosch LJ, et al. Are atraumatic spinal needles as efficient as traumatic needles for lumbar puncture? Neurol Sci. 2014;35(12):1997–9. Available from: https://pubmed.ncbi.nlm.nih.gov/25139108/.
16. Sjövall S, Kokki M, Turunen E, Laisalmi M, Alahuhta S, Kokki H. Postdural puncture headache and epidural blood patch use in elderly patients. J Clin Anesth. 2015;27(7):574–8. Available from: https://pubmed.ncbi.nlm.nih.gov/26286134/.
17. Davis A, Dobson R, Kaninia S, Espasandin M, Berg A, Giovannoni G, et al. Change practice now! Using atraumatic needles to prevent post lumbar puncture headache. Eur J Neurol. 2014;21(2):305–11. Available from: https://pubmed.ncbi.nlm.nih.gov/24320927/.
18. Honarbakhsh S, Osman C, Teo JT, Gabriel C. Ultrasound-guided lumbar puncture as a diagnostic aid to reduce number of attempts and complication rates. Ultrasound. 2013;21(4):170–5. Available from: http://journals.sagepub.com/doi/10.1177/1742271X13504332.

19. Darrieutort-Laffite C, Bart G, Planche L, Glemarec J, Maugars Y, Le Goff B. Usefulness of a pre-procedure ultrasound scanning of the lumbar spine before epidural injection in patients with a presumed difficult puncture: a randomized controlled trial. Joint Bone Spine. 2015;82(5):356–61. Available from: https://pubmed.ncbi.nlm.nih.gov/25764916/.
20. Ausman JI. Open Access SNI: general neurosurgery, a supplement to Surgical Neurology International. 2016. Available from: http://www.surgicalneurologyint.com.
21. Sukul V, Lynch T, Loftus CM. Optimal approaches to skin preparation prior to neurosurgery. US Neurol. 2010;06(02):14.
22. Ahmed SV, Jayawarna C, Jude E. Post lumbar puncture headache: diagnosis and management [Internet]. Postgrad Med J. BMJ Publishing Group. 2006;82:713–6. Available from: https://www.ncbi.nlm.nih.gov/pmc/articles/PMC2660496/.

Intracranial Access

Michael Ortiz Torres and Steven B. Carr

1 Introduction

Accessing the intracranial space for both diagnostic and therapeutic purposes has been attempted for thousands of years. Archaeological evidence exists that even ancient human civilizations performed rudimentary intracranial access [1]. In the modern era, our efforts are more informed and refined, and these interventions are performed safely by thousands of practitioners worldwide. Although some surgeons and interventionalists perform these procedures in the operating room, all the procedures described in this chapter are safely, effectively, and routinely performed at the bedside as well. This chapter seeks to clearly outline safe and effective practices regarding: (1) the indications for bedside intracranial access procedures, (2) the steps and important technical points for those procedures, and (3) common pitfalls and difficulties that can be faced.

Elevated intracranial pressure (ICP) can be a dangerous condition, and typically requires treatment. As a result, ICP

M. O. Torres · S. B. Carr (✉)
Division of Neurosurgery, University of Missouri School of Medicine, Columbia, MO, USA
e-mail: ortiztorresm@health.missouri.edu;
carrsb@health.missouri.edu

© The Author(s), under exclusive license to Springer Nature Switzerland AG 2022
N. Arora (ed.), *Procedures and Protocols in the Neurocritical Care Unit*, https://doi.org/10.1007/978-3-030-90225-4_10

monitoring has become a critical component of the care of patients at risk for acutely pathological intracranial hypertension. The most common indication for invasive ICP monitoring is traumatic brain injury (TBI), however patients with a wide range of intracranial pathology can benefit from ICP monitoring, including intracranial hemorrhages, ischemic stroke, cerebral edema, tumors, aneurysmal rupture, hydrocephalus, and others. However, obviously not all patients with conditions such as those listed above require ICP monitoring, thus the important question to start with is not "which conditions require ICP monitoring", but rather "which patients require intracranial pressure monitoring?"

As in most situations in neurocritical care, much of the answer to this question depends on the clinical judgment of an experienced physician who is capable of assessing and integrating all the relevant clinical and radiographic factors to make a decision. However, in the modern era we do have evidence to help inform these decisions, and general guidelines and principles to ensure we provide appropriate care. Perhaps the most appropriate place to begin the discussion on the indications for intracranial pressure monitoring is in the setting of traumatic brain injury.

The Brain Trauma Foundation has undertaken the task of performing systematic reviews of the literature and has synthesized recommendations related to ICP monitoring based on different levels of evidence. Their most recent recommendations have been published as part of the Guidelines for Management of Severe Traumatic Brain Injury, 4th edition [2]. While there is currently no Level I or II A evidence to recommend ICP monitoring as standard of care, there is Level II B evidence for using ICP monitoring information to reduce in-hospital and 2-week post-injury mortality in patients with severe TBI. Level II B evidence suggests that ICP above 22 mm Hg is the recommended threshold for treatment as it is associated with increased mortality, and Level III evidence suggests that a combination of ICP values, clinical data, and brain CT findings may be used to make management decisions. The inconclusiveness of this data suggests that the practitioner should take into consideration all available data to make a patient-specific decision. It also raises the point that the heterogeneity of the trauma population and diseases makes standardizing treatment decisions a very challenging task.

These concepts can be extrapolated to other conditions as well: patients with enlarged ventricles and a concerning neurologic exam may require cerebrospinal fluid (CSF) diversion and ICP monitoring. These two goals are closely related, but mentioned separately here because external ventricular drain (EVD) placement can be both diagnostic (measuring ICP, sampling CSF) and therapeutic (draining CSF, ability to administer intrathecal medications). However, an ICP monitor ("Camino®" [Natus Medical Inc.; California, USA] or "bolt") is purely diagnostic and lacks any direct treatment benefit from the intervention. Both an EVD and an ICP monitor are effective for measuring intracranial pressure, the decision of which option to use depends on multiple factors. Our priority for the following discussion is to provide practical guidance on using and interpreting these devices.

2 Intracranial Pressure Monitoring

Indications
While other modalities we will discuss exist to reliably achieve the same goal, a well fluid-coupled EVD is considered the standard of care for measuring intracranial pressure. An EVD is a narrow catheter placed through the skull and brain parenchyma in order to situate the tip of the catheter inside the ventricular system at the foramen of Monroe, roughly the center of the intracranial space. It is tunneled out through the skin and attached to a bedside drainage system. This drainage system is leveled at the tragus, which is an approximation for where the tip of the catheter is in order to avoid the siphon or antisiphon effects of gravity with the fluid column. The drainage system ("Becker drain") can be attached to a transducer and an ICU bedside monitor to

continuously measure ICP and then visualize the pressure waveform, however this requires drainage to be turned off. Conversely, the drainage system can also be left open to drain if the pressure exceeds a pressure set manually on the Becker drain, however this sacrifices continuous monitoring.

When open to drain, the Becker drain can be used to manually check a pressure by raising the setting to the maximum number and making note of where the meniscus of the fluid column settles relative to the scale at the side, similar in concept to measuring a pressure with a lumbar puncture manometer. Pressures are generally measured either in millimeters of mercury (mmHg) or centimeters of water (cmH2O), and most Becker drains have both scales on the drainage system chamber. Both scales are valid, however we recommend routinely using one scale for consistency and clarity at an institution, and having a quick way to convert to the other system as needed. So-called "normal" ranges are roughly 5–20 mmHg, or 10–27 cmH2O. A "quick and dirty" way to convert mmHg numbers to cmH2O is to be able to quickly approximate what 5, 10, 15, and 20 mmHg correlate to in cmH2O. In fact, for these four values, remembering "2, 4, 6, 8" can be a useful mnemonic, as adding 2 to 5 mmHg, adding 4 to 10 mmHg, adding 6 to 15 mmHg, and adding 8 to 20 mmHg roughly correlates with what the number would be in cmH2O.

As one might expect, significant variability in practice patterns exist about how frequently an EVD (as opposed to an ICP monitor or Licox) is used as the ICP monitoring modality, and depends on comfort level, experience, risks, and clinical factors. A patient with acute symptomatic hydrocephalus and dilated ventricles may need continuous CSF diversion more than intracranial pressure monitoring, whereas a patient without mass hematoma, but diffuse cerebral edema and slit-like ventricles may not get as much benefit from having even a perfectly placed catheter in collapsed ventricles, from a CSF diversion standpoint. The Neurocritical Care Society [3] and Society for Neuroscience in Anesthesiology and Critical Care [4] have issued a consensus statements which include evidence-based recommendations regarding EVD placement and management, and inform our institutional practice as described.

2.1 External Ventricular Drain Placement

Technique/Method

1. *Positioning*

    The patient should be supine with the head midline (not turned), and the head of bed elevated to 30°. If done at the bedside, the bed should be moved away from the wall to provide adequate space to efficiently maneuver and maintain a sterile field. A bedside table should be easily accessible for the instruments and equipment, and the Becker drain should be set up prior to the procedure.

2. *Preparation*

    The cranial access kit (Fig. 1a) and EVD catheter (Fig. 1b) are opened in sterile fashion to create a sterile field on the bedside table. A generous sterile prep is per-

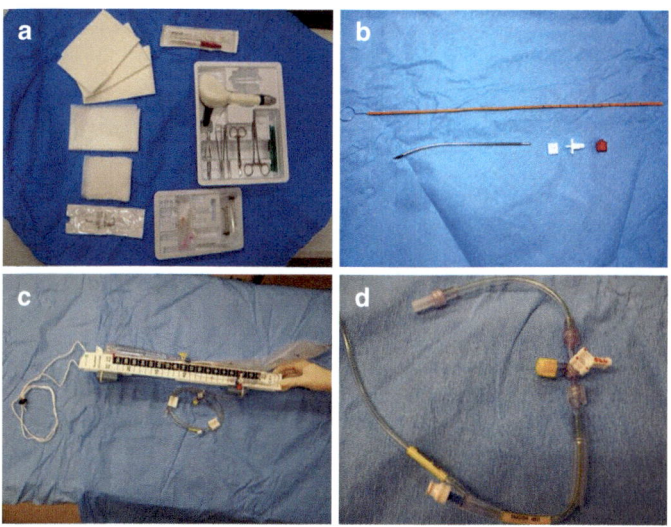

FIGURE 1 External ventricular drain equipment

formed of the frontal region, at which point the proceduralist should don a hat, mask, sterile gown, and sterile gloves. A standard cranial access kit comes with 3 paper sterile white drapes, which can be placed on either side of the patient's head, and at the top of the head where the proceduralist stands. Then the clear plastic drape is placed over the patient's frontal region at Kocher's point. Using the sterile ruler, measurements are made 11 cm posterior to the nasion and 3 cm lateral to the midline, where a mark is placed, and a 2–3 cm planned incision line is made oriented anterior to posterior, centered over Kocher's point. This point should lie at the intersection of the midpupillary line and the midpoint between the lateral canthus and external auditory meatus, 1 cm anterior to coronal suture (Fig. 2a–c). Local anesthesia with lidocaine with or without

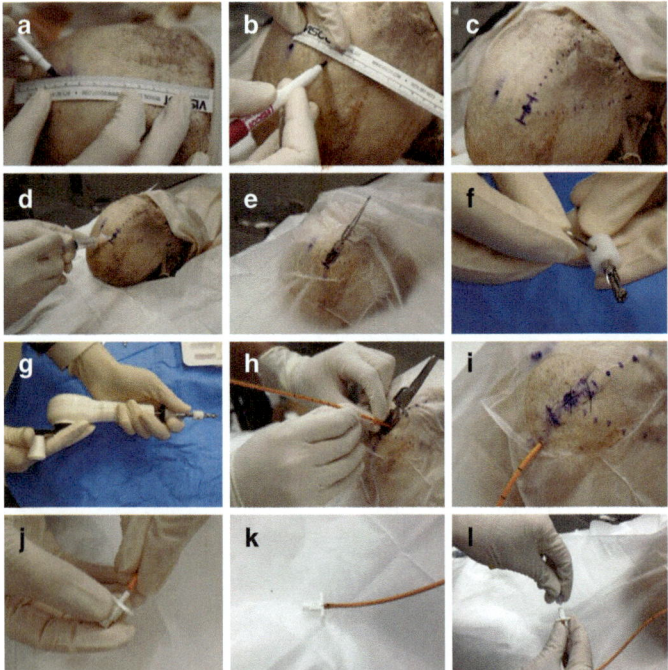

FIGURE 2 EVD placement steps

epinephrine 1:2000,000 is routinely provided and infiltrated using a small-bore needle (Fig. 2d). Prior to making incision, ensure the twist drill is assembled and the guide is set to ~1.5 cm, and all instruments are ready to use (Fig. 2f, g). Since local anesthetic takes a few minutes to reach peak effect, this is a good time to prepare the sterile instruments and equipment.

3. *Procedure: Obtaining intracranial access*

    An incision is made with the 15 blade scalpel down to the skull and the belly of the scalpel blade can be used to scrape back and forth on the skull to elevate the pericranium. A small Heiss self-retaining retractor is provided in a standard cranial access kit, and can be used to keep the scalp open and skull exposed if needed (Fig. 2e). Hemostasis can be achieved either by scalp tension produced by retractor placement, or if bleeding obscuring the field is still present, using hemostats, irrigation, or a disposable pen bovie. The twist drill is brought into the field and the tip is placed on the skull, perpendicular to the surface of the skull, pointed at the center of the head. Steady and firm, but not hard pressure is applied while rotating the drill handle forward. Three different bone consistencies are typically felt during drilling – the first being the hard cortical bone, followed by the softer/more irregular cancellous bone, then inner cortical bone again, until the drill feels like it starts to "catch" a bit. This means the drill bit is starting to breach the inner cortex, which is a good time to stop drilling. Our technique is to then manually twist the silver drill head forward slowly with your hand, as the drill head will be "pulled" in more rapidly with rotation at this point, but a clear and full inner breach is necessary. Once the drill is all the way through, continue to slowly twist forward (to avoid bone dust/material from being delivered from the drill bit into the intracranial space) as you pull the drill out. The burr hole is rinsed with saline. At this point, use the blunt allen wrench provided to probe the hole to feel for whether the dura still needs to be opened. If so, one can use the 18-gauge needle to puncture and open the dura.

4. *Procedure: Passing the catheter*

Once confident the dura is open, bring the EVD catheter (antibiotic-impregnated Bactiseal® [Codman Integra; San Diego, CA, USA] catheters are associated with lower risk of infection [5]) with the stylet in place into the sterile field. We favor tunneling the trocar posteromedially 5 cm away to lower the risk of infection [6], avoid a possible VP shunt tract, and avoid the contralateral side in case of a procedure is required contralaterally. If the trocar is placed through the skin prior to passing the EVD catheter, it can help minimize the potential inadvertent advancement/displacement of the catheter that can happen with placing the EVD catheter prior to tunneling the trocar, which requires some degree of force and catheter manipulation. The EVD with the stylet is brought in and oriented so that the numbers (centimeters of length) are visible to the proceduralist. The EVD is then passed perpendicular to the skull, directed toward the contralateral medial canthus (Fig. 2h). The catheter should not be "hard passed" (with the stylet in place) more than 5–6 cm. When CSF egress is returned, the stylet is removed, the catheter can be soft passed another centimeter in depth, and the end of the catheter is pinched while the other hand should use a forceps to grab the catheter at the skull entrance to hold it in place. The catheter is attached to the trocar end, and the trocar pulls it through the skin. Make note of the number (depth) at the skull, as well as the number at the skin exit site to ensure that the catheter does not advance or back out during securing.

5. *Procedure: Securing the catheter*

We recommend cutting the catheter with a scissors from the trocar, and then attaching the white Luer lock adapter (Fig. 2j) with the Luer lock cap in place, and a tie should be secured around the connection to the adapter (Fig. 2k), and a cap placed on the Luer lock until ready to connect the catheter to the Becker drain. A running 3-0 nylon suture is used to close the incision (Fig. 2i); a separate galeal closure is not typically done for this procedure.

A second 3-0 nylon is used to secure the catheter, we find the most reliable method to secure the catheter and avoid the catheter from unintentionally being advanced or backed out is a U-stitch surrounding the exit site, snug without pinching off the catheter, followed by a modified Roman sandal technique [7].

6. *Procedure: Completion*

At this point, an assistant should pass the clamped Becker drain drainage catheter (Fig. 1c, d) to the proceduralist with the cap removed, being careful not to touch the sterile connection tip, and the proceduralist removes the Luer lock cap and attaches the Becker drain tubing to the sterile EVD catheter Luer lock adapter (Fig. 2l). The drain should be ensured to be leveled correctly at the tragus, hung from/attached to an IV pole, and then unclamped to measure an opening pressure and ensure patency of the system.

Pearls and Pitfalls
- Preoperative platelet count and coagulation profile should be optimized and blood thinning medications assessed prior to placement to minimize risk of iatrogenic intracranial hemorrhage
- Adequate space and attention to set-up can make maintaining a sterile field and efficiency more smooth
- Ensuring the twist drill craniotomy hole is oriented in the exact direction the catheter needs to be passed is crucial for accurate placement, as the hole represents a cylinder which can deflect the bendable catheter as it passes through the skull
- Making note of the numbers showing the length at the exit points from the skull and skin can help ensure the catheter does not advance or retract during post-placement maneuvers
- Having multiple methods for identifying Kocher's point is useful to confirm appropriate entry point, as head shapes and available landmarks can vary

- If spontaneous CSF egress is not encountered by the time the catheter has been passed 5 cm, a syringe can be placed on the EVD end and gently aspirated to encourage or confirm CSF flow
- Generally, no more than 3 passes are attempted prior to leaving the catheter in place and sending the patient for CT scan to evaluate catheter position
- The procedure note should include number of passes, opening pressure, and appearance of CSF as relevant findings

2.2 Fiberoptic Intracranial Pressure Monitor (Camino, or "bolt")

Technique/Method

1. *Positioning*

   Positioning is identical to EVD placement. The patient should be supine with the head midline and the head of bed elevated to 30°. If done at the bedside, the bed should be moved away from the wall to provide adequate space to efficiently maneuver and maintain a sterile field. A bedside table should be easily accessible for the instruments and equipment.

2. *Preparation*

   Procedural preparation is identical to EVD and Licox placement, with the exception that a ventricular catheter is not used. A separate ICP monitor kit (Fig. 3) is used with a cranial access kit, and a nonsterile bedside monitoring box. Of note, the twist drill bit is smaller for an ICP monitor compared to the bit provided in the cranial access kit to place an EVD, thus the drill bit from the ICP monitor kit is used instead. The nonsterile bedside ICP monitor box should be attached to an IV pole and turned on and ensured to be functioning.

3. *Procedure: Obtaining Intracranial Access*

   Using the correct drill bit, the cranial access process is identical to that of an EVD/Licox placement.

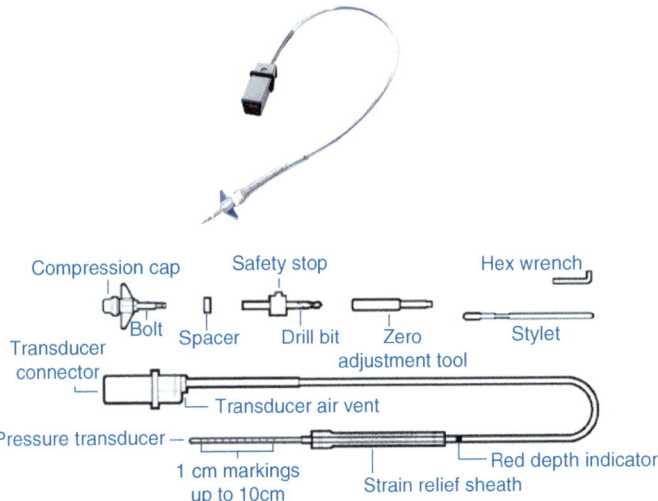

FIGURE 3 Intracranial pressure monitor (Camino [8]) equipment

4. *Procedure: Monitor Placement*

The ICP monitor housing often comes with a white washer screwed on the tip which is used for infants. This should be removed for non-infant patients. When the dura is confirmed to be penetrated, the monitor housing is screwed into the skull until finger tight. The white plastic should be twisted to loosen, and the blunt metal stylet should be advanced to ensure clear passage, and resecured. At this point, an assistant (or nurse) at the bedside holds the cord plug adaptor in close proximity to the proceduralist, and the proceduralist stays sterile but advances the black fiberoptic plug into the female end of the cord system the nurse holds. There is a small screw on this component that should face upward, which should stay sterile. A small plastic screwdriver is included in the ICP monitor set, and is used to gently twist the screw slightly in either direction necessary to zero the system. The white screw top on the monitor housing is then loosened, the metal stylet removed, and the fiberoptic catheter is advanced until the

double hatch marks are at the level of the white screw top, and the screw top is tightened. Ensure the pressure has a good waveform and makes sense with the patient's situation, then advance the plastic sheath over the white screw top.
5. *Procedure: Conclusion*

    An untied 3-0 nylon U-stitch can be left untied in place and wrapped around the ICP monitor to save a separate suture at the time of removal. The base of the housing can be wrapped with sterile petroleum, chlorhexidine, or betadine-soaked gauze, and the components can be wrapped with sterile Tegaderm to prevent nonsterile entry into adjoining components (housing, sheath, fiberoptic).

Pearls and Pitfalls
- The most difficult part of ICP monitor placement is getting the fiberoptic system zeroed and placed, which can require very subtle changes to the adjustment screw and a steady hand from the assistant
- Giving the fiberoptic cord a gentle 180° turn and securing across it with tape can help to ensure that during patient turning/moving for scans, routine nursing care that the catheter being occasionally tugged will not pull the fiberoptic straight out.
- Pressure drift can occur over time, thus ICP monitors' pressure reading should be read with some skepticism the longer a monitor has been in place (generally greater than a week)

2.3 Brain Oxygenation Monitoring (Licox®, Integra; San Diego, CA, USA)

Indications

Patients with elevated intracranial pressure may lose cerebral autoregulation which could lead to decreased perfusion and oxygen delivery [2]. This can result in metabolism fails and cell death. Although brain tissue oxygenation monitoring is not standard of care, there are some studies [9–11] that suggest improved outcomes when brain tissue oxygen monitoring is used to detect tissue hypoxia and treat accordingly. The Licox system is used to monitor the perfusion status of cerebral tissue local to sensor placement.

Technique/Method

1. *Positioning*

    Positioning is identical to EVD placement. The patient should be supine with the head midline and the head of bed elevated to 30°. If done at the bedside, the bed should be moved away from the wall to provide adequate space to efficiently maneuver and maintain a sterile field. A bedside table should be easily accessible for the instruments and equipment.

2. *Preparation*

    The intracranial access kit and Licox kit are opened in sterile fashion to create a sterile field on the bedside table. A generous sterile prep is performed of the frontal region The Licox monitor is usually placed at Kocher's point, although placement may vary based on the specific area that would like to be monitor. Local anesthesia is infiltrated using a small-bore needle. Prior to making incision, ensure the twist drill is assembled and the guide is set to ~1.5 cm, and all instruments are ready to use.

3. *Procedure: Obtaining intracranial access*

    Obtaining intracranial access via twist drill craniotomy is identical to EVD placement.

4. *Procedure: Monitor placement*

    The bolt is placed into the skull and secured. The stylet is passed through the bolt to probe the space and ensure a clear path. The introducer is inserted in the burr hole and secured to the bolt. The guidewire is removed from the oxygen monitor introducer and the Licox oxygen monitoring probe is placed into the introducer and 2 cm deep into the intracranial space. The probe is then secured to the introducer with the compression cap. Care must be taken to not overtighten to cap as this may fracture the probe - finger

tight should be enough. A 3-0 nylon suture can be used in a figure of eight fashion around the bolt entry site to approximate the skin and obtain hemostasis, if necessary.
5. *Procedure: Completion*
   Petroleum impregnated gauzes are wrapped around the bolt over the skin to maintain the area occluded and moist. 4x4's is then opened and wrapped over the screw and silicone tubing attachment and then secured with tape.

Pearls and Pitfalls
- The practitioner must be cognizant that the parameters obtained by the monitor reflect only those of the tissue local to the sensor
- Care must be taken to avoid overtightening of the compression cap as this may fracture the probe. Conversely, a loose cap may allow for movement of the sensor and provoke a so-called "drift effect" where the sensor moves along its parenchymal tract and provides variable, and possibly unreliable values.

3 Subdural Drainage

Indications
Patients with symptomatic subdural hematomas (SDH) producing pathologic mass effect can benefit from evacuation of the hematoma. While acute hemorrhages consist of firm or formed clot and generally require craniotomy for evacuation when necessary, over time the hematoma breaks down and liquifies, and liquid subacute to chronic subdural hematomas can often be drained through a twist drill craniostomy and either subdural drain placement or subdural evacuating port system (SEPS) placement. Typically, subdural drains and SEPS are only used for chronic or late subacute SDH, which are hypodense to brain on CT and ideally homogeneous in density, as mixed density SDH are less likely to be successfully evacuated via this method [12]. The indications for either subdural drain placement or SEPS drain placement are essentially the same.

3.1 Subdural Drain

Technique/Method

1. *Positioning*

    Essentially identical to EVD placement. The patient should be supine with the head turned 30° to the contralateral side and the head of bed elevated to 30°. If done at the bedside, the bed should be moved away from the wall to provide adequate space to efficiently maneuver and maintain a sterile field. A bedside table should be easily accessible for the instruments and equipment, and the Becker drain should be set up and primed with sterile saline prior to the procedure.

2. *Preparation*

    The cranial access kit and EVD catheter are opened in sterile fashion to create a sterile field on the bedside table. A generous sterile prep is performed of the frontal region, at which point the proceduralist should don a hat, mask, sterile gown, and sterile gloves. A standard cranial access kit comes with 3 paper sterile white drapes, which can be placed on either side of the patient's head, and at the top of the head where the proceduralist stands. Then the clear plastic drape is placed over the patient's frontal region. Generally, the entry point for the drain will be at the level of the superior temporal line and 0–1 cm anterior to the coronal suture. This may vary depending on the location of the hematoma. Local anesthesia is infiltrated using a small-bore needle. Prior to making incision, ensure the twist drill is assembled and the guide is set to ~1.5 cm, and all instruments are ready to use.

3. *Procedure: Obtaining intracranial access*

    An incision is made with the scalpel down to the skull and the belly of the scalpel blade can be used to scrape back and forth on the skull to elevate the pericranium. A small Heiss self-retaining retractor is provided in a standard cranial access kit, and can be used to keep the scalp exposure open and skull exposed if needed. Hemostasis can be achieved either after retractor placement tension, or if bleeding obscuring the field is still present, using hemostats, irrigation, or a disposable pen bovie. The twist drill is brought into the field and the tip is placed on the skull, perpendicular to the surface of the skull, pointed at the center of the head. Steady and firm, but not hard pressure is applied while rotating the drill handle forward. Three different consistencies are typically felt – the first being the hard cortical bone, followed by the softer/more irregular cancellous bone, then inner cortical bone again, until the drill feels like it starts to "catch" a bit. This means the drill bit is starting to breach the inner cortex, which is a good time to stop drilling. Once the outer cortex is breached, the hand drill can be angled approximately 45° posteriorly to create an angled twist drill hole. This allows the catheter to enter the intracranial space tangentially, avoiding unintentional catheter penetration of the cortex. Once the drill is all the way through, continue to slowly twist forward (to avoid bone dust/material from being delivered from the drill bit into the intracranial space) as the drill is pulled out. The craniostomy hole is rinsed with saline. At this point, the blunt allen wrench provided is used to probe the hole to feel for whether the dura still needs to be opened. If so, one can use the 18-gauge needle to puncture and open the dura.

4. *Procedure: Passing the catheter*

An EVD catheter is used as a subdural drainage catheter, but instead of the holes in the tip draining CSF from the ventricle, the catheter is placed in the subdural space. With the stylet inserted all the way down the catheter, the tip can be slightly bent to create a "hockey-stick" angle. The tip of the catheter is then inserted through the twist drill hole with the stylet in to provide rigidity. Once the catheter tip is passed into the subdural space the stylet is stabilized with the non-dominant hand and the dominant hand is used to slowly advance the catheter over the stylet and into the subdural space. Minimal to no resistance should be felt when advancing the catheter. Resistance may indicate intraparenchymal passage or passage into the epidural space. The catheter length advanced into the subdural space depends on the posterior extent of the subdural collection relative to the catheter's entry point. The catheter end is then placed below the level of the head to test for fluid egress. Usually, dark, so-called "motor oil" fluid is drained. The trocar is then used to create a posteromedial subcutaneous tunnel with the exit site approximately 5 cm away from the entry site. The catheter is attached to the trocar and, while securing the catheter at its entry point to avoid pull-out, is then advanced through the subcutaneous tunnel. Make note of the number (depth) at the skull, as well as the number at the skin exit site to ensure that the catheter does not advance or back out during securing.

5. *Procedure: Securing the catheter*

    Identical to that of EVD placement. We recommend cutting the catheter with a scissors from the trocar, and then attaching the white Luer lock adapter with the Luer lock cap in place, and a suture should be used around the connection to the adapter. A running 3-0 nylon suture can be used to close the incision, a separate galeal closure is not typically done for this procedure. A second 3-0 nylon is used to secure the catheter, we find the most reliable method to secure the catheter and avoid the catheter from unintentionally being advanced or backed out is a U-stitch surrounding the exit site, snug without pinching off the catheter, followed by a modified Roman sandal technique [7].

6. *Procedure: Completion*

    At this point, an assistant should pass the clamped Becker drain drainage catheter to you with the cap removed, being careful not to touch the sterile connection tip, and the proceduralist removes the Luer lock cap and attaches the Becker drain tubing to the sterile EVD catheter Luer lock adapter. The chamber is usually set approximately 20 cm below the tragus to create a siphon effect and facilitate drainage.

3.2 Subdural Evacuating Port System (SEPS) Placement

Technique/Method
1. *Positioning*
   Positioning is identical to that of a subdural drain and EVD placement.
2. *Preparation*
   Preparation for the procedure is identical to that of a subdural drain, with the exception being SEPS drain kits (Fig. 4a–c) contain the necessary instruments and equipment, and one does not require a ventricular catheter or separate cranial access kit. Of note, the twist drill for a SEPS drain is larger bore than that of a standard cranial access kit (Fig. 4b).
3. *Procedure: Obtaining intracranial access*
   Obtaining intracranial access via twist drill craniostomy is identical to that of a subdural drain – however the twist drill hole is placed perpendicular to the skull and not angled as in a subdural drain (Fig. 4d–g).

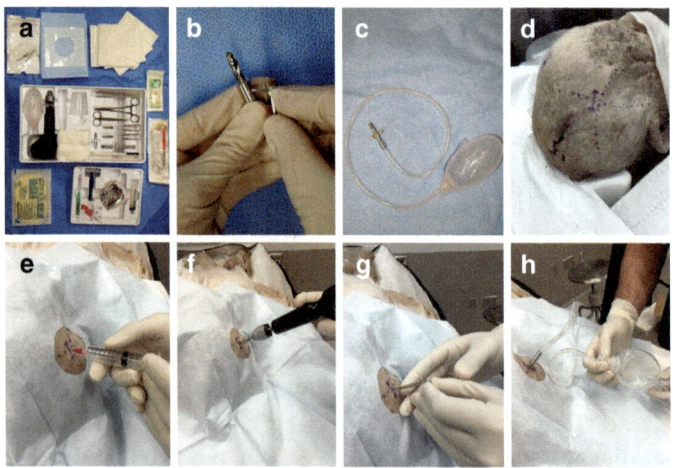

FIGURE 4 SEPS drain equipment & placement steps

4. *Procedure: Screw placement*

   Once the dura is confirmed to be open, the SEPS screw is then placed inside the burr hole and turned clockwise until finger tight. The silicone tubing is then placed on the screw. The suction reservoir bulb is attached, compressed, and then closed (Fig. 4h). A 3-0 nylon suture can be used in a figure of eight fashion around the screw entry site to approximate the skin and obtain hemostasis, if necessary.

5. *Procedure: Completion*

   Petroleum impregnated gauzes are wrapped around the screw over the skin to maintain the area occluded and moist. 4×4's is then opened and wrapped over the screw and silicone tubing attachment and then secured with tape.

Pearls and Pitfalls

Subdural drain

- Tangential entry into the subdural space avoids intraparenchymal passage.
- As the practitioner becomes more experienced, a certain "feel" for accessing the subdural space is developed. This helps to ensure safe catheter placement.
- Despite no definitive guidelines for chamber leveling, the practitioner must keep in mind that decompression that is too rapid may create a sudden pressure differential which may cause contralateral SDH or even upward herniation. Nausea/vomiting, bradycardia, diaphoresis, and any change in neurologic exam should prompt immediate CT imaging.

SEPS drain

- The threaded end of the SEPS screw housing is slightly tapered, which means that the same twist drill hole cannot be re-used if initial screw placement is unsuccessful.
- Inappropriate position and ineffective dural opening are the most common causes of SEPS failure, along with loculation of the SDH
- SEPS may also be used to relieve tension pneumocephalus after intracranial surgery

References

1. Clower WT, Finger S. Discovering trepanation: the contribution of Paul Broca. Neurosurgery. 2001;49(6):1417–25; discussion 25–6. https://doi.org/10.1097/00006123-200112000-00021.
2. Carney N, Totten AM, O'Reilly C, Ullman JS, Hawryluk GW, Bell MJ, et al. Guidelines for the management of severe traumatic brain injury, Fourth Edition. Neurosurgery. 2017;80(1):6–15. https://doi.org/10.1227/neu.0000000000001432.
3. Fried HI, Nathan BR, Rowe AS, Zabramski JM, Andaluz N, Bhimraj A, et al. The insertion and management of external ventricular drains: an evidence-based consensus statement : a statement for Healthcare Professionals from the Neurocritical Care Society. Neurocrit Care. 2016;24(1):61–81. https://doi.org/10.1007/s12028-015-0224-8.
4. Lele AV, Hoefnagel AL, Schloemerkemper N, Wyler DA, Chaikittisilpa N, Vavilala MS, et al. Perioperative management of adult patients with external ventricular and lumbar drains: guidelines from the Society for Neuroscience in anesthesiology and critical care. J Neurosurg Anesthesiol. 2017;29(3):191–210. https://doi.org/10.1097/ana.0000000000000407.
5. Bayston R, Lambert E. Duration of protective activity of cerebrospinal fluid shunt catheters impregnated with antimicrobial agents to prevent bacterial catheter-related infection. J Neurosurg. 1997;87(2):247–51. https://doi.org/10.3171/jns.1997.87.2.0247.
6. Omar MA, Mohd Haspani MS. The risk factors of external ventricular drainage-related infection at hospital kuala lumpur: an observational study. Malays J Med Sci. 2010;17(3):48–54.
7. Whitney NL, Selden NR. Pullout-proofing external ventricular drains. J Neurosurg Pediatr. 2012;10(4):320–3. https://doi.org/10.3171/2012.7.Peds1280.
8. Intracranial Pressure Monitoring Systems & Catheters. Natus Medical Incorporated. Retrieved Feb 23, 2021 via the WWW: https://neuro.natus.com/products-services/intracranial-pressure-monitoring-systems-catheters.
9. Lee HC, Chuang HC, Cho DY, Cheng KF, Lin PH, Chen CC. Applying cerebral hypothermia and brain oxygen monitoring in treating severe traumatic brain injury. World Neurosurg. 2010;74(6):654–60. https://doi.org/10.1016/j.wneu.2010.06.019.

10. Spiotta AM, Stiefel MF, Gracias VH, Garuffe AM, Kofke WA, Maloney-Wilensky E, et al. Brain tissue oxygen-directed management and outcome in patients with severe traumatic brain injury. J Neurosurg. 2010;113(3):571–80. https://doi.org/10.3171/2010.1.Jns09506.
11. Narotam PK, Morrison JF, Nathoo N. Brain tissue oxygen monitoring in traumatic brain injury and major trauma: outcome analysis of a brain tissue oxygen-directed therapy. J Neurosurg. 2009;111(4):672–82. https://doi.org/10.3171/2009.4.Jns081150.
12. Kenning TJ, Dalfino JC, German JW, Drazin D, Adamo MA. Analysis of the subdural evacuating port system for the treatment of subacute and chronic subdural hematomas. J Neurosurg. 2010;113(5):1004–10. https://doi.org/10.3171/2010.5.Jns1083.

Point of Care Ultrasound

Armin Krvavac, Ramya Gorthi, Jennifer Minoff, and Rajamurugan Subramaniyam

1 Introduction

Point-of-care ultrasound (POCUS) is a term used to describe bedside ultrasound examination performed by healthcare providers with the goal of answering specific diagnostic questions to guide management or successful completion of an invasive procedure. The incorporation of POCUS in nearly every medical and surgical specialty has revolutionized medicine over the past decade. It has dramatically expanded in use and is now routinely employed to aid clinical decision making for a variety of clinical situations. Unlike standard ultrasonography where performance of the scan and interpretation of the results is delayed, intensivists utilizing POCUS are able to immediately obtain, interpret, and apply their findings to treat critically ill patients at the bedside. In 2011, the Expert Round Table on Ultrasound in ICU unanimously agreed that general critical care ultrasound and "basic" critical care echocardiography should be mandatory in the curriculum of intensive care unit physicians [1]. The Accreditation Council

---

A. Krvavac (✉) · R. Gorthi · J. Minoff · R. Subramaniyam
Department of Internal Medicine, Saint Louis University School of Medicine, St. Louis, MO, USA
e-mail: krvavaca@health.missouri.edu;
Armin.krvavac@health.slu.edu

for Graduate Medical Education (ACGME) now mandates knowledge of POCUS as part of critical care fellowship training.

2 Basics of Ultrasonography

2.1 Echogenicity

Basic understanding of ultrasonography starts with familiarization of ultrasound terminology and knobology. Echogenicity refers to the ability of a tissue to reflect or transmit ultrasound waves. A visible contrast in echogenicity between two adjacent structures allows for identification of specific anatomy [2]. Various anatomic structures can be characterized based on the echogenicity as either anechoic, hyperechoic, or hypoechoic (Table 1).

2.2 Probe Selection

Most of the POCUS machines interface with at least two different types of probes (linear and phased array). It is important to understand the function and limitations of each probe before selecting a probe for a specific examination. The most important difference between the linear and phased array probes is the frequency of ultrasound waves arising from the probe (Table 2). The linear probe emits a higher frequency that results in greater detail of imaged structures but a significant decrease in tissue penetration. This makes it an ideal

TABLE 1 Echogenicity

Echogenicity	Appearance on ultrasound	Example anatomic structures
Anechoic	black on screen	Veins, Arteries
Hyperechoic	white on screen	Pleura
Hypoechoic	gray on screen	Adipose tissue

TABLE 2 Probe selection

Probe	Linear	Phased array	Curvilinear
Frequency	5–15 MHz	1–5 MHz	2–5 MHz
Depth of penetration	Poor	Good	Good
Footprint	Moderate	Small	Large
Resolution	Good	Poor	Moderate
Photo of probe			
Photo of US beam			

probe for visualization of superficial structures such as vessels and the pleura. The phased array emits a much lower frequency that allows significantly deeper tissue penetration with much less detail. This makes the phased array ideal for evaluation of deeper structures such as the heart. A curvilinear probe has become increasingly popular, but is not available on all ultrasound machines. The curvilinear probe provides reasonably good tissue penetration like the phased array but also has a much larger footprint that allows for easy scanning [3, 4].

2.3 Positioning and Probe Control

When performing POCUS examination, the ultrasound machine is placed on the same side of the patient as the examiner. This allows for easier operation and adjustment of the controls with the free hand. The probe is applied to the patient with sufficient gel for adequate conduction of sound waves. The base of the hand applying the probe rests on the patient to help stabilize the ultrasound image. Modern POCUS machines automatically set gain, which controls the brightness of the image by amplifying the ultrasound signal. Despite automatic adjustment by the machine, occasional adjustment of gain is necessary to enhance the ultrasound image. The appropriate depth is adjusted to place the anatomic target in the center of the screen [4, 5]. There are four terms that describe adjustment of the probe in the topographic plane (Fig. 1) [5].

3 Vascular Ultrasound

Vascular POCUS, including techniques using ultrasound to guide vascular access procedures and deep vein thrombosis detection, can be particularly useful to minimize complications and guide therapeutic decisions [6–8]. The linear probe should be used for vascular POCUS. High-frequency from the linear probe provides a high level of detail that is necessary for proper evaluation of superficial vascular structures.

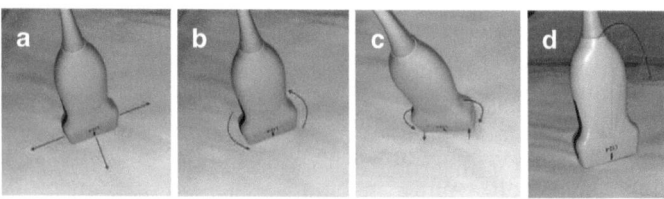

FIGURE 1 Probe movement: (**a**) sliding, (**b**) rotating, (**c**) tilting, (**d**) rocking

3.1 Vascular Access

The use of ultrasound guidance for central venous access has become a standard of care that is supported by multiple guidelines [9, 10]. Ultrasound guided placement of internal jugular and femoral vein catheters reduced failure rates and complications whilst improving patient comfort [6–8]. The vascular ultrasound may be employed to mark the site prior needle stick or in real-time to guide the needle. We will focus on preferred technique of real-time ultrasound use throughout the insertion and cannulation of vessel as it is associated with lower failure rates and complications [11]. A brief ultrasound inspection of the target vessel and surrounding structures prior to attempted central venous access procedure can help identify the best location and possible contraindications. These may include the presence of a venous thrombus in the vein, overlying soft tissue infection, or unfavorable anatomy. Once the appropriate site is selected, it should be sterilely prepped and the ultrasound probe draped in a sterile sheath.

For internal jugular central venous access, the ultrasound is performed with the proceduralist at the head of the bed looking towards the feet with the patient in a Trendelenburg position, to maximize the diameter of the vein and reduce the risk of air embolism. The ultrasound probe is held in the non-dominant hand, allowing the dominant hand to perform the other parts of the procedure. The probe is placed on the anterior neck at the junction of the sternal head of the sternocleidomastoid muscle and the clavicle. Then the probe is slid cephalad to find the best view and approach (i.e., identifying vein lateral to the artery rather than on top of the artery). To obtain a transverse or short-axis view of the vessel, the probe marker is pointed towards the midline of the patient. The longitudinal or long-axis view is obtained by identifying the internal jugular vein in transverse view and then rotating the probe 90° until it runs parallel to the vein.

Appropriate identification of the internal jugular vein is confirmed by applying gentle pressure to the neck with the probe. Pressure results in collapse of the internal jugular vein

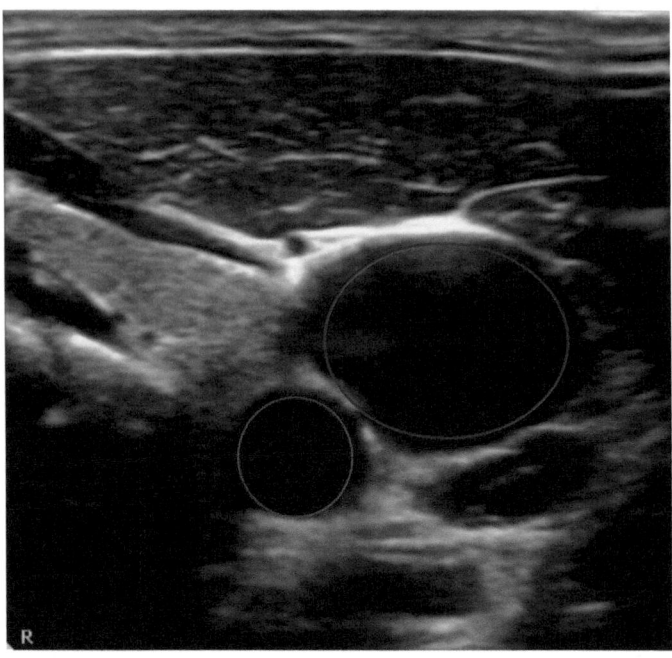

FIGURE 2 Ultrasound examination of internal jugular vein. *Red Circle: Right Common Carotid Artery; Blue Circle: Right Internal Jugular Vein*

while the carotid artery remains round and pulsatile (Fig. 2). Under ultrasound guidance, the site is anesthetized before advancing the needle into the internal jugular under direct ultrasound visualization. As the needle is advanced, negative pressure is applied in order to aspirate venous blood once the vessel wall is punctured. The combination of concurrent aspiration of blood and direct visualization of the needle within the vessel lumen indicate successful cannulation. The probe is often set aside briefly at this point, while the guidewire is advanced through the needle, in the usual fashion.

At this point, the ultrasound probe is employed once again to visualize the vasculature and confirm accurate positioning of the guidewire. Confirmation of appropriate guidewire position is vital to verify that vein rather than artery has been cannulated before dilation and insertion of the central venous catheter. Ideally the guidewire is traced from the skin entry site down by sliding and tilting the probe caudally along the vessel until it dives under the clavicle. Once the central venous access line has been inserted and the wire withdrawn, a lung ultrasound can be performed to rule out complication pneumothorax. This is discussed further later in this chapter.

The same technique can also be used for femoral and subclavian venous access with real-time ultrasound guidance to improve success rate [6–8, 12]. The common femoral vein is best imaged in the transverse or short access just below the inguinal ligament. It should be visualized medially to the artery (in contrast to the internal jugular which is lateral to the artery), but can run posteriorly to the artery as we move further from the inguinal ligament. The subclavian vein can be visualized in the transverse and longitudinal axis. However, unlike the internal jugular and common femoral veins, it may not be easily compressible. In these cases, scanning for venous valves, observation of respirophasic changes, or Doppler scanning with compression of the ipsilateral arm can assist in proper distinction of the vein and artery.

Lastly, real-time ultrasound guidance can also be expended to patients with difficult peripheral intravenous catheter and arterial catheter placement. Ultrasound guidance improves success rate in both and reduced complication rates in arterial catheter placement [13, 14].

3.2 Deep Venous Thromboembolism Screening and Diagnosis

The immediate assessment of veins for potential deep venous thrombosis (DVT) can be particularly helpful for clinicians when a pulmonary embolism (PE) is suspected. Evidence of DVT is confirmed in 70% of cases with positive angiographic evidence of PE, although only 50% of patients with DVT are diagnosed with PE [15]. An emergency department study utilizing combination of vascular, lung, and cardiac POCUS yielded a 90% sensitivity and 86.2% specificity in diagnosis of PE [16]. Similarly, an inpatient study utilizing the same combination of POCUS examinations, noted a potential decrease in the need for CT pulmonary angiography (gold standard for diagnosis of PE) by 58.3% [17]. Therefore, the use of POCUS by trained intensivists to assess for DVT can provide useful and immediate information about the possibility of PE.

3.3 Two-Point DVT Screen

The two-point DVT screen provides immediate feedback with a high accuracy to aid in therapeutic decision-making [18]. A comparison of two-point DVT POCUS performed by trained critical care physicians and fellows versus a formal vascular studies yielded a 95% diagnostic accuracy and reduced time-delay by an average of 13.8 h [19]. The two-point DVT screen is performed with the same linear probe as used to obtain vascular access. As described by the name, the two-point DVT screen involves scanning of only two high yield points (the common femoral vein and the popliteal vein). Although not as rapid, a three point DVT screen or more extensive screening can be done to slightly improve diagnostic accuracy [18, 20].

The leg is externally rotated with the patient in supine position. The two-point DVT screen starts with evaluation of the common femoral vein (CFV). The vein is scanned in the transverse axis with the transducer placed perpendicular to the skin and centered over the vein (Fig. 3a). It is important to scan below the inguinal ligament so that compression will be possible. Once properly identified the vein is scanned for echogenic structure within the lumen. If no echogenic structure is evident to suggestive of thrombus then, a compression maneuver is performed. Sufficient compression should be applied to deform the adjacent artery with the transducer perpendicular to the skin and centered over the vein (Fig. 3b).

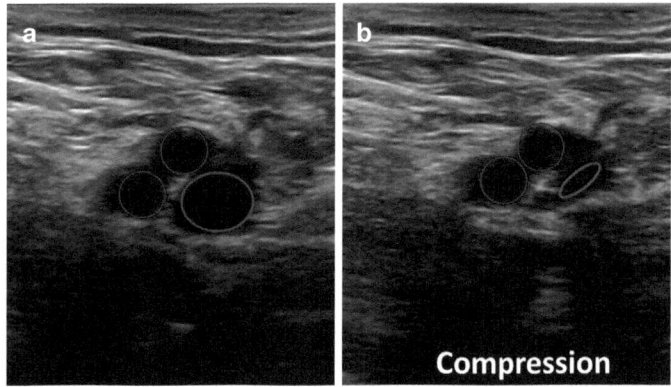

FIGURE 3 Common femoral vein and artery. (**a**) *Without compression;* (**b**) *With Compression; Red Circle: Artery; Blue Circle: Vein*

A normal vein should be completely compressible. In a patient with a symptomatic DVT, inability to compress the vein portends a positive predictive value of 94–97%, while full compression of both sites nearly excludes DVT with a negative predictive value of 98–99% [21, 22]. Although the addition of Doppler is common place in formal vascular studies, it does not add significant improvement in accuracy over compression in POCUS and is therefore not routinely used [23].

After scanning the CFV, the second point to be evaluated in a two-point DVT screen is the popliteal vein (PV). The knee is flexed approximately 45–60° with the leg remaining externally rotated with the patient in supine position. The probe is placed in the popliteal fossa and the vein is scanned in the transverse axis with the transducer placed perpendicular to the skin and centered over the vein (Fig. 4a). Anatomically, the PV is superficial to the popliteal artery. The PV is properly identified and scanned for echogenic structure within the lumen before compression testing is performed in similar fashion (Fig. 4b).

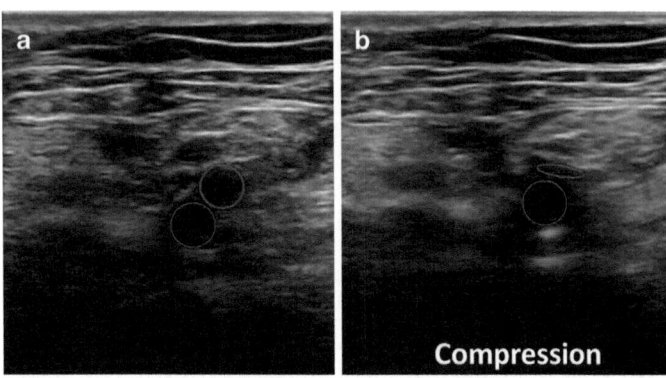

FIGURE 4 Popliteal vein and artery. (**a**) *Without compression;* (**b**) *With Compression; Red Circle: Artery; Blue Circle: Vein*

4 Lung Ultrasound

Ultrasound utilizes the variation in acoustic impedance of different tissues for direct visualization. Acoustic impedance is a measure of resistance of particles to mechanical vibrations such as ultrasound waves [2]. When ultrasound waves reach the interface between different mediums such as fluid and soft tissue, some of the waves are absorbed while some are reflected. The interface between soft tissue and air reflects almost 99.9% of the ultrasound waves due to vast difference in the acoustic impedance between these surfaces, making it virtually impenetrable to US waves [2]. Hence structures beneath the pleural surface in the air-filled lung are not directly visualized and results in reverberation artifacts. The difference in the acoustic impedance and greater fraction of reflection results in a hyperechoic image. Hence, the interface between pleural surface and air-filled lung appears hyperechoic (white band) as seen in Fig. 5.

Most lung POCUS is performed with the phased array as the small footprint allows the probe to fit in between rib spaces to image the lung. However, the detail provided by the linear probe is the preferred method for imaging of the pleural surface.

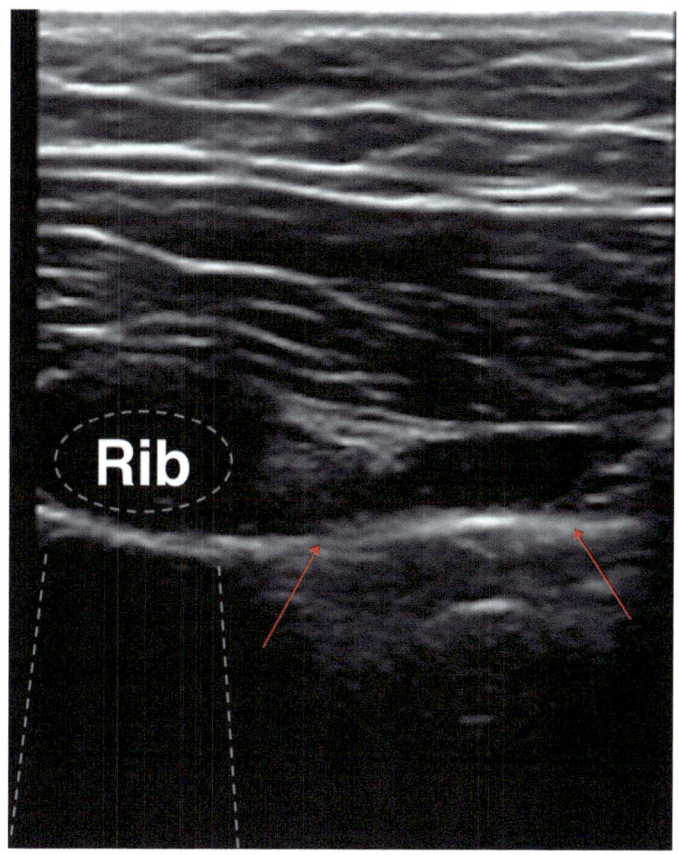

FIGURE 5 Lung ultrasound: pleural line. *Dotted line: Rib Shadow; Red arrow: Pleural Line*

4.1 Normal Lung Ultrasound Patterns

4.1.1 Lung Sliding

As detailed above, the interface of the pleural surface and the lung air boundary appears hyperechoic (as a white band) [3]. This is referred to as the pleural line and represents the apposition of the parietal and visceral pleura. The dynamic motion of the visceral and parietal pleura with respirations gives the appearance of "lung sliding". M-mode image at the location of lung sliding will present the "seashore sign" [2] M-mode is a time motion display of ultrasound waves along the set one-dimensional line. When utilized to image the pleura, M-mode will reveal horizontal straight lines generated by the motionless layers of subcutaneous tissue above the pleural line and a sandy appearance beneath the pleural line is caused by the motion of lung sliding (Fig. 6a). M-mode image in location without lung sliding reveals horizontal straight lines throughout and is referred to as "stratosphere sign" (also called "barcode sign") (Fig. 6b) [2, 24].

4.1.2 A-Lines

The reverberating artifacts described above produced by bouncing of echo between the pleural line and probe result in A-lines when normally aerated lung is scanned. A-lines are gradually fading, regularly spaced (equal to the distance between the skin and the pleural space), horizontal, motionless lines like the pleural lines (Fig. 7) [2, 3]. However, since A-lines are produced by the presence of air beneath the pleural surface, they are seen in both normally aerated lung as well as pneumothorax.

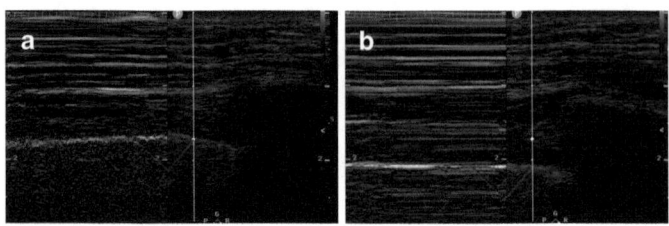

FIGURE 6 M-Mode of pleura. (**a**) Seashore sign indicating normal lung sliding; (**b**) Stratosphere sign/Barcode sign – indicating lack of pleural apposition i.e. Pneumothorax. *Blue arrows: Pleural Line*

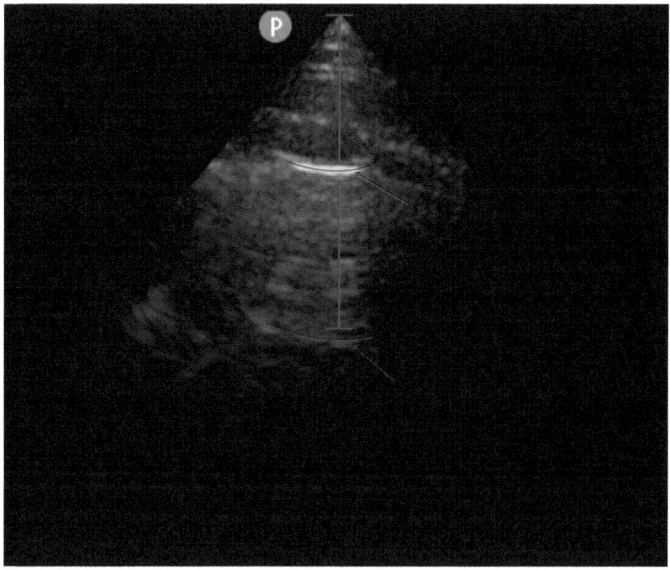

FIGURE 7 A-Lines. A-line measures equal distance from pleural line as probe from pleural line. *Red Line and Arrow: Pleural Line; Blue Line and Arrow: A-Line*

4.2 Abnormal Lung Ultrasound Patterns

4.2.1 Pneumothorax

The first reported use of ultrasound in the detection of pneumothorax was published by Wernicke in 1987 [24]. Today, POCUS is widely adopted in emergency departments and intensive care units for evaluation of pneumothorax. Even the Focused Assessment with Sonography in Trauma (FAST) has now been modified to E-FAST (Extended FAST) to include lung ultrasound. This is largely because POCUS has been demonstrated to be superior to chest radiography for detection of pneumothorax. A meta-analysis of reviewing role of ultrasound and chest radiography in the diagnosis of pneumothorax showed that ultrasound had a pooled sensitivity of 78.6% and specificity of 98.4% while chest radiography had a pooled sensitivity of only 39.8% and specificity of about 99.3% [25].

As noted previously, the linear probe is most helpful in evaluating superficial structures such as pleural lines and should therefore be utilized when using POCUS to rule out pneumothorax. Air in a pneumothorax will typically rise to the least dependent area of the chest and scanning should therefore be performed in the anterior region of chest between the second to fourth intercostal spaces in the midclavicular line in a supine patient or semi-recumbent patient. The Probe is placed in the sagittal plane with the indicator pointing cephalad and the chest region is scanned cephalocaudal starting from the second intercostal space.

The presence of lung sliding and/or M-mode with "seashore sign" effectively rules out pneumothorax with a negative predictive value of about 99–100% [26–28]. However, the absence of lung sliding does not automatically confirm pneumothorax. Lung sliding is absent in conditions where the pleural surfaces are not opposed such as pneumothorax. But, absence of lung sliding can also occur with pathologies that result in reduced air entry into the lung such as acute respiratory distress syndrome, status asthmaticus, or occlusion of a mainstem bronchus. Furthermore, lung sliding can be absent when the pleural surfaces are adhered to each other (i.e. pleurodesis). Using POCUS presence of a lung-point can be identified on occasion to confirm the diagnosis of pneumothorax. Lung-point is the border of the pneumothorax where normal lung sliding is noted. It can be identified laterally in patients with large pneumothorax after scanning of the anterior chest revealed absence of lung sliding. Lung point has a 100% specificity, effectively ruling in pneumothorax [28, 29].

4.2.2 B-Lines

B-lines are produced by the difference of acoustic impedance of an object compared to its surroundings. They are vertical artifacts projecting from the pleural surface to the bottom of the ultrasound screen (comet-tail artifact or laser beam artifact) (Fig. 8) [30]. This sonographic entity is caused by the juxtaposition of alveolar air and septal thickening. Up to two

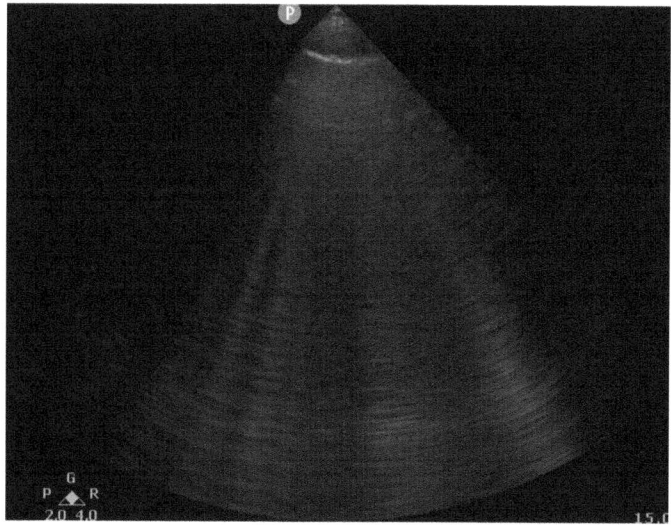

Figure 8 B-Lines

B-lines can normally be seen moving synchronously with pleural sliding in each intercostal space. The finding of three or more B-lines in an intercostal space indicates a pathologic process resulting in thickening of the septum between the secondary pulmonary lobules.

The pathology can be narrowed depending on the distribution of pulmonary B-lines. For example, lobar pneumonia exhibits increased B-lines in the affected lung while pulmonary edema or ARDS results in a diffuse increase in B-lines in both lungs. In cardiogenic pulmonary edema, the number of B-lines directly correlates with the severity of pulmonary edema [2]. B-lines are usually homogeneously distributed, with no significant pleural abnormalities and with associated pleural effusions when caused by cardiogenic pulmonary edema. Non-cardiogenic pulmonary edema conditions such as ARDS results in areas of the lung with B-lines interspersed with areas of consolidation and normal lung.

Due to the accumulation of air within the pleural space, B-lines or comet-tail artifacts are absent in pneumothorax.

Therefore, evidence of B-lines like the presence of pleural siding can be used to rule out pneumothorax. The presence of at least one B-line has a negative predictive value of 98–100%, effectively ruling out pneumothorax [29, 31].

4.2.3 Pleural Effusions

The space between the visceral and parietal pleura contains a minimal amount of pleural fluid under normal circumstances. Accumulation of excess fluid in the pleural space can result in respiratory failure, especially in critically ill patients. Common causes of pleural effusion in critically ill patients include decompensated congestive heart failure, volume overload, pulmonary infections, malignancies, and decompensated cirrhosis [32]. Although the diagnosis can be made by physical examination, patient factors such as obesity, positioning, and mechanical ventilation can pose a challenge. In these cases, lung ultrasound plays a crucial role in the timely diagnosis of pleural effusion.

POCUS helps with the confirmation, quantification, and characterization of pleural effusions. Pleural effusions are typically represented by an anechoic space between the pleural lines (Fig. 9). However, various pathologies can result in a more complex appearance on POCUS as a result of fibrin strands or increased echogenic densities [33]. For example, long standing pleural effusions commonly seen with congestive heart failure, cirrhosis or nephrosis can develop complex appearance without septa referred to as echogenic swirling [34]. Conversely, the presence of infection in the pleural space resulting in an empyema displays a complex appearance with thick septa and fibrin strands.

After prompt identification of pleural effusion or pneumothorax, POCUS can be used for guidance of thoracentesis or chest tube placement. Utilization of POCUS increases the rate of success and reduces the frequency of complications [35, 36].

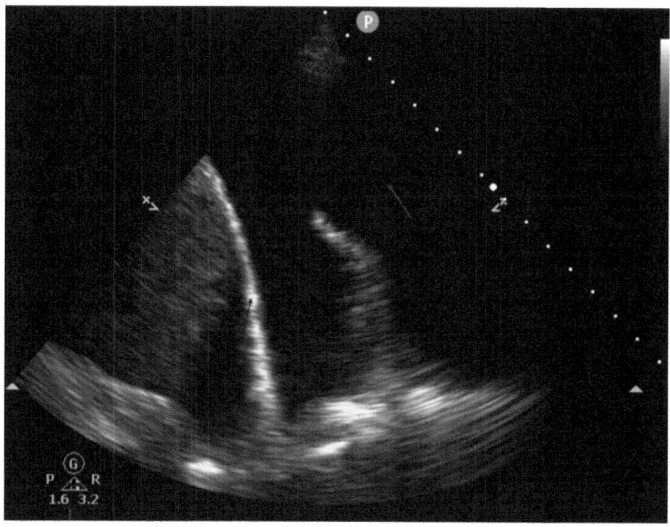

FIGURE 9 Pleural effusion. *Red arrow: Diaphragm. Blue arrow: Pleural Effusion*

4.2.4 Consolidation

Alveolar consolidation is identified by two signs on POCUS. An image resembling the appearance of liver beneath the pleural line is referred to as "hepatization" or "tissue sign." This is primarily seen in trans-lobar consolidation. Scanning consolidated lung may reveal a fractal line, an irregular hyperechoic line separating the consolidated and normally aerated lung. When present, this is referred to as "shred sign" and indicates non-trans lobar consolidation [37]. Scanning may also reveal linear hyperechoic artifacts within the consolidation, representing air bronchograms. The centrifugal movement of air bronchogram of more than 1 millimeter defines dynamic air bronchograms. Dynamic air bronchogram are suggestive of inflamed lungs likely in the setting of pneumonia. The presence of heterogeneous echotexture of lung, thickened pleura, B-lines and consolidated lung with shred sign is suggestive of multifocal pneumonia with acute respiratory distress syndrome [37, 38].

Consolidated appearance of the lung is also seen in atelectasis. Atelectasis can result from external compression such as a pleural effusion (compressive atelectasis) or as a result of endobronchial obstruction (resorptive atelectasis). The appearance of atelectatic lung may be difficult to distinguish from consolidated lung. Atelectatic lung is associated with lack of lung sliding and presence of lung pulse, from transmission of cardiac rhythm vibrations across the poorly aerated lung [38].

4.2.5 BLUE Protocol

Bedside lung ultrasound in emergencies (BLUE) protocol was developed by French intensivist Daniel Lichtenstein [39]. It is a fast protocol (less than 3 min) implemented to elicit the etiology of acute respiratory failure. The patient is examined in a semi-recumbent position and three points are scanned on each side of the lung. The points can be identified by laying two hands across the patient's chest as seen in Fig. 10. The first is the upper anterior point which corresponds to the base of the ring and middle finger of the upper hand and overlies the upper lobe. The second is the lower anterior point which corresponds to the middle of the palm of the lower hand and overlies the middle lobe/lingual. The third is the posterior lateral alveolar pleural point which corresponds to the intersection of horizontal line at the lower anterior point and vertical line at the posterior axillary line and overlies the lower lobe [39].

The lungs are evaluated for presence or absence of lung sliding, A-lines, B-lines, pleural effusions, and consolidations. BLUE protocol offers an overall accuracy of 90.5% in determining etiology of acute respiratory failure [39].

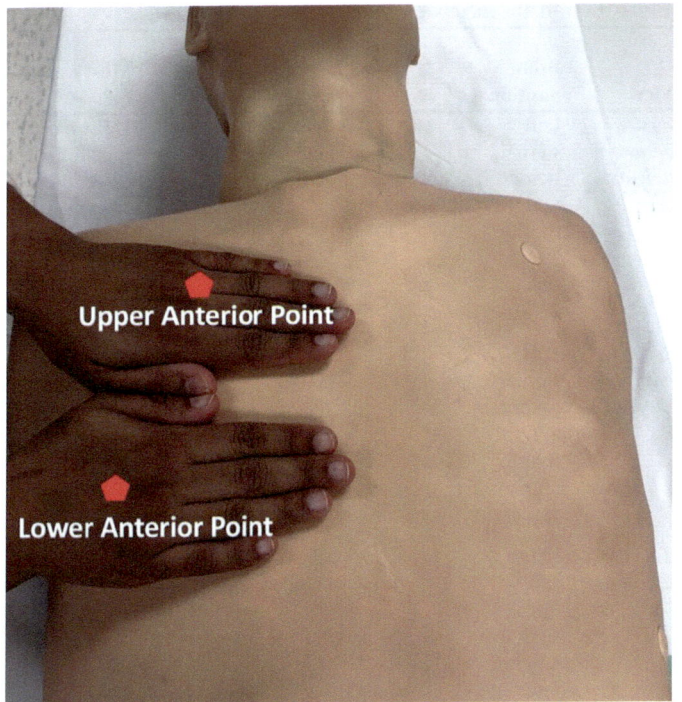

FIGURE 10 BLUE protocol scanning points

5 Cardiac Ultrasound

Basic critical care echocardiography is an integral part in the evaluation and management of critically ill patients. It allows critical care physicians to qualitatively evaluate cardiac function and anatomy to answer very specific clinical questions with immediate clinical implications such as cardiac tamponade, right ventricular strain, and left ventricular systolic function [40]. The American College of Chest Physicians identifies five standard views for basic critical care echocardiography which are discussed in the detail below (Table 3).

Critical care echocardiography is performed with a phased array probe. The probe marker is placed on the right side of

TABLE 3 Transthoracic views

View	Probe position	Probe marker position	Imaging plane of heart	Most useful for
First parasternal long-axis	Left sternal border at third to fifth intercostal space	Right shoulder	Sagittal plane	LV size and function LV outflow tract diameter Pericardial effusion Evaluate MV and AV
Second parasternal short-axis	Left sternal border at third to fifth intercostal space	Left shoulder	Transverse plane	Evaluate MV LV function RV volume and pressure
Third apical four-chamber	Mid-axillary line at sixth to seventh intercostal space	Left shoulder	Coronal plane	LV, RV size and function LV/RV ratio Evaluate MV and TV LVOT VTI -estimates stroke volume (*apical five-chamber view)
Fourth subcostal long-axis	Inferior to the xiphoid process/sternum	Left	Coronal plane	LV and RV function Pericardial effusions Accessible during CPR and may be only view in patients with difficult body habitus
Fifth inferior vena cava longitudinal	Inferior to the xiphoid process/sternum	Cephalad	"Transverse plane of IVC"	Volume status Fluid responsiveness

the ultrasound screen. On most newer POCUS machines, this is done by changing the exam mode to cardiac. The patient is positioned in supine or slight left lateral decubitus position when possible. The complete examination should be performed in the described sequence below. Some views may fail due to patient position, body habitus, or operator skill. Nevertheless, all views should be attempt as on may yield critical data even if others cannot be obtained.

5.1 Transthoracic Views

5.1.1 Parasternal Long-Axis View

The probe is placed at the left sternal border between the third to firth intercostal space with the probe marker pointing towards the right shoulder. The intercostal space yielding best images depends on patient body habitus and anatomy. The probe is adjusted by tilting so that the image bisects the aortic valve (AV), mitral valve (MV), and left ventricle (LV) in the long axis. In many instances the right ventricular (RV) outflow tract is also visualized at the base of the ultrasound image. The various structures are labeled below in Fig. 11.

5.1.2 Parasternal Short-Axis View

From the parasternal long-axis view, the probe is rotated 90° in a clockwise fashion so that the probe marker is pointing towards the left shoulder to obtain the parasternal short-axis view. This reveals a cross-sectional view of the LV at the papillary muscle level (transverse plane of the heart). By tilting the probe on an axis between the left hip and right shoulder, cross-sectional views are obtained at different levels of the heart, from the aorta to the LV apex. For example, tilting all the way to the aortic level reveals the RV outflow tract and can be used to visualize clots in transit. The mitral valve level reveals the fish-mouth appearing MV. The papillary muscle level reveals the round LV cavity with its papil-

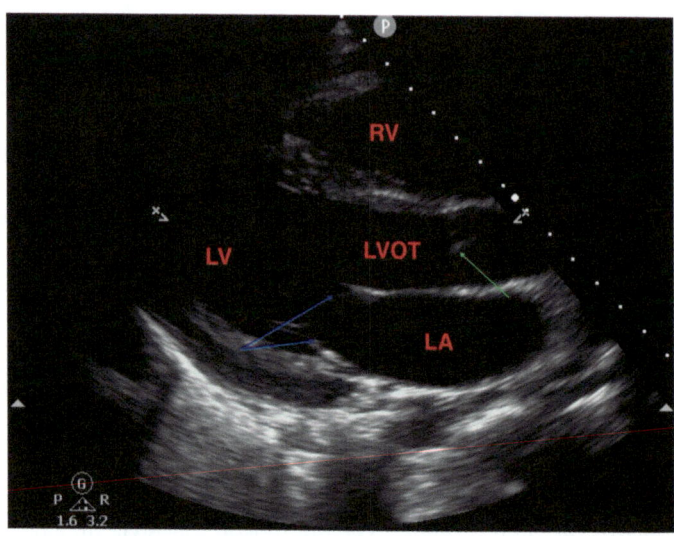

Figure 11 Parasternal long-axis. *RV: Right Ventricle, LV: Left Ventricle, LVOT: Left Ventricular Outflow Tract, LA: Left Atrium. Blue Arrows: Open Mitral Valve Leaflets. Green Arrow: Closed Aortic Valve*

lary muscles at the 4 and 7 o'clock positions and crescent shaped RV cavity. The various structures described are labeled below in Fig. 12.

5.1.3 Apical Four-Chamber View

The probe is slid from the previous position down and laterally to the midclavicular line at approximately the sixth-seventh intercostal space. With the probe marker still pointing towards the left shoulder, the probe is slowly tilted and rocked until the intraventricular septum is oriented vertically on the ultrasound image. Next, the probe can be rotated slightly to open up the widest diameter of both ventricles and obtain an optimal apical four-chamber view. In this coronal plane of the heart the two ventricles, two atria, MV, and tri-

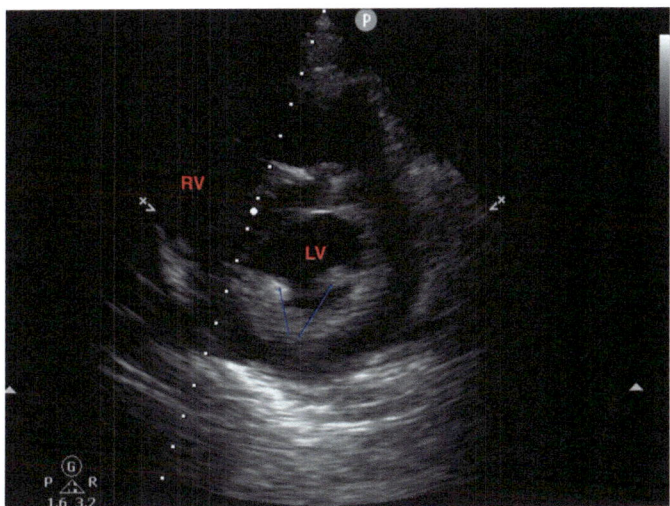

FIGURE 12 Parasternal short-axis. *RV: Right Ventricle, LV: Left Ventricle. Blue Arrows: Papillary Muscles*

cuspid valve (TV) can be visualized and evaluated. The various structures described are labeled below in Fig. 13. Tilting down slightly more reveals the LV outflow tract (apical five-chamber view), which is used to evaluate stroke volume and fluid responsiveness.

5.1.4 Subcostal Long-Axis View

The probe is slid just inferior to the xiphoid process with the prober marker pointing towards the patients left side. Some pressure may need to be applied as the probe is tilted down below the xiphoid process/sternum to obtain the subcostal long-axis view. The view is adjusted by tilting and rotating until all four chambers can be visualized. However, in this case the RV will be the base of the ultrasound image. The various structures described are labeled below in Fig. 14. The subcostal long-axis view is ideal to visualize pathologies involving the pericardial space.

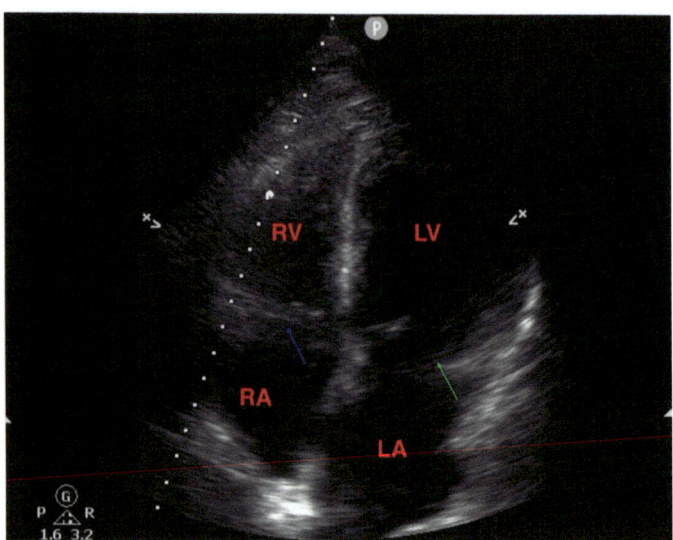

FIGURE 13 Apical four-chamber view. *RV: Right Ventricle, LV: Left Ventricle, RA: Right Atrium, LA: Left Atrium. Blue Arrow: Tricuspid Valve. Green Arrow: Mitral Valve*

5.1.5 Inferior Vena Cava Longitudinal View

The last view is obtained by tilting the probe back up to a perpendicular position from the subcostal long-axis view. Next, the probe is rotated counterclockwise at the same position (inferior to the xiphoid process) until the probe marker is pointing towards the patient's head. The probe is slightly tilted to the right from this position to obtain a longitudinal view of the inferior vena cava (IVC). This view is used to assess IVC for volume status and fluid responsiveness. Rocking the probe slightly inferiorly may reveal IVC emptying into the right atrium. The various structures described are labeled below in Fig. 15.

Point of Care Ultrasound 219

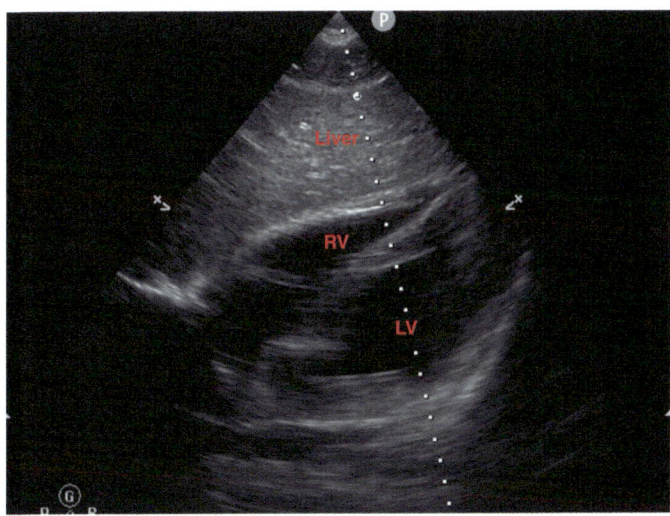

FIGURE 14 Subcostal long-axis view

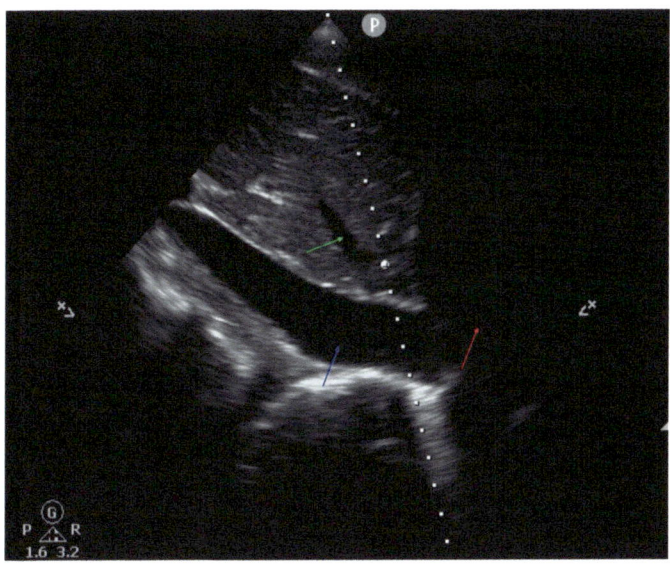

FIGURE 15 Inferior vena cava longitudinal view. *Blue Arrow: Inferior Vena Cava. Red Arrow: Right Atrium. Green Arrow: Hepatic Vein*

5.2 Utility of Cardiac POCUS

The introduction of bedside ultrasound allows critical care physicians to immediately identify and potentially intervene on life threatening causes of shock. Emergencies such as tamponade, massive pulmonary embolism, and severe valve or left ventricular failure can be identified in minutes so that lifesaving treatment can be initiated. Furthermore, cardiac ultrasound can be used to categorize shock (hypovolemic, distributive, obstructive, or cardiogenic) and guide management.

5.2.1 Left Ventricular Systolic Function

A global assessment of left ventricular systolic function can be inferred from the degree of inward LV wall motion, myocardial thickening, longitudinal motion of the mitral annulus, and overall geometry of the LV. The left ventricular ejection fraction (LVEF) is often used as a surrogate for global LV function and is defined as the LV stroke volume divided by LV end-diastolic volume **[Ejection Fraction % (EF%) = Stroke Volume (SV)/End-Diastolic Volume (EDV) × 100%]**. LVEF is assessed in a semi-quantitively way in basic critical care echocardiography using visual estimation. In this case the LV function is described as hyperdynamic (EF ≥70%), normal (EF = 55–69%), or reduced (EF <55%). When LVEF is depressed, the dysfunction is further described as mild (45–54%), moderate (30–44%), or severe (<30%) (Table 4).

TABLE 4 LV systolic function

LV systolic function	LVEF % (estimated or measured)
Hyperdynamic	≥70
Normal	55–69
Mildly reduced	45–54
Moderately reduced	30–44
Severely reduced	<30

LV left ventricle, *LVEF* left ventricular ejection fraction

Although visual estimation of EF from multiple views is sufficient for most clinical scenarios in the intensive care unit, certain occasions or inability to obtain multiple views call for different assessment. Global assessment of LV function can also be obtained from single linear measurements in the parasternal long-axis and apical four-chamber views [41].

In the parasternal long-axis view, a gross assessment of LV function can be measured by measuring fractional shortening (FS) of the left ventricle. This is done by using M-mode on the LV cavity to measure the left ventricular end-diastolic diameter (LVEDD) and left ventricular end-systolic diameter (LVESD) (Fig. 16). Fractional shortening is then calculated as follows **[FS% = (LVEDD − LVESD)/LVEDD × 100%]**. In men, a FS of 25–43% is normal and FS of <15% indicates severely impaired LV function. In women, a FS of 27–54% is normal and FS of <16% indicates severe impairment [42]. Multiplying the fractional shortening percentage by 2 will give a rough estimation of the LVEF.

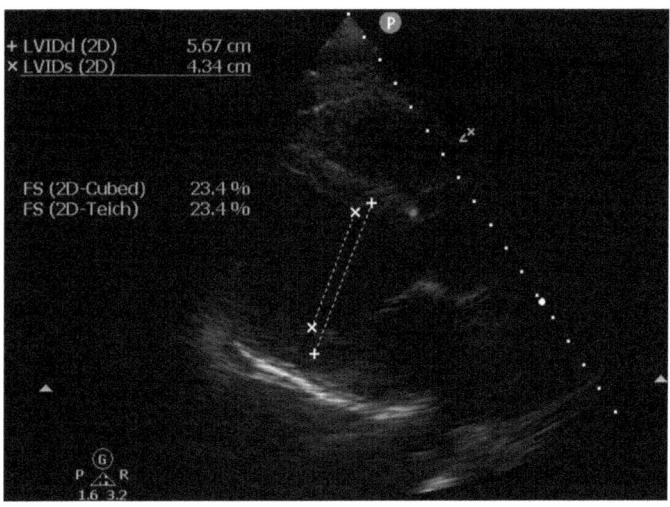

FIGURE 16 Fractional Shortening in parasternal long-axis view. *LVIDd: Left Ventricular End-Diastolic Diameter, LVIDs: Left Ventricular End-Systolic Diameter. FS: Fractional Shortening*

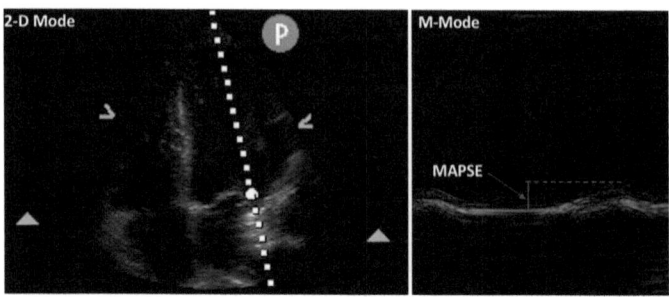

FIGURE 17 Mitral annular plane systolic excursion (MAPSE) in apical four-chamber view

In the apical four-chamber view, the mitral annular plane systolic excursion (MAPSE) can be measured using M-mode to estimate LV function. MAPSE is obtained by directing the M-mode pick at the septal (lateral) mitral annulus and measuring the apical excursion in millimeters (mm) (Fig. 17). A MAPSE of >10 mm correlates with a normal EF of >55% [43].

Limitations of linear measurements such as FS and MAPSE include regional wall motion abnormalities, off axis measurements, and angulation of the intraventricular septum in elderly patients.

5.2.2 Fluid Responsiveness

Cardiac POCUS is used to measure both static and dynamic parameters to help determine volume status and guide resuscitation. Although static parameters are useful in determining volume status, they do not predict fluid responsiveness and should therefore be substituted with dynamic measurements to guide resuscitation. Furthermore, the POCUS findings should be taken within the clinic context. Fluid responsiveness should not imply need for fluids in an otherwise stable patient.

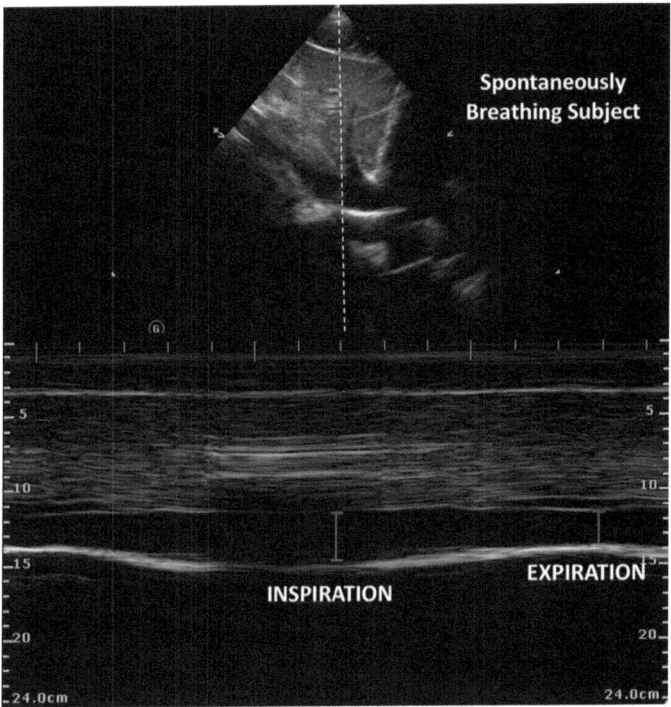

Figure 18 Inferior vena cava diameter

Static Parameters:
The simplest POCUS measurement in assessment of volume status is the inferior vena cava (IVC) diameter. The IVC diameter is measured from the inferior vena cava longitudinal view in either 2-D or M-mode. The diameter is measured perpendicular to the long axis of the IVC proximal to the hepatic vein (approximately 1–3 cm from the RA) (Fig. 18). Once a good image is obtained the IVC diameter is measured during exhalation in spontaneously breathing patient. Then the patient is asked to sniff so that that collapse of the IVC with decrease in intrathoracic pressure can be evaluated to estimated right atrial (RA) pressure (Table 5) [44].

Static measurements of the IVC diameter have important limitations. IVC diameter may be dilated in young athletic

TABLE 5 Estimated right atrial Pressure based on IVC diameter

IVC diameter	% Collapse of IVC with sniff	Estimated RA pressure
Spontaneous respirations		
<2.1 cm	>50%	3 (0–5) mmHg
>2.1 cm	<50%	15 (10–20) mmHg
Positive-pressure ventilation		
≤1.2 cm		<10 mmHg

IVC inferior vena cava

patients and correlation with CVP in mechanically ventilated patients is poor. Nevertheless, a significant decrease in IVC diameter of <1.2 cm and collapsibility of the IVC does suggest hypovolemia in patients undergoing positive-pressure ventilation [45]. These static measurements do not predict fluid responsiveness but changes in IVC diameter can be used as a dynamic measure to assess fluid responsiveness in patients with positive-pressure ventilation. Fluid responsiveness assessments are performed to predict the efficacy of intravenous volume expansion on improvement in stroke volume.

Dynamic Parameters:

The IVC distensibility index is the simplest dynamic measurement to predict fluid responsiveness in mechanically ventilated patients. It is calculated by measuring the IVC diameter during inspiration and expiration in a patient with positive-pressure ventilation and passive inspiration/full synchrony with the ventilator. Additional requirements before measurements are obtained include: tidal volume of ≥8 mL/kg, sinus rhythm, and absence of right heart failure. The IVC diameter measurements are obtained in the same manner as described above and IVC distensibility is calculated as follows: **IVC Distensibility Index = [(IVC Diameter$_{Inspiration}$ − IVC Diameter$_{Expiration}$)/(IVC Diameter$_{Expiration}$)] × 100%**. In this case an index >18% predicts fluid responsiveness [46].

Aortic blood flow changes before and after passive leg raising is another dynamic measurement used to predict fluid responsiveness. Although it is more cumbersome and technically challenging to perform, it offers more valuable information (estimated stroke volume) and can be used for both spontaneously breathing and mechanically ventilated patients. The stroke volume (SV) can be calculated by measuring the LVOT cross-sectional area (CSA) and LVOT velocity-time integral (VTI) **[SV = LVOT CSA × LVOT VTI]** [47].

LVOT CSA is calculated by obtaining the diameter of the LVOT in the parasternal long-axis view during mid systole. The measurement should be taken at the junction of the aortic valve cusps and LVOT as shown in Fig. 19. [LVOT CSA = (Diameter $_{LVOT}$/2)^2 × π] or [LVOT CSA = (Diameter $_{LVOT}$)^2 × 0.785].

The LVOT VTI is measured in the apical five-chamber view. This view can be obtained by tilting the probe down in the apical four-chamber view until the LVOT opens as pictured in Fig. 20. Once obtained, the pulse wave (PW) Doppler

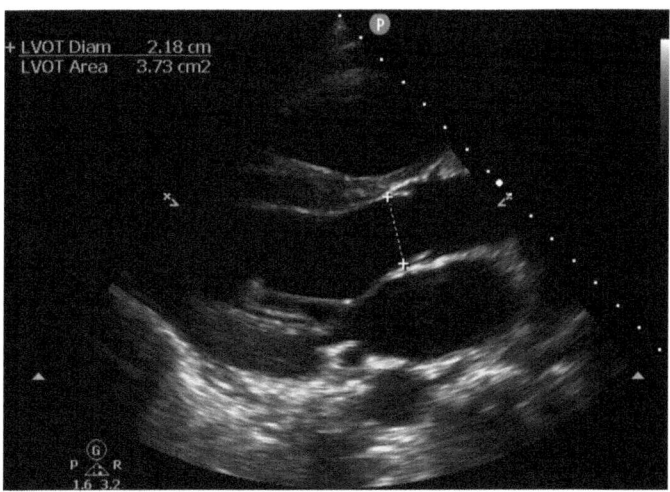

FIGURE 19 Measuring LVOT diameter

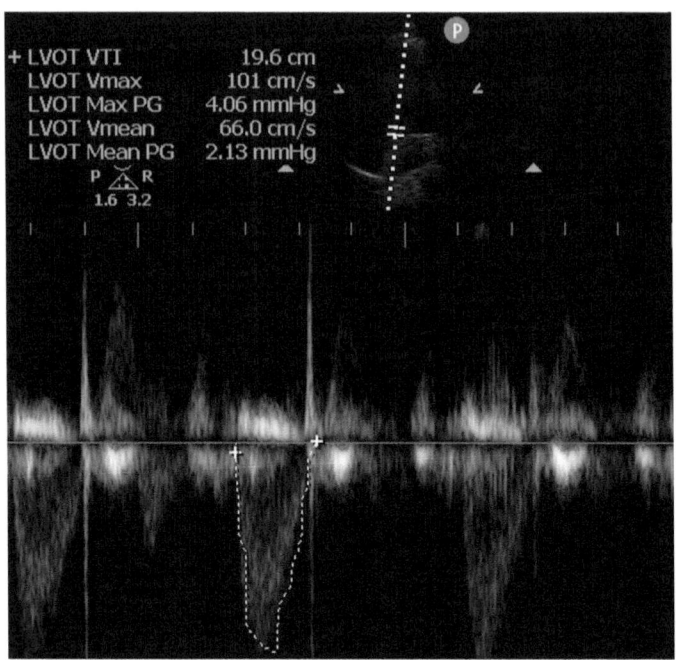

FIGURE 20 Measuring LVOT velocity-time integral

is placed near the aortic annulus with the beam aligned as close as possible to direction of flow. Incomplete alignment of >20° can significantly alter the results. Once properly positioned the LVOT tracing is obtained as shown in Fig. 20.

Once both measurements are obtained, stroke volume can be quickly calculated. The cardiac output can then be calculated as follows: **[Stroke Volume (SV) × Heart Rate (HR) = Cardiac Output (CO)]**. Furthermore, the LVOT VTI can be used as a dynamic measurement to predict volume responsiveness. In this case, the LVOT VTI is measured before and after a passive leg raise (PLR). The PLR mobilizes blood from the lower limbs, increases venous return and increases SV that is reflected in a change of the LVOT VTI. Increases in LVOT VIT or SV by more than 12.5% during PLR predict increase in SV with further intravenous fluid bolus (i.e. fluid responsiveness) [48, 49]. As mentioned previously, this aortic blood flow variability can be used in spontaneously breathing and mechanically ventilated patients. However, PLR can be difficult to perform in patients with lower extremity bandages or fractures. Furthermore, pregnancy or abdominal compartment syndrome resulting in compression of the IVC will blunt venous return of blood during PLR and limit validity of the results.

5.2.3 Tamponade

Tamponade is a clinical diagnosis that is established by combining multiple sources of information. Clinical signs include tachycardia, tachypnea, hypotension, pulsus paradoxus (or reverse pulsus paradoxus in positive pressure ventilation), electrical alternans, and low voltage on electrocardiograms. Tamponade is a direct result of increased intrapericardial pressure that leads to the collapse of cardiac chambers and decreased venous return. Systolic right atrial systolic and diastolic right ventricular collapses occur when intrapericardial pressures exceed in intracavitary pressures [50].

Pericardial effusions are the most common cause of tamponade. Acute development of pericardial effusion results in a more significant increase in intrapericardial pressure due to lower pericardial compliance. A chronic increase in intrapericardial fluid allows for higher pericardial compliance due to the slow increase in pericardial pressure. Therefore, acute pericardial effusion or more likely to lead to the development of tamponade. The evaluation of pericardial effusion can be done immediately with the use of cardiac POCUS. A pericardial effusion can be distinguished from a pleural effusion by locating the aorta. Effusions that are in between the aorta and cardiac free wall are pericardial in origin.

Echocardiographic criteria for the diagnosis of tamponade include right atrial systolic collapse, right ventricular diastolic collapse, and variation in left and right ventricular inflow velocities during respiration. Evaluation of atrial collapse is summarized in Table 6.

Table 6 Right atrial and right ventricular collapse in cardiac tamponade

	Cardiac cycle:	Best view:
RA collapse	Early systole collapse of RA (>30% collapse, lasting >1/3 of systole)	Apical four-chamber Alternative: *Subcostal long-axis*

| RV collapse | Early diastolic collapse of RV | Subcostal long-axis
Alternative: Parasternal long-axis or short-axis | 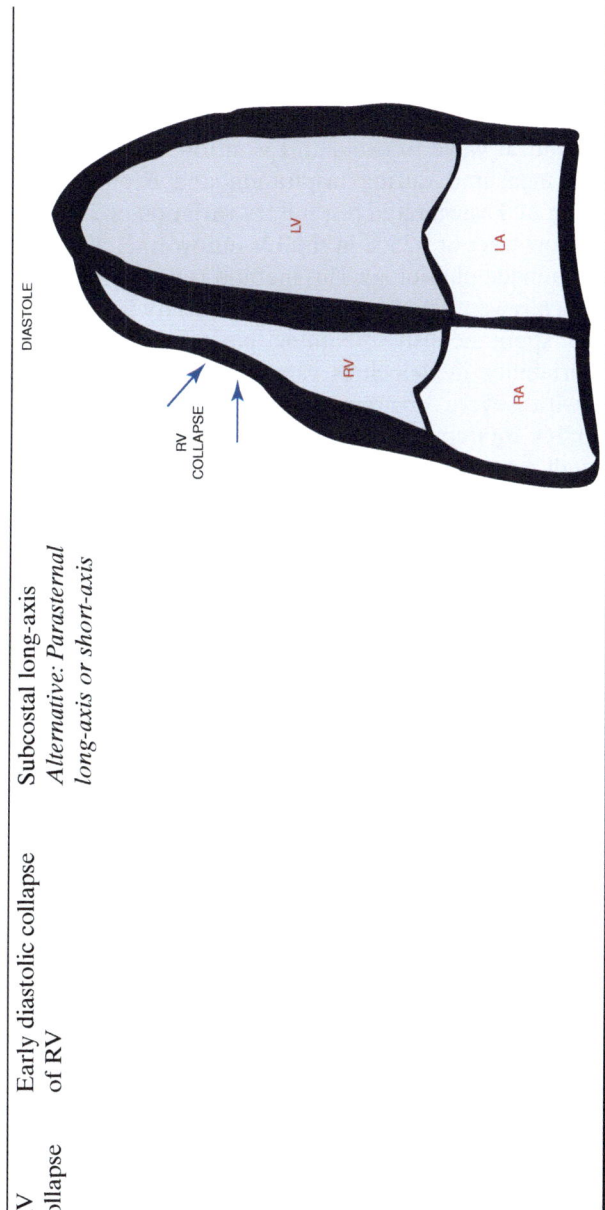 |

RV right ventricle, *LV* left ventricle, *RA* right atrium, *LA* left atrium

Variation in left and right ventricular inflow velocities during respiration is performed with pulse wave (PW) doppler. In the apical four-chamber view, the PW doppler is placed over the tricuspid valve to evaluate RV inflow velocities and above the mitral valve to evaluate LV inflow velocities. The velocity is measured during inspiration and expiration as noted in Fig. 21. Exaggerated respiratory variation of >40% in the RV inflow tract or >25% in the LV inflow tract is indicative of tamponade physiology. This method is not well studied in mechanically ventilated patients and its utility is therefore limited to spontaneously breathing patients. Additionally, similar variability in velocities can sometimes be seen in patients with severe obstructive lung disease, pulmonary embolism, RV infarction, or profound hypovolemia [50, 51].

Although echocardiographic criteria for the evaluation of tamponade is helpful it is by no means necessary to make a diagnosis.

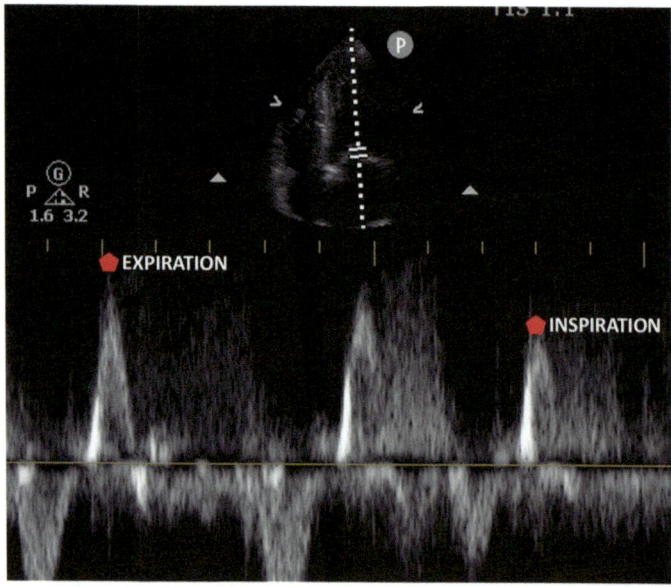

FIGURE 21 Pulse Wave (PW) Doppler of mitral inflow for evaluation of cardiac tamponade

5.3 Right Ventricular Function and Pulmonary Embolism

POCUS is frequently utilized in patients with known acute pulmonary embolism (PE) to guide therapy. Furthermore, evaluation of the RV for significant strain and impaired function can be used to work up undifferentiated shock or raise concern for acute PE. POCUS or formal echocardiography is rarely diagnostic of PE, unless a clot is visualized in the right sided chambers or pulmonary artery. Evaluation of the right ventricular focuses on morphology and function.

RV morphology is best evaluated from the apical four-chamber view. The relative RV/LV area ratio is ≤0.6. An RV/LV area ratio ≥ 1.0 indicates severe RV dilation. The parasternal short-axis is also used to evaluate RV morphology and can give some insight into RV volume and/or pressure overload when abnormal. The RV shares the intraventricular septum with the dominant LV. The relationship between LV and RV pressure can alter the appearance of the septum in the parasternal short-axis as depicted in Fig. 22. RV volume

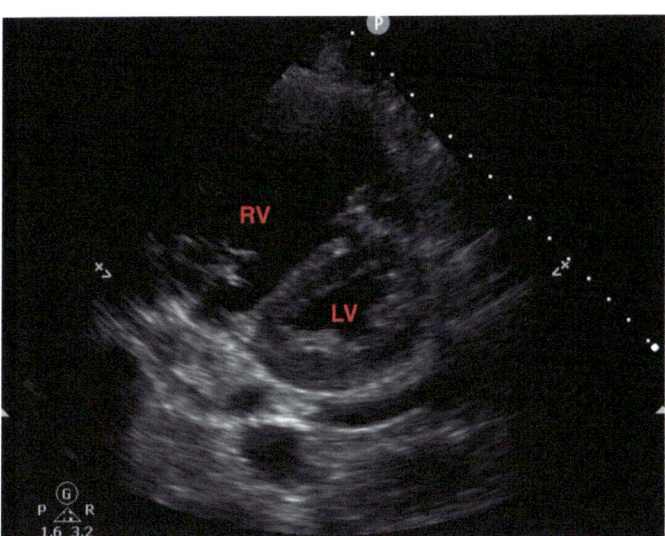

FIGURE 22 Flattening of the intraventricular septum

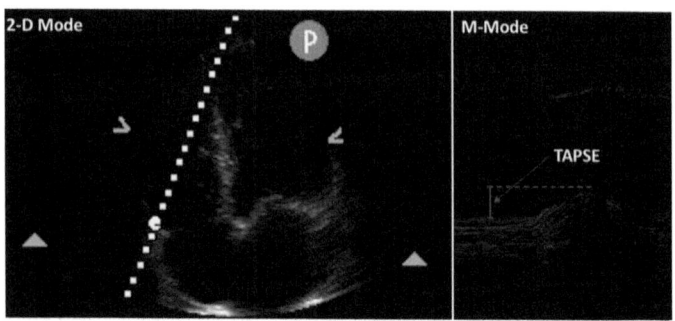

FIGURE 23 Tricuspid Annular Plane Systolic Excursion (TAPSE) in apical four-chamber view

overload results in septal flattening (leftward shift of the septum resulting in D-shaped LV) only during diastole. On the other hand, RV pressure overload results in persistent septal flattening during both systole and diastole.

The RV function can be evaluated with POCUS when morphology is abnormal or PE is suspect. In the apical four-chamber view, measurement of the tricuspid annular plane systolic excursion (TAPSE) is performed using M-mode to estimate RV function. TAPSE is obtained by directing the M-mode pick at the septal (lateral) tricuspid annulus and measuring the apical excursion in millimeters (mm) (Fig. 23). A TAPSE of <1.6 cm correlates with abnormal or decreased RV function [44].

6 Focused Assessment Sonography in Trauma (FAST)

FAST is an ideal POCUS exam that is performed in order to quickly detect pneumothorax or free fluid in the chest and abdomen. It is indicated in patients with blunt or penetrating trauma to the thorax or abdomen. FAST can also be utilized in the intensive care unit to evaluate critically ill patients with unexplained hypotension. In comparison to CT, FAST is cost-effective, portable, rapid, and easily repeatable for serial monitoring. However, it is less accurate in diagnosis of specific etiologies and extensive bowel gas, subcutaneous air, and patient body habits increase difficult of the exam [52].

FAST is performed with the low frequency probe (phased array or preferably curvilinear array because of its larger footprint) with the patient in the supine position. The exam mode is set to abdomen. This is important as probe and marker orientation are 180° opposite in abdomen and cardiac modes. The classic FAST, utilized in the evaluation of trauma patients, includes four views: subxiphoid, right upper quadrant, left upper quadrant, and pelvis. The extended FAST, which is outlined in detail below, also incorporates scanning of the anterior chest. Extended FAST (Table 7) is more com-

TABLE 7 Extended focused assessment sonography in trauma views

View	Probe position	Structures seen	Pathologies found
Anterior chest (extended FAST)	Anterior chest on each side at second or third intercostal space Slide caudally M-mode if no lung sliding evident	Pleural line/lung sliding	B-lines Absent lung sliding barcode sign
Subxiphoid	Inferior to xiphoid process/sternum Probe marker to left shoulder (opposite of subcostal long-axis)	Cardiac chambers	Pericardial effusion
Right upper quadrant	Right midaxillary line Probe maker cephalad Slide cephalad and rotate counterclockwise (scan below and above diaphragm)	Liver Right Kidney Right hemi-diaphragm	Pleural effusion Consolidated lung Free fluid in Morison's Pouch (in between right kidney and liver)

(continued)

TABLE 7 (continued)

View	Probe position	Structures seen	Pathologies found
Left upper quadrant	Left posterior axillary line Probe maker cephalad Slide cephalad and rotate clockwise (scan below and above diaphragm)	Spleen Left Kidney Left hemi-diaphragm	Pleural effusion Consolidated lung Free fluid around spleen
Pelvis	Above the pubic bone Probe maker cephalad (longitudinal view) Slide probe slightly cephalad and rotate 90° (transverse view)	Bladder Pouch of Douglas (females) Recto-vesical pouch (males)	Free fluid posterior to bladder

monly utilized in the evaluation of hemodynamically unstable patients in the intensive care unit [53]. All views should be scanned when performing the exam and serial examination should be performed if patient clinical condition continues to deteriorate.

7 Conclusion

POCUS can provide intensivists with rapid answers to specific diagnostic questions, guide management, and improve successful completion of invasive procedures. Once mastered, POCUS can be used to obtain difficult venous access, screen and diagnose venous thromboembolism, elicit etiology of respiratory failure, evaluate cardiac function, and identify causes of hemodynamic instability. These broad applications with important clinical implications have led to a rapidly expanding incorporation of POCUS in intensive care units.

References

1. Cholley B, Mayo P, Poelaert J, et al. Expert round table on ultrasound in ICU, international expert statement on training standards for critical care ultrasonography. Intensive Care Med. 2011;37:1077–83.
2. Miller A. Practical approach to lung ultrasound. BJA Educ. 2015;16:39–45.
3. Saraogi A. Lung ultrasound: present and future. Lung India. 2015;32:250–7.
4. Ihnatsenka B, Boezaart AP. Ultrasound: basic understanding and learning language. Int J Shoulder Surg. 2010;4(3):55–62.
5. Zander D, Huske S, Hoffmann B, Cui XW, Dong Y. Ultrasound image optimization ("Knobology"): B-mode. Ultrasoung Int Open. 2020;6(1):E14–24. https://doi.org/10.1055/a-1223-1134.
6. Brass P, Hellmich M, Kolodziej L, Schick G, Smith AF. Ultrasound guidance versus anatomical landmarks for internal jugular vein catheterization. Cochrane Database Syst Rev. 2015;1:Cd006962.
7. Brass P, Hellmich M, Kolodziej L, Schick G, Smith AF. Ultrasound guidance versus anatomical landmarks for subclavian or femoral vein catheterization. Cochrane Database Syst Rev. 2015;1:Cd011447.
8. Saugel B, Scheeren TWL, Teboul JL. Ultrasound-guided central venous catheter placement: a structured review and recommendations for clinical practice. Crit Care. 2017;21(1):225. https://doi.org/10.1186/s13054-017-1814-y. PMID: 28844205; PMCID: PMC5572160.
9. Lamperti M, Bodenham AR, Pittiruti M, et al. International evidence-based recommendations on ultrasound-guided vascular access. Intensive Care Med. 2012;38(7):1105–17.
10. Troianos CA, Hartman GS, Glas KE, et al. Guidelines for performing ultrasound guided vascular cannulation: recommendations of the American Society of Echocardiography and the Society of Cardiovascular Anesthesiologists. J Am Soc Echocardiogr. 2011;24(12):1291–318.
11. Milling TJ Jr, Rose J, Briggs WM, et al. Randomized, controlled clinical trial of point-of-care limited ultrasonography assistance of central venous cannulation: the Third Snography Outcomes Assessment Program (SOAP-3) Trial. Crit Care Med. 2005;33(8):1764–9.
12. Prabhu MV, Juneja D, Gopal PB, et al. Ultrasound-guided femoral dialysis access placement: a single-center randomized trial. Clin J Am Soc Nephrol. 2010;5(2):235–9.

13. McCarthy ML, Shokoohi H, Boniface KS, et al. Ultrasounography versus landmark for peripheral intravenous cannulation: a randomized controlled trial. Ann Emerg Med. 2016;68(1):10–8.
14. Shiloh AL, Eisen LA. Ultrasound-guided arterial catheterization: a narrative review. Intensive Care Med. 2010;36(2):214–21.
15. Chang A, Eisen L, Rhamanian M. Imaging of the critically ill patient: bedside ultrasound. In: Oropello JM, Pasores SM, Kvetan V, editors. Critical care. McGraw-Hill; 2021.
16. Nazerian P, Vanni S, Volpicelli G, et al. Accuracy of point-of-care multiorgan ultrasonography for the diagnosis of pulmonary embolism. Chest. 2014;145(5):950–7.
17. Koenig S, Chandra S, Alaverdian A, et al. Ultrasound assessment of pulmonary embolism in patients receiving CT pulmonary angiography. Chest. 2014;145(4):818–23.
18. Lee JH, Lee SH, Yun SJ. Comparison of 2-point and 3-point point-of-care ultrasound techniques for deep vein thrombosis at the emergency department: a meta-analysis. Medicine (Baltimore). 2019;98(22):e15791.
19. Kory PD, Pellecchia CM, Shiloh AL, et al. Accuracy of ultrasonography performed by critical care physicians for the diagnosis of DVT. Chest. 2011;139(3):538–42.
20. Zuker-Herman R, Ayalon Dangur I, Berant R, et al. Comparison between two-point and three-point compression ultrasound for the diagnosis of deep vein thrombosis. J Thromb Thrombolysis. 2018;45(1):99–105.
21. Talbot SR. Venous imaging technique. In: Talbot SR, Oliver MA, editors. Techniques of venous imaging. Pasadena: Appleton Davies, Inc; 1992. p. 59–118.
22. Cronan JJ, Dorfman GS, Scola FH, Schepps B, Alexander J. Deep venous thrombosis: US assessment using vein compression. Radiology. 1987;162:191–4.
23. Frazee BW, Snoey ER, Levitt A. Emergency department compression ultrasound to diagnose proximal deep vein thrombosis. J Emerg Med. 2001;20(2):107–12.
24. Wernecke K, Galanski M, Peters PE, Hansen J. Pneumothorax: evaluation by ultrasound – preliminary results. J Thorac Imaging. 1987;2:76–8.
25. Alrajab S, Youssef AM, Akkus NI, Caldito G. Pleural ultrasonography versus chest radiography for the diagnosis of pneumothorax: review of the literature and meta-analysis. Crit Care. 2013;17:R208.

26. Husain LF, Hagopian L, Wayman D, Baker WE, Carmody KA. Sonographic diagnosis of pneumothorax. J Emerg Trauma Shock. 2012;5:76–81.
27. Volpicelli G. Sonographic diagnosis of pneumothorax. Intensive Care Med. 2011;37(2):224–32.
28. Lichtenstein D, Meziere G, Biderman P, et al. The "lung point": an ultrasound sign specific to pneumothorax. Intensive Care Med. 2000;10:1434–40.
29. Lichtenstein DA, Mezière G, Lascols N, Biderman P, Courret JP, Gepner A, Goldstein I, Tenoudji-Cohen M. Crit Care Med. 2005;33(6):1231–8.
30. Raheja R, Brahmavar M, Joshi D, Raman D. Application of lung ultrasound in critical care setting: a review. Cureus. 2019;11:e5233.
31. De Luca C, Valentino M, Rimondi M, Branchini M, Baleni MC, Barozzi L. Use of chest sonography in acute-care radiology. J Ultrasound. 2008;11:125–34.
32. Brogi E, Gargani L, Bignami E, et al. Thoracic ultrasound for pleural effusion in the intensive care unit: a narrative review from diagnosis to treatment. Crit Care. 2017;21:325.
33. Yang PC, Luh KT, Chang DB, Wu HD, Yu CJ, Kuo SH. Value of sonography in determining the nature of pleural effusion: analysis of 320 cases. AJR Am J Roentgenol. 1992;159:29–33.
34. Chen HJ, Tu CY, Ling SJ, Chen W, Chiu KL, Hsia TC, Shih CM, Hsu WH. Sonographic appearances in transudative pleural effusions: not always an anechoic pattern. Ultrasound Med Biol. 2008;34:362–9.
35. Kanji HD, McCallum J, Sirounis D, et al. Limited echocardiography-guided therapy in subacute shock is associated with change in management and improved outcome. J Crit Care. 2014;29(5):700–5.
36. Mayo PH, Goltz HR, Tafreshi M, et al. Safety of ultrasound-guided thoracentesis in patients receiving mechanical ventilation. Chest. 2004;125(3):1059–62.
37. Lichtenstein DA. Lung ultrasound in the critically ill. Ann Intensive Care. 2014;4:1.
38. Lichtenstein DA, Mezière GA, Lagoueyte JF, Biderman P, Goldstein I, Gepner A. A-lines and B-lines: lung ultrasound as a bedside tool for predicting pulmonary artery occlusion pressure in the critically ill. Chest. 2009;136:1014–20.

39. Lichtenstein DA, Mezière GA. Relevance of lung ultrasound in the diagnosis of acute respiratory failure: the BLUE protocol. Chest. 2008;134:117–25.
40. Andrus P, Dean A. Focused cardiac ultrasound. Glob Heart. 2013;8(4):299–303.
41. Silverstein JR, Laffely NH, Rifkin RD. Quantitative estimation of left ventricular ejection fraction from mitral valve E-point to septal separation and comparison to magnetic resonance imaging. Am J Cardiol. 2006;97(1):137–40.
42. Weekes AJ, Reddy A, Lewis MR, Norton HJ. E-point septal separation compared to fractional shortening measurements of systolic function in emergency department patients: prospective randomized study. J Ultrasound Med. 2012;31(12):1891–7.
43. Hu K, Liu D, Herrmann S, Niemann M, Gaudron PD, Voelker W, Ertl G, et al. Clinical implication of mitral annular plane systolic excursion for patients with cardiovascular disease. Eur Heart J Cardiovasc Imaging. 2013;14(3):205–12. https://doi.org/10.1093/ehjci/jes240.
44. Rudski LG, et al. Guidelines for the echocardiographic assessment of the right heart in adults: a report from the ASE. J Am Soc Echocardiogr. 2010;23:685–713.
45. Jue J, et al. Does inferior vena cava size predict right atrial pressure in patients receiving mechanical ventilation? J Am Soc Echocardiogr. 1992;5:613–9.
46. Barbier C, et al. Respiratory changes in IVC diameter are helpful in predicting fluid responsiveness in ventilated septic patients. Intensive Care Med. 2004;2004:1740–6.
47. Blanco P. Rational for using the velocity-time integral and the minute distance for assessing the stroke volume and cardiac output in point-of-care settings. Ultrasound J. 2020;12:21.
48. Maizel J, et al. Diagnosis of central hypovolemia by using passive leg raising. Intensive Care Med. 2007;33(7):1133–8.
49. Lamia B, et al. Echocardiographic predictions of volume responsiveness in critically ill patients with spontaneously breathing activity. Intensive Care Med. 2007;33(7):1125–32.
50. Kearns MJ, Walley KR. Tamponade: hemodynamic and echocardiographic diagnosis. Chest. 2018;153(5):1266–75.
51. Smith AT, Watnick C, Ferre RM. Cardiac tamponade diagnosed by point-of-care ultrasound. Pediatr Emerg Care. 2017;33(2):132–4.

52. Scalea TM, et al. Focused Assessment with Sonography for Trauma (FAST): results from an international consensus conference. J Trauma. 199;46(3):466–72.
53. Montoya J, Stawicki SP, Evans DC, et al. From FAST to E-FAST: an overview of the evolution of ultrasound-based traumatic injury assessment. Eur J Trauma Emerg Surg. 2016;42(2):119–26.

Transcranial Doppler Ultrasound

Nanda Thimmappa

1 Introduction

Transcranial Doppler (TCD) is a valuable imaging tool in the assessment of wide variety of intracranial pathologies such as stenosis or occlusion within major intracranial vessels, evaluation of sickle cell disease to determine stroke risk, detection of right to left Cardiac shunt, evaluation of collateral pathways of intra cranial blood flow and arteriovenous malformations pre and post neurointervention, assessment of cerebral hemodynamics after trauma, stroke or migraine, and as an adjunct to the clinical diagnosis of brain death. Most common indication of transcranial Doppler is in the detection and follow up of vasospasm involving the cerebral vessels after subarachnoid hemorrhage (SAH) due to aneurysm rupture. Serial transcranial Doppler ultrasonographic examinations accurately detect the presence of vasospasm and allow for optimizing of medical therapy for vasospasm before the patient becomes symptomatic [1].

CT Angiography (CTA), MR Angiography (MRA) and Ultrasound (US) are all utilized for evaluation of cerebral vessels. Non contrast CT is routinely used of diagnosis of

N. Thimmappa (✉)
University of Missouri, Columbia, MO, USA
e-mail: thimmappan@health.missouri.edu

subarachnoid hemorrhage. CT has higher resolution, provides rapid diagnosis, lower cost than MRA, and wider availability but requires radiation exposure. CT is the largest contributor to medical radiation exposure among the U.S. population [2]. In addition, repetitive administration of iodinated intravenous (IV) contrast can have deteriorating effect on the kidneys [3]. Digital subtraction angiography considered the gold standard for diagnosis of vasospasm, is however invasive, cannot be performed bedside, associated with radiation and nephrotoxic effects from IV contrast and cannot be frequently repeated [4]. MRI is expensive and is not readily available compared with CT and US. MRI also requires long scan times that can last up to an hour with some patients needing anesthesia which has its own risks. It may be challenging for acutely ill patients to remain immobile during the duration of the scan leading to motion artifacts and a nondiagnostic study.

For these reasons US should be considered when appropriate for follow-up studies. US is radiation free, inexpensive and well-tolerated by patients. Most importantly, ultrasound is portable and can be performed bedside.

In this chapter we will discuss the basic principles of Doppler ultrasound, compare the imaging and nonimaging transcranial Doppler equipment currently available, protocols and techniques for performing transcranial Doppler imaging as well as avoiding potential pitfalls. We will discuss important clinical applications of transcranial Doppler, with emphasis on evaluation of cerebral vasospasm following SAH.

2 Doppler Ultrasound Concepts

'Ultrasound' is sound at frequencies above the upper limit of human hearing (approximately 0.02 MHz). Diagnostic US imaging involves frequency range of 2 to 18 megahertz [5]. In creating an ultrasound image, sound pulses are transmitted into tissue by a 'transducer', where they reflect from various structures, the extent depending to various factors including the density of the structure and are captured by the same transducer, postprocessed to form an image. 'Grey scale images' consist of different shades of brightness proportional to the extent of signal received from various structures.

If the reflecting source is in motion either toward or away from the transducer, the frequency of the sound waves received will be higher or lower than the frequency at which they were emitted, respectively called 'Doppler Shift' [6]. A Doppler shift equation is utilized by the machine to indirectly calculate the velocity of the blood [6]. This information can also be used to create color blood flow maps of the vasculature.

A spectral Doppler waveform (Fig. 1) is a visual display of blood flow velocities within a small sample volume within a blood vessel on transcranial color Doppler technique that is represented as a time velocity curve throughout the cardiac cycle [7]. Peak Systolic Velocity (PSV), End Diastolic Velocities (EDV) can be measured from the waveform and these values are used to calculate the Mean Flow Velocity [MFV=PSV+(EDV × 2)/3] and Resistive Index [RI = (PSV − EDV)/PSV] [8]. Resistive Index is a measure of resistance to

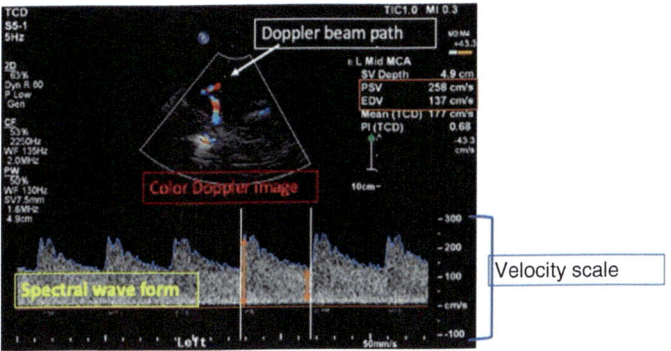

FIGURE 1 Components of Transcranial Color Doppler (TCCD). Peak systolic and diastolic velocities (orange arrows) are calculated from spectral waveform and displayed on right top corner (orange box)

the flow of blood into an organ. Low-resistance spectral waveforms are characterized by continued forward diastolic flow throughout the cardiac cycle with a slower increase in flow velocity with the onset of systole [7] (Fig. 2). Arteries that supply vital organs such as cerebral arteries characteristically have a low-resistance waveform.

Angle of insonation: The angle between the direction of the ultrasound beam and the in-line axis of the vessel is 'angle of insonation' (Fig. 3). Blood flow velocity is most accurate when this angle is zero. This is impossible to achieve unless an intra vascular probe is used and angles between zero and 60° are considered acceptable. Increasing insonation angles is associated with false decrease in recorded velocities. Angle correction can be applied to compensate for decreases in velocity [6]. It should be noted that velocities obtained with Doppler imaging equipment may be lower than those obtained with non-imaging equipment. Per ACR–AIUM–SPR–SRU

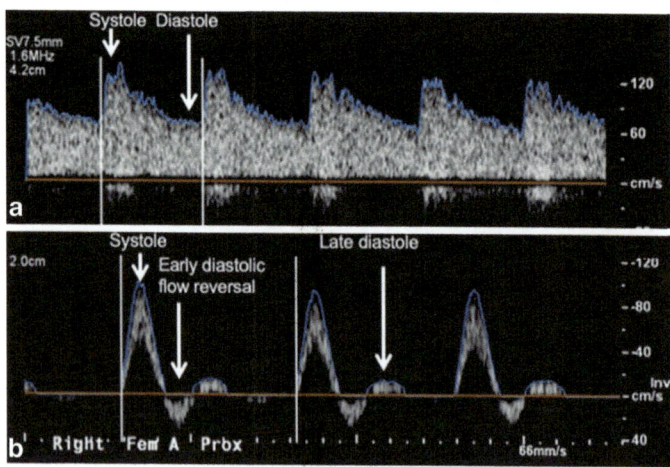

FIGURE 2 Low resistance waveforms are seen in intracranial vessels where forward flow during diastole is essential (**a**). Note the entire flow in systole and diastole is above the baseline. High resistance waveform is seen in extremities where there is reversal of flow during diastole (**b**)

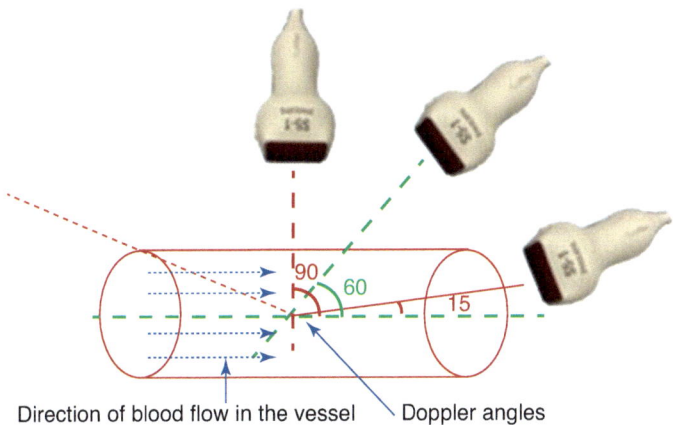

FIGURE 3 Doppler angle-the angle between the direction of blood Flow and the direction of transmitted sound wave should be 30–60°. Less than 30° can cause reflection of sound waves and no Doppler shift is recorded at 90°

practice parameter for the performance of transcranial Doppler ultrasound, angle correction should not be applied if velocity reference standards have been previously acquired with nonimaging TCD methods which are not angle corrected [9].

Pulsatility index (PI): the Gosling PI (Systolic Flow Velocity – Diastolic Flow Velocity/Mean Flow Velocity) [10] is based on the fact that when Intra Cranial Pressure (ICP) increases, diastolic flow velocity is affected more than systolic flow velocity, hence increase in PI. Many authors have indicated that PI is not reliable in assessing ICP and can be influenced by many extracranial factors [11, 12]. PI is influenced by cerebral perfusion pressure (CPP), pulse amplitude of arterial pressure, cerebrovascular resistance and heart rate. PI Is considered to describe CPP more accurately than ICP [13]. In general, if PI >2.0, with normal Mean Arterial Pressure and $PaCO2$ >30, there is a concern for elevated ICO [14, 15].

3 TCD Equipment and the Technique

Two types of TCD equipment are currently available: non-duplex (non-imaging) and duplex (imaging) devices. Nonduplex TCD technique is performed without visual guidance but with well-established criteria to identify vessels of interest, using a pulsed wave adjustable 2-MHz transducer to record range-gated velocity measurements at selected depths within the skull [16]. Machines post process the measurements to display a color-coded spectral analysis of the vessel being interrogated, but no image of the vascular anatomy is produced (Fig. 4a). These machines are used for bedside US in neuro ICU.

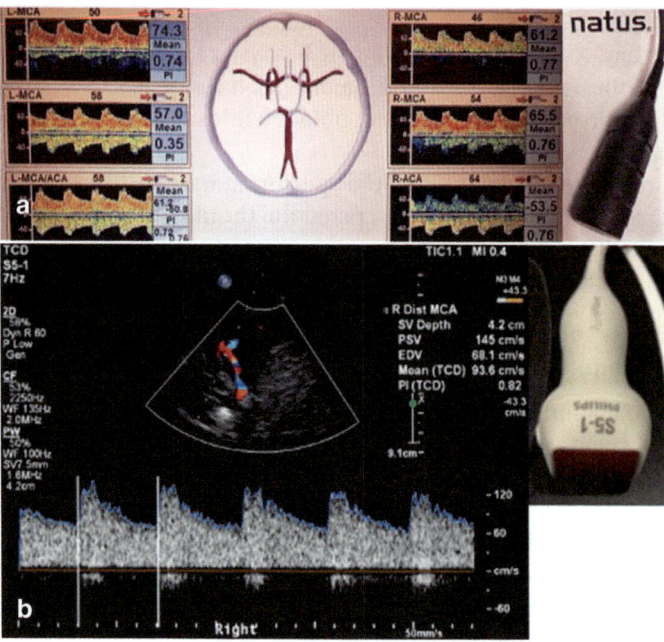

FIGURE 4 (**a**) Transcranial Doppler images obtained with Natus® nonduplex, 2 MHz, 'pencil' TCD transducer. (**b**) Transcranial Color Doppler images obtained with Phillips D5–1, duplex, phased-array, 2–3-MHz, sector transducer. This transducer has larger footprint and heavier than Natus® nonduplex, 2 MHz, TCD transducer

Duplex imaging devices also called Transcranial Color Doppler (TCCD). Circle of Willis can be directly visualized, and individual vessels can be selected to obtain blood flow velocity and spectral waveform. This mode of transcranial Doppler is performed in the Radiology Department on their dedicated machines with a specific post processing software to display real time color Doppler image of the vessels. A phased- array, 2- to 3-MHz, sector transducer is used (Fig. 4b).

3.1 Comparison of TCD to TCCD

Both doppler devices are compared on Table 1. TCD transducer is lightweight and the controls on the monitor are simple. TCCD is more complex to perform with the investigator continuously handling the knobs to freeze, analyze, and store velocity measurements, while holding the transducer steady with the other hand. TCD examinations take less time than TCCD examinations. Neish AS et al. have reported that, the average TCD took 29 min, compared with an average of 43 min for TCCD [17]. Benefits of TCCD includes shorter learning curve relative to TCD, greater confidence to the interpreting physician as the vessels are directly visualized and may reveal incidental findings such as vascular malformation or aneurysm.

Time- averaged mean maximum velocity (TAMM) is obtained on TCD machines by calculating the mean of the maximum velocities within an envelope trace over numerous cardiac cycles [18]. TAMM is usually higher than the mean maximum velocities recorded on TCCD (time average of the maximum -TAMx, time average peak -TAP) [19]. Although angle-corrected velocity measurements obtained with TCCD may be more accurate than non- angle-corrected velocity measurements obtained with TCD, it is important to consider that, for some applications, such as evaluating children with sickle cell anemia, clinical guidelines regarding normal versus abnormal or conditional velocities were validated in large clinical trials using TCD. For this reason, if comparing

TABLE 1 Comparison of non-imaging TCD and imaging TCCD techniques (Refs. [16, 17])

Transcranial Doppler (TCD)	Transcranial Color Doppler (TCCD)
Smaller footprint lightweight transducer	Wider 2.5 cm foot print, Bulkier
Easy controls on monitor	More effort to analyze and save velocity measurements.
Shorter duration study	10–15 more minutes of acquisition and postprocessing than TCD (17)
Blind approach, investigator relies on an audible Doppler signal and continuous velocity readout to optimize the angle of insonation and maximize the velocity measurement. Because there is no image of the vessel being interrogated, angle correction is not possible.	Vessels can be directly visualized. Information for the waveform is obtained from a small sample volume that is placed in the center of the vessel by the sonographer. Optimization of the angle of insonation, and angle correction can be performed to get accurate velocities.
Time- averaged mean maximum velocity (TAMM) is recorded.	Time average of the maximum -TAMx and/or Time Average Peak -TAP measurements are recorded.
Validated velocity-based stroke-risk categorizations, through large prospective clinical trials were performed using TCD equipment	Measurements obtained on TCCD cannot be compared to results described on literature. Velocities obtained TCCD may be lower than those obtained with TCD. Velocities obtained without angle correction may be close to standardized values.

TCCD measurements with TCD becomes necessary to assess disease stability angle correction on TCCD should not be performed [9, 16].

4 Technique

Performing TCD and TCCD ultrasonography requires expertise obtained by training and practice. The examination can be performed at the bedside or dedicated ultrasound examination room with the operator seated at the head of the bed. Patient is requested to lie still in supine position or turn head to the side if necessary.

In infants open fontanelles provides excellent acoustic window for visualization of intracranial circulation (Fig. 5). Higher frequency (5–15 MHz) sector, curvilinear or linear probes are used to perform doppler. TCCD is preferred over TCD in children for precise localization of targeted intracranial vessels. Criteria for localization and depth of intracranial vessels to be visualized via TCD are not well established for children.

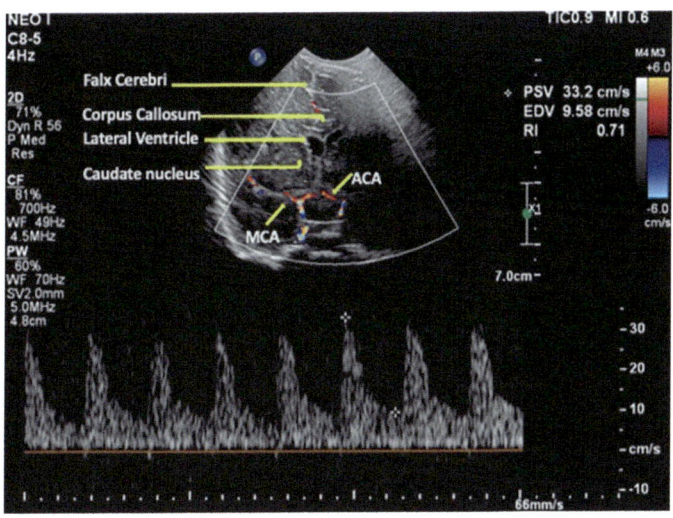

FIGURE 5 TCCD images in infants through anterior fontanelle shows excellent visualization of intracranial arteries as well as superior grayscale visualization of intracranial structures

After fontanelle closure, the 2 available acoustic windows are the temporal bone and the foramen magnum. The transtemporal window allows optimal visualization of the circle of Willis; the Middle Cerebral Artery (MCA), Anterior cerebral artery (ACA), posterior cerebral artery (PCA) and the distal internal carotid artery (ICA). Optimum location to scan is the thinnest portion of the temporal bone (the pterion), cephalad to the zygomatic arch and anterior to the ear [8, 9]. We perform TCCD examinations using a 6-mm sample volume to obtain atleast 3 velocity measurements along the Proximal, mid and distal MCA, at 2 depths within the ACA, PCA, the distal ICA (Fig. 6a).

The transducer is placed in the midline below the occiput and angled cephalad to allow visualization of the Vertebral and Basilar arteries via the Foramen Magnum for transforaminal approach (Fig. 6b). Sometimes the transducer is placed on the closed eyelid for visualization of occipital artery and cavernous portion of the ICA -transorbital approach (Fig. 6c) [8, 19].

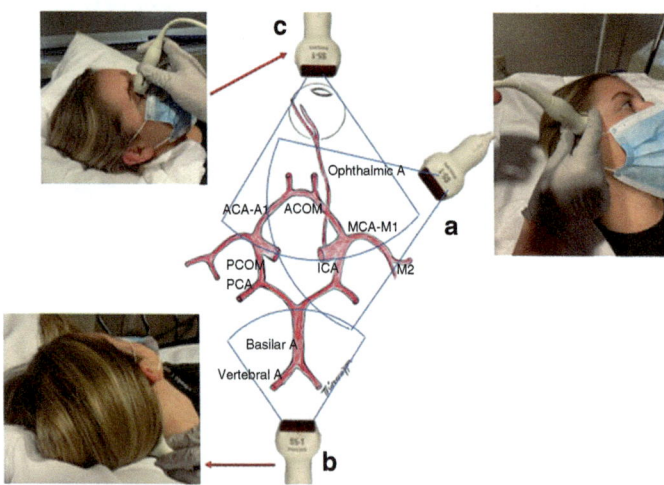

FIGURE 6 Acoustic windows for imaging intracranial vessels after fontanelle closure: Transtemporal (**a**), Trans occipital (**b**), Transorbital (**c**)

As mentioned before, TCD is performed without vessel visualization. The operator relies on an audible Doppler signal and continuous velocity readout to optimize the angle of insonation and maximize the velocity measurement. Because the actual vessels are not visualized, correction for angle of insonation cannot be applied. Since the MCA and PCA course towards the transducer, the angle of insonation is small and it is no significant effect on velocity is obtained [20]. However, ACA courses perpendicular to the angle of insonation and velocities obtained from this vessel are not accurate on TCD [16]. Normal velocities of the visualized cerebral vessels and expected depth of the vessels are detailed on Table 2.

Despite excellent safety profile, there are a few biosafety concerns related to diagnostic ultrasound use that the operator needs to be aware of. Focused energy deposition from the ultrasound beam can result in increased temperature within the tissues as well as mechanical injury to the cells.

Table 2 On non-imaging TCD vessels are identified by approximate depth and the directionality of blood flow through the given acoustic window (Ref. [8])

Artery	Acoustic window	Transducer orientation	Depth in mm	Flow direction
MCA	Transtemporal	Neutral, Facing Forward	35–60	Toward
ACA	Transtemporal	Anterior	60–75	Away
PCA	Transtemporal	Posterior	60–75	Toward
VA	Transforaminal	Superior, oblique	45–75	Away
BA	Transforaminal	Superior	70–120	Away
OA	Transorbital	Slightly Medial	40–50	Toward

MCA middle cerebral artery, *ACA* anterior cerebral artery, *PCA* posterior cerebral artery, *VA* vertebral artery, *BA* basilar artery, *OA* occipital artery

This concern is even higher with transorbital imaging where the eye because of relatively low perfusion and slow dissipation of heat is at higher risk of thermal injury. Machine settings should be maintained at lowest output power without compromising the diagnostic quality of the images and scanning times should be kept short [21].

5 Clinical Applications of TCD

5.1 Vasospasm

Vasospasm is a secondary consequence of SAH and is associated with high mortality and morbidity [22]. Additional sequala of SAH and vasospasm is delayed cerebral infarction (DCI) also associated with disability and death [23]. Cerebral vasospasm—the narrowing of the cerebral arteries after SAH—is a common complication that occurs in up to 70% of patients and can be seen with radiographic and ultrasound imaging [24]. Cerebral vasospasm may be present in some patients as early as in the first 24 h of SAH but more frequently begins 3–4 days after an aneurysm rupture, reaching a peak after 7–10 days and resolving spontaneously after 21 days [25] (Fig. 7). Bedside TCD and TCCD can detect vasospasm before the patient develops ischemic neurological deficits or cerebral infarction. Elevated TCD velocities initiate and guide, treatment of vasospasm [26]. In addition, it is important to remember that multiple intracranial vessels may be affected by vasospasm and both anterior and posterior circulation should be interrogated.

The pooled sensitivity of TCD for the detection of vasospasm has been reported to be 67% and 82% for TCCD per metaanalysis published by Mastantuono JM et al. [27]. Increases in flow velocity correspond to cross-sectional diameter decreases in vessel lumen resulting from vasospasm. The more severe the vasospasm, the higher the flow velocity. Threshold PSV and MFV values for Mild, Moderate and Severe vasospasm on TCCD used in our institution are

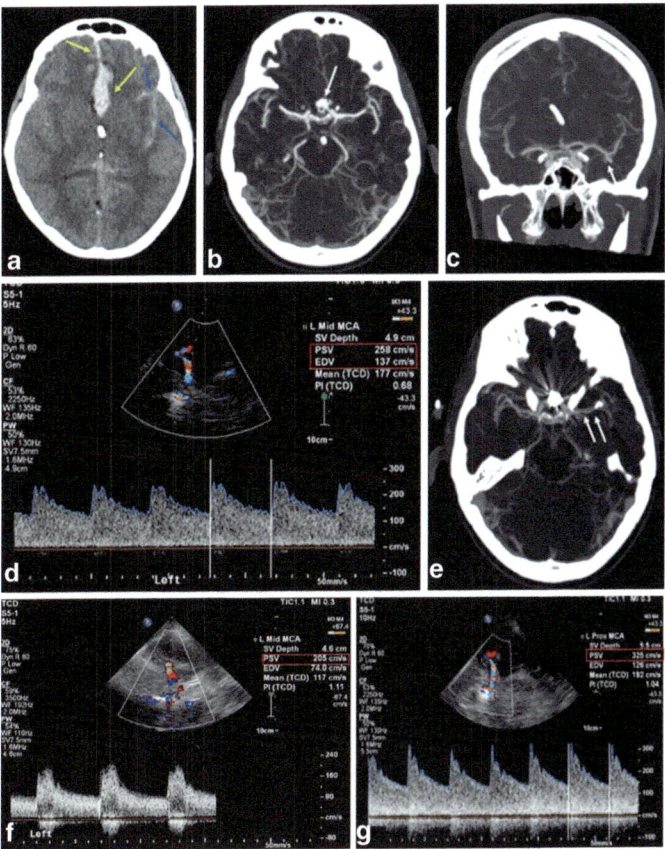

FIGURE 7 39 years old women with subarachnoid hemorrhage- seen on non-contrast CT (**a**) as high-attenuation blood in the Sylvian fissures (yellow arrows) and the interhemispheric fissure (blue arrows). Post contrast maximum intensity projection (MIP) axial images show a ACOM artery saccular aneurysm (arrow on image **b**) and a smaller aneurysm arising from M2 (arrow on image **c**). Patient demonstrated moderate spasm of left MCA on TCCD on day 4 (**d**), which was also seen on CTA head from the same day. See narrowed MCA vessels compared to CTA from day 1 (arrows on image **e**). The patient also demonstrated mild vasospasm and severe vasospasms on serial TCCD's performed over 14 days post initial diagnosis (**f, g**)

TABLE 3 Vasospasm criterias for intracranial vessels (Refs. [8, 28–31])

Artery	PSV (cm/sec)	MFV (cm/sec)	Ratios
MCA	Mild 200–250 Moderate 250–300 Severe >300	Mild: 120–150 Moderate: 150–200 Severe >200	Lindegaard Ratio (MFV MCA/MFV EICA: Mild: 3–4.5 Moderate 4.5–6.0 Severe >6
ACA	>120	>80	Sloan ratio (MFV ACA/MFV EICA) >4.0
PCA	>120	>85	
VA		>60	
BA		>50	Soustiel's posterior circulation index >2.0 (MFV BA/MFV EICA)

adapted from the article published by Kirsch et al. and shown in Table 3 [8]. Apart from vessel narrowing, flow velocity obtained on TCCD is also influenced by patient factors such as hypertension, hypervolemia and hyperemia [4]. Ratio between the MFV of the middle cerebral artery and extracranial internal carotid artery, also called Lindegaard ratio was developed to correct for these confounders [28]. These ratios take precedence over the absolute values of MFV in assessment of vasospasm. A Lindegaard ratio of 3–6 is indicative of mild to moderate vasospasm, and a ratio greater than 6.0 is indicative of severe vasospasm (Table 3, Fig. 8). Cutoff PSV and MFV values for anterior and posterior circulation is shown on Table 3 (Figs. 9 and 10). Additional ratios have been developed for anterior and posterior circulation to exclude the effect of confounders. Sloan's hemispheric ratio, is the ratio of MFV of the ACA to MFV of distal ICA. A ratio of =/>4 is highly concerning for vasospasm [29]. Soustiel's posterior circulation index is calculated as the ratio of the MFV of the basilar artery to MFV of the extracranial vertebral artery. A ratio =/> 2 is considered concerning for vasospasm [30].

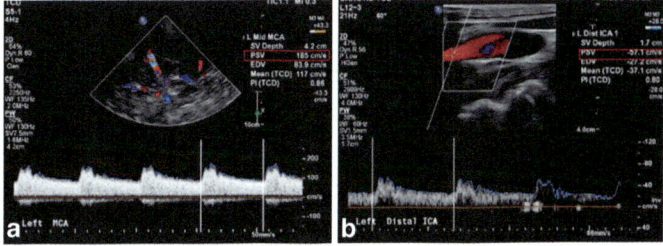

Lindegaard ratio: MFV MCA/MFV Extracranial ICA = 185/57=3.2

FIGURE 8 In this patient with hypovolemia, the absolute MCA velocity is not indicative of vasospasm (**a**). However, Lindegaard ratio is 3.2 is indicative of mild to moderate vasospasm. Note, although visually the waveforms look similar for both MCA and ICA (**b**), the scales are set differently, the velocities of MCA are significantly higher than ICA

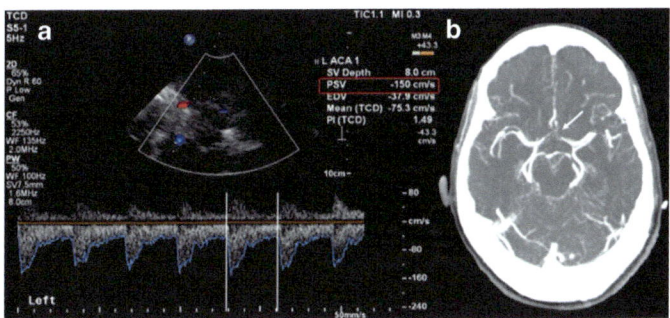

FIGURE 9 Patient with subarachnoid hemorrhage and ACA velocities of 150 cm/s, consistent with vasospasm (**a**). Which was seen on CTA performed subsequently (arrow) (**b**)

A baseline TCD and TCCD are obtained after initial diagnosis of SAH on CT or MRI. In our institution daily follow-up of US via bedside TCCD is performed for 14 days after initial diagnosis of SAH. As mentioned previously, given the differences in recorded mean velocities between TCD and TCCD, the measurements obtained by imaging and non imaging techniques should not be compared, instead individual trends on TCD and TCCD should be monitored separately.

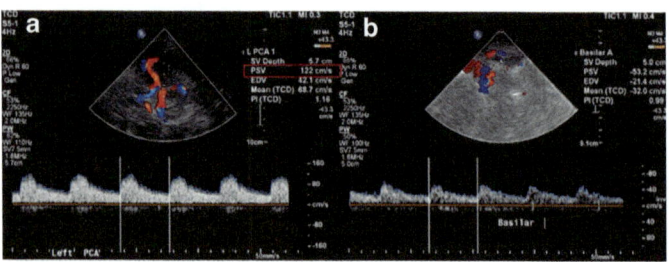

FIGURE 10 Patient with subarachnoid hemorrhage and PCA velocities of 122 cm/s, consistent with vasospasm (**a**). Normal basilar artery waveform seen in the same patient (**b**)

5.2 Stenosis

TCD is a great adjunct to DSA or CTA for diagnosis and follow-up of major intra cranial vessels diagnosis before and after neurointervention. The MFV thresholds and ratio's to diagnose 50% stenosis with high accuracy is not well established. The Stroke Outcomes and Neuroimaging of Intracranial Atherosclerosis (SONIA) trial compared the performance of TCD against invasive angiography for identification of ≥50% intracranial stenosis and demonstrated that TCD could reliably exclude the presence of intracranial stenosis (negative predictive value >80%) (Fig. 11). The following MFV cut-offs on TCD were used for identification of ≥50% stenosis (SONIA criteria) for MCA: MFV >100 cm/s and VA/BA MFV >80 cm/s [32]. The commonly used cut-off values for the diagnosis of moderate (>50%) stenosis in various intracranial arteries is published by Bathala et al. [31].

5.3 Acute Ischemic Stroke

TCD has application in both diagnosis and management of acute ischemic stroke. For the diagnosis of acute ischemic stroke, the sensitivity and specificity of TCD depends on the

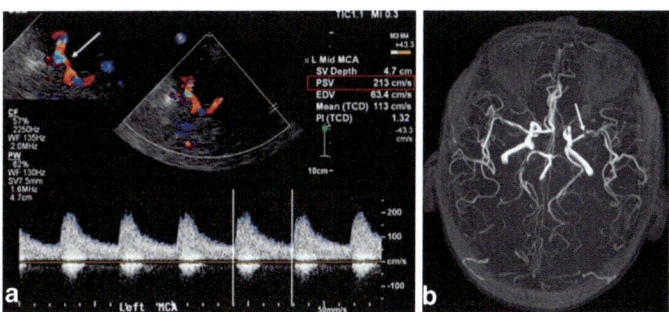

FIGURE 11 Left mid MCA demonstrates persistent narrowing (arrow) with elevated velocities (red box), consistent with stenosis (**a**). Moderate stenosis of MCA was seen on MIP axial MRA (**b**)

location of circulatory deficit. Most reliable results are noted in the anterior circulation. Demchuk et al., [33] noted an overall sensitivity of 83% and specificity of 94% in angiographic confirmed arterial occlusion. The sensitivity of TCD in diagnosing ischemic stroke was 94% for proximal ICA, 93% for MCA, 56% for terminal VA and 60% for BA.

After the initial MRA and thrombolytic therapy for acute stroke, there is no good mechanism to monitor flow. TCD can monitor and grade residual blood flow after thrombolytic therapy using the Thrombolysis in Brain Ischemia (TIBI) grading system. (0 = absent, 1 = minimal, 2 = blunted, 3 = dampened, 4 = stenotic, 5 = normal). Stolz et al., [34] in their meta-analysis noted that clinical improvement at 48 h correlates with recanalization on TCD measurements. Correlation was also noted with improved functional capacity at 3 months. Mortality benefit was also noted with patent MVA as opposed to occluded MCA 2 h after thrombolytic therapy. Alexandrov et al., [35] demonstrated that TIBI grading system on TCD can also detect early post thrombolytic re-occlusion (<2 h) which can occur in a third of the patients. Such early re-occlusion after thrombolysis is associated with higher inpatient mortality and poor functional outcomes at 3 months.

5.4 Traumatic Brain Injury

Mild CT findings associated with a reduced Diastolic Flow Volume (Fd) <25 cm/s and/or increased PI values >1.25 on TCD at the time of admission indicated a high risk of neurological deterioration within the first week after Traumatic Brain Injury in study conducted by Bauzat et al. [36]. These cut offs accurately predicted neurologic worsening with 90% sensitivity and 91% specificity [36]. TCD as a bedside monitoring tool compliments initial CT scan and could improve the early screening of mild to moderate TBI patients in the emergency setting, thus allowing the initiation of appropriate treatment and management [11].

5.5 Brain Death Evaluation

Brain stem death is usually a clinical diagnosis utilizing clinical examination and confirmatory testing such as EEG. Occasionally, circumstances such as brain stem injury, paralytics, sedative medications, or hypothermia may pose challenges to accurate clinical examination [37]. Under such circumstances, TCD may be used as a confirmatory test for cerebral circulatory arrest which precedes brain stem death.

For confirmation of cerebral circulatory arrest, one of the following waveforms must be observed in the BA, bilateral ICA, and bilateral MCA on two examinations at least 30 min apart [38] (Fig. 12):

1. An oscillating waveform (zero net flow)
2. Small systolic spikes of <200 ms duration and <50 cm/s PSV with no diastolic flow
3. Disappearance of previously registered Doppler flow signals

It must be mentioned that operator experience is important in reliably deriving conclusions using TCD for cerebral circulatory arrest. A good acoustic window may sometimes be obtained by repeated attempts at testing even if the initial attempt demonstrated suboptimal window.

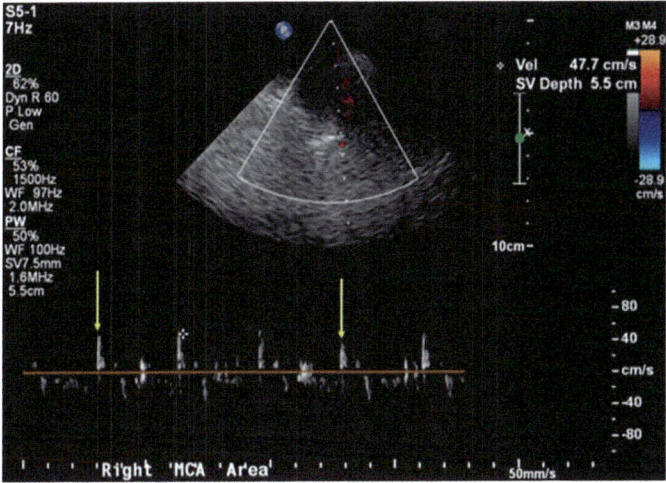

FIGURE 12 In a patient suspected with brain death, TCCD in right MCA area demonstrates an oscillating waveform (arrow) with small systolic spikes of <50 cm/s and no definite diastolic flow

Sensitivity and specificity of TCD for cerebral circulatory arrest have been shown to be 89–100% and 97–100%, respectively [29, 39].

5.6 Sickle Cell Disease

Patients with sickle cell disease (SCD) may have neurologic injury in the form of infarction or intracranial bleed. The pathophysiology is stenosis and occlusion of distal ICA, proximal MCA and ACA by sickle cells and their adherence to the vascular endothelium. TCD can be particularly helpful in subclinical infarction (Fig. 13). Asymptomatic children with SCD with CBF-V >200 cm/s have been shown to have an increased risk of stroke [40]. Blood transfusion in such children may reduce the risk of stroke by >90% [41]. TCD screening of children with SCD aged 2–6 years is recommended every 6–12 monthly. Involving measurement of the time-

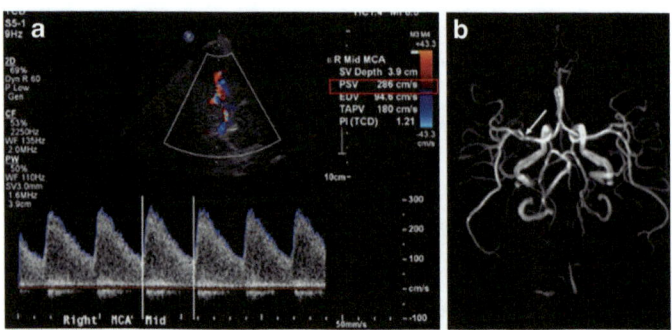

FIGURE 13 In a 3-year-old with Sickle Cell Disease demonstrates elevated velocities in Right MCA on TCCD (**a**) with stenosis demonstrated on MRA (arrow) (**b**)

averaged mean maximum CBF-V in bilateral MCA, bifurcation, distal ICA, ACA, PCA, and BA [42]. Patients with a time averaged mean maximum CBF-V of >200 cm/s in bilateral MCA, distal ICA, ACA, PCA and BA are recommended to receive blood transfusion to prevent stroke [42, 43].

6 Conclusion

TCD and TCCD (imaging) techniques allow measurement of blood flow velocity in the major intracranial vessels. Both techniques offer unique advantages and can complement each other along with other imaging modalities for detection and follow-up of cerebral vasospasm. For successful performance and accurate interpretation, the operator should be empowered with adequate training, understanding the concepts of Doppler and working knowledge of TCD equipment. Because not all vasospasm is necessarily symptomatic, the finding must be correlated with a clinical neurologic examination to determine the appropriate therapy.

References

1. Krejza J, Kochanowicz J, Mariak Z, Lewko J, Melhem ER. Middle cerebral artery spasm after subarachnoid hemorrhage: detection with transcranial color-coded duplex US. Radiology. 2005;236(2):621–9.
2. https://www.cancer.gov/about-cancer/causes-prevention/risk/radiation/pediatric-ct-scans. Accessed 01/02/2021.
3. Davenport MS, Perazella MA, Yee J, et al. Use of intravenous iodinated contrast media in patients with kidney disease: consensus statements from the American College of Radiology and the National Kidney Foundation. Radiology. 2020;294(3):660–8.
4. Samagh N, Bhagat H, Jangra K. Monitoring cerebral vasospasm: how much can we rely on transcranial Doppler. J Anaesthesiol Clin Pharmacol. 2019;35(1):12–8.
5. Carovac A, Smajlovic F, Junuzovic D. Application of ultrasound in medicine. Acta Inform Med. 2011;19(3):168–71. https://doi.org/10.5455/aim.2011.19.168-171.
6. Bushberg JT, Anthony Seibert J, Leidholdt EM, Boone JM. The essential physics of medical imaging. 3rd ed. Philadelphia: Lippincott Williams and Wilkins; 2012.
7. McNaughton DA, Abu-Yousef MA. Doppler US of the liver made simple. RadioGraphics. 2011;31(1):161–88.
8. Kirsch JD, Mathur M, Johnson MH, Gowthaman G, Scoutt LM. Advances in transcranial Doppler US: imaging ahead. RadioGraphics. 2013;33(1):E1–E14.
9. https://www.acr.org/-/media/ACR/Files/Practice-Parameters/us-transcranial.pdf?la=en. Accessed 01/02/2021.
10. Michel E, Zernikow B. Gosling's Doppler pulsatility index revisited. Ultrasound Med Biol. 1998;24(4):597–9.
11. Behrens A, Lenfeldt N, Ambarki K, et al. Transcranial Doppler pulsatility index: not an accurate method to assess intracranial pressure. Neurosurgery. 2010;66:1050–7.
12. Bauzat P, Almeras L, Manhes P, et al. Transcranial Doppler to predict neurological outcome after mild to moderate traumatic brain injury. Anesthesiology. 2016;125:346–54.
13. De Riva N, Budohoski KP, Smielewski P, et al. Transcranial Doppler pulsatility index: What it is and what it isn't. Neurocrit Care. 2012;17:58–66.
14. http://www.neurosurg.cam.ac.uk/files/2017/09/18.-TCD-Pulsatility-index.pdf.

15. Sierra J, Hanel R, Mooney L, Freeman W. Differential considerations of TCD pulsatility (Gosling's) and resistance (Pourcelot) indices after AVM surgery. J Vasc Interv Neurol. 2014;7(4):41–3.
16. McCarville BM. Transcranial Doppler ultrasonography: comparison of duplex and nonduplex. Ultrasound Q. 2008;24:167–71.
17. Neish AS, Blews DE, Simms CA, et al. Screening for stroke in sickle cell anemia: comparison of transcranial Doppler imaging and nonimaging US techniques. Radiology. 2002;222:709–14.
18. Taormina MA, Nichols FT III. Use of transcranial Doppler sonography to evaluate patients with cerebrovascular disease. Neurosurg Clin N Am. 1996;7:589–603.
19. Blanco P. Volumetric blood flow measurement using Doppler ultrasound: concerns about the technique. J Ultrasound. 2015;18(2):201–4.
20. Lupetin AR, Davis DA, Beckman I, et al. Transcranial Doppler sonography. Part 2. Evaluation of intracranial and extracranial abnormalities and procedural monitoring. Radiographics. 1995;15:193–209.
21. Ter Haar G. Ultrasonic imaging: safety considerations. Interface Focus. 2011;1(4):686–97. https://doi.org/10.1098/rsfs.2011.0029.
22. Opancina V, Lukic S, Jankovic S, Vojinovic R, Mijailovic M. Risk factors for cerebral vasospasm in patients with aneurysmal subarachnoid hemorrhage. Open Med (Wars). 2020;15(1):598–604. Published 2020 July 3. https://doi.org/10.1515/med-2020-0169.
23. Francoeur CL, Mayer SA. Management of delayed cerebral ischemia after subarachnoid hemorrhage. Crit Care. 2016;20(1):277. Published 2016 Oct 14. https://doi.org/10.1186/s13054-016-1447-6.
24. Diringer MN, Bleck TP, Hemphill JC, et al. Critical care management of patients following aneurysmal subarachnoid hemorrhage: recommendations from the Neurocritical Care Society's Multidisciplinary Consensus Conference. Neurocrit Care. 2011;15(2):211–40.
25. Psychogios K, Tsivgoulis G, Subarachnoid hemorrhage, vasospasm, and delayed cerebral ischemia. Pract Neurol. 2019. https://practicalneurology.com/articles/2019-jan/subarachnoid-hemorrhage-vasospasm-and-delayed-cerebral-ischemia/pdf.
26. Topcuoglu MA. Transcranial Doppler ultrasound in neurovascular diseases: diagnostic and therapeutic aspects. J Neurochem. 2012;123(Suppl. 2):39–51.
27. Mastantuono JM, Combescure C, Elia N, Tramèr MR, Lysakowski C. Transcranial Doppler in the diagnosis of cerebral

vasospasm: an updated meta-analysis. Critical Care Medicine. 2018;46(10):1665–72.
28. Lindegaard KF, Nornes H, Bakke SJ, Sorteberg W, Nakstad P. Cerebral vasospasm diagnosis by means of angiography and blood velocity measurements. Acta Neurochir. 1989;100(1–2):12–24.
29. Sloan MA, Alexandrov AV, Tegeler CH, et al. Assessment: transcranial Doppler ultrasonography: report of the Therapeutics and Technology Assessment Subcommittee of the American Academy of Neurology. Neurology. 2004;62:1468–81.
30. Soustiel JF, Shik V, Shreiber R, Tavor Y, Goldsher D. Basilar vasospasm diagnosis: investigation of a modified "Lindegaard Index" based on imaging studies and blood velocity measurements of the basilar artery. Stroke. 2002;33:72–7.
31. Bathala L, Mehndiratta MM, Sharma VK. Transcranial doppler: technique and common findings (Part 1). Ann Indian Acad Neurol. 2013;16(2):174–9. https://doi.org/10.4103/0972-2327.112460.
32. Feldmann E, Wilterdink JL, Kosinski A, et al. The Stroke Outcomes and Neuroimaging of Intracranial Atherosclerosis (SONIA) trial. Neurology. 2007;68(24):2099–106.
33. Demchuk AM, Christou I, Wein TH, et al. Accuracy and criteria for localizing arterial occlusion with transcranial Doppler. J Neuroimaging. 2000;10(1):1–12.
34. Stolz E, Cioli F, Allendoerfer J, Gerriets T, Sette MD, Kaps M. Can early neurosonology predict outcome in acute stroke?: a metaanalysis of prognostic clinical effect sizes related to the vascular status. Stroke. 2008;39(12):3255–61.
35. Alexandrov AV, Grotta JC. Arterial reocclusion in stroke patients treated with intravenous tissue plasminogen activator. Neurology. 2002;59(6):862–7.
36. Bouzat P, Francony G, Declety P, et al. Transcranial Doppler to screen on admission patients with mild to moderate traumatic brain injury. Neurosurgery. 2011;68(6):1603–10.
37. Panerai RB. Assessment of cerebral pressure autoregulation in humans—a review of measurement methods. Physiol Meas. 1998;19(3):305–38.
38. Ducrocq X, Braun M, Debouverie M, Junges C, Hummer M, Vespignani H. Brain death and transcranial Doppler: experience in 130 cases of brain dead patients. J Neurol Sci. 1998;160(1):41–6.
39. Monteiro LM, Bollen CW, van Huffelen AC, Ackerstaff RGA, Jansen NJG, van Vught AJ. Transcranial Doppler ultrasonogra-

phy to confirm brain death: a meta-analysis. Intensive Care Med. 2006;32(12):1937–44.
40. Adams RJ, McKie VC, Carl EM, et al. Long-term stroke risk in children with sickle cell disease screened with transcranial Doppler. Annals of Neurology. 1997;42(5):699–704. [PubMed] [Google Scholar].
41. Adams RJ, McKie VC, Hsu L, et al. Prevention of a first stroke by transfusions in children with sickle cell anemia and abnormal results on transcranial Doppler ultrasonography. N Engl J Med. 1998;339(1):5–11.
42. Platt OS. Prevention and management of stroke in sickle cell anemia. Hematology. 2006;2006(1):54–7.
43. Adams RJ. TCD in sickle cell disease: an important and useful test. Pediatr Radiol. 2005;35(3):229–34.

Cervical Traction

Michael Ortiz Torres and Steven B. Carr

1 Introduction

Cervical traction is a cornerstone for the treatment of acute cervical spine injuries. Providing weighted traction to the cervical spine can reduce fracture/dislocations, restore and maintain normal spinal alignment as well as temporally immobilizing the spine until definitive treatment can be performed, whether that be open reduction and fixation or prolonged halo vest immobilization [1]. The endpoint of cervical traction is to decompress the spinal cord and nerve roots in order to prevent secondary, delayed spinal cord injury related to spinal instability.

2 Indications, Contraindications, and Caveats

- A patient with an unstable cervical spinal injury must be immobilized by external orthoses or sandbags until cervical traction can be performed.

M. O. Torres · S. B. Carr (✉)
Division of Neurosurgery, University of Missouri School of Medicine, Columbia, MO, USA
e-mail: ortiztorresm@health.missouri.edu;
carrsb@health.missouri.edu

- Cervical traction is indicated for immobilization and/or reduction of an unstable cervical spinal injury (displaced fracture, unilateral/bilateral facet fracture/dislocations, ligamentous injury), as well as for decompression of the spinal cord or nerve roots secondary to spinal misalignment [1].
- The patient must be awake and cooperative. Neurological examination during traction is essential to ensure weight tolerance and prevent the development of a new neurologic deficit.
- Concomitant radiographs are necessary to sequentially assess traction/reduction and to correlate imaging to the patient's neurological exam during the procedure.
- Pin sites should not be over skull fractures or prior skull defects.
- Cervical traction should not be performed if: (1) there is another unstable injury rostral to the target level, (2) there is a significant traumatic disc herniation with associated neurological deficit, and (3) if there is a definitive, complete ligamentous injury at any cervical spine level [2–5]. MRI should be obtained when appropriate to rule out a compressive lesion which could put the patient at risk for neural element impingement with traction
- Traction can be applied using either Gardner-Wells tongs or a halo ring; generally in patients who are going to be treated long term or post-operatively with halo fixation, a halo ring is used as the traction modality, otherwise Gardner-Wells tongs are used

3 Procedure: Cervical Traction/Closed Reduction with Garner-Wells Tongs

1. *Pre-medication*

Short-acting opiates and muscle relaxants should be available and may be used. Opiates will ameliorate pain related to manipulation of the acute injured spine while muscle relaxants can "loosen" spasmodic spine musculature to allow for easier manipulation. The authors prefer the use of IV fentanyl and IV valium for this phase of the procedure.

2. *Preparation*

Necessary supplies include: gloves, clippers, betadine ointment, local anesthetic and a cervical traction cart or the equivalent for your institution. For Gardner-Wells tongs (Fig. 1), necessary equipment consists of: tongs and rope, bed frame bars, pulley, pins, and weight.

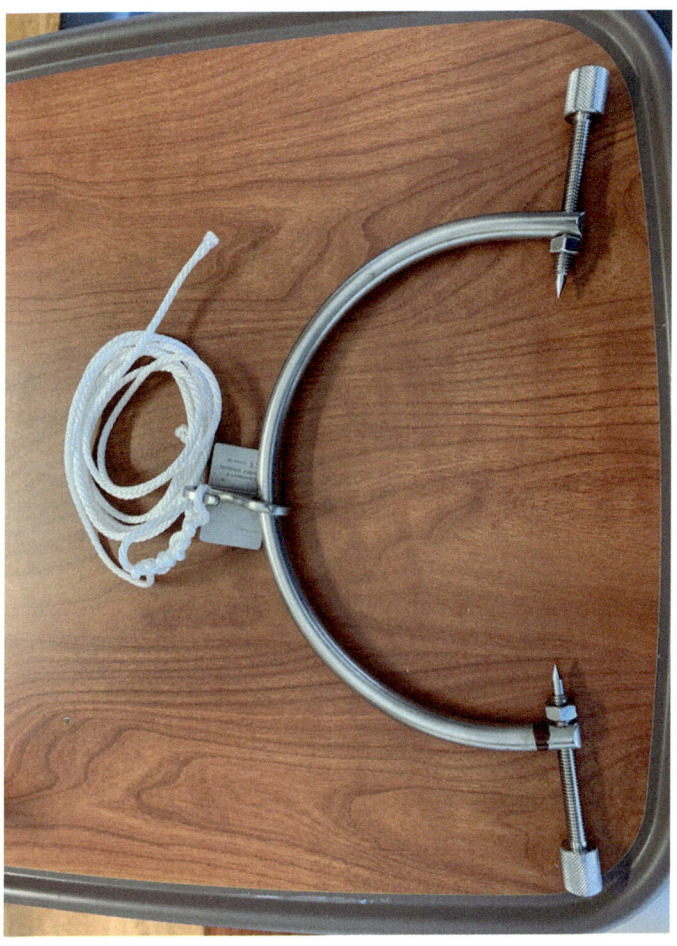

FIGURE 1 Gardner-Wells tongs

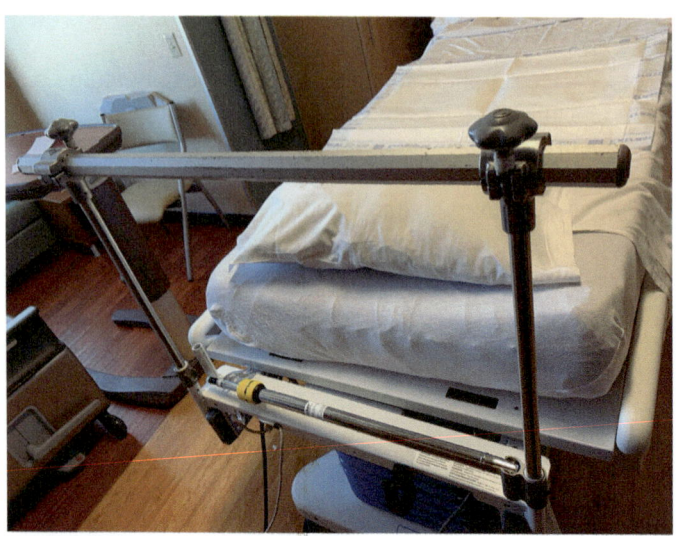

FIGURE 2 Step 1: Bed frame base

Start by placing the vertical bars on each side of the bed attachments and connect the vertical bars with a horizontal bar (Fig. 2). Apply another bar perpendicular to the horizontal bar (this will act as a pivot point to rotate and adjust the angle of the pulley, we will refer to this as the pivot bar) and apply a short bar perpendicular to that bar (this will serve as the pulley attachment point, we will refer to this as the pulley bar) (Fig. 3). Attach the pulley (Fig. 4).

3. *Patient positioning*

The patient is positioned supine in bed with the neck in the neutral position. Now, adjust the pivot bar and the pulley bar until the pulley is parallel to the horizontal axis of the patient's spine. This will be, in most instances, the starting position.

Cervical Traction 269

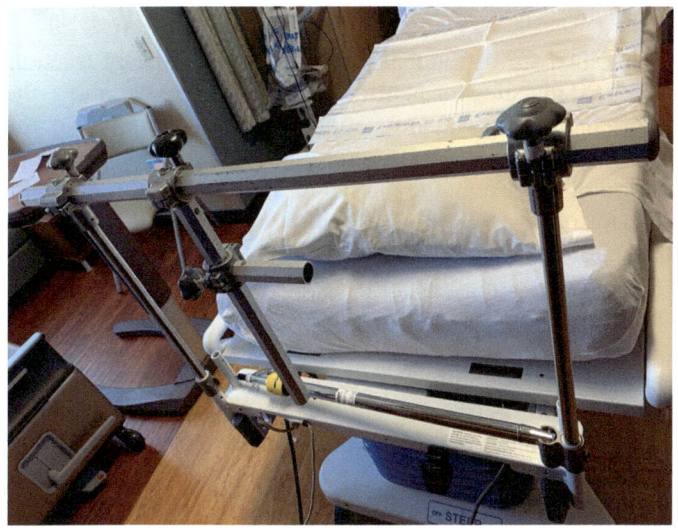

FIGURE 3 Step 2: Pivot bar and pulley bar in place

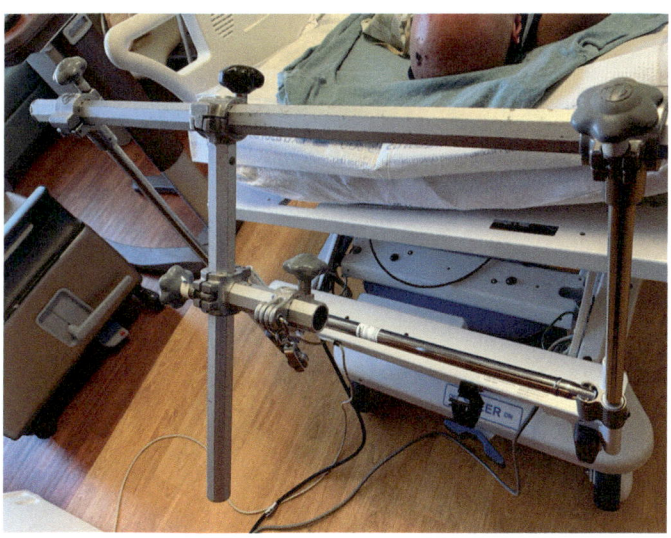

FIGURE 4 Step 3: Pulley attached

4. *Pin placement*

Pin sites are dependent on the intended type of traction. The ideal pin sites for neutral traction are directly above the external auditory meatus, approximately 3 cm above the pinna, at the superior temporal line. If attempting to induce flexion or extension, the pins should be placed either 2–3 cm anterior or posterior to that point, respectively [6]. Once the adequate site is identified, the area is cleaned with alcohol prep followed by iodine prep. The area is infiltrated with local anesthetic. The authors prefer a 2.5 cc infiltration of 1% lidocaine at each pin site. The pins are covered with iodine ointment and screwed into placed. Both pins are tightened at the same time until an adequate level of torque is achieved, in which the tongs are tightly secured to the patient's head. The rope from the tongs is then passed through the pulley and secured to the weight hanger with a knot (Fig. 5).

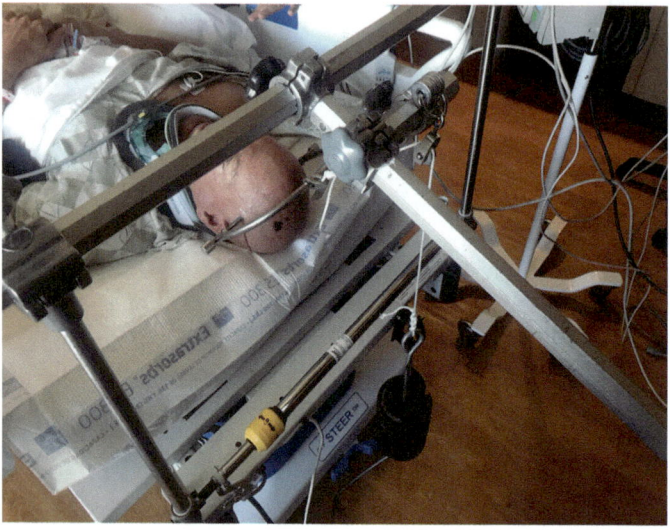

FIGURE 5 Step 4: Tongs secured

5. *Traction/reduction*

Start the critical portion of the procedure by obtaining a baseline lateral x-ray. As a general rule of thumb, initial weight is dependent on the level of injury and is calculated as (3–5 lbs × # of cranial levels) [1]. This initial weight can be added, a neurologic exam is done, and an x-ray is obtained to evaluate the alignment. Additional weight can be added every 10–15 min. It is our practice to add weight in increments of 2.5 lbs and to not surpass more than 5 lbs per number of level treated. Despite that, definitive consensus on the ideal weight per level or a maximum amount of weight has not been established. The pulley angle can be adjusted to modify the amount of flexion/extension added and the amount of weight can be adjusted to increase distraction. It is important to obtain X-rays after every adjustment to ensure distraction is being applied safely. Once adequate traction/reduction is achieved, the patient is left in the supine position with the adequate weight. We routinely obtain repeat x-rays 2 h post-procedure as changes in muscle tone may induce delayed motion of the cervical spine and may altered the traction/reduction.

4 Post-procedural Care

- Patients must be admitted to a neurological ICU and should have frequent neurological checks (every hour).
- Adequate pain control is essential.
- Repeat imaging should be routinely obtained, including any time there is patient transfer or adjustments in weight or pulley angle.
- Inspect pin torque daily and adjust as necessary. Generally the pins are re-tightened the day after placement to ensure they remain secure
- Routinely clean the pin sites with hydrogen peroxide twice a day.
- Beware of pressure injuries related to patient immobilization (especially the occiput which can be pulled against the bed) in the supine position and treat accordingly.

5 Case Presentation

A 62 y/o gentleman presented to our institution after suffering a ground level fall while hunting. CT of the cervical spine revealed a comminuted Hangman's fracture with resultant grade 2 anterolisthesis of C2–3 (Fig. 6a and b). He was neurologically intact but had severe neck pain. Gardner-Wells tongs were placed with the intention to distract and extend the neck in order to rotate C2 anteriorly in a sagittal plane, hence the pins where placed 3 cm above the EAM and 2 cm anterior. The pre-traction x-ray is presented in Fig. 7a. 6 lbs (3 lbs × 2 levels) was selected as the initial weight (Fig. 7b). Weight was sequentially increased, and the pulley was adjusted as to increasingly distract and flex the spine to revert the misalignment (Fig. 7c). The patient tolerated traction well, and no changes in alignment were obtained past 16 lbs,

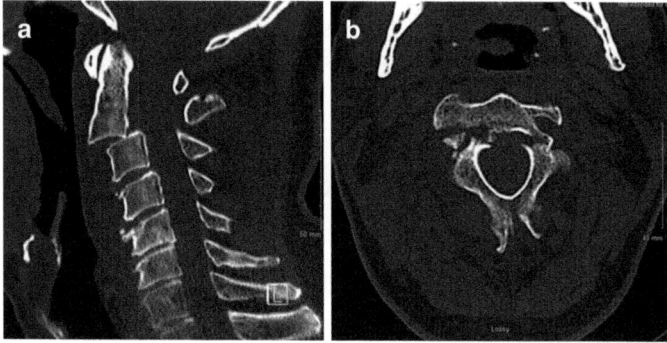

FIGURE 6 (**a**) Sagittal CT cervical spine bone window without contrast demonstrating unstable C2 injury with grade anterolisthesis at C2–3. (**b**) Axial CT cervical spine bone window without contrast demonstrating bilateral C2 pedicle fractures as classically described for Hangman's fracture

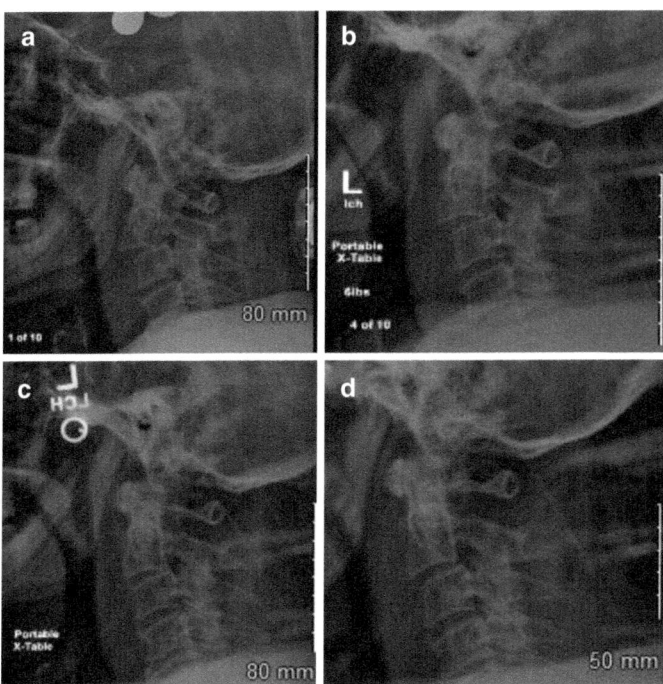

FIGURE 7 (a) Pre-traction lateral cervical spine x-ray with Gardner-Wells tongs in place. Notice grade 2 spondylolisthesis of C2–3. (b) Initial 6 lbs of weight have been added. Notice reduction of spondylolisthesis to grade 1. (c) A total of 10 lbs have been added, as well as slight flexion of the neck. (d) Final x-ray demonstrating adequate reduction and near-normal alignment at the C2–3 level

so this was deemed our final weight (Fig. 7d). The patient had immediate improvement of his neck pain and remained neurologically intact post-operatively. He later underwent posterior cervical instrumentation and fusion from C1 to C3, traction was removed, and he did not require external orthoses for stabilization.

References

1. Hadley MN, Walters BC, Grabb BC, Oyesiku NM, Przybylski GJ, Resnick DK, et al. Initial closed reduction of cervical spine fracture-dislocation injuries. Neurosurgery. 2002;50(3 Suppl):S44–50. https://doi.org/10.1097/00006123-200203001-00010.
2. Doran SE, Papadopoulos SM, Ducker TB, Lillehei KO. Magnetic resonance imaging documentation of coexistent traumatic locked facets of the cervical spine and disc herniation. J Neurosurg. 1993;79(3):341–5. https://doi.org/10.3171/jns.1993.79.3.0341.
3. Maiman DJ, Barolat G, Larson SJ. Management of bilateral locked facets of the cervical spine. Neurosurgery. 1986;18(5):542–7. https://doi.org/10.1227/00006123-198605000-00005.
4. Lee AS, MacLean JC, Newton DA. Rapid traction for reduction of cervical spine dislocations. J Bone Joint Surg Br. 1994;76(3):352–6.
5. Crutchfield WG. Skeletal traction in treatment of injuries to the cervical spine. J Am Med Assoc. 1954;155(1):29–32. https://doi.org/10.1001/jama.1954.03690190035010.
6. Ullman JS, Raskin PB. Application of closed spinal traction. In: Atlas of emergency neurosurgery. Thieme Medical; 2015. p. 170–8.

Part II
Protocols

Sedation and Analgesia Management

Kathryn E. Qualls and Francisco E. Gomez

1 Introduction

Analgo-sedation in the NCCU is a challenging proposition given conflicting objectives and varied indications [1], needing to balance an adequate sedation depth with preservation of the capacity to perform neurological examinations. Furthermore, patients with cognitive dysfunction are more prone to restlessness and agitation [1]. It is indeed a fine line as both over- and under-sedation incur complications and there is no evidence to support any particular sedation protocol over another, if at all [2]. Further confounding the issue, most existing research on analgesia and sedation in the critical care setting have included general intensive care unit (ICU) patients with different pathophysiologies from those with neurological injury [3].

K. E. Qualls (✉) · F. E. Gomez
Pharmacy Department, University of Missouri Health Care, Columbia, MO, USA
e-mail: quallske@health.missouri.edu; quallske@umsystem.edu; fegyr7@missouri.edu

2 Indications

Indications for analgesia and sedation in the NCCU can be subdivided into general indications and neuro-specific indications. The former comprises indications generalizable to all ICU patients such as: pain reduction, anxiolysis, ventilator synchrony, hemodynamic stabilization or blunting of stress response [4]. The latter includes conditions wherein sedatives are a treatment upon itself, such as status epilepticus or ICP crises [5] (Table 1).

A majority of critically ill patients will suffer pain and anxiety [6, 7] during their admission, which if uncontrolled may lead to long term complications such as post-traumatic stress disorder, chronic pain and lower quality of life even years after discharge [6]. It is recommended to attempt analgesia prior to sedation, as pain itself may be a cause for agitation [6, 8].

Table 1 Analgo-sedation indications, general vs neurocritical specific [5–7]. Pathologies such as traumatic brain injury, increased intracranial pressure and status epilepticus may require deep sedation or induced coma as therapy and are discussed elsewhere in this text

General indications	Neurocritical specific indications
Anxiety	Status epilepticus
Intubation	Intracranial pressure (ICP) crisis
Ventilator dys-synchrony	Paroxysmal sympathetic hyperactivity
Prior to painful interventions	
Pain (with or without attendant catecholaminergic response)	
Paralytic administration	
Targeted temperature management	

3 Drug Selection

The ideal regimen in the NCCU would achieve the minimum analgosedation necessary to ensure care delivery, patient comfort and pain minimization [6, 8]. Of note, sedation intensity carries a dose-dependent relationship with delirium, mortality and prolonged intubation [4, 6], while light sedation leads to decreased rates of tracheostomy, and length of mechanical ventilation [6]. In the interest of preserving the neurological exam, the ideal regimen would preferably exhibit short onset and offset and have a short terminal half-life [6]. Thus, drug selection is an exquisite affair in the NCCU wherein mechanisms of action, half-lives, side effects and metabolic pathways of elimination are to be accounted for when selecting an agent.

Ketamine, a nonbarbiturate phencyclidine derivative has gained recent attention due to opioid-sparing effect and ability to provide neuroprotection with minimal side effects in the NCCU. Analgesic effects are observed at lower plasma concentrations than those that produce psychomimetic effects. At lower doses, ketamine has little effect on blood pressure [9]. The fear that ketamine could raise the ICP in brain injured patients has been disproved in some clinical studies and has been utilized as part of an ICP management protocol in others [10].

Benzodiazepines deserve special mention, as they are noted to have high tissue accumulation and may prolong awakening times [5]. Thus, some consider dexmedetomidine or propofol preferable agents [6]. The authors usually employ midazolam when there is a clear primary indication i.e. neuro-specific conditions.

4 Pharmacological Agents for Sedation and Analgesia

When starting medications for analgesia or sedation, patient specific factors should be taken into account. These include but are not limited to hepatic, cardiac, and kidney function at the time of initiation. Select agents are listed in Table 2 with

TABLE 2 Continuous doses of analgesia or sedation agents and pharmacokinetic properties [1, 3, 11–16]

Agent	Initial dose	Titration	Maximum dose	Mechanism of action	Half life elimination	Common adverse effects
Fentanyl	25–50 mcg/h	Increase by 25 mcg/kg/h every 30 min to 1 h	250 mcg/h	Mu receptor agonist	2–4 h	Respiratory depression and gastric dysmotility
Remifentanil	0.5–2 mcg/kg/h	0.5–15 mcg/kg/h	15 mcg/kg/h	Mu receptor agonist	10–20 min	Respiratory depression, hypotension, gastric dysmotility
Midazolam	0.5–1 mg/h	Increase 1 mg/h every 30 min to 1 h	20 mg/h	GABA-a receptor agonist	3–4 h	Respiratory depression and hypotension

Propofol	5 mcg/kg/min	Increase 5 mcg/kg/min every 10 min	80 mcg/kg/min	Unclear; possibly GABA-a receptor agonist and NMDA receptor antagonist	Biphasic; initially 40 min with terminal 4 to 7 h	Hypotension, respiratory depression, hypertriglyceridemia, propofol infusion syndrome
Ketamine	0.1–0.5 mg/kg/h	Increase by 0.25–0.5 mg/kg/h every 30 min	4.5 mg/kg/h	Noncompetitive NMDA receptor antagonist	10–15 min	Tachycardia, increased saliva, emergence reactions
Dexmedetomidine	0.2 mcg/kg/h	Increase by 0.1 mcg/kg/h every 30 min	1.7 mcg/kg/min	Selective alpha2 agonist	30 min to 3 h	Bradycardia and hypotension

their pharmacologic properties as well as adverse effects. Choosing which agent to start is part of practicing medicine in the grey zone as there is no clear cut answer for NCCU patients.

5 Tools for Objective Measuring of Sedation and Analgesia

The Richmond Agitation and Sedation Scale (RASS) [17] and the Riker Sedation-Agitation Scale (SAS) [18] are commonly utilized for sedation scoring in the NCCU. The RASS (see Table 3) is commonly utilized as this scale included NCCU patients at its inception [17]. Most sedation policies or procedures titrate sedative medication based on a RASS goal, which may aid in the minimization of total dosage [19]. The RASS or SAS goal is determined based on patient specific factors and should be defined in medication orders.

The most common pain scores utilized in mechanical ventilated ICU patients include the behavioral pain scale (BPS)

TABLE 3 Richmond agitation and sedation score [17]

Score	Term
+4	Combative
+3	Very agitated
+2	Agitated
+1	Restless
0	Alert and calm
−1	Drowsy
−2	Light sedation
−3	Moderate sedation
−4	Deep sedation
−5	Unarousable

Table 4 Critical care pain observation tool [21]

Indicator	Score	Description
Facial expression	0	Relaxed, neutral
	1	Tensed
	2	Grimacing
Body movements	0	Absence of movements
	1	Protection
	2	Restlessness
Compliance with ventilator OR Vocalization	0	Tolerating ventilator
	1	Coughing but tolerating
	2	Fighting ventilator
	0	Talking in normal tone or no sound
	1	Sighing, moaning
	2	Crying out, sobbing
Muscle tension	0	Relaxed
	1	Tense, rigid
	2	Very tense or rigid

[20] and the Critical Care Pain Observation Tool (CPOT) [21]. When using the BPS, it is suggested to treat pain greater than or equal to six. Severe or unacceptable pain is a score greater than two in the CPOT score (see Table 4). These scoring tools can be utilized for initiation of medications on an as needed basis or for use when titrating continuous infusions.

6 Sedation Interruptions

Sedation interruptions have been described as safe [19], however conflicting data has emerged when comparing said interventions to targeted light sedation [6] and notably major studies on daily sedation interruption involved patients receiving primarily benzodiazepines [22]. Furthermore, most studies on sedation interruptions have not included patients with acute brain injury, on which data on sedation interruptions is scant [23].

There are cases wherein abrupt sedative cessation may be deleterious, e.g. ICP crisis. In one study, sedation interruption led to increased ICP and lactate to pyruvate ratio as per microdialysis in subarachnoid hemorrhage and traumatic brain injury patients [23]. Some authors have found in favor of targeted minimal sedation for these patients [19].

7 Pitfalls

Analgosdation in the NCCU is a balancing act. Over-sedation is associated with increased lengths of stay and mortality, as well as worse long term recovery [2], while under-sedation may lead to long-term sequelae [6, 8]. The former also mars the neurological exam, which may lead to underdetection of neurological complications.

Additionally, sedatives are noted to decrease cerebral blood flow, this is often accompanied with a commensurate decrease in $CMRO_2$. However, systemic effects of several sedatives and analgesics include systemic hypotension which may exacerbate secondary injury [5], thus careful monitoring of vital signs is paramount in order to avoid complications.

8 Summary

- The goal of sedation in the NCCU is to achieve patient comfort and optimal care delivery while administering the least amount of analgosedation possible.
- Drug selection must take patient factors such as primary indication, mechanisms of action and elimination, half-life and therapeutic goal, e.g. RASS −1 to 0.
- A common side effect of sedatives or analgesic is hypotension, which is to be promptly treated in order to avoid complications such as secondary brain injury.

References

1. Makii JM, Mirski MA, Lewin JJ. Sedation and analgesia in critically ill neurologic patients. J Pharm Pract. 2010;23(5):455–69.
2. Aitken LM, Bucknall T, Kent B, Mitchell M, Burmeister E, Keogh SJ. Protocol-directed sedation versus non-protocol-directed sedation in mechanically ventilated intensive care adults and children. Cochrane Database of Syst Rev. 2018;11(11):CD009771.
3. Opdenakker O, Vanstraelen A, De Sloovere V, Meyfroidt G. Sedatives in neurocritical care: an update on pharmacological agents and modes of sedation. Curr Opin Crit Care. 2019;25(2):97–104.
4. Vanaclocha N, Chisbert V, Quilis V, Bilotta F, Badenes R. Sedation during neurocritical care. J Neuroanaesthesiol Crit Care. 2019;6:56–61.
5. Oddo M, Crippa IA, Mehta S, Menon D, Payen JF, Taccone FS, Citerio G. Optimizing sedation in patients with acute brain injury. Crit Care. 2016;20(1):128.
6. Devlin JW, Skrobik Y, Gélinas C, Needham DM, Slooter AJ, Pandharipande PP, et al. Clinical practice guidelines for the prevention and management of pain, agitation/sedation, delirium, immobility, and sleep disruption in adult patients in the ICU. Crit Care Med. 2018;46(9):e825–73.
7. Paul BS, Paul G. Sedation in neurological intensive care unit. Ann Indian Acad Neurol. 2013;16:194–202.
8. Caballero J, García-Sánchez M, Palencia-Herrejón E, Muñoz-Martínez T, Gómez-García JM, Ceniceros-Rozalén I. Oversedation Zero as a tool for comfort, safety and management in the intensive care unit. Med Intensiva (Engl Ed). 2020;44(4):239–47.
9. Oddo M, Crippa IA, Mehta S, et al. Optimizing sedation in patients with acute brain injury. Crit Care. 2016;20:128. https://doi.org/10.1186/s13054-016-1294-5.
10. Eriksen N, Rostrup E, Fabricius M, Scheel M, Major S, Winkler MKL, Bohner G, Santos E, Sakowitz OW, Kola V, Reiffurth C, Hartings JA, Vajkoczy P, Woitzik J, Martus P, Lauritzen M, Pakkenberg B, Dreier JP. Early focal brain injury after subarachnoid hemorrhage correlates with spreading depolarizations. Neurology. 2019;92(4):e326–41. https://doi.org/10.1212/WNL.0000000000006814.
11. Fentanyl. In: Specific Lexicomp Online Database [database on the Internet]. Hudson (OH): Lexicomp Inc.; 2021 [updated 05

Mar. 2021; cited 10 Mar. 2021]. Available from: http://online.lexi.com. Subscription required to view.
12. Remifentanil. In: Specific Lexicomp Online Database [database on the Internet]. Hudson (OH): Lexicomp Inc.; 2021 [updated 01 Feb. 2021; cited 10 Mar. 2021]. Available from: http://online.lexi.com. Subscription required to view.
13. Midazolam. In: Specific Lexicomp Online Database [database on the Internet]. Hudson (OH): Lexicomp Inc.; 2021 [updated 03 Mar. 2021; cited 10 Mar. 2021]. Available from: http://online.lexi.com. Subscription required to view.
14. Propofol. In: Specific Lexicomp Online Database [database on the Internet]. Hudson (OH): Lexicomp Inc.; 2021 [updated 05 Mar. 2021; cited 10 Mar. 2021]. Available from: http://online.lexi.com. Subscription required to view.
15. Ketamine. In: Specific Lexicomp Online Database [database on the Internet]. Hudson (OH): Lexicomp Inc.; 2021 [updated 01 Mar. 2021; cited 10 Mar. 2021]. Available from: http://online.lexi.com. Subscription required to view.
16. Dexmedetomidine. In: Specific Lexicomp Online Database [database on the Internet]. Hudson (OH): Lexicomp Inc.; 2021 [updated 19 Feb. 2021; cited 10 Mar. 2021]. Available from: http://online.lexi.com. Subscription required to view.
17. Sessler CN, Gosnell MS, Grap MJ, Brophy GM, O'Neal PV, Keane KA, et al. The Richmond Agitation-Sedation Scale: validity and reliability in adult intensive care unit patients. Am J Respir Crit Care Med. 2002;166(10):1338–44.
18. Riker R, Picard J, Fraser G. Prospective evaluation of the Sedation-Agitation Scale for adult critically ill patients. Crit Care Med. 1999;27(7):1325–9.
19. Nassar AP, Junior PM. Sedation protocols versus daily sedation interruption: a systematic review and meta-analysis. Rev Bras Ter Intensiva. 2016;28(4):444–51.
20. Payen JF, Bru O, Bosson JL, et al. Assessing pain in critically ill sedated patients by using a behavioral pain scale. Crit Care Med. 2001;29(12):2258–63.
21. Gélinas C, Fillion L, Puntillo KA, Viens C, Fortier M. Validation of the critical-care pain observation tool in adult patients. Am J Crit Care. 2006;15(4):420–7.

22. Kress JP, Pohlman AS, O'Connor MF, Hall JB. Daily interruption of sedative infusions in critically ill patients undergoing mechanical ventilation. N Engl J Med. 2000;342(20):1471–7.
23. Helbok R, Kurtz P, Schmidt MJ, Stuart MR, Fernandez L, Connolly SE, et al. Effects of the neurological wake-up test on clinical examination, intracranial pressure, brain metabolism and brain tissue oxygenation in severely brain-injured patients. Crit Care. 2012;16(6):R226.

Intracranial Hypertension in Intensive Care Unit

Niraj Arora and Chandra Shekar Pingili

1 Introduction

Intracranial Hypertension (IH) is a commonly encountered condition in the Neuro-critical Care Unit (NCCU). Left untreated, it carries a high mortality (80–100%) [1]. Normal values of Intracranial Pressure (ICP) vary with age. Most adults and older children have values of 10–15 mmHg, while that of young children and infants ranges between of 3–7 mmHg and 1.5–6 mmHg, respectively [2]. As per recent Brain Trauma Foundation guidelines, ICP values higher than 22 mmHg are s associated with high mortality and warrant treatment [3]. However, a temporal component of the area under curve may also play a role, one study found ICP more than 20 mmHg for more than 20% of the monitoring time could be a more accurate definition for IH [4]. Persistent elevation in ICPs more than 40 mmHg is life threatening. Therefore, urgent, and timely intervention is a keystone for management.

N. Arora (✉)
Department of Neurology- Neurocriticalcare unit, University of Missouri, Columbia, MO, USA
e-mail: arorana@health.missouri.edu

C. S. Pingili
Dayton Lung and Sleep Medicine, Inc, Dayton, OH, USA

© The Author(s), under exclusive license to Springer Nature Switzerland AG 2022
N. Arora (ed.), *Procedures and Protocols in the Neurocritical Care Unit*, https://doi.org/10.1007/978-3-030-90225-4_15

1.1 Pathophysiology of Raised ICP

The Brain is encased within the rigid calvarium, with very little reserve (60–80 mL in young, 100–140 mL in elderly) [2] for expansion (Fig. 1). Based on the Monro-Kellie doctrine [1, 2, 5], the sum volume of brain, CSF and blood is constant and any increase in one component must cause a proportional decrease in the other component. During the initial phase of injury, up to 30 mL of intracranial volume expansion is compensated by CSF and venous blood movement out of the cranial vault. Intracranial compliance is determined by the compressibility of the expanding constituents. Blood and CSF are non-compressible (as in intracranial haemorrhage or acute hydrocephalus) and cause rapid rise in intracranial pressure however, brain parenchyma is more compressible and the rise in ICP happens gradually (as in tumours or other space occupying lesions).

The ICP waveform (Fig. 2) is pulsatile with respiratory and cardiac cycle correlates. Amplitude of respiratory waves varies between 2 and 10 mmHg due to changes in intrathoracic pressure and the variation is obscured with elevated ICP. Amplitude of the cardiac component of the ICP wave varies between 1 and 4 mmHg due to pressure dynamics and forms three waveforms. When ICP is elevated (Fig. 3), P2

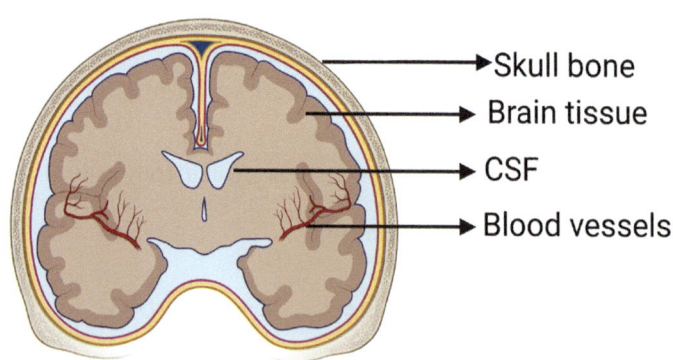

FIGURE 1 Normal intracranial contents: Brain tissue, CSF and Blood

Intracranial Hypertension in Intensive Care Unit 291

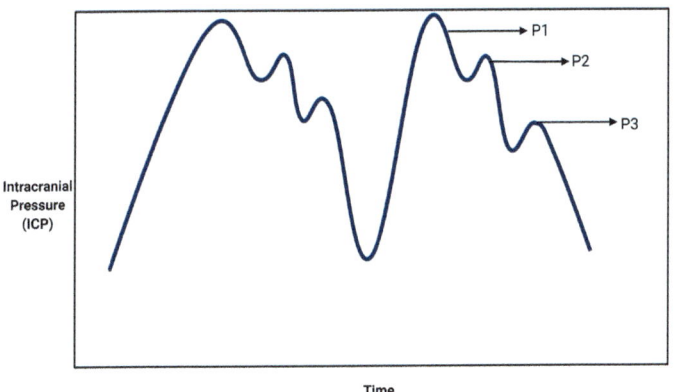

FIGURE 2 Normal ICP waveform

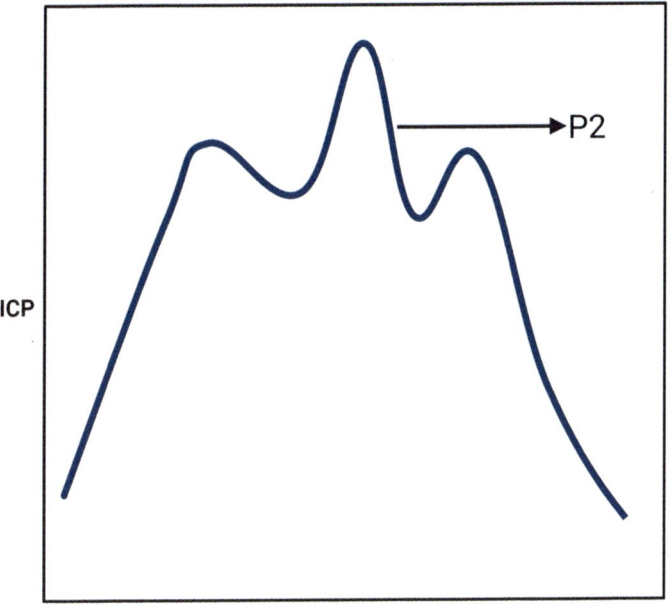

FIGURE 3 Waveform in elevated ICP

component is elevated and assumes the shape of arterial pulse (P2 > P1), also the cardiac waveform amplitude increases while the respiratory waveform amplitude decreases along with rounding off the waveform. Due vigilance to such changes in waveforms can lead to early intervention and timely management.

Historically, elevated ICP can lead to characteristic waveforms known as Lundberg A, B and C waves (Fig. 4). These waveforms are not seen frequently in the bedside monitors as they are plotted over time and are not the individual waveform patterns. The goal is not to wait for pathological waveforms to develop to initiate treatment but to treat the underlying cause of raised ICP and prevent brain herniation. Lundberg C waves are related to blood pressure variation and are of no pathological significance.

While ICP monitoring is a useful tool to measure cerebral compliance, the necessity is to maintain cerebral perfusion pressure (CPP) in the brain. CPP is the difference between the mean arterial pressure (MAP) and the Intracranial Pressure (ICP). (CPP = MAP-ICP). It is recommended to maintain a CPP goal of 50–70 mmHg. The cerebral circulation is capable of self regulation in which there is a change in the intracranial vessel diameter to maintain a constant cerebral blood flow (CBF) over a wide range of cerebral perfusion pressure (CPP) and metabolic factors especially PaCO2 (Fig. 5).

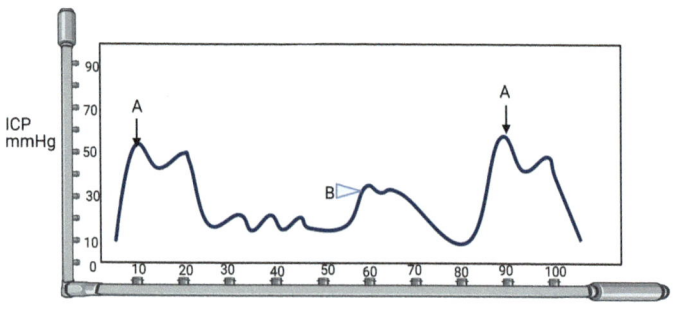

FIGURE 4 Elevated ICP with characteristic waveforms

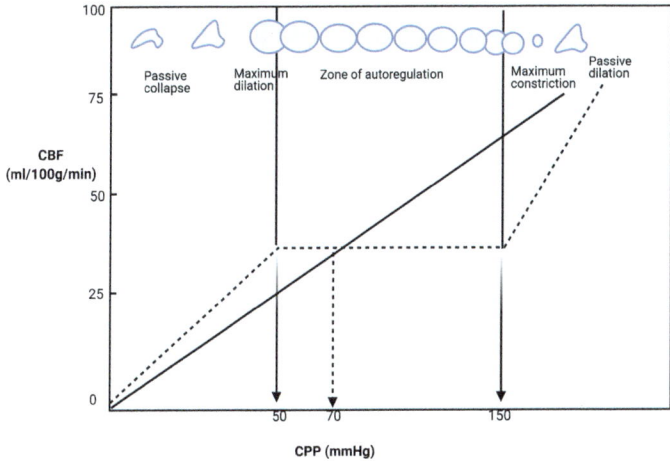

FIGURE 5 Cerebral autoregulation curve

In the absence of available CBF monitoring, CPP is used as a surrogate marker for CBF [2, 3]. Overtreatment of CPP could lead to hyperaemia and vasogenic edema while undertreatment could lead to ischemia especially when autoregulation has failed due to underlying brain injury.

Metabolic factors regulating the CBF are CO_2, potassium, adenosine, nitric oxide and prostaglandins. Elevated CO_2 causes lowering of pH which leads to arteriolar dilation which in turn increases CBF and raises ICP [2]. For every 1 mmHg rise in the $PaCO_2$, CBF increases by 4%. On the other hand, hypoxia with PaO_2 below 50 mmHg and hypoglycaemia decreases cerebral blood flow [6] Statins have been proven to improve autoregulation of the nitric oxide reserves [7].

1.2 Etiology of Elevated ICP: [8–12]

There are multiple causes of elevated ICP as However, in the acute setting the most common cause of elevated ICP is cerebral edema from traumatic brain injury, ischemic or hemorrhagic stroke (Table 1).

TABLE 1 Causes of raised ICP

1. Increased brain volume
  (A) Cerebral edema from strokes, trauma
  (B) Hyperammonemia
  (C) Uremia
  (D) Hyponatremia
  (E) Rapid correction of hypernatremia

2. Increased blood flow:
  (A) Hypercarbia causing vasodilation
  (B) Hyperdynamic circulations
  (C) Arterio-venous malformations
  (D) Venous stasis from thrombus, tumors, and epidural or subdural bleeds

3. Increased csf production:
  (A) Ependymal tumors

4. Decreased CSF absorption:
  (A) Obstructive hydrocephalus
  (B) Ventriculitis/meningitis
  (C) Blood clots
  (D) Granulomatous inflammation
  (E) Spinal tumors

5. Mass affects:
  (A) Tumors
  (B) Abscess
  (C) Bleeds
  (D) Blood clots

6. Other causes: Generally seen in the outpatient set up
  (A) Idiopathic hydrocephalus-
  (B) Tetracyclines
  (C) Oral contraceptives
  (D) Hypervitaminosis A
  (E) Craniosynostosis

1.3 Clinical Features: Table 2 [13–15]

Clinical features in raised ICP vary according to the cause and location of the acute setting; clinical features are common, irrespective of the mechanism of injury. Nausea and

TABLE 2 Symptoms and signs in raised ICP

Symptoms	Comments
Headaches	Worse in the morning hours and with bending, coughing/straining
Nausea/vomiting	Projectile vomiting
Diplopia and/or anisocoria	Due to sixth and/or third nerve palsy
Papilledema	May not develop for several days
Downward deviation of eyeballs (Sunset eyes)	Due to lesion in dorsal midbrain
Cushing's triad: Elevated blood pressure, bradycardia, and abnormal breathing pattern.	Brain herniation (Usually a late sign)

vomiting, dizziness, headache and blurred vision are early symptoms of raised ICP. New anisocoria >1 mm, dilated pupils, lateral rectus palsy and worsened weakness or ataxia are also the early signs. Decreasing level of consciousness related to compression upon thalamus and brainstem is an alarming sign of potentially life threatening raised ICP due to cerebral edema. Focal deficits (hemiplegia, global or expressive aphasia, severe dysarthria, neglect, gaze preference, and a visual field defect) results from direct insults to the cortex or subcortical areas. Herniation syndromes are the worst dreadful complications of the elevated ICP, and immediate treatment is essential to prevent irreversible damage (Tables 3 and 4).

1.4 ICP Monitoring: [1, 2, 8, 13, 16]

ICP monitoring serves as the cornerstone for better management of acute neurological injuries. The ideal system should be simple, inexpensive, accurate, reliable and with minimal complications. The **invasive transducer monitoring system**

TABLE 3 Herniation syndromes

Type of herniation/definition	Structures involved	Symptoms/signs
1. Sub-falcine Herniation (herniation of anterior fossa contents under falx)	Cingulate gyrus	Asymptomatic Headache Loss of attention and apathy. Contralateral leg weakness due to ACA circulation kinking is a late finding. Measured radiologically by shift of septum pellucidum away from midline.
2. Descending central herniation (Structures move down through the tentorium cerebelli)	Diencephalon Uncus Pituitary stalk Bilateral PCA	Central DI Posturing (flexion/extension) Cortical blindness Duret hemorrhages (due to shearing of perforators from basilar artery) Periodic breathing pattern
3. Ascending central herniation (infratentorial lesions cause structures to move upwards)	Thalami Midbrain SCAs Cerebral aqueduct	Posturing Acute hydrocephalus Asymmetric pupils
4. Trans-calvarial herniation (Brain mater herniates through defect in skull)	Vary according to site	Vary according to site involved

TABLE 3 (continued)

Type of herniation/ definition	Structures involved	Symptoms/signs
5. Uncal herniation or Lateral trans-tentorial herniation (medial temporal lobe herniates further medially)	Third nerve Crus cerebri PCAs	First, compress the ipsilateral third nerve (parasympathetic) leading to the dilated pupil. Later, compress the motor part of the ipsilateral third nerve: leading to downward and outward gaze from fourth and sixth nerve activity. Ipsilateral crus cerebri compression leads to contralateral weakness. Contralateral cerebral crus compression leads to false localizing signs of ipsilateral weakness. (Kernohan's phenomenon) Ipsilateral PCA involvement with contralateral homonymous hemianopsia: usually not apparent due to altered mentation. Brain stem compression with worsening pressure: Flexion posturing.

(continued)

TABLE 3 (continued)

Type of herniation/ definition	Structures involved	Symptoms/signs
6. Tonsillar herniation (terminal result of any type of herniation)	Cerebellar tonsils herniate through the foramen magnum Medulla	Respiratory arrest Cushing's triad

ACA anterior cerebral artery, *PCA* posterior cerebral artery, *SCA* superior cerebellar artery, *DI* diabetes insipidus

with use of EVD with catheter placement in the ventricular system is considered the gold standard. Detailed discussion about the ICP monitoring system and EVD placement is done in a separate chapter. Other invasive systems with catheter placement in subarachnoid, epidural or subdural locations have less utility in clinical practice. Main complication of invasive systems is the risk of infection and hemorrhage and antibiotic and silver impregnated catheters have been developed to mitigate that risk. **Non-invasive monitoring systems** using ultrasound technique measuring optic nerve sheath diameter, use of transcranial doppler, pupillometry or EEG are some of the techniques which have some evidence for ICP estimation but would need long term validation in clinical trials (Table 5).

1.5 Indications for ICP Monitoring Devices [3]

Considerable variability exists in the clinical practice about the placement of ICP monitoring devices. However, it is generally accepted that severe acute neurological injury with the potential to raise ICP merits ICP monitoring. Specific guidelines have been published for severe traumatic brain injury. In severe TBI cases with a normal CT scan, ICP monitoring is indicated if two or more of the following features are noted at admission: (1) Age over 40 years, (2) Unilateral or bilateral motor posturing, or (3) Systolic blood pressure <90 mmHg.

TABLE 4 Stages of central and lateral transtentorial herniation

	Uncal herniation (lateral transtentorial)			Central transtentorial herniation			
	Stages			Stages			
Clinical Features	Early third nerve	Late third nerve	Midbrain-Pons	Diencephalic	Midbrain-Upper pons	Lower pons-Upper Medullar	Medullar
Consciousness	May be normal. Not a reliable sign	Stupor or coma		Altered (agitation, stupor or coma)	Comatose	Comatose	Comatose
Pupils	Ipsilateral dilating pupil (may be sluggish)	Ipsilateral dilated	Contralateral pupil dilated and then bilateral pupil dilated (5–6 mm)	Small (1–3 mm) but Reactive. May develop Perinaud's syndrome	Midposition (3–5 mm), fixed	Midposition (3–5 mm), fixed	Dilated (>5 mm)
Oculomotor	Doll's eye: normal or dysconjugate. CWC: slow ipsilateral deviation	External oculomotor ophthalmoplegia	External oculomotor ophthalmoplegia	Doll's eyes: conjugate. CWC positive.	Dysconjugate eye movements, impaired Doll's eyes and CWC.	Absent Doll's eyes and CWC.	Absent Doll's eyes and CWC.
Respirations	Normal Appropriate response.	Hyperpnea (CNH)	Hyperpnea (CNH)	Sighs, yawns and later Chyne-Stokes.	Chyne-Stokes or sustained tachypnea	Tachypnea but shallow breathing	Ataxic breathing

(continued)

TABLE 3 (continued)

Clinical Features	Uncal herniation (lateral transtentorial)				Central transtentorial herniation			
	Stages				Stages			
	Early third nerve	Late third nerve	Midbrain-Pons		Diencephalic	Midbrain-Upper pons	Lower pons-Upper Medullar	Medullar
Motor	Contralateral Babinski positive	Contralateral hemiplegia. May develop ipsilateral hemiplegia (Kernohan's phenomenon) and then bilateral decerebration.	Bilateral decerebrate posturing		Early: appropriate motor response, Upper motor neuron signs. Later: Motionless and then decorticate posturing	Decorticate and then bilateral decerebrate	Flaccid. Occasional Triple flexion to pain	No response. Occasional Triple Flexion to pain.

TABLE 5 Non-invasive modalities for ICP estimation

Technique	Rationale
Optic Nerve Sheath diameter (ONSD): Measured with linear transducer probe (13–7.5 MHz) positioned over closed eyelid and at 3 mm depth from posterior pole of eyeball. Diameter of 4.5–5.5 mm indicates raised ICP.	Screening tool
Transcranial Doppler (TCD)	Based on Gosling's Pulsatility Index (PI), ICP can be calculated. ICP = $10.93 \times PI - 1.28$.
Near Infra-red Spectroscopy (NIRS)	Based on principle of light absorption to detect changes in concentration of oxygen and deoxyhemoglobin. More evidence is needed before its use is justified.
Electroencephalogram (EEG)	Neurophysiological changes precede ICP changes and certain components of EEG power spectrum analysis may be useful in correlating with ICP prediction
Pupillometry	There is an inverse association between ICP and pupillary reactivity exists. Cannot provide direct ICP value.
Visual Evoked Response (VER): N2 wave found at 70 ms represent cortical phenomenon.	Relationship between raised ICP and a shift in latency of the N2 wave.

(continued)

TABLE 5 (continued)

Technique	Rationale
Venous Opthalmodynamometry	CRV pressure measurement or ophthalmodynamometry showed good correlation with invasive ICP monitoring but it was not useful for continuous monitoring.
Tympanic membrane displacement (TMD): Cochlear fluid would affect stapedial excursions and TMD measured in response to auditory stimulation would represent the ICP.	Screening tool. Does not provide specific ICP value. Need intact middle ear apparatus.
Radiological techniques	CT/MRI criteria

1.6 Role of Fundoscopy: [17–22]

Fundoscopy for detection of papilledema is a fundamental ophthalmologic technique a neurologist should know. Papilledema is the bulging of the optic disc which can be acute or chronic. Non-ICP related pathologies such as central retinal arterial or venous occlusion, congenital anomalies, and optic neuritis from infectious and inflammatory causes can also cause papilledema. For the purpose of this chapter, the discussion of papilledema would be limited to ICU related conditions only. Fundoscopic examination of the retina for papilledema is one useful, non-invasive bedside test to screen for elevated ICP and recurrence of ICP after discontinuation of an EVD or after hemicraniectomy. Papilledema can often be a delayed clinical sign from ICP especially in patients with epidural hematoma involving the vertex region compressing the superior sagittal sinus. Not all patients with ICP will have papilledema. Papilledema can be unilateral or bilateral. In patients with brain bleeds, especially from aneurysmal bleeds, papilledema can happen within hours (16%) and is most of the time ipsilateral. Ironically, TBI patients only have a 3.5% chance of having papilledema despite elevated ICP, and the absence of a swollen disc doesn't correlate with the existing ICP. Papilledema can often be delayed by 2 weeks in TBI patients, usually a consequence of hydrocephalus and cerebral edema.

1.7 Management: [3, 23–28]

The management of raised ICP requires timely vigilance and due diligence to prevent the ongoing secondary injury. For a list of possible interventions for ICP management see Table 6.

TABLE 6 General measures for management of raised ICP

Measures	Method	Rationale
Bed position	30–45° HOB elevation	Increases venous return outflow from cranial vault and also reduces mean carotid pressure but no net change in CBF
Neck Position	Keep neck straight, avoid tight ties around neck	Avoid constriction of jugular venous outflow
Maintain airway and adequate oxygenation, intubation if need.	Goal PaO2 >60 mmHg or O2 saturation >90%	Hypoxia causes further ischemic brain injury
Temperature modulation (Goal: Normothermia-37–37.5 °C)	Acetaminophen Cooling measures (Non-invasive devices or invasive devices)	Maintain normothermia. Fever increases metabolic demand and increases CBF and ICP which in turn exacerbates cerebral edema.

(continued)

TABLE 6 (continued)

Measures	Method	Rationale
Hyperventilation	Mechanical ventilation with goal PaCO2 30–35 mmHg	Lowers ICP by reducing PaCO2 which causes cerebral vasoconstriction thus reducing the cerebral blood volume (CBV) and cerebral blood flow (CBF) [29]. Use briefly for clinical evidence of raised ICP (neurologic deterioration) or chronically for documented raised ICP unresponsive to other measures.
Glucose control (Goal 140–180 mg%)	Insulin therapy	Hyperglycemia causes increased oxidative load, cerebral edema and hemorrhagic transformation of ischemic stroke and inflammation. Hyperglycemia exacerbates cerebral edema and perihematomal cell death in ICH which leads to worse clinical outcomes.

TABLE 6 (continued)

Measures	Method	Rationale
Antiepileptic therapy	Antiepileptic drugs	Decrease cortical irritability in high risk injuries
Treatment of hypotension (Goal SBP >90 mmHg)	Norepinephrine, Phenyleprine, Epinephrine	Normalize intravascular volume and maintain euvolemia
Treatment of Malignant hypertension	Labetalol, Nicardipine, Hydralazine	Treatment of underlying condition for goal SBP.

These measures are based on simple rationales and cannot replace the more definitive therapies. Definitive treatment of the underlying cause is pivotal to successful management of elevated ICP (Table 7). CSF diversion with EVD placement allows CSF drainage and decreases intracranial volume. Surgical approach in the form of hemicraniectomy has been shown to decrease mortality in the short term but no long-term difference [3]. Tiered approach to the ICP management is shown in the Fig. 6. The strategy is three-pronged (1) Maintain ICP less than 22 mmHg (2) Definite treatment of underlying cause (Tumor, hemorrhage, hematoma) (3) Maintain CPP >50–70 mmHg. The latter is achieved with MAP augmentation with fluids, pressors, oral midodrine, and reducing the PEEP on the ventilator.

1.8 Surgery [30–32]

Decompressive hemicraniectomy and surgical evacuation of the inciting aetiologies will be the key treatment strategies in the management of elevated ICP especially in patients with compressive tumours and hemispheric strokes with a positive

TABLE 7 Definitive measures for management of raised ICP

Measures	Drugs	Rationale
Sedation, analgesia with or without paralytics	Combination of short acting opioid (Fentanyl or remifentanil), propofol +/− vecuronium/ rocuronium	Reduce agitation which decreases metabolic demand, improves ventilator synchrony, decreases sympathetic responses (hypertension and tachycardia)
Osmotic therapy (Goal serum osmolality up to 320 mmol/L)	Mannitol Hypertonic saline (3%, 23%)	Expands plasma volume, improves rheologic properties of blood, cause fluid shift into intravascular space via osmotic gradient.
CSF diversion with EVD insertion	none	Decrease the CSF volume
Surgical treatment (Hemicraniectomy/ Craniotomy)	none	Specific indications per pathological condition
Medical Coma (Complete cerebral activity suppression)	Pentobarbital	Decrease metabolic rate and CBV and hence ICP reduction. Continuous EEG monitoring is a must.
Abdominal Decompression	Laparotomy	Help in ICP reduction in some cases when other measures fail [28]

impact on the short term and long-term prognosis. Decompression surgeries have improved survival in ICH patients too but its effects on long-term prognosis are still debated.

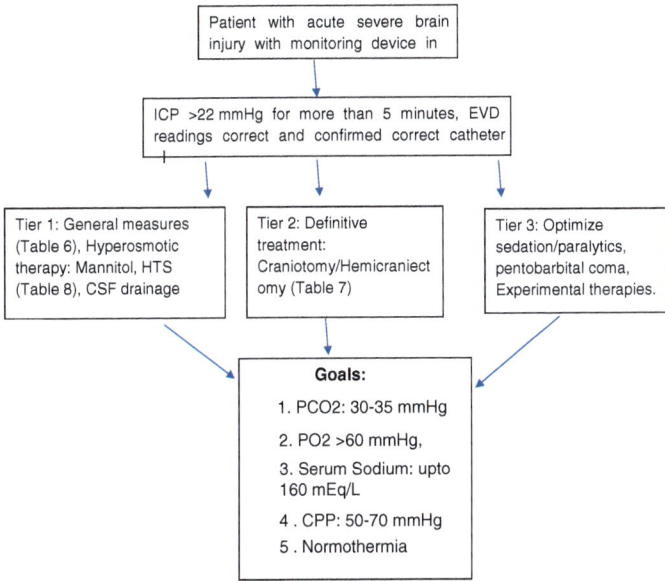

FIGURE 6 Simplified tiered management protocol for raised ICP. In practice, combination of approaches is used to appropriately control ICP. Role of multimodal monitoring is not included in the current practice

1.9 Mannitol [33–35]

Mannitol is a sugar alcohol that is filtered at the glomerulus and not reabsorbed from the renal tubules. It acts like an osmotic diuretic i.e.; it leads to free water clearance and increases serum osmolality. Mannitol reduces the blood viscosity and causes expansion of plasma which in turn decreases cerebral oxygen delivery (rheological effect). Since mannitol does not cross the blood-brain barrier, there is an osmotic gradient between the brain and intravascular space which leads to reduction in brain tissue volume. Effects can be seen as early as within 10–15 min, peak in 20–120 min and lasts for

1–5 h. This drug is contraindicated in patients with acute kidney injury with oliguria or anuria, pulmonary edema (osmotic diuresis could flood the low-pressure chambers in the pulmonary venous system), severe dehydration, acute congestive heart failure, allergy to mannitol. There is a risk of crystal deposition in-vivo which is eliminated using an 0.22 micron in-line filter. It is advised to taper this drug instead of abruptly stopping the scheduled infusions. Mannitol can cross the placenta and to date, there are no recommendations to and against the use of this drug in the pregnant population. Dosing for mannitol is given in Table 8.

Hypertonic Saline (HTS): [34, 36] HTS works by creating the osmotic fluid shifts from intracellular space to intravascular space with subsequent expansion of the intravascular volume, this increases blood pressure, cardiac output and cerebral blood flow. Normal plasma osmolarity is 280–295 mOsm/L while HTS osmolarity is 1026–8008 mOsm/L depending on the concentration (3–23.4%). HTS has better short-term outcomes in controlling ICP but over all there is no long-term difference in the clinical outcomes as compared to mannitol. It can be given as a bolus or continuous infusion and both have been found to be effective. However, in emergency situations like transtentorial herniation and elevated ICP, a bolus of 23.4% was found to be most effective. Commonly, bolus of 3% 250 mL HTS is given, followed by continuous infusion of 3% HTS at 50–100 mL per hour, with a goal of increasing the serum sodium by approximately 5 mEq/L in the first hour and maintaining the serum sodium between 145 and 155 mEq/L thereafter. For practical purposes, the maximum allowed serum sodium is 160 mEq/L. Hyperchloremia is associated with renal complications and must be avoided where possible. There is a risk of rapid correction of hyponatremia and pontine myelinolysis too. Like mannitol, HTS is also considered a category C drug in pregnancy and should be used only if really needed.

Table 8 Commonly used medications with doses

Medication/Route/Duration	Dose and monitoring	Side effects/complications
Mannitol (20% or 25%)/peripheral access/90 min–6 h	1 g/kg bolus (0.5–1.5 g/kg) over 5–15 min followed by 0.5 g/kg q4–6 h. Monitor serum osmolality.[a]	Dehydration Hypotension Acute kidney injury Rebound ICP elevation Electrolyte disturbances
Hypertonic saline (HTS)[b]/central access/90 min–4 h	3%: 5 mL/kg bolus over 5–20 min (central line preferred) 23%: 30 mL over 5–10 min (only through central line)	Pulmonary edema Heart failure Acute kidney injury Hypernatremia, hyperchloremia acidosis. Osmotic demyelination with rapid sodium increase
Pentobarbital/central or peripheral/long acting	3–7 mg/kg bolus followed by 1–5 mg/kg/h continuous infusion	Hypotension Inability to follow neurological examination. Respiratory depression and mucus plugging

[a]Mannitol should be avoided when serum osmolality becomes >320 mOsm/L or specifically if osmolar gap >20. Osmolar gap = calculated osmolality (mOsm/kg) - measured osmolarity (mOsm/L). It is a measure of serum mannitol level and its clearance. Calculated Osmolality = (Na × 2 + glucose/18) + (blood urea nitrogen [BUN]/2.3)
[b]HTS is available in 2%, 3%, 7.5% and 23.4% concentrations

There is a potential role of osmolytes such as 8.4% sodium bicarbonate and hypertonic lactate in the management of elevated ICP. However, further research is warranted before these could be used in clinical practice [37, 38].

1.10 Sedation: [16, 27, 39]

Pain, agitation, seizures, fevers, and shivering all contribute to elevated ICP. While opiates have been proven to increase ICP in patients with intact cerebrovascular autoregulation, fentanyl has an analgesic and sedative property with a short half-life and is a useful drug in the management of ICP surges. Propofol is another drug used in the NCCU with sedative and antiepileptic properties. Both these mechanisms are exploited by clinicians in the management of ICP surges. Propofol however has no benefit on 6-month survival or neurological outcome. Cisatracurium [29] as a bolus or as an infusion is a well-tested strategy in the management of ICP surges. Ketamine will not worsen the ICP and on the other hand has good neuroprotective, antiseizure, analgesic, and sedative properties [40]. Pentobarbital coma is often used as a last resort in the management of refractory ICP. Less than 20% of all NCCU admits with ICP issues end up on this protocol. Barbiturates work by reducing brain metabolism and oxygen consumption and decreasing not just the CPP but also the ICP. However, there is no long-term clinical benefit from this protocol. Pentobarbital can complicate the clinical picture with hypotension, bone marrow suppression, severe ileus, and dilated cardiomyopathy. Propylene glycol is one additive in the pentobarbital infusion that will contribute to high anion gap acidosis [41, 42]. Midazolam also works by reducing cerebral metabolism and antiseizure properties and helps reduce the ICP [43]. Most of the sedatives and analgesics reduce the MAP and CPP. This will be counterproductive as this will worsen cerebral perfusion. MAP augmentation should be achieved with fluid boluses and maintenance doses, as-needed use of vasopressor drugs, oral midodrine. PEEP on the ventilator should theoretically increase the intrathoracic pressures and reduce the venous return from the brain and indirectly contribute to ICP surges. However, a search of literature doesn't reveal any direct correlation between higher PEEP and ICP surges.

1.11 Temperature Modulation

Hypothermia is well known to reduce the ICP, but the overall prognosis is not altered [44]. Normothermia is recommended in the management of ICP. Therapeutic hypothermia reduces ICP but leads to high mortality and poor functional outcome.

2 Lumbar Drain (LD)

An external lumbar drain can be used to estimate and control the ICP. There are case reports that support the use of LD with a good neurological outcome at 6 months. The risk of infection is around 4% [45].

2.1 Future Directions

The management of ICP continues to evolve but not much therapeutic advances have been made in this field. Multimodality monitoring could potentially modulate the outcomes as more targeted physiology directed treatments are provided. Threshold to initiate such treatments can vary from patient to patient which could provide a more personalised approach to medicine [46, 47]. One of the important randomized clinical trial determining the comparative effectiveness of ICP and brain tissue oxygen (PbtO2) in patient with TBI is underway [48].Whether multimodality monitors comprising of ICP, CBF, $PbtO_2$, cerebral metabolism, and electrocortical activity have a role in patient management still needs to be determined in large clinical trials however as per the current evidence these modalities improve the neurologic variables without any improvement in patient outcomes [49, 50].

References

1. Bumberger A, Braunsteiner T, Leitgeb J, Haider T. Intracranial pressure monitoring following traumatic brain injury: evaluation of indications, complications, and significance of follow-up imaging—an exploratory, retrospective study of consecutive patients at a level I trauma center. Eur J Trauma Emerg Surg. 2020:1–8. https://doi.org/10.1007/s00068-020-01570-3.
2. Nag DS, Sahu S, Swain A, Kant S. Intracranial pressure monitoring: gold standard and recent innovations. World J Clin Cases. 2019;7(13):1535–53. https://doi.org/10.12998/wjcc.v7.i13.1535.
3. Carney N, et al. Guidelines for the management of severe traumatic brain injury, fourth edition. Neurosurgery. 2017;80(1):6–15. https://doi.org/10.1227/NEU.0000000000001432.
4. Crippa IA, Creteur J, Smielewski P, Taccone FS, Czosnyka M. Delay of cerebral autoregulation in traumatic brain injury patients. Clin Neurol Neurosurg. 2021;202:106478. https://doi.org/10.1016/j.clineuro.2021.106478.
5. Bugedo G, Santis C. Intracranial hypertension and deep sedation. Crit Care. 2019;23(1):342. https://doi.org/10.1186/s13054-019-2578-3.
6. Silverman A, Petersen NH. Physiology, cerebral autoregulation. In: StatPearls. Treasure Island (FL): StatPearls Publishing; 2020.
7. Rasmusen C, Cynober L, Couderc R. Arginine and statins: relationship between the nitric oxide pathway and the atherosclerosis development. Ann Biol Clin (Paris). 2005;63(5):443–55.
8. Pinto VL, Tadi P, Adeyinka A. Increased intracranial pressure. In: StatPearls. Treasure Island (FL): StatPearls Publishing; 2020.
9. Lin AL, Avila EK. Neurologic emergencies in the cancer patient: diagnosis and management. J Intensive Care Med. 2017;32(2):99–115. https://doi.org/10.1177/0885066615619582.
10. Zhao P-P, et al. Increased intracranial pressure in Guillain–Barré syndrome. Medicine (Baltimore). 2018;97(30):e11584. https://doi.org/10.1097/MD.0000000000011584.
11. Elgallab J, Graber J. Hydrocephalus in Neurofibromatosis-Three cases with different etiologies. (P2.104). Neurology. 2015;84(14 Supplement):P2.104. Accessed: Dec. 28, 2020. [Online]. Available: https://n.neurology.org/content/84/14_Supplement/P2.104.
12. Tofteng F, Hauerberg J, Hansen BA, Pedersen CB, Jørgensen L, Larsen FS. Persistent arterial hyperammonemia increases the concentration of glutamine and alanine in the brain and

correlates with intracranial pressure in patients with fulminant hepatic failure. J Cereb Blood Flow Metab. 2006;26(1):21–7. https://doi.org/10.1038/sj.jcbfm.9600168.
13. Schizodimos T, Soulountsi V, Iasonidou C, Kapravelos N. An overview of management of intracranial hypertension in the intensive care unit. J Anesth. 2020;34(5):741–57. https://doi.org/10.1007/s00540-020-02795-7.
14. Frank JI. Large hemispheric infarction, deterioration, and intracranial pressure. Neurology. 1995;45(7):1286–90. https://doi.org/10.1212/wnl.45.7.1286.
15. Hacke W, Schwab S, Horn M, Spranger M, De Georgia M, von Kummer R. 'Malignant' middle cerebral artery territory infarction: clinical course and prognostic signs. Arch Neurol. 1996;53(4):309–15. https://doi.org/10.1001/archneur.1996.00550040037012.
16. Hawryluk GWJ, et al. A management algorithm for patients with intracranial pressure monitoring: the Seattle International Severe Traumatic Brain Injury Consensus Conference (SIBICC). Intensive Care Med. 2019;45(12):1783–94. https://doi.org/10.1007/s00134-019-05805-9.
17. Rajajee V, Fletcher JJ, Rochlen LR, Jacobs TL. Comparison of accuracy of optic nerve ultrasound for the detection of intracranial hypertension in the setting of acutely fluctuating vs stable intracranial pressure: post-hoc analysis of data from a prospective, blinded single center study. Crit Care. 2012;16(3):R79. https://doi.org/10.1186/cc11336.
18. Marotta G, De Bernardo M, Vitiello L, Rosa N. Ocular Ultrasonography to Detect Intracranial Hypertension in Subarachnoid Hemorrhage Patients. Neurocrit Care. 2020;33(3):855–6.
19. Rajajee V, Vanaman M, Fletcher JJ, Jacobs TL. Optic nerve ultrasound for the detection of raised intracranial pressure. Neurocrit Care. 2011;15(3):506–15. https://doi.org/10.1007/s12028-011-9606-8.
20. Yaqub MA, Mehboob MA, Islam QU. Efficacy and safety of optic nerve sheath fenestration in patients with raised intracranial pressure. Pak J Med Sci. 2017;33(2):471–5.
21. Du J, Deng Y, Li H, Qiao S, Yu M, Xu Q, Wang C. Ratio of optic nerve sheath diameter to eyeball transverse diameter by ultrasound can predict intracranial hypertension in traumatic brain injury patients: a prospective study. Neurocrit Care. 2020;32(2):478–85.

22. Richards E, Mathew D. Optic Nerve Sheath Ultrasound. [Updated 2021 Jul 31]. In: StatPearls [Internet]. Treasure Island (FL): StatPearls Publishing; 2021 Jan-. Available from: https://www.ncbi.nlm.nih.gov/books/NBK554479/.
23. Arora NA, O'Phelan KH. Cerebral edema in stroke. Springer Publishing Company; 2021.
24. Ragland J, Lee K. Critical care management and monitoring of intracranial pressure. J Neurocrit Care. 2016;9(2):105–12. https://doi.org/10.18700/jnc.160101.
25. Chen H, et al. Effects of increased positive end-expiratory pressure on intracranial pressure in acute respiratory distress syndrome: a protocol of a prospective physiological study. BMJ Open. 2016;6(11):e012477. https://doi.org/10.1136/bmjopen-2016-012477.
26. Caricato A, et al. Effects of PEEP on the intracranial system of patients with head injury and subarachnoid hemorrhage: the role of respiratory system compliance. J Trauma. 2005;58(3):571–6. https://doi.org/10.1097/01.ta.0000152806.19198.db.
27. Robba C, Citerio G. How I manage intracranial hypertension. Crit Care. 2019;23(1):243. https://doi.org/10.1186/s13054-019-2529-z.
28. Dorfman JD, Burns JD, Green DM, DeFusco C, Agarwal S. Decompressive laparotomy for refractory intracranial hypertension after traumatic brain injury. Neurocrit Care. 2011;15(3):516–8. https://doi.org/10.1007/s12028-011-9549-0.
29. Schramm WM, Jesenko R, Bartunek A, Gilly H. Effects of cisatracurium on cerebral and cardiovascular hemodynamics in patients with severe brain injury. Acta Anaesthesiol Scand. 1997;41(10):1319–23. https://doi.org/10.1111/j.1399-6576.1997.tb04651.x.
30. Yang X, et al. Is decompressive craniectomy for malignant middle cerebral artery infarction of any worth? J Zhejiang Univ Sci B. 2005;6(7):644–9. https://doi.org/10.1631/jzus.2005.B0644.
31. Kilincer C, et al. Factors affecting the outcome of decompressive craniectomy for large hemispheric infarctions: a prospective cohort study. Acta Neurochir (Wien). 2005;147(6):587–94; discussion 594. https://doi.org/10.1007/s00701-005-0493-7.
32. Mendelow AD, et al. Early surgery versus initial conservative treatment in patients with spontaneous supratentorial intracerebral haematomas in the International Surgical Trial in Intracerebral Haemorrhage (STICH): a randomised trial. Lancet. 2005;365(9457):387–97. https://doi.org/10.1016/S0140-6736(05)17826-X.

33. Shawkat H, Westwood M-M, Mortimer A. Mannitol: a review of its clinical uses. Cont Educ Anaesthesia Crit Care Pain. 2012;12(2):82–5. https://doi.org/10.1093/bjaceaccp/mkr063.
34. Fink ME. Osmotherapy for intracranial hypertension: mannitol versus hypertonic saline. Continuum (Minneap Minn). 2012;18(3):640. https://doi.org/10.1212/01.CON.0000415432.84147.1e.
35. García-Morales EJ, Cariappa R, Parvin CA, Scott MG, Diringer MN. Osmole gap in neurologic-neurosurgical intensive care unit: Its normal value, calculation, and relationship with mannitol serum concentrations. Crit Care Med. 2004;32(4):986–91. https://doi.org/10.1097/01.CCM.0000120057.04528.60.
36. Mangat HS. Hypertonic saline infusion for treating intracranial hypertension after severe traumatic brain injury. Crit Care. 2018;22(1):37. https://doi.org/10.1186/s13054-018-1963-7.
37. Arifianto M, Ma'ruf A, Ibrahim A, Bajamal A. Role of hypertonic sodium lactate in traumatic brain injury management. Asian J Neurosurg. 2018;13(4):971. https://doi.org/10.4103/ajns.AJNS_10_17.
38. Bourdeaux CP, Brown JM. Randomized controlled trial comparing the effect of 8.4% sodium bicarbonate and 5% sodium chloride on raised intracranial pressure after traumatic brain injury. Neurocrit Care. 2011;15(1):42–5.
39. Oddo M, et al. Optimizing sedation in patients with acute brain injury. Crit Care. 2016;20(1):128. https://doi.org/10.1186/s13054-016-1294-5.
40. Pfenninger E, Himmelseher S. Neuroprotection by ketamine at the cellular level. Anaesthesist. 1997;46(Suppl 1):S47–54. https://doi.org/10.1007/pl00002465.
41. Kim Y-I, Park S-W, Nam T-K, Park Y-S, Min B-K, Hwang S-N. The effect of barbiturate coma therapy for the patients with severe intracranial hypertension: a 10-year experience. J Korean Neurosurg Soc. 2008;44(3):141–5. https://doi.org/10.3340/jkns.2008.44.3.141.
42. Majdan M, Mauritz W, Wilbacher I, Brazinova A, Rusnak M, Leitgeb J. Barbiturates use and its effects in patients with severe traumatic brain injury in five European countries. J Neurotrauma. 2013;30(1):23–9. https://doi.org/10.1089/neu.2012.2554.
43. George SE, Mathew JE. Midazolam is effective in controlling intracranial pressure in severe traumatic brain injury. CHRISMED J Health Res. 2019;6(4):242. https://www.cjhr.org/

article.asp?issn=2348-3334;year=2019;volume=6;issue=4;spage=242;epage=247;aulast=George. Accessed 1 Nov 2020.
44. Andrews PJ, et al. Therapeutic hypothermia to reduce intracranial pressure after traumatic brain injury: the Eurotherm3235 RCT. Health Technol Assess. 2018;22(45):1–134. https://doi.org/10.3310/hta22450.
45. Abadal JM, Llompart-Pou JA, Homar J, Molina M, Pérez-Bárcena J. Lumbar drainage for intracranial pressure. JNS. 2009;111(6):1295. https://doi.org/10.3171/2009.6.JNS09873.
46. Frontera J, et al. Regional brain monitoring in the neurocritical care unit. Neurocrit Care. 2015;22(3):348–59. https://doi.org/10.1007/s12028-015-0133-x.
47. Zygun D. Can we demonstrate the efficacy of monitoring? Eur J Anaesthesiol Suppl. 2008;42:94–7. https://doi.org/10.1017/S026502150700347X.
48. Barsan W. Brain oxygen optimization in severe TBI (BOOST3): a comparative effectiveness study to test the efficacy of a prescribed treatment protocol based on monitoring the partial pressure of brain tissue oxygen. clinicaltrials.gov, Clinical trial registration NCT03754114, Mar. 2020. Accessed: Feb. 14, 2021. [Online]. Available: https://clinicaltrials.gov/ct2/show/NCT03754114.
49. Roh D, Park S. Brain multimodality monitoring: updated perspectives. Curr Neurol Neurosci Rep. 2016;16(6):56. https://doi.org/10.1007/s11910-016-0659-0.
50. Ruhatiya RS, Adukia SA, Manjunath RB, Maheshwarappa HM. Current status and recommendations in multimodal neuromonitoring. Indian J Crit Care Med. 2020;24(5):353–60. https://doi.org/10.5005/jp-journals-10071-23431.

Sepsis and Fever in the Neuro-Critical Care Unit (NCCU)

Chandra Shekar Pingili and Niraj Arora

1 Introduction

Sepsis is one of the most common causes of morbidity and mortality in patients admitted to the ICU [1]. It is essential to recognize the early signs of sepsis and manage the patients in a timely manner before irreversible multi-organ dysfunction ensues [2, 3]. In simple terms, when one mentions sepsis, it becomes indispensable to look for the source of infection. Management of sepsis is challenging in NCCU as drugs should be able to cross the blood-brain barrier and the medication doses should be adjusted. Quite often, the therapy is initiated empirically and later on tapered according to the specific organisms cultured. Neuro-intensivist is often faced with the complex issue of differentiating nosocomial infections related to the neurosurgical procedures from other non-infectious causes. This requires due diligence on the part of

---

C. S. Pingili (✉)
Department of Neurocritical Care, University of Missouri, Columbia, MO, USA
e-mail: cpygd@health.missouri.edu;

N. Arora
Department of Neurology- Neurocriticalcare unit, University of Missouri, Columbia, MO, USA
e-mail: arorana@health.missouri.edu

the neuro-intensivist to be familiar with the various sources of infections and choosing the right antibiotics.

1.1 Definitions

- **Fever in the Intensive Care Unit (ICU):** Any temperature that exceeds the normal daily diurnal variation could be considered as fever. However, fever in ICU is measured numerically as body temperature more than 38.3 °C (101 °F) in immunocompetent patients and more than 38 °C (100.4 °F) for immunocompromised patients [4].
- **Systemic Inflammatory Response Syndrome (SIRS):** Table 1

    Physiologic response of the host to noxious processes either infectious or non-infectious (trauma, surgery, acute inflammation, ischemia or reperfusion, or malignancy) which helps to limit and possibly eliminate the source of the process [5]. The incidence of SIRS is more than 80% in the medical or surgical intensive care unit [3]. The exact incidence of SIRS in NCCU is still unknown however it can be implied that the incidence could be much higher.
- **Sepsis:** Life-threatening organ dysfunction caused by a dysregulated host response to infection [1]. The latest definition of sepsis excludes SIRS from the definition because of the overall prevalence of SIRS in the hospitals, irrespective of the patient's location. Also, the all-cause adjusted mortality rate for sepsis with and without SIRS is identical [2].

    In the critically ill patients with suspected sepsis in medical or surgical intensive care units, SIRS criteria have been compared to the Logistic Organ Dysfunction system

TABLE 1 Systemic Inflammatory Response Syndrome (SIRS)

Body temperature >38 or <36 °C
Heart rate more than 90 beats/min
Respiratory rate more than 20 breaths/min or pCO_2 <32 mmHg
White Cell Count >12,000 or <4,000/μL or over 10% immature forms or bands

SIRS is defined as presence of any 2 or more of the above criteria

TABLE 2 Quick Sequential Organ Failure Assessment (qSOFA) score (1 point for each)

Respiratory Rate ≥22/min

Change in mental status

Systolic Blood Pressure ≤100 mmHg

(LODS) and Sequential Organ Failure Assessment (SOFA) score. SOFA score has been found superior to SIRS criteria and relatively easier to calculate compared to LODS. An increase in the SOFA score with the first 2 days of admission carries an increased mortality rate of 50% [6]. A modified version of the SOFA score called Quick SOFA (qSOFA) has been developed to identify organ dysfunction. However, the utility of this score is questionable in NCCU since most patients present with altered mental status satisfying one of the three criteria mentioned (Table 2). Since the qSOFA score cannot be applied as a gold standard in NCCU because most of the patients present with low GCS and tachypnea, to begin with, the author encourages to apply SOFA score, clinical exam, sequential inflammatory markers, radiology, and microbiological analysis to make a true determination about sepsis.

- **Neurogenic fever (NF) or Central fever** [7]: Non-infectious cause of elevated body temperature found in patients with neurological injuries. The exact pathophysiology of neurogenic fever is still unknown but it is presumed to be due to injury in the hypothalamus which disrupts the set-point temperature. It is reported that patients with NF have a high temperature which is resistant to common antipyretic medications and have relative bradycardia, absence of perspiration, no diurnal variation in the temperature curve (Plateau-like temperature curve) that could continue for a few days to weeks. Patients could have altered mentation with varying degrees of unawareness during this time and may have fluid-electrolyte disturbance related to diabetes insipidus. Infectious causes of fever should be ruled out before considering this diagnosis.
- **Sympathetic storming** [7, 8]: In patients with severe brain injury, especially in severe traumatic brain injury, there is

an exaggerated response of the hypothalamic mediated sympathetic activation leading to a surge of catecholamine. This phenomenon happens episodically and causes a calm individual to turn into a chaotic state. There is an alteration in consciousness, diaphoresis, tachycardia, tachypnea, hyperthermia, posturing, and agitation.

2 Measurement of Body Temperature [9, 10]

Fever is the most common sign in NCCU. More than 75% of the NCCU admissions have a fever during their ICU stay. While mentioning fever, it is essential to mention the location where the temperature is taken. Surface body temperature is a less reliable source than the core body temperature. To define fever a T_{max} above 37.5 °C is fever. Temperature below 35 °C is hypothermia. T_{max} more than 41 °C is called hyperpyrexia. A pulmonary artery thermistor is the most sensitive tool to detect body temperature. A probe on the eardrum will give an exact temperature of the hypothalamus. However, both are invasive. A probe in the Foley catheter is equally effective as any other invasive tool and the detection of temperature is independent of urine output. Rectal temperatures are a few tenths slower than the core temperature [1, 2].

It is essential to treat patients with fever without delay. Identifying true sepsis is challenging in NCCU due to the presence of various non-infectious causes of fever. However, one must not delay the investigations to the diagnosis of sepsis and timely initiation of life-saving antibiotics. Every hour of delay in antibiotics increases mortality by 8% [2].

3 Causes of Fever in Intensive Care Unit (ICU)

Fever in ICU could be due to infectious or noninfectious causes. Infectious causes require early identification and prompt treatment to improve the outcome. Below we discuss in detail about important causes of fever, appropriate antibiotics and the certain clinical pearls which are important during the management of fever.

4 Infectious Causes of Fever (Table 3)

1. Meningitis: [11, 12]
Meningitis is an inflammatory disease of the leptomeninges (arachnoid and pia mater), characterized by an abnormal number of white blood cells in the cerebrospinal fluid (CSF). Meningitis in NCCU could be either community-acquired or nosocomial.

(a) Community-acquired meningitis (CAM): The common pathogens causing CAM are listed in the Tables 4, 5 and 6. CAM pathogens are usually classified on the age of the host but these pathogens usually exhibit a crossover into all age groups. Comorbid conditions that make a host immunocompromised like diabetes, organ transplants hosts,

TABLE 3 Infectious causes of fever [10]

1. Meningitis: (a) Community-acquired (Bacterial, Viral, Fungal) (b) Nosocomial (related to EVD, VPS, post-operative) (c) Traumatic Brain Injury related

2. Sinopulmonary infections

3. Oropharyngeal infections

4. Cardiovascular infections: Endocarditis

5. Intra-abdominal infections

6. Genito-urinary tract infections

7. Musculoskeletal infections: (a) Septic arthritis (b) Osteomyelitis (c) Cellulitis (d) Necrotizing fasciitis

8. Bloodstream infection: Catheter-related

9. Skin and soft tissue infection

Table 4 Common causes of CAM (bacterial) in adults [11, 12] and associated risk factors

Agent	Source	Age	Comments
Streptococcus pneumoniae	Nasopharynx colonization followed by invasion.	All ages except <1 month old. Most common cause	Incidence decreasing due to availability of 7 valent pneumococcal conjugate vaccine.
Neisseria meningitidis	Nasopharynx colonization followed by invasion.	All ages. Second most common in adults	Complement defects are a risk factor.
Group B streptococci (*S. agalactiae*)	Nasopharynx colonization followed by invasion.	Less than 1 month age child	
Haemophilus influenzae	Nasopharynx	Any age-especially infants and children-not vaccinated	Decreased humoral immunity is a risk factor
Listeria monocytogenes	Gastrointestinal tract	Older adults, neonates.	Immunocompromised hosts, chronic kidney disease, Cell-mediated defects, pregnancy, alcoholism, liver disease, and malignancy are major risk factors

Mycobacterium tuberculosis	Air borne infection BCG irrigation of the bladder	Any age	Bovine TB in patients who get BCG bladder irrigation for bladder cancer. AIDS patients and patients from high risk countries any cause of T cell lymphopenia
Staphylococcus aureus	Bacteremia	Any age	Endocarditis, skin and soft tissue infections, hardware, decubitus ulcer.
Borrelia burgdorferi	Lyme infection from tick bites in endemic areas – mostly in wisconsin, michigan and eastern states	Any age – but mostly teens and adults with risk of tick exposure	meningitis-meningoencephalitis – cranial nerve palsy

TABLE 5 Common causes of Viral Meningitis [13, 14]

COMMON VIRUSES: (a) Herpesvirus 1 and 2 (b) Enterovirus (most common) (c) Epstein-Barr virus (EBV) (d) Varicella Zoster virus (VZV) (e) HIV (f) Lymphocytic Choriomeningitis Virus (LCV) – the patient is exposed to rodent droppings

IMMUNOCOMPROMISED PATIENTS : Cytomegalovirus (CMV)

TRAVEL ASSOCIATED VIRUSES: (a) St. Louis encephalitis virus (b) West Nile virus (c) Tick Borne encephalitis virus

BLOOD TRANSFUSION/ORGAN TRANSPLANT: West Nile virus, Rabies virus

and patients on biologics are all at risk of bacterial, viral and fungal meningitis.

The majority of the cases of CAM are managed on the medical floors or in the medical ICU. If there is a concern about patients developing hydrocephalus, increased intracranial pressure along with clinical symptoms like altered mentation or seizures, such patients are better served in NCCU where they could be monitored and frequent neurological examinations performed. Though rare, vasculopathy is one of the complications of infectious meningitis which could cause ischemic strokes [19].

- **Bacterial Meningitis:** In the United States and Europe, the incidence of bacterial meningitis has declined in the past 10–20 years to 0.7–0.9 per 100,000 persons per year [11]. The incidence of meningococcal meningitis has decreased following the introduction of serogroup A and C meningococcal vaccines, however, in spite of pneumococcal conjugate vaccine, incidence of pneumococcal meningitis has not decreased due to serotype replacement [20]. Table 4 [11, 12] shows the common causes of bacterial meningitis along with associated risk factors.
- **Viral meningitis** [13, 14]**:** Unlike bacterial meningitis where the etiological agent varies with age and immune status of the patient, viral meningitis on the other hand

generally affects the pediatric and younger group of the patient population and the risk comes down as age advances. Most cases of viral meningitis resolve as aseptic meningitis with no residual sequelae but some strains like HSV-1/2 and West Nile virus can cause long-term disability. Table 5 shows the common viruses responsible for the community acquired viral meningitis.

- **Fungal Meningitis** [15–18]**:** Fungal Meningitis is a very rare phenomenon and the exact incidence of these infections is still unknown. Fungal infections usually are indolent to begin with and difficult to eradicate unless the source is removed. Common causes of fungal meningitis are described in Table 6 along with important features. Table 7 [21–23] shows the fungal pathogens, means of diagnosis and treatment strategy. Candida is the usual pathogen. IV

TABLE 6 Common causes of Fungal Meningitis [15–18]

Agent	Source	Comments
Cryptococcus	Infected bird droppings or unwashed raw fruit.	Immunocompromised state is a major risk factor.
Coccidioides	Infected bird droppings.	More common in Southwestern US. Life threatening disease and fatal without treatment.
Histoplasma	Infected bird or bat droppings.	More common in Ohio and Mississippi River basins. Spore inhalation causes pulmonary symptoms. Hematogenous spread to CNS.
Aspergillus	Decaying leaves and compost	Invades tissues and vessels. More common in immunocompromised
Mucormycosis	Decaying leaves and compost	Invades blood vessels (angio-invasive). Diabetes and immunocompromised patients is a risk factor. Rhinocerebral disease is more common.

Table 7 Fungal Meningitis [21–23] pathogens, means of diagnosis and treatment strategy

Fungal Species and important facts	Diagnosis	Treatment facts
Candida species Device removal is mandatory C. krusei and tropicalis is resistant to azoles C. auris is an emerging infection – resistant to all antifungal agents.	Diagnosis is based on cultures (CSF/blood)	The common cause of device-associated NVM. Initial treatment is with IV amphotericin and flucytosine followed by long-term oral fluconazole.
Histoplasma History of bird droppings and bats exposure. Central and the eastern USA.	CSF/serum/urine antigen testing Serum or CSF antibody test Blood/CSF/Bone marrow biopsy cultures	Itraconazole/Posaconazole is the drug of choice. H.capsulatum is resistant to Echinocandins High dose fluconazole can be used Voriconazole – less effective than itraconazole
Blastomyces More prevalent in midwestern USA	CSF/Blood cultures Skin biopsy Serology is not useful Urine and serum antigen	For CNS infections: IV liposomal Amphotericin for 6 weeks then AZOLE drug for 1 year

TABLE 7 (continued)

Fungal Species and important facts	Diagnosis	Treatment facts
Coccidioidomycosis More prevalent in Southern California/ Arizona (Sandiego and Tucson area)	Antigen in serum/ urine/CSF CSF/blood/urine cx Serological testing with EIA followed by confirmation with ICA Immunodiffusion tests	High dose fluconazole orally Itraconazole Intrathecal amphotericin in the first trimester of pregnancy because azoles are teratogenic in the first trimester This fungus is resistant to echinocandins.
Aspergillus	CSF culture Serum/BAL galactomannan has diagnostic and prognostic value	IV Amphotericin for CNS infections followed by voriconazole as a step-down Posaconazole, Itraconazole are alternative agents
Mucormycosis Affects immunocompromised and Diabetics, IV drug users Generally spreads as severe Rhino-orbital-cerebral invasive infections Very high mortality		Needs surgical debridement IV Amphotericin with either Echinocandin or posaconazole

Liposomal amphotericin and IV flucytosine is the suggested initial regimen followed by oral azole drugs as a step-down therapy. Amphotericin can cause chills. Rigors, renal failure, hyponatremia, hypokalemia, hypomagnesemia, and hypocalcemia [24]. Liposomal amphotericin, flucytosine, and azole group of drugs achieve very good CSF levels. Echinocandins on the other hand have no CSF penetration [25]. **Candida lusitaniae** is universally resistant to amphotericin [26]. **Candida tropicalis** and **Candida krusei** are resistant to fluconazole [27]. Voriconazole achieves good CSF penetration and is the drug of choice for invasive aspergillosis [28]. However, if a patient cannot tolerate this drug, then liposomal amphotericin can be used. Transient visual disturbances, renal failure, and hyper or hypokalemia are few observed side effects besides drug-drug interactions. **Candida auris** is an emerging infection and the organism is universally resistant to all antifungal drugs known to us [29].

5 Management of Bacterial Meningitis

Bacterial meningitis carries a very high mortality (70%) and morbidity [11]. Streptococcus pneumoniae, Neisseria meningitidis and Haemophilus influenzae are the leading cause of meningitis in most of the patient population with the exception of the neonates [12]. These three pathogens spread from person to person in close vicinity and colonize the nasal and oral mucosa, from where they spread to the blood brain barrier. Streptococcus pneumoniae is the leading pathogen in this group and its CSF MIC is different from that of the peripheral cultures. Table 8 [30, 31] provides a detailed approach to the antimicrobial selection for the various bacterial pathogens. The incidence of later two microbes ebbed significantly with universal vaccination precautions. Meningococcus (MCM) has a more fulminant course of all the known pathogens and patients often decompensate within a few hours. Bacteremia is the major issue with CNS

Table 8 Treatment of bacterial meningitis [30, 31]

Microbes	Diagnosis	Antimicrobial of choice	Alternative drugs
Streptococcus pneumoniae (MIC <0.1 μg/mL)	CSF PCR Blood cultures QTL Urine antigen	IV Penicillin, IV Ampicillin	Ceftriaxone, Cefotaxime Vancomycin
Penicillin resistant (MIC >0.1 μg/mL), third-generation cephalosporin susceptible (MIC <2 μg/mL)		IV Ceftriaxone/IV Cefotaxime	Vancomycin, Cefepime, Meropenem, Levofloxacin/Moxifloxacin
Cephalosporin resistant (MIC ≥2 μg/mL)		IV Vancomycin Alone IV Vancomycin + Ceftriaxone 2 g twice daily Linezolid	Meropenem/Quinolones Other Than Ciprofloxacin IV Dexamethasone For 4 Days [32]
Haemophilus influenzae	CSF PCR Blood cultures QTL	IV Ceftriaxone	Quinolones Doxycycline Macrolides IV Dexamethasone For 4 Days [32]

(continued)

TABLE 8 (continued)

Microbes	Diagnosis	Antimicrobial of choice	Alternative drugs
Neisseria meningitidis MIC <0.1 MIC: 0.1 TO 1 Intolerant To Beta Lactams	CSF PCR Blood cultures	IV Penicillin High Dose IV Penicillin Or Ceftriaxone Use Chloramphenicol	Ceftriaxone
MSSA	CSF PCR/ Cultures Blood cultures	Nafcillin	Ceftriaxone, Cefotaxime, Vancomycin
MRSA Vancomycin MIC <2 Vancomycin MIC >2	CSF PCR Cultures Nasal swab PCR Blood cultures	IV Vancomycin with a trough level >15 Use IV Linezolid, Daptomycin With Rifampin OR can be used intrathecal, IV sulfamethoxazole-trimethoprim	IV Linezolid, Daptomycin With Rifampin or can be used intrathecal, IV sulfamethoxazole-trimethoprim

Listeria Monocytogenes	CSF PCR/ Cultures Blood cultures	IV Penicillin – even if a patient has PNC anaphylaxis – we suggest to desensitize the patient and use PNC	Sulfonamides, IV Vancomycin Aminoglycosides Moxifloxacin
Pseudomonas	CSF PCR/ Cultures Blood cultures	IV Cefepime, Iv Meropenem	IV Aztreonam, IV Quinolones
Amp-C Organisms (MYSPACE) **M**organella, **Y**ersenia enterocolitica, **S**erratia, **P**roteus vulgaria, **P**rovidentia, **A**cinetobacter, **E**nterobacter	CSF PCR/ Cultures Blood cultures	IV Cefepime, Iv Quinolones	IV Sulfonamides, IV Carbapenems
Strongyloides	Serology Stool nucleic acid amplification Blood cultures for secondary infections	Ivermectin	

and systemic manifestations. The latter usually manifests as systemic shock, multi-organ dysfunction and adrenal gland hemorrhage with antecedent Addisonian crisis. Meningococcus B and C are the common stereotypes to infect American children and adolescents. There are two vaccines approved to date. One is the meningococcal conjugate vaccine and the other is the serogroup B vaccine (MENB). CDC recommends a conjugate vaccine at the age of 11 or 12 years and a booster dose at 16 years. MENB vaccine can be given as a single dose between 16–23 years of age. Patients with complement deficiencies (C5-C9, properdin, factor H, factor D, or are taking a complement inhibitor such as Eculizumab or Ravulizumab-cwvz) and those with functional or anatomic asplenia will need a booster dose every 3 years with the MENB vaccine. Household contacts and other close contacts of patients with meningococcal meningitis should be treated with post exposure prophylaxis with ceftriaxone or ciprofloxacin or rifampin [33]. Patients with MCM should be kept in droplet isolation for 24 h after which the isolation can be safely discontinued because the antimicrobials will effectively bring down the nasopharyngeal bacterial colonial burden.

Two types of vaccines against *Streptococcus pneumoniae* are available: older pneumococcal polysaccharide vaccine (PPSV) and newer pneumococcal conjugate vaccines (PCV). PPSV is composed of 23 pneumococcal capsular polysaccharides, and it covers the most antigens of streptococcus pneumoniae. However, since children less than 2 years of age do not respond to it, it is not suitable for them. PCV contains pneumococcal capsular polysaccharides linked to a carrier protein that allows the immune system of infants to produce antibodies. The recommendation is to use PCV in the children's routine immunizations. There are two types of PCV available with a different number of serotypes: PCV10 and PCV13. The efficacy of these vaccines is about 75% [34].

Haemophilus influenzae (Hib) like Streptococcus pneumoniae not only cause meningitis but also sino-pulmonary infections and also fatal epiglottitis in pediatric patients. The polysaccharide protein conjugate vaccine has eliminated this menace. To date there is no strain replacement in the Hib group making the vaccine offer stable herd immunity, which so far is not possible with the meningococcal and streptococcal species.

Lumbar puncture (LP) is a mandated procedure in the management of CAM. Administration of IV antibiotics should not be delayed for the sake of an LP as it takes nearly 4 half-lives of the antibiotics to achieve therapeutic levels in the CSF and early antibiotics will not significantly alter the CSF chemistry and microbiology. There is no cut off for the WBC count to clinch a diagnosis of meningitis but counts greater than 500 cells/mm^3 with neutrophil predominance, a low CSF glucose with CSF glucose, serum glucose ratio less than 0.5 and elevated protein greater than 45 mg% with a positive gram stain and cultures are the defining features of bacterial meningitis [35]. Table 9 shows the CSF findings

TABLE 9 CSF findings based on the etiological agent [11–18]

Etiology	WBC × 10^6	Cell type dominating	CSF: Serum glucose ratio (normal >0.5)	Protein (mg%) (Normal 15–45 mg%)
Bacterial	100 – 5k	Polymorphs	<0.5	50–200
Viral	10–300	Polymorphs in the early course. But mostly Monocytes. CSF could be bloody with HSV	>0.5	40–800
Cryptococcus	10–200	Monocytes	<0.5	50–300
Parasite-migrating larvae carry bacteria with them		Eosinophilic plus high polys. CSF culture is usually polymicrobial		

based on the etiologic agent. The risk of serious complications including brain herniation with the LP is around 1.2%. A routine CT scan of the brain is not needed in every patient with CAM. Only those patients with new onset seizures, focal neurological deficits, papilledema, immunocompromised hosts and those with a history of known CNS lesions should undergo a screening CT scan before an LP.

Listeria is one organism that can infect patients at their extreme ages but also any immunocompromised host. Contrary to the convention, this microbe gains entry into the host's CNS by the oral route [36]. Meat, poultry, coleslaw, unpasteurized milk and produce contaminated in the soil are all responsible for outbreaks of Listerial meningitis. Pregnant patients are one special group at risk and the pathogen can cross the placenta. Ampicillin with or without gentamycin is the drug of choice and the author of this text recommends to desensitize the patients if there is a documented history of IGE mediated life threatening reaction to Penicillins. IV vancomycin, Meropenem and Sulfonamides are the other options. Limited research supports the use of linezolid and rifampin [11, 36–39].

The use of IV Dexamethasone is highly debated in the management of meningitis. Literature supports the use of IV dexamethasone for 4 days only in proven cases of Streptococcus pneumoniae and Hib meningitis. Steroids should preferably be given before the first dose of the antibiotics. Steroids confer a very poor prognosis in the Listeria meningitis.

Regardless of the etiology, all patients with CAM should receive blanket coverage with IV Ceftriaxone, IV Vancomycin and IV Acyclovir +/− IV ampicillin awaiting CSF results. In patients with life threatening allergies to Penicillins, the alternatives are IV Meropenem, IV levofloxacin, IV Sulfonamides. Antibiotics are then tailored based on the CSF yield. Final duration of antibiotics usually varies from a week to a few months depending on the presence or absence of ventriculitis, meningoencephalitis, rhombencephalitis and intracranial abscesses. Tuberculous meningitis is usually treated for a year.

Unless there is no clinical improvement or worsening of the clinical symptoms, there is no need for a repeat LP and or imaging [20, 40, 41]. Table 10 [36–39] shows the CSF penetration of different antibiotics along with common side effects.

Table 10 Antibiotics and CSF penetration

Class of antibiotics	CSF penetration	Side effects to monitor
Sulfonamides- oldest available antibiotics	Best CSF penetration of all drugs	Hyperkalemia Hepatitis Pancreatitis Renal failure Bone marrow suppression Steven Johnson syndrome/ Toxic epidermal necrolysis
Beta Lactams	Drugs of choice Good levels achieved at higher doses without side effects Piperacillin/ Tazobactam has poor CSF penetration	Hepatitis Interstitial nephritis Bone marrow suppression Anaphylaxis Fevers 33% risk of clinical seizures Imipenem, Aztreonam and Cefazolin are the major epileptogenic beta lactams Cefepime rarely causes encephalopathy with EEG changes of triphasic waves Symptoms resolve after withdrawing the drug

(continued)

TABLE 10 (continued)

Class of antibiotics	CSF penetration	Side effects to monitor
Fluoroquinolones	Lipophilic drugs with good CSF penetration irrespective of the meningeal inflammatory state MOXIFLOXACIN – has no renal penetration	Seizures risk is lower compared to beta-lactams QTc prolongation with Macrolides, Amiodarone and other antiarrhythmic drugs. Tendon rupture Aortic aneurysm rupture Exacerbation of myasthenia gravis
Macrolides	Lipophilic drugs with high molecular mass inhibit CSF penetration	Arrhythmias
Tetracyclines	Lipophilic drugs Doxycycline and Minocycline have good CSF penetration Tigecycline has poor CSF penetration and no renal penetration	Photosensitivity even after discontinuation of the drugs Fatal hepatitis in pregnant patients Intracranial hypertension Severe GERD
Vancomycin	Good penetration	Renal failure Thrombocytopenia Vasculitis
Tiecoplanin	Poor	Not recommended for CNS infections

TABLE 10 (continued)

Class of antibiotics	CSF penetration	Side effects to monitor
Linezolid	Good	Bone marrow suppression Peripheral neuropathy Optic neuropathy SSRI syndrome
Daptomycin	Poor – but can be used at higher doses for MRSA infections	Inactivated by surfactant and is not used for pneumonia treatment
Metronidazole	Good	Irreversible peripheral neuropathy Pontine damage
Clindamycin	Good	Clostridium difficile diarrhea
Azoles	Good	QTc Prolongation Hepatic inhibition
Echinocandins	Poor	No renal penetration
Amphotericin	Good	Renal failure Hypotension Electrolyte abnormalities shivering
Acyclovir/Ganciclovir	Moderate	Renal failure – can be prevented with IV Fluids Bone marrow suppression
Cidofovir	Poor	Not recommended for CNS infections

(b) Nosocomial ventricular meningitis (NVM) [12, 21–23, 42–46]

NVM is a complication following neurological surgeries, TBI, EVD insertions, spine surgeries with retained hardware and prosthetic device implants in the spine (3.6–20%). Insertion of external ventricular drainage (EVD) is a very common procedure performed in the NCCU for the management of hydrocephalus and intracranial pressure monitoring in patients with acute neurological or neurosurgical injuries. A major complication of this procedure is nosocomial meningitis or ventriculitis (NVM) with a reported incidence of 2–27% [47, 48]. Infection of the skin and soft tissues at the EVD insertion site is more common than meningitis/ventriculitis. One needs to be aware that true ventriculitis is a potentially life-threatening condition with a very high mortality rate. The risk of NVM increases with the frequency of catheter flushing and manipulation and the insertion technique itself. Catheter leaks and repositioning on the other hand is not a proven risk of contracting NVM. The longer the EVD stays in situ, the higher the risk of NVM with a peak incidence occurring from day 7 to day 14. EVD complication is not only permitted to NVM but also cerebritis, and brain abscess formation. Contamination, EVD catheter colonization, and a full-blown NVM is the usual clinical spectrum observed with these devices. The most common causative pathogens for NVM are listed in Table 11. Diagnosing NVM is a clinical challenge and clinicians should be aware of the concepts of contamination, colonization, and a culture proven true NVM (Table 12). A **contaminated sample** usually has an isolated positive growth with no CSF or clinical findings of infection. **Colonization** on the other hand will have positive cultures with borderline CSF findings but no clinical manifestations other than fevers. NVM will have CSF changes and positive cultures and there will be clinical decline too. Most of the NCCU patients' CSF is hemorrhagic, to begin with, and this is usually complicated with an inflammatory leukocytosis. The latter is a universal finding complicating CSF analysis in these groups of patients. A CSF should be sent for analysis on

TABLE 11 Common organisms causing NVM [12, 21–23, 42–46]

Agent	Source	Comments
Coagulase-negative staphylococci *(Staphylococcus epidermidis)*	Skin flora	Most common
Staphylococcus aureus	Skin flora	Along with S.epidermidis, account for 70% of NVM
Gram-negative rods (Klebsiella, E. coli, Pseudomonas, enterobacter, acinetobacter)	Various routes	Increasing prevalence due to antibiotic useNeonates and adults
Anaerobes	Aspiration	Rare cause
Candida spp	Skin or mucosa	Very rare cause, more common in immunocompromised patients

TABLE 12 Correlation of evidence of NVM with symptoms, signs, laboratory and imaging findings [12, 21–23, 42–46]

Nosocomial ventriculitis/meningitis	Correlation with ventriculitis/meningitis
SYMPTOMS New-onset Headaches, nausea, lethargy or change in GCS, seizures	Strong/moderate
SIGNS Erythema, tenderness over the shunt site, peritonitis in patients with VP shunts, pleuritis in patients with VPl shunts, bacteremia in a patient with VA shunts	Strong/Weak
Cell counts, protein, and sugars in the CSF	Weak/Moderate
CSF cultures Cultures should be held for 10 days for *Propionibacterium acnes*	Strong/Moderate

(continued)

TABLE 12 (continued)

Nosocomial ventriculitis/meningitis	Correlation with ventriculitis/meningitis
Shunt or drain cultures if removed for infection	Strong/Moderate
Shunt or drain cx if removed for some other reason	Weak/Moderate
Blood cultures in VA shunts	Strong/High
Blood cultures in VP and Pleural shunts	Weak/Low
LABORATORY: CSF pleocytosis with positive cultures Hypoglycorrhachia and elevated CSF protein Growth of a contaminant (e.g., coagulase-negative staphylococcus) in enrichment broth only or on just 1 of multiple cultures in a patient with normal CSF and no fevers CSF sample growing staph, fungus, and gram negative rods CSF galactomannan and Beta-D-glucan for fungal infections CSF lactate and procalcitonin Detection of β-D-glucan and galactomannan in CSF may be useful in the diagnosis of fungal ventriculitis and meningitis	Strong/High Strong/High Weak/Low Strong/Moderate Strong/Moderate Weak/Moderate Strong/Moderate
IMAGING: MRI with contrast CT abdomen/USG in patients with V-P shunts and abdominal symptoms	Strong/Moderate Strong/Moderate

all patients with suspected NVM and repeat samples at least twice a week or more as the clinical situation demands.

Initiation of antibiotics is almost always empirical as is the practice elsewhere. Early initiation of broad-spectrum antibiotics should be based on the patient's immune status and facility's antibiogram. Every 1 h delay in initiating the right antibiotics carries a mortality rate of 8% [49]. NVM doesn't cause significant meningeal inflammation; hence antibiotics should be given based on CNS dosing. Initial antibiotics should cover MRSA and gram-negative rods including the AMP-C group of microbes. To start with, IV Vancomycin and IV Cefepime should cover the majority of the pathogens excluding Stenotrophomonas. The latter is usually sensitive to sulfonamides, levofloxacin, ceftazidime, and minocycline. Patients with hemodynamic instability are better started on a combination of IV Vancomycin and IV Meropenem. Anaerobic coverage is rarely needed. Imipenem-cilastatin is generally not a preferred drug given the risk of seizures. Patients with a severe allergy to Penicillin (PNC) should receive IV quinolones instead of cefepime. The rate of cross-reaction between PNC and carbapenems is usually minimal and not prohibitive [50, 51]. Aztreonam on the other hand has no beta-lactam ring in its chemical structure and the risk of a cross-reaction with PNC is negligible. Aztreonam on the other hand shares the same side chain as ceftazidime and clinicians are advised not to use either of these drugs if the patient has a documented IgE mediated reaction to one of these drugs [52, 53]. For patients allergic to vancomycin, the other options will be high dose daptomycin [54], sulfamethoxazole-trimethoprim, linezolid, and doxycycline.

If CSF cultures are positive, antibiotics should be tailored based on cultural sensitivities. MRSA cultures are usually positive within the first 48 h unless the patient received prior anti-MRSA coverage. If the CSF cultures are positive for MRSA and the MIC for vancomycin <2, then the patient can be treated with IV vancomycin aiming for a trough of 15–20. If the MIC of the microbe >2, then the MRSA is considered resistant to vancomycin. Linezolid/Daptomycin/Sulfamethoxazole-Trimethoprim/Doxycycline can be tried. Clinicians should be aware that daptomycin has variable penetration into the blood-brain barrier and blood CSF barrier even in inflamed meninges. If a patient never received anti-MRSA coverage and the CSF cultures are negative for MRSA, then Vancomycin can be safely discontinued. Patients on IV vancomycin should be monitored for renal dysfunction, dropping platelets, and a vasculitis rash. Ceftaroline is a fifth-generation cephalosporin with anti-MRSA activity but is mainly approved for skin and soft tissue infections and MRSA pneumonia. This drug has been tried in combination with other drugs for MRSA endocarditis but to date, there are no documented clinical trials [30].

If the gram-positive cocci turns out to be MSSA, then vancomycin can be switched to IV ceftriaxone 2 gm twice a day. Patients who grow streptococcus in the CSF should be treated based on the MIC to the antibiotics. A MIC≤0.06 for PNC, it is considered to be a sensitive strain. If the MIC is >0.06, the strain should be considered PNC resistant and must be treated with a third-generation cephalosporin or vancomycin if the patient is allergic to cephalosporins. If the MIC ≤0.5 for cephalosporins then the strain is considered sensitive and resistant if the MIC >1, in the latter case, the microbe should be treated with vancomycin, linezolid, doxycycline [31, 32]. IV dexamethasone 0.15 mg/kg every 6 h for four days can be used for the first 4 days of infection with streptococcus, but this generally applies to CAM [55–57]. Cephalosporins can cause encephalopathy, neuropathy, myelosuppression, hepatitis, rash, fevers, and interstitial nephritis [58].

Gram-negative rod NVM is often caused by Pseudomonas, Klebsiella, and the AMP-C group of organisms [45]. CNS doses of Cefepime covers the entire spectrum of microbes stated above except Stenotrophomonas [59]. Quinolones achieve excellent CSF penetration and cover the entire spectrum of gram-negative rods stated above [21]. Contrary to the belief, the risk of seizures is less frequent with quinolones compared to beta-lactams. Quinolones on the other hand can prolong QT_C when given with other QTc prolonging drugs. Quinolones can cause phototoxicity, tendon ruptures, seizures, peripheral neuropathy, aortic dissection, dysglycemia, and C.difficile infection [59, 60]. Quinolones are generally contraindicated in pregnancy and pediatric patients.

Sulfonamides are the oldest antibiotics in the market with broad-spectrum activity and most of the nosocomial pathogens are still sensitive to this class of drugs. This class of drugs is still efficacious in treating AMP-C organisms [61]. Of all classes of antibiotics, the Sulfonamide group achieves the highest CSF concentrations. However, sulfonamides are given in a dextrose solution which is not encouraged in the NCCU. Besides this, sulfonamides can cause life-threatening Stevens-Johnson reactions and hyperkalemia. Hyponatremia, myelosuppression, hepatitis, pancreatitis, and renal failure are other side effects of the sulfa group [62].

Device removal will enhance the pace of microbial clearance, achieving CSF sterility, and clinical improvement. However, this may not be possible in every clinical scenario. Patients with coagulase negative staphylococcal infection can be managed with EVD retention and CNS dosing of antibiotics. However if the CSF cultures continue to stay positive and the patient continues to stay symptomatic, then device removal is a rule rather than an exception. EVD should be removed in all patients with gram-negative rods infection and fungal NVM [45]. The decision for EVD reimplantation is based on a case by case basis and if needed can be reinserted on the same day of explanation. There's no consensus on the total duration of treatment and is a very debated topic. Primary ventriculitis is usually treated for 2–3 months like brain abscess but NVM on the other hand is treated for 10 to 14 days clubbed with clinical, chemical, and microbiological improvement [45, 63]. The use of antibiotic-impregnated catheters is a highly debated topic and to date, there is no consensus on the clinical benefits of these catheters in reducing the incidence of NVM [64–66]. The 2017 IDSA guidelines have outlined a systemic approach to this problem based on the strength of recommendations and quality of evidence using the GRADE (Grading of Recommendations Assessment, Development, and Evaluation) system [67]. Table 12 shows the IDSA recommendations on the evidence of clinical features, laboratory studies and imaging on the

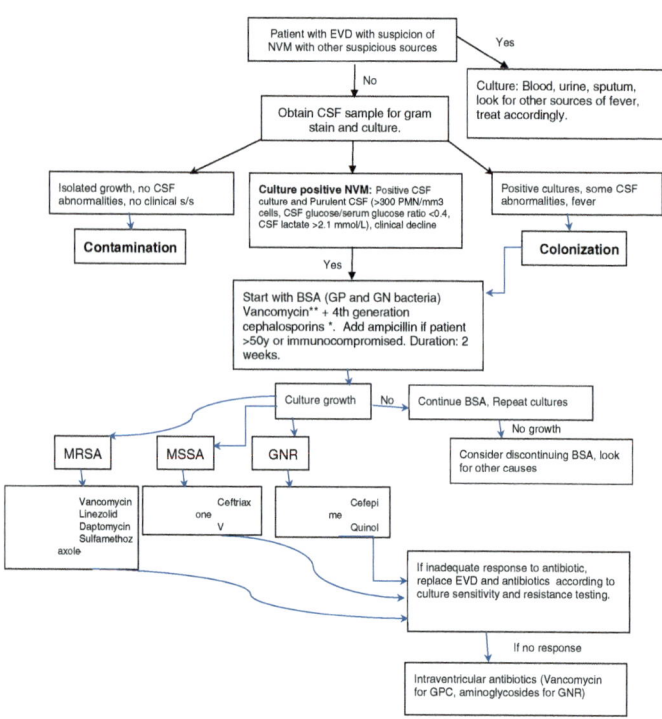

Figure 1 Approach to a patient with suspected NVM

NVM management. Figure 1 shows the flowchart for the management of the NVM.

6 AMP-C Group of Organisms

AMP-C groups of microbes are gram-negative rods that belong to the Enterobacteriaceae family. Clinicians often encounter these pathogens in the NCCU. Microbiologically they look sensitive to the third generation cephalosporins like ceftriaxone, ceftazidime, cefotaxime, and cefixime. However, this is only in-vitro susceptibility, and in vivo these microbes develop resistance to the third-generation cephalosporins. The ideal regimen for these microbes should be Cefepime, carbapenems, quinolones, and sulfamethoxazole-trimethoprim. These microbes are remembered by the acronym **MYSPACE** (Table 8).

(c) Traumatic Brain injury related Meningitis [13, 45]:

4% of all head injuries end up with basilar skull fractures. This represents a fourth of all the skull fractures. Otorrhoea and rhinorrhoea is CSF leak from the ear and the nose respectively. 45% of the basilar skull fractures are associated with CSF leak but the risk of meningitis is 5% and prophylactic antibiotics have no clinical significance unless the patient is getting an ICP monitoring device or unless the CSF leak is prolonged with clinical deterioration. CSF leak can occur any time from day 1 to day 3 and the risk of meningitis is high during the first week. Cases of meningitis after TBI have been documented months to years after the initial insult [68, 69]. Fever, nuchal rigidity, and altered sensorium is the clinical triad used for the diagnosis of meningitis, but these signs are all non-specific in patients with TBI or those with SAH. CSF lactate is a better indicator of meningitis than the CSF WBC, but lactate is also elevated in other clinical conditions like seizures and strokes. A sensitivity of 98% for the CSF lactate comes down to 45% with the use of antibiotics. A CSF lactate of 35 mg/dl has been postulated as a cut off to differentiate between bacterial and aseptic meningitis. Antibiotic administration before LP will raise the sugars and bring down the protein levels but the leucocytosis and the neutrophil count are usually not altered. Gram stain and culture sensitivities are all affected by prior use of antibiotics before LP, but this should not be a reason to hold the antibiotics PCR is 100% sensitive and specific for most of the causative pathogens even in those on antibiotics. Since PCR will not include all the microbes, it should not replace CSF cultures [31, 42, 67].

Acute traumatic CSF fistulae carry a very high meningitis risk of 30.6% before surgical correction of the dura mater with a cumulative risk of 80% at 10 years follow up.

Recurrence of CSF leak is 7% after surgical repair but the risk of recurrent meningitis is very high in this group at 30%. This is one subgroup of patients where the risk of infection is significantly improved with prophylactic antibiotics [68].

2. Sino-pulmonary infections

Sinusitis can develop from prolonged use of a nasogastric tube, gingivitis, dental abscesses and retropharyngeal abscesses. Lemierre's syndrome is thrombosis of the internal jugular vein (IJV) with septic metastasis and is usually a complication of sino-pharyngeal infections. It is often overlooked in NCCU patients, especially the intubated ones. Orotracheal infections carry a lesser risk of sino-pulmonary infections compared to nasotracheal intubations. Pseudomonas and other gram-negative pathogens are the major culprits [55]. CT angiogram of the neck will show filling defects in the internal jugular vein. Fusobacterium necrophorum is the usual pathogen and is inherently resistant to metronidazole despite being an anaerobe. This bacterium usually responds well to 4–6 weeks of IV ampicillin-sulbactam combination. Hypercoagulable states should be ruled out and the patient should be anticoagulated for 4 to 6 weeks [56, 57]. The retropharyngeal abscess is either a complication of an upper respiratory tract infection (URTI) or from pharyngeal trauma and needs surgical correction followed by a 7–10 day course of antibiotics based on the culture sensitivities [58, 70].

Pulmonary infections are the major sites of infection in clinical practice including the NCCU. 20% Of the community-acquired pneumonia patients end up in the ICU and the risk of ventilator-associated pneumonia (VAP) is 3% per day on the ventilator and the mortality rate with VAP is almost 70%. Patients with low GCS have a high risk of aspiration, compounded by cranial nerve palsies, prolonged Intubations, nasogastric feeds, clinical and subclinical seizure activity, Percutaneous feeding tube placements, and overall debilitation. The above-mentioned clinical picture also predisposes them to nosocomial infections. A full-blown respiratory tract infection usually presents with fever, increased endotracheal secretions, increasing need for a higher FiO2 on the ventilator, tachypnoea, hypotension, and worsening leukocytosis. Blood cultures are rarely positive in less than 10% of patients. Blood cultures are still recommended because when positive will decide the exact duration of antibiotics. Parapneumonic effusions if exudative will need aggressive antibiotics and a bedside chest tube or surgical drainage. Daptomycin is inhibited by the surfactant of the alveoli and is contraindicated in the management of pneumonia and is not proven effective even in patients with septic metastasis to the lungs [61]. Aspiration pneumonia is usually treated with drugs with significant anaerobic coverage like Ampicillin/Sulbactam or Piperacillin/Tazobactam or clindamycin. However, the latest data suggests no additional benefit from anaerobic coverage unless there is a complication like an empyema or abscess formation. Aspiration pneumonitis on the other hand is treated conservatively and doesn't mandate antibiotic coverage [62–65].

The MRSA PCR assay demonstrated 88.0% sensitivity and 90.1% specificity, with a positive predictive value of 35.4% and a negative predictive value of 99.2%. Any patient with pneumonia and a negative MRSA PCR on the nasal swab need not be treated with an anti-MRSA regimen. On the other hand, any patient with multilobar pneumonia and significant pleural effusion In summer should be treated as a case of MRSA pneumonia until proven otherwise [66, 67].

Pleural effusions are either transudative or exudative and at times inconclusive. Fluid analysis is based on the Light's criteria or the two-point or three-point criteria in the clinical context [25, 71] Table 6. Treatment of empyema usually mandates surgical wash followed by antibiotics. Antibiotics should never be delayed for the planned surgery. Post obstructive Pneumonia from a lung mass requires anaerobic coverage. Lung abscess is usually a complication of aspiration. Besides Staphylococcus, Streptococci, and gram negative rods, anaerobes like peptostreptococcus, Bacteroides, Fusobacterium, and Prevotella [26, 28].

3. Oro-pharyngeal infections: Sinusitis from a Nasogastric tube, gingivitis, dental abscesses and retropharyngeal abscesses, Internal jugular vein thrombosis (Lemierre's syndrome) from recent oropharyngeal infections are often overlooked in NCCU patients, especially the intubated ones. Orotracheal infections carry a lesser risk of sino-pulmonary infections compared to naso-tracheal intubations. Pseudomonas and other gram-negative pathogens are the major culprits [31, 32, 55]. Lemierre's syndrome is thrombosis of the internal jugular vein with septic Mets and is usually a complication of nasopharyngeal infections. CT angiogram of the neck will show filling defects. Fusobacterium necrophorum is the usual pathogen and is inherently resistant to metronidazole despite being an anaerobe. This bacterium usually responds well to 4–6 weeks of IV Ampicillin/Sulbactam. Hypercoagulable states should be ruled out and the patient should be anticoagulated for 4 to 6 weeks [56, 57]. Retro pharyngeal abscess is either a complication of a URTI or from pharyngeal trauma and needs surgical correction followed by a 7–10 day course of antibiotics based on the culture sensitivities [58, 70].

4. Infective endocarditis (IE) is not a common complication in the NCCU.. However, patients with IE often present with septic metastasis to the brain and spine. Staphylococcus and Pseudomonas coverage is mandated in addition to anaerobic coverage in any brain abscess patient. Despite medical advancements, IE carries a mortality of 25%. Clinicians should be watchful for tetanus and botulism in IV drug users (using black tar heroin). Botulism presents with descending, symmetric paralysis, diplopia, dysarthria, dysphagia, and respiratory failure with diaphragmatic palsy but sparing of the sensory system. Tetanus usually presents with a stiff neck and trismus. Respiratory muscle spasticity is the cause of mortality.

The Duke's criteria are still applicable in the diagnosis of IE (Table 13) [14, 69].

TABLE 13 Modified Duke's Criteria [14, 69]

Confirmed clinical IE: Presence of only 2 Major Criteria OR 1 Major Criteria and 3 Minor Criteria OR only 5 Minor Criteria
Possible IE: Presence of 1 major and 1 minor criterion or 3 minor clinical criteria
Rejected IE: Definite alternate diagnosis made OR Resolution of clinical symptoms after <= 4 days of treatment OR No pathological evidence of IE is noted at pathology or autopsy with <= 4 days of treatment OR clinical criteria for definitive or possible IE not met
Definite diagnosis of IE based on pathological findings: vegetations or valvular abscess seen OR microbiological cultures or histology of vegetation

Major criteria

1. Positive blood culture for typical infective endocarditis organisms (S. viridans or S. bovis, HACEK organisms, S. aureus without other primary site, Enterococcus), from 2 separate blood cultures or 2 positive cultures from samples drawn >12 h apart, or 3 or a majority of 4 separate cultures of blood (first and last sample drawn 1 h apart)
2. Echocardiogram with oscillating intracardiac mass on valve or supporting structures, in the path of regurgitant jets, or on implanted material in the absence of an alternative anatomic explanation, or abscess, or new partial dehiscence of prosthetic valve or new valvular regurgitation
3. Single positive blood culture for Coxiella burnetii or anti-phase 1 IgG antibody titer >1:800

Minor criteria

1. Predisposing heart condition or intravenous drug use
2. Temperature >38 °C (100.4 °F)
3. Vascular phenomena: arterial emboli, pulmonary infarcts, mycotic aneurysms, intracranial bleed, conjunctival hemorrhages, Janeway lesions
4. Immunologic phenomena: glomerulonephritis, Osler nodes, Roth spots, rheumatoid factor
5. Microbiological evidence: positive blood culture but does not meet a major criterion as noted above or serological evidence of active infection with organism consistent with endocarditis (excluding coag neg staph, and other common contaminants)

5. Clostridium difficile induced diarrhea (CDI) is uncommon in the NCCU compared to the MICU. CDI is more common in the MICU with an overall incidence of roughly 4%. Up to 20% of ICU patients that develop the symptomatic disease will progress to fulminant colitis with a mortality rate of nearly 60%. The spores of *C. difficile* are difficult to eradicate and can be isolated from environmental swabs taken from a patient's room months after discharge. Every antibiotic including Metronidazole can put the patient at risk of CDI. Clindamycin and Quinolone exposure is the leading cause of CDI. Use of proton pump inhibitors, enteral feeding, and mechanical ventilation all increase the risk of CDI. Watery diarrhea is a universal clinical presentation with and without fever and or abdominal cramps. Cessation of diarrhea without treatment suggests an ominous sign of toxic megacolon. ELISA test for Toxin A and B is what should be ordered for confirmation and this test carries 90% sensitivity. ELISA test for the Glutamate dehydrogenase (GDH) is an indirect test with high specificity but if positive will need the toxin ELISA test for confirmation. Oral vancomycin is the drug of choice irrespective of the severity of clinical presentation, irrespective of the albumin levels, serum creatinine, and WBC count. IV Vancomycin achieves very poor stool concentrations. Oral/IV Metronidazole achieves good stool concentrations. Cessation of antibiotics if possible is important. Oral Vancomycin should be started at 125 mg q 6 hrs irrespective of the severity of the illness and can be escalated to 500 mg every 6 h for 2 weeks total. Recurrent CDI can retreat with oral vancomycin again with a tapering regimen. Oral Fidaxomicin is not inferior to oral vancomycin but is expensive. However, Fidaxomycin is bactericidal compared to oral Vancomycin which is bacteriostatic. Probiotics have no role in the management of CDI. Colectomy is suggested for patients with toxic megacolon. Use of oral cholestyramine for toxin debulking is not suggested as this will bind to the oral vancomycin and brings down the drug levels in the stool [65, 72–74].

Ascending cholangitis, cholecystitis, perforated viscus, diverticular abscess, tubo-ovarian abscess, Fournier's gangrene all require the prompt surgical evacuation of the source of infection. The latter needs toxin inhibiting drugs like clindamycin in addition to broad-spectrum beta-lactams and or quinolones combined with Metronidazole.

6. The risk of a urinary tract infection (UTI) increases by 5% per day with an indwelling Foley catheter. The incidence of UTI is almost up to 30% in hospitalized patients. Catheter-associated UTI (CAUTI) is a leading cause of morbidity, mortality and prolonged stay in the units. 50% of the patients will have asymptomatic bacteriuria and candiduria by the fifth day of catheter insertion. Fever, flank/suprapubic pain, urinary symptoms, hematuria and or pyuria, and a change in the GCS in patients aged above 65 should suggest CAUTI. Foley should be present for a minimum of 48 h for a diagnosis of CAUTI and at least 10^3 Colony-forming units of microbes in cultures. Avoiding or early discontinuation of the Foley catheter, closed drainage, and dependent drainage, and protecting the drainage port will help reduce the incidence of CAUTI in the units. These are all category 1B recommendations. Routine use of Foley catheter is not indicated even in patients with urinary incontinence (category 1 B). E Coli followed by candida and Enterococcus are the most common microbes cultured in the urine. A dipstick test is not a reliable indicator for CAUTI and the presence or absence of nitrite on the dipstick should not guide the antibiotic regimen because not all gram-negative rods test nitrite positive on the dipstick. Treating asymptomatic bacteriuria carries no clinical significance and there is no observed mortality benefit. Use external condom catheters and intermittent catheterizations in patients with spinal cord injuries, spastic bladders, and those with a meningomyelocele. Moxifloxacin, Tigecycline, and echinocandins have no UTI penetration and should not be used in the management of UTIs. Silver alloy urinary catheters have no impact on the incidence of CAUTI and so is the impact of Nitrofurazone coated catheters [75–77].

7. Musculoskeletal infections:

Septic joints are usually unusual in the NSICU. Fever with joint swelling, pain and tenderness with mobility or joint examination with elevated WBC are the usual findings. Bacteremia is unusual. Joint aspiration usually shows a cloudy synovial fluid with WBC >50 k and polymorphs predmoninance. Patients should be taken to the operating room for a joint wash followed by a week to 4 weeks of IV or oral antibiotics depending on the pathogen.

8. Catheter related bloodstream infections: [35–41]

Every febrile patient should have 2 sets of blood cultures drawn from two different sites of the body and never from the existing peripheral venous accesses. Both sets should be drawn as soon as possible and an intercultural delay between the two sets carries no clinical significance. The risk of contaminated blood cultures is as high as 20% if drawn from an existing peripheral venous access. If CVC is the suspected source of sepsis, then a set of blood cultures should be drawn from the CVC and one set from the periphery. At least 20 mL of blood should be drawn for each bottle. In patients with difficult venous access and limited blood, the draw is hardly possible, then it's better to culture the blood in the aerobic bottles because most of the clinically significant pathogens are facultative anaerobes. If blood cultures from the CVC site are positive 120 min earlier than the peripheral cultures, then CVC site infection is the cause of sepsis here. Otherwise routine culture of the catheter tips and CVC line cultures carries no clinical significance. More than 25% of the catheter tip cultures are just contamination. As long as the CVC insertion technique is sterile, the site of insertion does not influence the risk of line-related infections. CVC infections with yeast/MRSA and gram negative rods mandate device removal. An infection with other gram positive cocci is usually managed with device retention and frequent blood cultures to assess sterility and clinical improvement. We recommend all device removal in patients with line sepsis.

9. Skin and soft tissue infection: The overall incidence of skin and soft tissue infections (SSTI) getting admitted to the ICU is less than 7% and the exact numbers admitted to the NCCU is very low. Streptococci and Staphylococci are the common skin flora responsible for SSTI. Besides clostridial species, almost any other microbe can cause SSTI. Diabetic patients need additional pseudomonal coverage and patients with open wounds will need anaerobic coverage. Crepitus is a late sign and is found in only about 18% of cases of Necrotizing fasciitis (NF). Although crepitus and blistering are the most specific signs of necrotizing soft tissue infection, they are not sensitive. NF patients are disproportionately more toxic compared to the physical findings. Computed tomography and magnetic resonance imaging (MRI) might be useful in cases where a diagnosis is doubtful. Asymmetrical fascial thickening, fat stranding, and gas tracking along fascial planes are important imaging findings. Computed tomography scans are estimated to have a sensitivity of 80% for detecting necrotizing soft tissue infections. The sensitivity of MRI is 100% with a specificity of 86% in NF. NF patients need debridement and repeat debridement if needed based on the clinical course. The initial antibiotic regimen should include MRSA and other gram-positive and anaerobic coverage with toxin inhibiting antibiotics like clindamycin. Ceftaroline is the fifth generation cephalosporin approved for MRSA activity for SSTI [66].

Toxic shock syndromes (TSS) are usually either Staphylococcal or streptococcal. Staphylococcal toxic shock syndrome usually presents with a retained nasal or any other surgical packing or with the use of a tampon. An external sign of cellulitis is usually absent but skin rash will present as diffuse erythroderma and blood cultures are negative. Besides the removal of the offending agent, treatment usually includes an anti-MRSA regimen with either Clindamycin or linezolid for toxin inhibition and sometimes immunoglobulins. Streptococcal toxic shock syndrome on the other hand is a sequel to SSTI and is associated with bacteremia, multi-organ dysfunction, and carries higher mortality [78, 79].

7 Non-infectious Causes of Fever in NCCU

Non-infectious causes of fever need special attention in NCCU as 23–47% of the fevers in the NCCU could be non-infectious [80]. The Table 14 shows various non-infectious causes of fever.

Most noninfectious disorders except drug fever or transfusion reactions do not cause temperature rise more than 38.9 °C (102 °F); any temperature above this is considered infectious etiology, and diagnostic workup should be done.

Table 14 Non-infectious causes of fever [80]
Alcohol/drug withdrawal
Acalculous cholecystitis
Adrenal Insufficiency
Drug fever/Drug reaction
Deep Venous thrombosis
Decubitus ulcer
Fat emboli
Gout/pseudogout
Myocardial Infarction
Mesenteric Ischemia
Postoperative fever (48 h postoperative)
Post-transfusion fever
Pancreatitis
SIRS (Ischemic/Hemorrhagic stroke, SAH, TBI, malignancy)
Transplant rejection

Drug fever is quite uncommon in NCCU, this diagnosis is considered in unexplained fever in a patient receiving b-lactam antibiotics, procainamide, or diphenylhydantoin. It is characterized by high spiking temperatures, shaking chills, relative bradycardia, leukocytosis, and eosinophilia. Atelectasis in itself does not cause fever unless associated with pulmonary infection.

50% of the patients with ischemic stroke also suffer from hyperpyrexia. The latter carries a very poor prognosis. Central fevers are always a diagnosis of exclusion and are the most common aberration in the vitals noted in the NCCU. These fevers are persistent with no diurnal or nocturnal variation, persistently high grade, peaks higher compared to microbial fevers culminating in a higher fever burden. Patients on the other hand do not appear toxic. Brain bleed patients, especially those with intraventricular extension and patients with deeper grey matter bleeds and subarachnoid bleeders are at an exceedingly high risk of central fevers. Central fevers are often resistant to antipyretics [6, 8, 24, 35, 80–82]. Non-infectious causes of fever demand appropriate work up based on the suspected source of fever.

8 Protocol for Fever Management in NCCU

Figure 2 shows a simplified flowchart for fever management. Infectious or non-infectious causes should be thoroughly considered in order to provide the appropriate treatment.

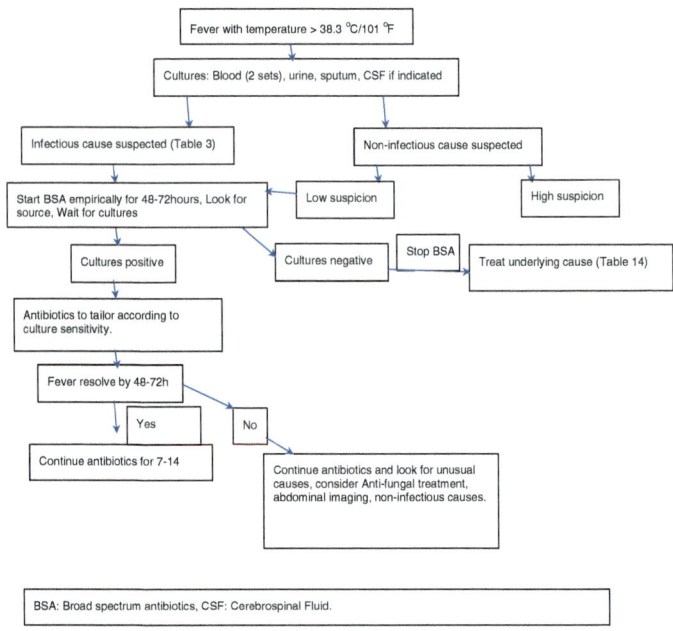

FIGURE 2 Approach to fever in NCCU

References

1. Sakr Y, et al. Sepsis in intensive care unit patients: worldwide data from the intensive care over nations audit. Open Forum Infect Dis. 2018;5(12):ofy313. https://doi.org/10.1093/ofid/ofy313.
2. Abe T, Yamakawa K, Ogura H, et al. Epidemiology of sepsis and septic shock in intensive care units between sepsis-2 and sepsis-3 populations: sepsis prognostication in intensive care unit and emergency room (SPICE-ICU). J Intensive Care. 2020;8:44.
3. Marik PE, Taeb AM. SIRS, qSOFA and new sepsis definition. J Thorac Dis. 2017;9(4):943–5. https://doi.org/10.21037/jtd.2017.03.125.
4. Ogoina D. Fever, fever patterns and diseases called 'fever' – a review. J Infect Public Health. 2011;4(3):108–24. https://doi.org/10.1016/j.jiph.2011.05.002.
5. Kaukonen K-M, Bailey M, Pilcher D, Cooper DJ, Bellomo R. Systemic inflammatory response syndrome criteria in defin-

ing severe sepsis. N Engl J Med. 2015;372(17):1629–38. https://doi.org/10.1056/NEJMoa1415236.
6. Ferreira FL. Serial evaluation of the SOFA score to predict outcome in critically ill patients. JAMA. 2001;286(14):1754. https://doi.org/10.1001/jama.286.14.1754.
7. Goyal K, Garg N, Bithal P. Central fever: a challenging clinical entity in neurocritical care. J Neurocrit Care. 2020;13(1):19–31. https://doi.org/10.18700/jnc.190090.
8. Hocker SE, Tian L, Li G, Steckelberg JM, Mandrekar JN, Rabinstein AA. Indicators of central fever in the neurologic intensive care UNIT. JAMA Neurol. 2013; https://doi.org/10.1001/jamaneurol.2013.4354.
9. Fever, fever patterns and diseases called 'fever' – a review. ScienceDirect. https://www.sciencedirect.com/science/article/pii/S1876034111000256. Accessed 21 Dec 2020.
10. Marik PE. Fever in the ICU. Chest. 2000;117(3):855–69. https://doi.org/10.1378/chest.117.3.855.
11. Bacterial Meningitis. https://www.idsociety.org/practice-guideline/bacterial-meningitis/. Accessed 31 Jan 2021.
12. Meningitis | Home | CDC. Apr. 22, 2020. https://www.cdc.gov/meningitis/index.html. Accessed 13 Oct 2020.
13. Eljamel MS, Foy PM. Acute traumatic CSF fistulae: the risk of intracranial infection. Br J Neurosurg. 1990;4(5):381–5. https://doi.org/10.3109/02688699008992759.
14. Nishimura RA, et al. 2014 AHA/ACC guideline for the management of patients with valvular heart disease: a report of the American College of Cardiology/American Heart Association Task Force on Practice Guidelines. J Am Coll Cardiol. 2014;63(22):e57–185. https://doi.org/10.1016/j.jacc.2014.02.536.
15. Agarwal R, Kalita J, Marak RSK, Misra UK. Spectrum of fungal infection in a neurology tertiary care center in India. Neurol Sci. 2012;33(6):1305–10. https://doi.org/10.1007/s10072-012-0932-1.
16. Salaki JS, Louria DB, Chmel H. Fungal and yeast infections of the central nervous system: a clinical review. Medicine (Baltimore). 1984;63(2):108.
17. Pfaller MA, et al. Candida krusei, a Multidrug-Resistant opportunistic fungal pathogen: geographic and temporal trends from the ARTEMIS DISK antifungal surveillance program, 2001 to 2005. J Clin Microbiol. 2008;46(2):515–21. https://doi.org/10.1128/JCM.01915-07.

18. Favel A, et al. Susceptibility of clinical isolates of Candida lusitaniae to five systemic antifungal agents. J Antimicrob Chemother. 2004;53(3):526–9. https://doi.org/10.1093/jac/dkh106.
19. Mook-Kanamori BB, Geldhoff M, van der Poll T, van de Beek D. Pathogenesis and pathophysiology of pneumococcal meningitis. Clin Microbiol Rev. 2011;24(3):557–91. https://doi.org/10.1128/CMR.00008-11.
20. Harrison LH, Trotter CL, Ramsay ME. Global epidemiology of meningococcal disease. Vaccine. 2009;27(Suppl 2):B51–63. https://doi.org/10.1016/j.vaccine.2009.04.063.
21. Safadi S, Mao M, Dillon JJ. Ceftriaxone-induced acute encephalopathy in a peritoneal dialysis patient. Case Rep Nephrol. 2014;2014:108185. https://doi.org/10.1155/2014/108185.
22. Triplett JD, Lawn ND, Chan J, Dunne JW. Cephalosporin-related neurotoxicity: metabolic encephalopathy or non-convulsive status epilepticus? J Clin Neurosci. 2019;67:163–6. https://doi.org/10.1016/j.jocn.2019.05.035.
23. Lengerke C, et al. Low tigecycline concentrations in the cerebrospinal fluid of a neutropenic patient with inflamed meninges. Antimicrob Agents Chemother. 2011;55(1):449–50. https://doi.org/10.1128/AAC.00635-10.
24. Nierman DM. Core temperature measurement in the intensive care unit. Crit Care Med. 1991;19(6):818–23. https://doi.org/10.1097/00003246-199106000-00015.
25. Leers MPG, Kleinveld HA, Scharnhorst V. Differentiating transudative from exudative pleural effusion: should we measure effusion cholesterol dehydrogenase? Clin Chem Lab Med. 2007;45(10):1332–8. https://doi.org/10.1515/CCLM.2007.285.
26. Chung and Goetz. Anaerobic infections of the lung. Curr Infect Dis Rep. 2000;2(3):238–44. https://doi.org/10.1007/s11908-000-0041-9.
27. Bartlett JG. How important are anaerobic bacteria in aspiration pneumonia: when should they be treated and what is optimal therapy. Infect Dis Clin N Am. 2013;27(1):149–55. https://doi.org/10.1016/j.idc.2012.11.016.
28. Baddour LM, et al. Infective endocarditis in adults: diagnosis, antimicrobial therapy, and management of complications: a scientific statement for Healthcare Professionals from the American Heart Association. Circulation. 2015;132(15):1435–86. https://doi.org/10.1161/CIR.0000000000000296.
29. Passaro DJ, Werner SB, McGee J, Mac Kenzie WR, Vugia DJ. Wound botulism associated with black tar heroin among

injecting drug users. JAMA. 1998;279(11):859–63. https://doi.org/10.1001/jama.279.11.859.
30. Widmer AF. Sterilization of skin and catheters before drawing blood cultures. J Clin Microbiol. 2003;41(10):4910;-author reply 4910. https://doi.org/10.1128/jcm.41.10.4910.2003.
31. van Zanten ARH, Dixon JM, Nipshagen MD, et al. Hospital-acquired sinusitis is a common cause of fever of unknown origin in orotracheally intubated critically ill patients. Crit Care. 2005;9(5):R583–90.
32. Salord F, et al. Nosocomial maxillary sinusitis during mechanical ventilation: a prospective comparison of orotracheal versus the nasotracheal route for intubation. Intensive Care Med. 1990;16(6):390–3. https://doi.org/10.1007/BF01735177.
33. Meningococcal Vaccination | CDC, Aug. 13, 2019. https://www.cdc.gov/vaccines/vpd/mening/index.html. Accessed 1 Feb 2021.
34. Mańdziuk J, Kuchar EP. Streptococcal Meningitis. In: StatPearls. Treasure Island (FL): StatPearls Publishing; 2020.
35. van de Beek D, et al. ESCMID guideline: diagnosis and treatment of acute bacterial meningitis. Clin Microbiol Infect. 2016;22:S37–62. https://doi.org/10.1016/j.cmi.2016.01.007.
36. Lecuit M. Understanding how Listeria monocytogenes targets and crosses host barriers. Clin Microbiol Infect. 2005;11(6):430–6. https://doi.org/10.1111/j.1469-0691.2005.01146.x.
37. Morosi S, Francisci D, Baldelli F. A case of rhombencephalitis caused by Listeria monocytogenes successfully treated with linezolid. J Infect. 2006;52(3):e73–5. https://doi.org/10.1016/j.jinf.2005.06.012.
38. Nguyen THM, et al. Dexamethasone in Vietnamese adolescents and adults with bacterial meningitis. N Engl J Med. 2007;357(24):2431–40. https://doi.org/10.1056/NEJMoa070852.
39. van de Beek D, de Gans J. Dexamethasone in adults with community-acquired bacterial meningitis. Drugs. 2006;66(4):415–27. https://doi.org/10.2165/00003495-200666040-00002.
40. Leimkugel J, et al. An outbreak of serotype 1 Streptococcus pneumoniae meningitis in northern Ghana with features that are characteristic of Neisseria meningitidis meningitis epidemics. J Infect Dis. 2005;192(2):192–9. https://doi.org/10.1086/431151.
41. Hsu HE, et al. Effect of pneumococcal conjugate vaccine on pneumococcal meningitis. N Engl J Med. 2009;360(3):244–56. https://doi.org/10.1056/NEJMoa0800836.

42. Viral meningitis: background, pathophysiology, etiology. Mar 2020 [Online]. Available: https://emedicine.medscape.com/article/1168529-overview. Accessed 13 Oct 2020.
43. Logan SAE, MacMahon E. Viral meningitis. BMJ. 2008;336(7634):36–40. https://doi.org/10.1136/bmj.39409.673657.AE.
44. Griffiths MJ, McGill F, Solomon T. Management of acute meningitis. Clin Med. 2018;18(2):164–9. https://doi.org/10.7861/clinmedicine.18-2-164.
45. La Russa R, et al. Post-traumatic meningitis is a diagnostic challenging time: a systematic review focusing on clinical and pathological features. Int J Mol Sci. 2020;21(11):4148. https://doi.org/10.3390/ijms21114148.
46. Nau R, Sörgel F, Eiffert H. Penetration of drugs through the blood-cerebrospinal fluid/blood-brain barrier for treatment of central nervous system infections. Clin Microbiol Rev. 2010;23(4):858–83. https://doi.org/10.1128/CMR.00007-10.
47. Beer R, Lackner P, Pfausler B, Schmutzhard E. Nosocomial ventriculitis and meningitis in neurocritical care patients. J Neurol. 2008;255(11):1617–24. https://doi.org/10.1007/s00415-008-0059-8.
48. Arabi Y, et al. Ventriculostomy-associated infections: incidence and risk factors. Am J Infect Control. 2005;33(3):137–43. https://doi.org/10.1016/j.ajic.2004.11.008.
49. Mimoz O, et al. Chlorhexidine compared with povidone-iodine as skin preparation before blood culture: a randomized, controlled trial. Ann Intern Med. 1999;131(11):834. https://doi.org/10.7326/0003-4819-131-11-199912070-00006.
50. Linsenmeyer K, Gupta K, Strymish JM, Dhanani M, Brecher SM, Breu AC. Culture if spikes? Indications and yield of blood cultures in hospitalized medical patients. J Hosp Med. 2016;11(5):336–40. https://doi.org/10.1002/jhm.2541.
51. Falagas ME, Kazantzi MS, Bliziotis IA. Comparison of utility of blood cultures from intravascular catheters and peripheral veins: a systematic review and decision analysis. J Med Microbiol. Jan. 2008;57(1):1–8. https://doi.org/10.1099/jmm.0.47432-0.
52. Blot F, et al. Earlier positivity of central-venous- versus peripheral-blood cultures is highly predictive of catheter-related sepsis. J Clin Microbiol. Jan. 1998;36(1):105–9. https://doi.org/10.1128/JCM.36.1.105-109.1998.
53. Gowardman JR, Robertson IK, Parkes S, Rickard CM. Influence of insertion site on central venous catheter colonization and blood-

54. Huber LC, Schibli A. Low yield, high costs. Chest. 2020;158(3):1284. https://doi.org/10.1016/j.chest.2020.04.014.
55. Stein M, Caplan ES. Nosocomial sinusitis: a unique subset of sinusitis. Curr Opin Infect Dis. 2005;18(2):147–50. https://doi.org/10.1097/01.qco.0000160904.56566.4a.
56. Eilbert W, Singla N. Lemierre's syndrome. Int J Emerg Med. 2013;6(1):40. https://doi.org/10.1186/1865-1380-6-40.
57. Ramirez S, et al. Increased diagnosis of Lemierre syndrome and other fusobacterium necrophorum infections at a children's hospital. Pediatrics. 2003;112(5):e380. https://doi.org/10.1542/peds.112.5.e380.
58. Jain H, Knorr TL, Sinha V. Retropharyngeal abscess. Treasure Island: StatPearls Publishing; 2021.
59. Kalanuria A, Zai W, Mirski M. Ventilator-associated pneumonia in the ICU. Crit Care. 2014;18(2):208. https://doi.org/10.1186/cc13775.
60. Zhang D, Yang D, Makam AN. Utility of blood cultures in pneumonia. Am J Med. 2019;132(10):1233–8. https://doi.org/10.1016/j.amjmed.2019.03.025.
61. Zainah H, Zervos M, Stephane W, Chamas Alhelo S, Alkhoury G, Weinmann A. Daptomycin failure for treatment of pulmonary septic emboli in native tricuspid and mitral valve methicillin-resistant Staphylococcus aureus endocarditis. Case Rep Infect Dis. 2013;2013:1–4. https://doi.org/10.1155/2013/653582.
62. Metlay JP, et al. Diagnosis and treatment of adults with community-acquired pneumonia. An official clinical practice guideline of the American Thoracic Society and Infectious Diseases Society of America. Am J Respir Crit Care Med. 2019;200(7):e45–67. https://doi.org/10.1164/rccm.201908-1581ST.
63. Müller F. Oral hygiene reduces the mortality from aspiration pneumonia in frail elders. J Dent Res. 2015;94(3 Suppl):14S–6S. https://doi.org/10.1177/0022034514552494.
64. Poster presentations – advanced trainee research. Australas J Ageing. 2016;35:42–59. https://doi.org/10.1111/ajag.12338.
65. Eljaaly K. Changes in therapy recommendations in the 2019 ATS/IDSA guidelines for community-acquired pneumonia. 2019.
66. Dangerfield B, Chung A, Webb B, Seville MT. Predictive value of Methicillin-Resistant Staphylococcus aureus (MRSA) nasal swab PCR assay for MRSA pneumonia. Antimicrob

Agents Chemother. 2014;58(2):859–64. https://doi.org/10.1128/AAC.01805-13.
67. Vardakas KZ, Matthaiou DK, Falagas ME. Incidence, characteristics and outcomes of patients with severe community acquired-MRSA pneumonia. Eur Respir J. 2009;34(5):1148–58. https://doi.org/10.1183/09031936.00041009.
68. Beeching NJ, Crowcroft NS. Tetanus in injecting drug users. BMJ. 2005;330(7485):208–9.
69. Habib G, et al. 2015 ESC Guidelines for the management of infective endocarditis: the Task Force for the Management of Infective Endocarditis of the European Society of Cardiology (ESC). Endorsed by: European Association for Cardio-Thoracic Surgery (EACTS), the European Association of Nuclear Medicine (EANM). Eur Heart J. 2015;36(44):3075–128. https://doi.org/10.1093/eurheartj/ehv319.
70. Chen XH, et al. The diagnosis and treatment strategy for patients with severemultispace abscesses in neck. Lin Chuang Er Bi Yan Hou Tou Jing Wai Ke Za Zhi. 2016;30(17):1388–93. https://doi.org/10.13201/j.issn.1001-1781.2016.17.012.
71. Light RW, Macgregor MI, Luchsinger PC, Ball WC. Pleural effusions: the diagnostic separation of transudates and exudates. Ann Intern Med. 1972;77(4):507–13. https://doi.org/10.7326/0003-4819-77-4-507.
72. Riddle DJ, Dubberke ER. Clostridium difficile Infection in the Intensive Care Unit. Infect Dis Clin N Am. 2009;23(3):727–43. https://doi.org/10.1016/j.idc.2009.04.011.
73. Honda H, Dubberke ER. The changing epidemiology of Clostridium difficile infection. Curr Opin Gastroenterol. 2014;30(1):54–62. https://doi.org/10.1097/MOG.0000000000000018.
74. Al Momani LA, Abughanimeh O, Boonpheng B, Gabriel JG, Young M. Fidaxomicin vs vancomycin for the treatment of a first episode of clostridium difficile infection: a meta-analysis and systematic review. Cureus. 2018;10(6):e2778. https://doi.org/10.7759/cureus.2778.
75. Hooton TM, et al. Diagnosis, prevention, and treatment of catheter-associated urinary tract infection in adults: 2009 International Clinical Practice Guidelines from the Infectious Diseases Society of America. Clin Infect Dis. 2010;50(5):625–63. https://doi.org/10.1086/650482.
76. Letica-Kriegel AS, et al. Identifying the risk factors for catheter-associated urinary tract infections: a large cross-sectional study

of six hospitals. BMJ Open. 2019;9(2):e022137. https://doi.org/10.1136/bmjopen-2018-022137.
77. Lam TBL, Omar MI, Fisher E, Gillies K, MacLennan S. Types of indwelling urethral catheters for short-term catheterisation in hospitalised adults. Cochrane Database Syst Rev. 2014;(9):CD004013. https://doi.org/10.1002/14651858.CD004013.pub4.
78. Ross A, Shoff HW. Toxic Shock Syndrome. In: StatPearls. Treasure Island (FL): StatPearls Publishing; 2020.
79. Schmitz M, Roux X, Huttner B, Pugin J. Streptococcal toxic shock syndrome in the intensive care unit. Ann Intensive Care. 2018;8:1–10. https://doi.org/10.1186/s13613-018-0438-y.
80. Rabinstein AA, Sandhu K. Non-infectious fever in the neurological intensive care unit: incidence, causes and predictors. J Neurol Neurosurg Psychiatry. 2007;78(11):1278–80. https://doi.org/10.1136/jnnp.2006.112730.
81. Simon LV, Newton EJ. Basilar skull fractures. In: StatPearls. Treasure Island (FL): StatPearls Publishing; 2020.
82. Sakushima K, Hayashino Y, Kawaguchi T, Jackson JL, Fukuhara S. Diagnostic accuracy of cerebrospinal fluid lactate for differentiating bacterial meningitis from aseptic meningitis: a meta-analysis. J Infect. 2011;62(4):255–62. https://doi.org/10.1016/j.jinf.2011.02.010.

Status Epilepticus

Kunal Bhatia and Komal Ashraf

1 Introduction

Status Epilepticus (SE) is a common medical and neurological emergency worldwide. Treatment is primarily aimed at aborting the seizures emergently and requires a targeted treatment approach to reduce patient morbidity and mortality [1]. Based on the population studies, SE has an incidence of 9.9 to 41 cases per 100,000 people annually in the US, with a bimodal distribution with peaks occurring at ages >50 years and in younger population <10 years of age [2, 3]. Depending on the etiology of SE, in-hospital mortality of SE ranges between 10–37%, and increases further up to 50% in those over 80 years of age [4]. According to the International League Against Epilepsy, the etiology of SE may be divided into two groups: (1) known or symptomatic and (2) unknown or cryptogenic [5]. The symptomatic group can be further

---

K. Bhatia (✉)
Department of Neurology, Division of Neurocritical Care, Washington University School of Medicine, St. Louis, MO, USA

K. Ashraf
Department of Neurology, University of Missouri, Columbia, MO, USA
e-mail: khazbb@missouri.edu

subdivided into acute and chronic. In general, acute symptomatic causes of SE are generally more common and tend to be associated with higher rates of morbidity and mortality than chronic etiologies [6]. Of the acute symptomatic etiologies, stroke followed by metabolic disturbances and hypoxia tends to be the most common. Whereas, chronic epilepsy, low antiepileptic drug levels, or medication noncompliance followed by a remote history of trauma, tumor, or chronic CNS infection are the most common causes of status epilepticus among chronic causes [1, 7]. Other less common but important etiologies include autoimmune disease, drug toxicity or withdrawal, and alcohol abuse [8].

Traditionally, SE was defined as continuous seizure activity lasting ≥30 min, or two or more seizures without recovery of consciousness lasting longer than 30 min [9]. However, most seizures are brief and last less than 5 min and resolve spontaneously [10]. Moreover, evidence from animal data has shown that permanent neuronal injury likely occurs after 30 min of continuous seizure activity as passed [11]. Similarly, pharmacoresistance, especially to benzodiazepines, increases as seizure duration increases [12, 13]. Therefore, a more operational definition of SE was proposed by International League against Epilepsy (ILAE) in 2015 – "SE is a condition resulting either from the failure of the mechanisms responsible for seizure termination or from the initiation of mechanisms which lead to abnormally prolonged seizures (after time point t1). It is a condition that can have long-term consequences (after time point t2), including neuronal death, neuronal injury, and alteration of neuronal networks, depending on the type and duration of seizures" [5]. For generalized convulsive status epilepticus (CSE), t1 is estimated to be 5 min, and t2 is 30 min. These time points are different for focal SE (t1 is considered 10 min and t2 is 60 min) and less clearly defined for absence SE. Hence, a more widely accepted definition of SE includes (i) continuous clinical and/or electrographic seizure activity, or (ii) recurrent seizure activity without recovery (returning to baseline) between seizures; lasting for ≥5 min [1].

Based on the seizure semiology, SE can broadly be categorized into two categories: Convulsive status epilepticus (CSE) and Non-convulsive status epilepticus (NCSE) [14]. CSE accounts for 37% to 70% of SE and includes generalized onset CSE, with recognized symmetrical tonic-clonic motor activity and impaired consciousness or may evolve from focal onset seizures to bilateral CSE [8]. One particular type of focal motor SE, called Epilepsia partialis continua (EPC), presents with focal motor seizures with preserved awareness. On the other hand, NCSE is characterized by a lack of convulsive motor movements as seen in CSE but presents with continuous or fluctuating alteration in mentation associated with evidence of characteristic electroencephalographic (EEG) patterns [1, 15]. CSE may evolve to NCSE in approximately 14–20% of patients with subsequent loss of clinical component [16, 17]. The prevalence of NCSE can be as high as 37% in patients who are evaluated for fluctuating levels of consciousness on continuous EEG monitoring [18].

SE can also be categorized based on the responsiveness to medications as Refractory Status epilepticus (RSE) and Super refractory status epilepticus (SRSE). RSE is defined as continuous seizure activity not controlled by appropriately chosen and dozed first-line (such as benzodiazepines) and second-line (such as fosphenytoin) antiepileptic drugs [19]. SRSE is defined either as status epilepticus not controlled by third-line intravenous (IV) anesthetic agents or as status epilepticus continuing for 24 h or longer after anesthesia is administered, or recurs after weaning anesthetic agents [20]. RSE is seen in approximately 9–43% of all cases of status epilepticus with a reported in-hospital mortality of 15–33% [19, 21, 22]. However, the exact incidence of SRSE cannot be determined accurately due to a low number of such patients and a lack of prospective studies. It has been observed that approximately 4–12% of patients with SE may eventually progress to SRSE with in-hospital mortality reported to be as high as 40–54% [23–25].

The urgency of treating SE is of paramount importance as the response to treatment and prognosis deteriorates with increased duration of seizure activity. Hence, the current chapter focuses on a stepwise approach and provides an algorithmic protocol for the management of SE, based on the available evidence and current clinical practices.

2 Treatment Algorithm for Management of Convulsive Status Epilepticus

The principal goal of management is to emergently abort both clinical and electrographic seizures, often warranting aggressive treatment. A staged approach to treatment has been advocated, with different drugs used in early (stage I), established (stage II), refractory (stage III), and super-refractory status epilepticus (stage IV) [26]. These stages overlap with phases of treatment defined by the American Epilepsy Society: 0–5 min identified as the patient stabilization phase, 5–20 min identified as the initial therapy phase, 20–40 min identified as the second therapy phase, and 40–60 min identified as the third therapy phase [14]. To limit morbidity and SE related adverse events, definitive control of SE should be established within 60 min of onset [1].

1. Stabilization phase: 0–5 min

    The initial management of SE includes an assessment of cardiorespiratory function in conjunction with measures to achieve seizure control. Treatment should mirror other resuscitation approaches like airway protection, hemodynamic resuscitation, intravenous access, along with direct and close supervision of the patient [27]. The following steps are recommended as part of the initial management of SE patients:

    - Evaluate and stabilize cardiocirculatory function
    - Ensure airway patency and administer supplemental oxygen via nasal cannula/mask (Airway protection may be facilitated by noninvasive methods initially, but early intubation can be performed based on the clinical necessity and acuity)
    - Obtain IV access

- Check fingerstick glucose
- Administer IV thiamine 100 mg × 1 before giving dextrose (in patients with suspected alcohol abuse or malnourished individuals)
- Give D50W 50 ml IV if low/unknown glucose
- Continuous monitoring: O2 saturation, HR, BP, EKG, ETCO2 (if possible)
- Order blood tests: complete blood count, comprehensive metabolic profile, creatine kinase, calcium, magnesium, phosphorus, troponin, blood gases, and hCG (in females)
- Consider toxicological screen (blood and urine) and drug level monitoring of antiepileptic drugs (AED) (if a patient is on known therapy)

Further studies should be guided by the diagnostic workup warranted and to rule out other treatable causes of SE. For example, in patients without a history of epilepsy or in whom seizures have occurred in conjunction with head trauma, computed tomography (CT) of the head should also be obtained once a patient is stable. Magnetic resonance imaging (MRI) of the brain with and without contrast (if possible) and diagnostic lumbar puncture along with early initiation of antibiotics, if indicated, can be considered once seizures have stopped and the patient is stable [28]. It is important to emphasize that these diagnostic studies are selected depending on the patient's history and physical examination and should be ordered based on the clinical situation.

2. Initial therapy phase: 5–20 min

    The initial therapy phase should begin when the seizure duration reaches 5 min and should conclude by the 20-min mark when a response (or lack of response) to initial therapy should be apparent. A benzodiazepine specifically IM midazolam (when IV access is not available), IV lorazepam, or IV diazepam is recommended as the initial therapy of choice, given their demonstrated efficacy, safety, and tolerability (Class of recommendation I, Level of evidence A) [14]. Initial therapy should be administered as an adequate single full dose rather than broken into multiple smaller doses, and should not be given twice except for IV lorazepam and diazepam. Benzodiazepines carry the risk of hypotension, excessive sedation, and decreased respiratory drive. Table 1 summarizes the first-line treatment options used during the initial therapy phase of SE.

- *Prehospital setting:*

  The recommendations for the management of epileptic seizures apply equally to the prehospital management of SE to ensure cardiorespiratory stability and to prevent or

TABLE 1 First line anti-epileptic drugs indicated for use in early Status Epilepticus

Drug of choice with IV access established	$T_{1/2}$ (h)	Alternative (No IV access)	Tmax (h)
1. IV lorazepam (0.1 mg/kg/dose, max: 4 mg/dose, can repeat dose once after 3–5 min), *or* 2. IV diazepam (0.15–0.2 mg/kg/dose, max: 10 mg/dose, can repeat dose once after 3–5 min)	1–20 40 (33–45)	1. IM midazolam (10 mg if body weight >40 kg, 5 mg if body weight 13–40 kg, single dose) 2. Rectal diazepam 0.2–0.5 mg/kg (maximum dose 20 mg). 3. Intranasal or buccal midazolam (10 mg, single dose).	0.25 (0.15–1.5) ~1.5 (1.18 ± 0.56) IN: 0.15 (0.1–0.35) Buccal: 0.5 (0.25–1.5)
If none of the above 2 options are available: 1. IV phenobarbital (15 mg/kg/dose, single loading dose)	~79 (53–118)		

$T_{1/2}$ Elimination half-life, *Tmax* time to maximum concentration, *IN* intranasal

minimize the risk of injuries [29]. Benzodiazepines, specifically IV lorazepam and IM midazolam, are safe and effective (Class of recommendation I, Level of evidence A) when administered by paramedics for the treatment of out-of-hospital SE in adults [30–32]. Other options available for use in the field or by family members at home include rectal diazepam (0.2–0.5 mg/kg, max dose 20 mg), buccal or nasal midazolam (5–10 mg) [29]. Use of benzodiazepines in the prehospital setting has been shown to terminate seizures in 43–59% cases with SE, en-route to the hospital, with less need for respiratory support on arrival to the emergency department and need for ICU subsequently [30].

If seizure activity persists despite treatment with benzodiazepines, the patient is considered to be in stage II or established SE, and a second-line IV AED should be initiated immediately.

3. Second therapy phase: 20–40 min

 The second-therapy phase should begin when the seizure duration reaches 20 min and should conclude by the 40-min mark when a response (or lack of response) to the second therapy should be apparent [14]. Approximately 40% of patients with convulsive SE do not respond to benzodiazepines and progress to established or stage II SE, which requires the use of second-line AEDs for the cessation of seizure activity. The following AEDs can be used, in no specific order, for the management of established SE:

- IV Fosphenytoin/phenytoin: 20 mg PE/kg IV at 150 mg/min; max 2000 mg. An additional dose of 5–10 mg/kg IV (max 500 mg) can be given if still seizing. If fosphenytoin is not available, IV phenytoin can be administered at a dose of 20 mg/kg IV at 50 mg/min; max 2000 mg.
- IV Valproic acid/Sodium Valproate: 40 mg/kg, max dose 3000 mg, should be administered over 5–10 min. If still seizing, an additional dose of 20 mg/kg IV (max 1500 mg).

- IV Levetiracetam: 40–60 mg/kg IV (over 15 min); max 4500 mg.
- IV Lacosamide: 200–400 mg in a single dose, administer over 10 min.
- Because of adverse events, IV phenobarbital is used as a reasonable second-therapy alternative if none of the above therapies are available. It is given at a dose of 15 mg/kg, max dose 1500 mg. If a patient is still seizing, an additional dose of 5–10 mg/kg can be administered.
- In patients with a known diagnosis of epilepsy, who have been on an AED at baseline, it is reasonable to administer an IV bolus of the same AED (if available) before initiating an additional agent. The rationale is to achieve higher than normal target concentrations of the AED, utilizing additional doses, to achieve the cessation of seizure activity.

Dosing considerations, mechanism of action, and adverse effects of second-line anti-epileptic drugs available for treating SE are summarized in Table 2.

4. Third therapy phase: 40–60 min

If seizure activity continues despite treatment with benzodiazepines and one second-line IV ASD, with or without additional doses, the patient is considered to be in refractory SE (RSE) or stage IV SE. Management of RSE is primarily composed of seizure suppression, treating the underlying etiology of the seizures, managing and preventing complications [33]. Continuous IV anesthetic agents are typically used to treat RSE. In general, the following principles should be applied for managing patients in RSE.

- It is recommended that patients be started on continuous EEG monitoring, if not on it already, especially while these medications are being used [34]. Initiation of continuous EEG monitoring within 1 h of onset of SE is recommended, especially if there is a concern that a patient is in NCSE or has failed to appropriately regain consciousness within 60 min after a convulsive event [1].

TABLE 2 Second line anti-epileptic drugs available for treating Established Status Epilepticus

Anti-epileptic drug	Mechanism of action	Dose	Half-life	Adverse effects/comments
Fosphenytoin/ Phenytoin	Blocks voltage-gated Na channels	IV 15–20 PE mg/kg at 150 mg/min; max dose 2000 mg (PHT is given at a max rate of 50 mg/min). May give an additional 5–10 mg/kg once	7–42 h	***Black box warning:*** rapid infusion related to cardiovascular effects, arrhythmia, hypotension, purple glove syndrome. ***Contraindications:*** atrioventricular blockade, bradycardia, severe hypotension.
Valproic acid	Na channel antagonism, GABA potentiation, T-type calcium channel blockade	IV 40 mg/kg; max 3000 mg. May give an additional 20 mg/kg once	3–16 h	Hyperammonemia, thrombocytopenia, hyponatremia, hepatotoxicity, acute hemorrhagic pancreatitis. ***Contraindications:*** liver impairment, mitochondrial diseases, liver porphyria

(continued)

TABLE 2 (continued)

Anti-epileptic drug	Mechanism of action	Dose	Half-life	Adverse effects/comments
Levetiracetam	SV2A modulation	IV 40–60 mg/kg; max 4500 mg	6–9 h	Agitation, psychosis, depression. **Contraindications:** Severe renal failure **Comments:** No cardiovascular side effects, no pharmacokinetic interactions
Lacosamide	Enhances the slow inactivation of voltage-gated Na channels and modulates CRMP2	IV 200–400 mg; max dose 600 mg	~13 h	PR prolongation, dizziness, abnormal gait, vertigo, abnormal hepatic dysfunction. **Contraindications:** II–III grade atrioventricular blockade. Monitor heart function if given concurrently with drugs that prolong PR interval.

Phenobarbital	Acts on GABA-A receptor to facilitate intrinsic Cl channel function	IV 15 mg/kg; Max rate 60 mg/min. May give an additional 5–10 mg/kg once	80–100 h	Respiratory depression, prolonged sedation, Stevens-Johnson syndrome, blood dyscrasias. **Contraindications:** porphyria, liver failure, severe heart disease.
Brivaracetam	SV2A modulation	IV 200 mg	7–8 h	Abnormal gait, vertigo, sedation
Topamax	Blocks voltage-gated Na channels, enhances GABA activity, antagonizes AMPA/kainite glutamate receptors, weakly inhibits carbonic anhydrase.	Initial dose: PO/NG 200–400 mg. Maintenance doses should be started 300–1600 mg/day (divided 2–4 times daily)	19–23 h	Metabolic acidosis. **Comments:** No IV formulation available

Status Epilepticus 375

- Another important aspect of management to be considered is airway protection. If the patient has not been intubated for airway protection by this point, it is reasonable to consider intubation (rapid sequence induction and intubation) to facilitate anesthetic management of ongoing seizures, as the use of anesthetic agents can cause respiratory depression [28].
- Cardiovascular monitoring is recommended with the use of continuous infusions of anesthetic agents. Vasopressor agents may be required due to the increased risk of hypotension and cardiopulmonary depression related to these medications [1].
- As far as duration of anesthetic treatment is concerned, it is not known for how long these agents should be administered to control seizures. However, it is recommended to maintain a continuous infusion for 24–48 h before weaning [1].
- The four major IV anesthetics used for refractory status epilepticus are midazolam, propofol, pentobarbital, and ketamine [1]. It should be noted that the drugs used in RSE have an insufficient level of evidence for use in RSE (level U) [29]. However, a combination of propofol and midazolam in continuous infusion may lower the required dose, hence reduces the risk of side effects without altering the efficacy of these agents for controlling seizures.
- If the continuous infusion of the first anesthetic agent chosen fails, then switching to a different agent is recommended.
- A second line AED started or chosen earlier should be continued.
- Patients who are hemodynamically stable and in nonconvulsive RSE (i.e. absence of prominent motor symptoms) or focal RSE can be managed less aggressively with the use of additional boluses of AEDs (valproate, levetiracetam, lacosamide, fosphenytoin) before starting continuous infusions of anesthetic agents.

- Continuous EEG monitoring should be used to guide drug titration towards a goal of electrographic seizure suppression or optimal duration of treatment.
- Due to the lack of prospective studies, there is no consensus with regards to the extent of seizure suppression needed to treat SE. Studies have shown inconsistent results on mortality, risk of breakthrough seizures, and functional outcome in patients treated for RSE with anesthetic agents with a goal for seizure suppression vs. burst suppression.
- In clinical practice, the goal is to achieve electrographic burst suppression, characterized by 1–2 s bursts of cerebral activity interspersed by 10 s interval of background suppression [35].
- Additional studies like lumbar puncture should be performed and both serum and CSF samples should be sent for autoimmune and paraneoplastic antibodies if no clear etiology can be found at this point.
- Fever should be treated appropriately.
- IV antibiotics can be started in case of high suspicion for infection.

Table 3 summarizes the mechanism of action, doses, and adverse effects of anesthetic agents used for the treatment of refractory and super-refractory status epilepticus.

5. Fourth therapy phase: >60 min

Stage IV SE or super refractory SE (SRSE) is defined as SE not controlled by third-line intravenous (IV) anesthetic agents and continues for 24 h or longer despite using appropriate doses of anesthetic agents, including those cases that recur upon reduction or withdrawal of anesthesia [20]. The primary aim of treatment during this phase is to control seizure activity, as in earlier stages of SE, along with limiting the effects of ongoing neurotoxicity from ongoing seizure activity. Another important aspect of management of SRSE includes avoiding or treating the systemic complications from prolonged unconsciousness due

TABLE 3 Drugs for management of Refractory and Super Refractory Status Epilepticus

Anti-epileptic drug	Mechanism of action	Dose	Half-life ($t_{1/2}$)	Adverse effects/comments
Midazolam	Enhances postsynaptic inhibitory GABA-A receptor	Initial dose: Load with 0.2 mg/kg IV; max 20 mg. Repeat 0.2–0.4 mg/kg boluses q5mins until seizures stop; max total load of 2 mg/kg. Continuous Infusion: start at 0.1 mg/kg/h; dose range 0.05–2 mg/kg/h; titrate to seizure suppression.	1–4 h, 6–50 h with continuous infusion	Respiratory insufficiency, hypotension, bronchospasm, delirium, hallucinations **Comments:** rapid action and good safety profile; may be associated with tachyphylaxis risk of accumulation in patients with renal failure, obesity, and elderly.

Propofol	GABA potentiation, NMDA antagonism, calcium modulation	Load dose: 1–2 mg/kg IV, may repeat every 5 min PRN until seizures stop (max dose 10 mg/kg) Continuous infusion: Initial rate 20 mcg/kg/min; continue at dose range 20–250 mcg/kg/min; titrate to seizure suppression	Initial: 40 min Terminal: 4–7 h, (after 10-day infusion, maybe up to 1–3 days)	Hypotension, apnea, arrythmia, involuntary movements, propofol infusion syndrome (shock, lactic acidosis, hypertriglyceridemia, rhabdomyolysis). ***Comments:*** Short-acting anesthetic, rapid action, and very short half-life; daily monitoring of pH, creatine kinase, and blood lactate levels is advised.

(continued)

TABLE 3 (continued)

Anti-epileptic drug	Mechanism of action	Dose	Half-life ($t_{1/2}$)	Adverse effects/comments
Pentobarbital	GABA potentiation, NMDA antagonism, calcium modulation	Load dose: 5 mg/kg IV, may repeat every 15–30 min PRN until seizures stop (max dose 20 mg/kg) Continuous infusion: start at 1 mg/kg/h; continue at dose range 1–10 mg/kg/h; titrate to seizure suppression or burst suppression.	15–50 h	Bradycardia, hypotension, angioedema, hepatotoxicity, paralytic ileus, immunosuppression, complete loss of neurological exam. ***Comments:*** reduces intracranial pressure and lowers body temperature; prone to accumulate which prolongs the duration of intubation and recovery time.
Ketamine	NMDA antagonist	Initial bolus: 0.5–4 mg/kg, may repeat every 5 min PRN (max 5 mg/kg). Continuous infusion rate: 0.3–5 mg/kg/h	Alpha phase: 10–15 min Beta phase: 45 min	Increased intracranial pressure, erythema, arrhythmia, apnea. ***Comments:*** Has sympathomimetic action, may induce tachycardia, hypertension, and increase intracranial pressure.

to continuous seizure activity and prolonged anesthesia [20]. A stepwise protocol for the management of SRSE, including alternative therapies available, has been mentioned below:
- Continue workup to identify the cause of SE, as treatment of underlying etiology can successfully terminate seizures.
- Neuroimaging, if not already performed, and preferably brain MRI should be obtained.
- With regards to medications, the first step should be to maximize the continuous infusions of anesthetic agents already being used, followed by adding or switching to another anesthetic agent. Pentobarbital and ketamine (refer to the doses mentioned in Table 3) are the most common medications used as continuous infusions during stage IV SE.
- Pentobarbital or ketamine dose should be titrated based on continuous EEG monitoring to achieve burst suppression.
- Due to the lack of prospective studies on the treatment of SRSE, the optimal duration of anesthesia is unknown. However, it is recommended to maintain patients in burst suppression on continuous EEG for a minimum of 24–48 h before beginning to wean off medications. If seizures recur then continuous infusion should be restarted and titrated again to achieve burst suppression.
- Attention should be paid to hemodynamic parameters, fluid balance, antithrombotic therapy, skincare, and respiratory care including chest physiotherapy.
- Anesthetic agents, particularly pentobarbital, can cause immunosuppression. Hence, patients should be monitored for nosocomial infections with a low threshold to initiate broad-spectrum antibiotics until culture results become available.
- Invasive BP and hemodynamic monitoring should be employed to guide therapy for the management of hypotension from prolonged use of anesthetic agents.

- If seizures continue to persist despite the above measures or tend to recur even after multiple attempts to withdraw or re-initiate therapy, one or more of the following alternative therapies can be used (no strong evidence to guide the best treatment is available):
    (i) Consider adding other AEDs
        - Clobazam (loading dose: 20–40 mg; maintenance dose: 20–60 mg/d divided BID) [36]
        - Topiramate (loading dose: 200–400 mg PO/NG; maintenance dose: 300–1600 mg/d) [37]
        - Perampanel (loading dose: 6–12 mg; maintenance dose: upto 12 mg/d) [38]
        - Oxcarbamazepine (loading dose: 600–1200 mg; maintenance dose: 600–2400 mg/d divided BID [36]
    (ii) Magnesium 4 g IV bolus followed by 2–6 g/h infusion (keep serum levels ~3.5 mmol/l) [39]
    (iii) Pyridoxine 100–400 mg/d IV or via orogastric tube [40]
    (iv) Immunotherapy: Methylprednisolone 1 g/d IV for 5 days followed by prednisone 1 mg/kg/d orally for 1 week. Alternatively, IVIg can be used 0.4 g/kg/d for 5 days or plasmapheresis for 5 sessions [41, 42]
    (v) Hypothermia: Therapeutic hypothermia with goal temp between 32–36 °C for <48 h. The target temperature can be achieved by the use of an endovascular cooling device [43, 44]. Cardiovascular and coagulation parameters, biochemistry and acid-base balance, serum lactate, and physical examination must be monitored carefully.
    (vi) Ketogenic diet: A 4:1 ketogenic diet is recommended (fat: carbohydrate) with total restriction of glucose initially. It is contraindicated in pyruvate carboxylase and β-oxidation deficiency [45–47]

(vii) Neurosurgical resection of the identifiable epileptogenic focus. Some success has been reported with urgent surgery (cortical or lobar resection, functional hemispherectomy, callosotomy, multiple subpial transections) for treating focal-onset SRSE [48, 49].
(viii) Electroconvulsive therapy: Daily sessions for 3–8 days [50]
(ix) Vagal nerve stimulation or deep brain stimulation or repetitive transcranial magnetic stimulation [51, 52].

- *Non Convulsive Status Epilepticus (NCSE)*
NCSE is treated on the same lines as CSE with a focus on suppressing seizures emergently to prevent secondary neuronal injury. Hence, it is important to utilize continuous EEG monitoring early to detect patients in NCSE due to a lack of motor symptoms [34]. There is no standard definition for NCSE that exists currently. However, a working definition has been recommended to diagnose NCSE based on electroclinical criteria, also called Salzburg criteria [15]. The electrographic criteria established for NCSE (in patients without known epileptic encephalopathy) is as follows: (1) epileptiform discharges >2.5 Hz or (2) epileptiform discharges at 0.5 to 2.5 Hz or rhythmic delta/theta activity (>0.5 Hz) and one of the following characteristics: (i) EEG and clinical improvement after a benzodiazepine or IV antiepileptic trial, or (ii) subtle clinical ictal phenomena during the EEG patterns mentioned above, or (iii) typical spatiotemporal evolution. In patients with known epileptic encephalopathy, a diagnosis of NCSE is assessed by either an increase in frequency or prominence of epileptiform features when compared with the patient's baseline EEG findings, or when epileptiform abnormalities occur with a clear change in clinical status. Regarding the use of medications, there is no strong evidence to guide the treatment of NCSE. However, benzodiazepines are recommended as first-line IV AEDs to control seizures as in CSE [18]. Once seizures become

prolonged and progress to refractory NCSE, despite using a benzodiazepine and another second line AED in appropriate doses, the decision to escalate treatment further should be made after weighing potential benefits of aggressive treatment (e.g. rapid termination of seizures, prevention of seizure-induced secondary brain injury) vs. potential risks (hypotension, prolonged mechanical ventilation, and risks of infection).

3 Drugs Used for Treatment of Status Epilepticus

Pharmacology of commonly used antiepileptic drugs, including the anesthetic agents used in refractory and super refractory SE, along with their doses and adverse effects have been discussed and summarized in Tables 1, 2, and 3. Other less studied drugs like IV magnesium sulfate, pyridoxine, and other AEDs (clobazam, topiramate, perampanel) have also been discussed earlier.

4 Current Evidence

Status epilepticus is a neurological emergency that requires immediate treatment to limit neurological injury from ongoing seizure activity. A staged approach for management of status epilepticus has been advocated by the Neurocritical care society (NCS), American Epilepsy Society (AES), and ILAE (see Fig. 1) [1, 14, 29]. As per the Neurocritical care society guidelines, IV benzodiazepines should be the agent of choice for emergent initial therapy. In the 1998 Veterans Affairs status epilepticus study, 4 drugs-lorazepam, phenobarbital, phenytoin, and diazepam followed by phenytoin, were studied and compared with each other for controlling seizures in overt or subtle SE [17]. The results showed that lorazepam was more successful than phenytoin in aborting status epilepticus in patients with CSE and no significant difference was observed in comparisons among other arms of

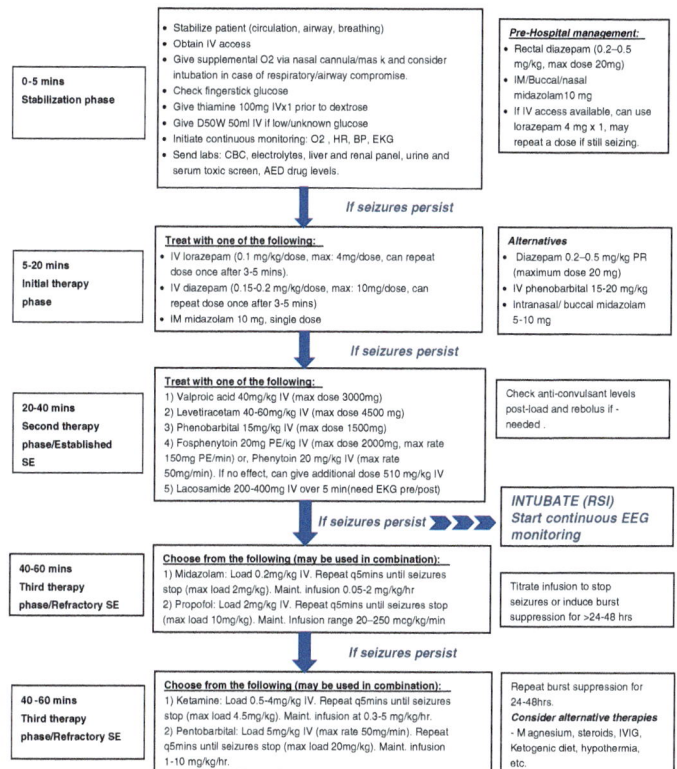

FIGURE 1 Status Epilepticus Treatment Protocol

the trial. In another study examining out-of-hospital use of benzodiazepines found that administration of IM midazolam was non-inferior to IV lorazepam in terminating seizures before arrival to the emergency department in patients with status epilepticus [31, 32]. However, IM midazolam was noted to be superior and more efficacious than IV lorazepam in patients without established IV access. Hence, in adults IM midazolam, IV lorazepam, IV diazepam (with or without phenytoin), and IV phenobarbital have been recommended as drugs of choice for stopping seizures lasting at least 5 min, with similar efficacy (level of evidence – A) [14].

The results of a meta-analysis, evaluating the efficacy of 5 different antiepileptic drugs (phenytoin, phenobarbital, valproic acid, levetiracetam, and lacosamide) for management of benzodiazepine resistant SE showed that the rate of seizure cessation was higher with valproate (75.7%) and phenobarbital (73.6%) as compared to levetiracetam (68.5%) and phenytoin (50.2%) [53]. As per the position statement by ILAE, phenytoin/fosphenytoin, phenobarbital, valproate, levetiracetam, and lacosamide; appear to be effective in the treatment of definite or established SE, with no clear indication for the preferred use of one drug over another [29]. In general, the efficacy of each subsequent AED added decreases after initiating the first AED. One randomized controlled trial showed that the efficacy of the first AED in aborting CSE was 55.5%, efficacy of the second AED 7.0%, and efficacy of the third AED was only 2.3%. In a more recent randomized controlled trial, the safety and efficacy of three different AEDs (levetiracetam, fosphenytoin, and valproate) were compared in patients with established status epilepticus. No statistically significant difference was observed in efficacy or primary safety outcomes within each group, and treatment success was seen in approximately 50% of patients [54]. Hence, any of the three drugs (levetiracetam, fosphyentoin, valproate) can be considered as a potential second-line drug for benzodiazepine-refractory SE. Physicians should choose AEDs based on the subtypes of SE – focal vs. generalized SE. Phenytoin/fosphenytoin, lacosamide, brivaracetam, carbamazepine have been noted to effective in suppressing focal seizures as compared to sodium valproate which is more efficacious in controlling generalized seizures. On the other hand, AEDs like levetiracetam, phenobarbital, and topiramate have been used for the management of both focal and generalized onset seizures. More recently, brivaracetam has been introduced as an adjunct AED in the management of focal epilepsy with anecdotal reports regarding its efficacy in the management of status epilepticus [55–57]. IV brivaracetam has shown to have a faster and unrestricted passage across the blood barrier accounting for faster onset of action with a peak in brain concentrations within minutes, as compared to levetiracetam [58, 59]. Also, brivaracetam has a 15- to 30-fold increased affinity for synaptic vesicle protein 2A (SV2A) as compared with levetiracetam, which accounts for its superior anticonvulsant efficacy and less psychiatric adverse effects [60]. However, further studies are required in a controlled setting to compare its efficacy as compared to levetiracetam in the management of status epilepticus.

With regards to the management of refractory and super-refractory SE, there is a lack of robust data supporting a specific anesthetic agent over another owing to the rarity of this condition and the difficulty of performing randomized trials. Alternatively, additional boluses of second line AEDs can be attempted before starting anesthetic agents. As per the Neurocritical care society guidelines for the management of SE, intermittent boluses of sodium valproate, levetiracetam, and phenytoin/fosphenytoin may be considered to suppress seizures if not previously used, before switching to continuous infusions of anesthetic agents [1]. Alternatively, the use of IV lacosamide at a loading dose of 200–400 mg, either as a single dose or intermittent boluses, has shown to be effective at stopping CRSE (Level of Evidence C) [61]. As per the ILAE, the choice of anesthetic agent should depend on patient characteristics, availability of medications, experience, and comfort level of the treating physician [29]. Midazolam is recommended as the first choice of agent in these patients, either as monotherapy or combined with propofol. Ketamine may also be useful, particularly in patients with hemodynamic compromise. Although ketamine is unlikely to suppress seizures when used as monotherapy, it is usually combined with another anesthetic agent for the treatment of RSE. Pentobarbital is often reserved as a last option for patients with RSE and SRSE due to its unfavorable safety and tolerability profile. There is also insufficient evidence for other AEDs (brivaracetam, levetiracetam, fosphenytoin) in the management of CRSE. Other alternative therapies like Adrenocorticotropic hormone, IVIg, corticosteroids, magnesium sulfate, and pyridoxine have been used in special situations but have not been studied for the management of CRSE.

5 Future Directions

Significant advances have been made in the management of status epilepticus in recent years. However, morbidity and mortality from status epilepticus continue to remain high. Future care of patients with SE can be improved by increasing awareness amongst physicians and paramedical staff about the importance of earlier detection and immediate treatment of seizures to prevent pharmacoresistance associated with prolonged seizures. Clinical research should be focused on early seizure termination in the prehospital setting to limit seizure duration and reducing the risk of progression to SE. Emphasis should be given towards conducting randomized trials focusing on the safety and efficacy of new drugs in patients with RSE and SRSE. Studies are needed to study the effects of early use of anesthetic agents, complications from prolonged use of such agents, defining and standardizing treatment goals including optimal duration of treatment to burst suppression vs. seizure suppression in refractory and super refractory SE.

References

1. Brophy GM, Bell R, Claassen J, et al. Guidelines for the evaluation and management of status epilepticus. Neurocrit Care. 2012;17(1):3–23.
2. Hesdorffer DC, Logroscino G, Cascino G, Annegers JF, Hauser WA. Incidence of status epilepticus in Rochester, Minnesota, 1965-1984. Neurology. 1998;50:735–41.
3. Dham BS, Hunter K, Rincon F. The epidemiology of status epilepticus in the United States. Neurocrit Care. 2014;20(3):476–83.
4. Sánchez S, Rincon F. Status epilepticus: epidemiology and public health needs. J Clin Med. 2016;5(08):71.
5. Trinka E, Cock H, Hesdorffer D, et al. A definition and classification of status epilepticus–Report of the ILAE Task Force on Classification of Status Epilepticus. Epilepsia. 2015;56(10):1515–23.

6. Lv RJ, Wang Q, Cui T, et al. Status epilepticus related etiology, incidence and mortality: a meta-analysis. Epilepsy Res. 2017;136:12–7.
7. DeLorenzo RJ, Pellock JM, Towne AR, Boggs JG. Epidemiology of status epilepticus. J Clin Neurophysiol. 1995;12:316–25.
8. Trinka E, Höfler J, Zerbs A. Causes of status epilepticus. Epilepsia. 2012;53(Suppl 4):127–38.
9. Recommendations of the Epilepsy Foundation of America's Working Group on Status Epilepticus. Treatment of convulsive status epilepticus. JAMA. 1993;270:854–9.
10. Jenssen S, Gracely EJ, Sperling MR. How long do most seizures last? A systematic comparison of seizures recorded in the epilepsy monitoring unit. Epilepsia. 2006;47(9):1499–503.
11. Meldrum BS, Horton RW. Physiology of status epilepticus in primates. Arch Neurol. 1973;28(1):1–9.
12. Jones DM, Esmaeil N, Maren S, Macdonald RL. Characterization of pharmacoresistance to benzodiazepines in the rat Li-pilocarpine model of status epilepticus. Epilepsy Res. 2002;50:301–12.
13. Kapur J. Rapid seizure-induced reduction of benzodiazepine and Zn2 sensitivity of hippocampal dentate granule cell GABAA receptors. J Neurosci. 1997;17(19):7532.
14. Glauser T, Shinnar S, Gloss D, et al. Evidence based guideline: treatment of convulsive status epilepticus in children and adults: report of the guideline committee of the American Epilepsy Society. Epilepsy Curr. 2016;16(1):48–61.
15. Beniczky S, Hirsch LJ, Kaplan PW, et al. Unified EEG terminology and criteria for nonconvulsive status epilepticus. Epilepsia. 2013;54(Suppl 6):28–9.
16. DeLorenzo RJ, et al. Persistent nonconvulsive status epilepticus after the control of convulsive status epilepticus. Epilepsia. 1998;39(8):833–40.
17. Treiman DM, et al. A comparison of four treatments for generalized convulsive status epilepticus. Veterans Affairs Status Epilepticus Cooperative Study Group. N Engl J Med. 1998;339(12):792–8.
18. Sutter R, Rüegg S, Kaplan PW. Epidemiology, diagnosis, and management of nonconvulsive status epilepticus: opening Pandora's box. Neurol Clin Pract. 2012;2(04):275–86.
19. Rossetti AO, Lowenstein DH. Management of refractory status epilepticus in adults: still more questions than answers. Lancet Neurol. 2011;10(10):922–30.

20. Shorvon S, Ferlisi M. The treatment of super-refractory status epilepticus: a critical review of available therapies and a clinical treatment protocol. Brain. 2011;134(Pt 10):2802–18.
21. Reznik ME, Berger K, Claassen J. Comparison of intravenous anesthetic agents for the treatment of refractory status epilepticus. J Clin Med. 2016;5(5):pii:E54.
22. Mayer SA, Claassen J, Lokin J, Mendelsohn F, Dennis LJ, Fitzsimmons BF. Refractory status epilepticus: frequency, risk factors, and impact on outcome. Arch Neurol. 2002;59(02):205–10.
23. Strzelczyk A, Ansorge S, Hapfelmeier J, Bonthapally V, Erder MH, Rosenow F. Costs, length of stay, and mortality of super-refractory status epilepticus: a population-based study from Germany. Epilepsia. 2017;58(09):1533–41.
24. Delaj L, Novy J, Ryvlin P, Marchi NA, Rossetti AO. Refractory and super-refractory status epilepticus in adults: a 9-year cohort study. Acta Neurol Scand. 2017;135(01):92–9.
25. Ferlisi M, Shorvon S. The outcome of therapies in refractory and super-refractory convulsive status epilepticus and recommendations for therapy. Brain. 2012;135(Pt 8):2314–28.
26. Trinka E, Kälviäinen R. 25 Years of advances in the definition, classification and treatment of status epilepticus. Seizure. 2017;44:65–73.
27. Grover EH, Nazzal Y, Hirsch LJ. Treatment of convulsive status epilepticus. Curr Treat Options Neurol. 2016;18(3):11.
28. Meziane-Tani A, Foreman B, Mizrahi MA. Status epilepticus: work-up and management in adults. Semin Neurol. 2020;40(6):652–60.
29. Minicucci F, Ferlisi M, Brigo F, Mecarelli O, Meletti S, Aguglia U, et al. Management of status epilepticus in adults. Position paper of the Italian League Against Epilepsy. Epilepsy Behav. 2020;102:106675.
30. Alldredge BK, Gelb AM, Isaacs SM, et al. A comparison of lorazepam, diazepam, and placebo for the treatment of out-of-hospital status epilepticus. N Engl J Med. 2001;345(09):631–7.
31. Silbergleit R, Lowenstein D, Durkalski V, Conwit R, Neurological Emergency Treatment Trials (NETT) Investigators. RAMPART (Rapid Anticonvulsant Medication Prior to Arrival Trial): a double-blind randomized clinical trial of the efficacy of intramuscular midazolam versus intravenous lorazepam in the prehospital treatment of status epilepticus by paramedics. Epilepsia. 2011;52(Suppl 8):45–7.

32. Silbergleit R, Durkalski V, Lowenstein D, Conwit R, Pancioli A, Palesch Y, et al.; NETT Investigators. Intramuscular versus intravenous therapy for prehospital status epilepticus. N Engl J Med. 2012;366(7):591–600.
33. Hocker S, Wijdicks EF, Rabinstein AA. Refractory status epilepticus: new insights in presentation, treatment, and outcome. Neurol Res. 2013;35(2):163–8.
34. Nelson SE, Varelas PN. Status epilepticus, refractory status epilepticus, and super-refractory status epilepticus. Continuum (Minneap Minn). 2018;24(6):1683–707.
35. Betjemann JP, Lowenstein DH. Status epilepticus in adults. Lancet Neurol. 2015;14(6):615–24.
36. Trinka E, Höfler J, Leitinger M, Brigo F. Pharmacotherapy for status epilepticus. Drugs. 2015;75(13):1499–521.
37. Brigo F, Bragazzi NL, Igwe SC, Nardone R, Trinka E. Topiramate in the treatment of generalized convulsive status epilepticus in adults: a systematic review with individual patient data analysis. Drugs. 2017;77(1):67–74.
38. Rohracher A, Höfler J, Kalss G, Leitinger M, Kuchukhidze G, Deak I, et al. Perampanel in patients with refractory and super-refractory status epilepticus in a neurological intensive care unit. Epilepsy Behav. 2015;49:354–8.
39. Visser NA, Braun KP, Leijten FS, van Nieuwenhuizen O, Wokke JH, van den Bergh WM. Magnesium treatment for patients with refractory status epilepticus due to POLG1-mutations. J Neurol. 2011;258:218–22.
40. Haenggeli C-A, Girardin E, Paunier L. Pyridoxine-dependent seizures, clinical and therapeutic aspects. Eur J Pediatr. 1991;150:452–5.
41. Nabbout R, Vezzani A, Dulac O, Chiron C. Acute encephalopathy with inflammationmediated status epilepticus. Lancet Neurol. 2011;10(1):99–108.
42. Gastaldi M, Thouin A, Vincent A. Antibody-mediated autoimmune encephalopathies and immunotherapies. Neurotherapeutics. 2016;13(1):147–62.
43. Rossetti AO. Treatment options in the management of status epilepticus. Curr Treat Options Neurol. 2010;12:100–12.
44. Corry JJ, Dhar R, Murphy T, Diringer MN. Hypothermia for refractory status epilepticus. Neurocrit Care. 2008;9(2):189–97.
45. Thakur KT, Probasco JC, Hocker SE, Roehl K, Henry B, Kossoff EH, et al. Ketogenic diet for adults in super-refractory status epilepticus. Neurology. 2014;82(8):665–70.

46. Cervenka MC, Hocker S, Koenig M, Bar B, Henry-Barron B, Kossoff EH, et al. Phase I/II multicenter ketogenic diet study for adult super refractory status epilepticus. Neurology. 2017;88(10):938–43.
47. Francis BA, Fillenworth J, Gorelick P, Karanec K, Tanner A. The feasibility, safety and effectiveness of a ketogenic diet for refractory status epilepticus in adults in the intensive care unit. Neurocrit Care. 2019;30(3):652–7.
48. Weimer T, Boling W, Palade A. Neurosurgical therapy for central area status epilepticus. W V Med J. 2012;108(5):20–3.
49. Ng YT, Kerrigan JF, Rekate HL. Neurosurgical treatment of status epilepticus. J Neurosurg. 2006;105(Suppl 5):378–81.
50. Kamel H, Cornes SB, Hegde M, Hall SE, Josephson SA. Electroconvulsive therapy for refractory status epilepticus: a case series. Neurocrit Care. 2010;12(2):204–10.
51. Shahwan A, Bailey C, Maxiner W, Harvey AS. Vagus nerve stimulation for refractory epilepsy in children: more to VNS than seizure frequency reduction. Epilepsia. 2009;50(5):1220–8.
52. Rotenberg A, Muller P, Birnbaum D, Harrington M, Riviello JJ, Pascual-Leone A, Jensen FE. Seizure suppression by EEG-guided repetitive transcranial magnetic stimulation in the rat. Clin Neurophysiol. 2008;119(12):2697–702.
53. Yasiry Z, Shorvon SD. The relative effectiveness of five antiepileptic drugs in treatment of benzodiazepine-resistant convulsive status epilepticus: a meta-analysis of published studies. Seizure. 2014;23(3):167–74.
54. Chamberlain JM, Kapur J, Shinnar S, Elm J, Holsti M, Babcock L, et al.; Neurological Emergencies Treatment Trials; Pediatric Emergency Care Applied Research Network Investigators. Efficacy of levetiracetam, fosphenytoin, and valproate for established status epilepticus by age group (ESETT): a double-blind, responsive-adaptive, randomised controlled trial. Lancet. 2020;395(10231):1217–24.
55. Strzelczyk A, Steinig I, Willems LM, et al. Treatment of refractory and super-refractory status epilepticus with brivaracetam: a cohort study from two German university hospitals. Epilepsy Behav. 2017;70:177–81.
56. Kalss G, Rohracher A, Leitinger M, et al. Intravenous brivaracetam in status epilepticus: a retrospective single-center study. Epilepsia. 2018;59(Suppl. 2):228–33.
57. Klein P, Schiemann J, Sperling MR, et al. A randomized, double-blind, placebo- controlled, multicenter, parallel-group study to

evaluate the efficacy and safety of adjunctive brivaracetam in adult patients with uncontrolled partial-onset seizures. Epilepsia. 2015;56:1890–8.
58. Klitgaard H, Matagne A, Nicolas JM, et al. Brivaracetam: rationale for the discovery and preclinical profile of SV2A ligand for epilepsy treatment. Epilepsia. 2016;57:538–48.
59. Gillard M, Fuks B, Leclercq K, et al. Binding characteristics of brivaracetam, a selective, high affinity SV2A ligand in rat, mouse and human brain: relationship to anti-convulsant properties. Eur J Pharmacol. 2011;664:36–44.
60. Nicolas JM, Hannestad J, Holden D, et al. Brivaracetam, a selective high-affinity synaptic vesicle protein 2A (SV2A) ligand with preclinical evidence of high brain permeability and fat onset of action. Epilepsia. 2016;57:201–9.
61. Vossler DG, Bainbridge JL, Boggs JG, Novotny EJ, Loddenkemper T, Faught E, et al. Treatment of refractory convulsive status epilepticus: a comprehensive review by the American Epilepsy Society Treatments Committee. Epilepsy Curr. 2020;20(5):245–64.

Targeted Temperature Management

Francisco E. Gomez, Jesyree Veitia, and David Convissar

1 Introduction

Several detrimental metabolic and inflammatory processes occur within the brain secondary to elevated temperatures, including but not limited to oxidative stress [1] local ischemia, inflammation, DNA damage, thermal pooling, apoptosis, and protein denaturation [2, 3], extending the lesioned area [4] likely leading to worse outcomes over several outcome measures [5].

Hypothermia has been shown to decrease the incidence of said detrimental processes as well as that of resulting seizures [2] While the initial neurologic insult is destructive to cerebral parenchyma, secondary injury prevention is one of the tenets of neurocritical care [6, 7] which may be in part mediated by hyperthermia [2].

F. E. Gomez (✉)
Department of Neurology, University of Missouri Health Care, Columbia, MO, USA
e-mail: fegyr7@umsystem.edu

J. Veitia
Yale University, New Haven, CT, USA

D. Convissar
Harvard University, Boston, MA, USA

© The Author(s), under exclusive license to Springer Nature Switzerland AG 2022
N. Arora (ed.), *Procedures and Protocols in the Neurocritical Care Unit*, https://doi.org/10.1007/978-3-030-90225-4_18

2 Indications and Contraindications (Table 1)

Targeted temperature management offers benefits in several neurological injury states. Therapeutic hypothermia is indicated in patients not following commands after cardiac arrest, regardless of presenting rhythm [8, 11–13] as well as for reactive control of medically resistant intracranial pressure in TBI [4].

Induced normothermia or hypothermia have also shown benefit in several neurological injuries [9, 14] such as: ischemic stroke and hepatic encephalopathy. Induced normothermia has shown benefit in SAH [9, 14] sepsis [15] and may decrease inflammatory related injury in the lung [2].

Contraindications include significant hemorrhage or infection, hemodynamic instability despite vasopressors, underlying terminal condition, patient awakens and follows commands [16, 17]. Other considerations include pre-existing illness precluding meaningful recovery or if continuing care would not be within the patient's wishes [16].

Table 1 Indications and contraindications for targeted temperature management [8–10]

Indications for Therapeutic Hypothermia	Indications for Therapeutic Normothermia	Contraindications for Therapeutic Hypothermia
Cardia carrest regardless of presenting rhythm	Acute ischemic stroke	Against patient's stated wishes
Medically refractory ICP in TBI	Subarachnoid Hemorrhage	Patient awakens and follows commands
	Intracerebral Hemorrhage	Severe sepsis or hemodynamic instability despite pressors
		Pre-existing or terminal illness precluding meaningful recovery

3 Techniques for Targeted Temperature Management

Hypothermia and rewarming are achieved through a variety of heat exchange methods [18]. There is no established superiority of surface vs endovascular cooling in outcomes or side effects [18]. Servo-controlled, self-adjusting mechanisms which adjust cooling fluid temperature in accordance to target and core temperatures are preferable [4, 10].

4 Conventional Methods

Cold crystalloid infusion is a cost-effective and readily available method to induce hypothermia. However it is not as effective for maintenance of a set temperature, there is a risk for overshooting the set cooling target [19] and risk of fluid overload [4]. A 30 cc/kg up to 2 L bolus of 4° saline or Ringer's lactate [4, 19] in addition to ice packs or cold compresses may be utilized as a coadjuvant during the induction phase.

5 Surface Cooling (SFC)

SFC consists of applying cooling pads directly on the patient's skin [18, 20]. Air cooling and cooling blankets are inefficacious [16, 20]. Adjustable temperature feedback-loop systems with liquid recirculating pads are commercially available. Devices include, but are not limited to: Arctic Sun (Bard, Medivance, Louisville, CO) Criticool (Belmont Medical Technologies, Billerica, Massachusstes), and STX surface pad system (Zoll, Pittsburgh, Pennsylvania). SFC can be readily initiated, and cooling rates are estimated about 1.5 °C/h with closed loop water recirculation systems [20].

SFC is a relatively simple procedure, necessitating only the application and connection of cooling pads to the patient and connecting the tubing to the appropriate console [21]. Complications include possible increased risk for skin damage due to immobility and thermal injury [22]. Additionally SFC is slowed in obese patients due to insulating properties of adipose tissue and an increased mass to surface area ratio [20].

6 Endovascular Cooling

EVC involves central vein cannulation with a specialized catheter (Figs. 1 and 2) equipped with a fluid-circulating heat exchanger connected to a matching console [8] EVC cooling speed is estimated at about 1.2 °C/h [12] Some of the major endovascular cooling systems on the market include the InnerCool RTx® Endovascular cooling system (Phillips Healthcare, Andover, Massachusetts) and the Thermoguard XP system as well as the Zoll The Thermogard XP® (Zoll, Pittsburgh, Pennsylvania) [23, 24].

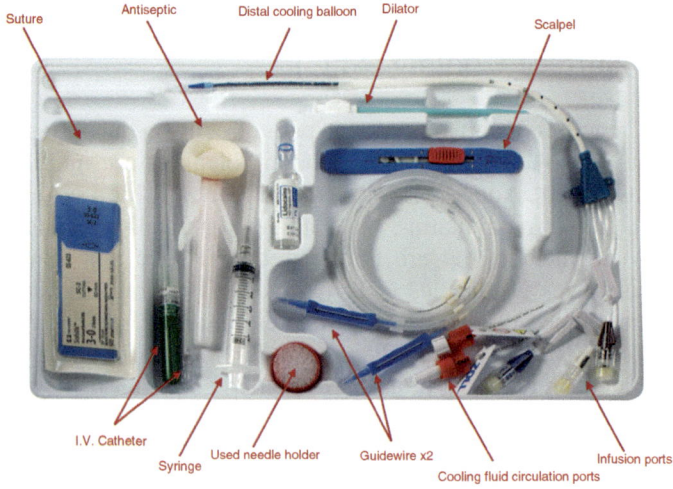

Figure 1 Intravascular cooling catheterkit

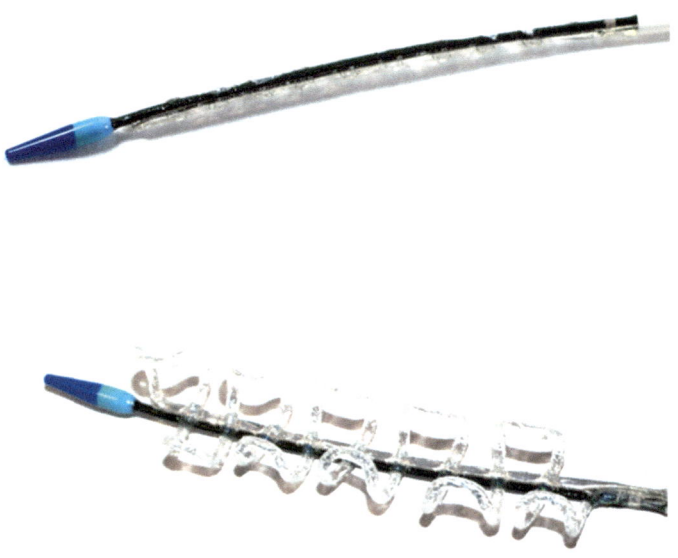

FIGURE 2 A serpentine balloon above, collapsed, below deployed, thus increasing surface area available for heat exchange. Photo Courtesy Joanne Neubauer

Advantages of EVC involve less temperature variability [22, 25–27], one meta analysis showing a trend towards improved outcomes [28], notwithstanding more frequent post-hypothermia fever [18]. Techniques and complications of central catheter placement may be found elsewhere in this text (chapter Vascular Access).

7 Other Methods

Procedures such as extracorporeal membrane oxygenation or hemodialysis incur in heat loss from the circulating extracorporeal blood, and have been deployed as TTM devices with success [29, 30]. Esophageal cooling devices also have shown promise and have been FDA approved [31]. New methods are being developed non-invasive Intranasal cooling and automated cold peritoneal lavage are currently under investigation [30, 32, 33].

8 Protocol

TTM is best applied as a protocol drive therapy [34], and can be divided into 3 distinct phases; induction, maintenance and rewarming, each presenting distinct management challenges (Fig. 3).

8.1 Induction

The induction phase comprises the beginning of therapeutic hypothermia induction up to the achievement of goal temperature.

TTM is to be initiated as soon as patient eligibility is determined [36, 37]. Combining cooling methods provides the

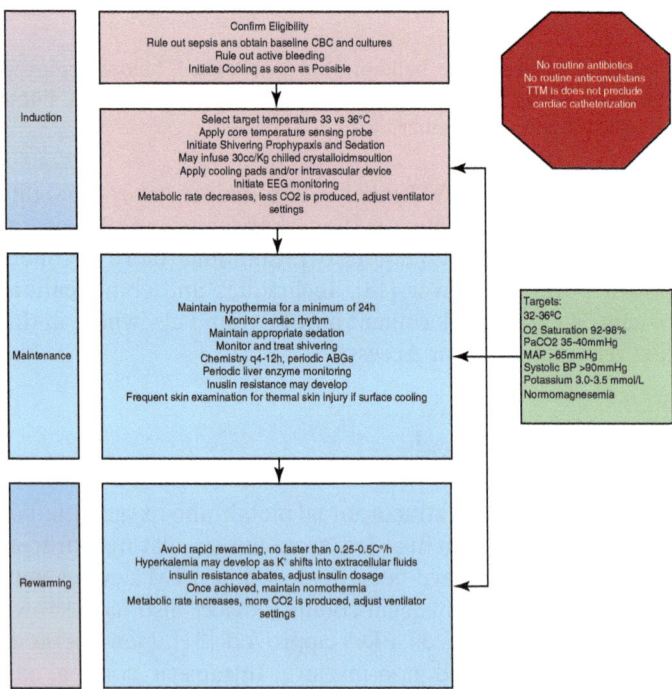

FIGURE 3 Hypothermia protocol [11, 14, 17, 35, 36]

most rapid induction, such as a rapid infusion of 30–40 cc/kg 4 °C crystalloid in combination with initiating SFC or EVC with a feed-back loop regulated device [16]. As surface temperature is unreliable in these patients core temperature monitored in these patients via bladder, esophageal, endovascular, or rectal probe [36].

Of note, shivering and peripheral vasoconstriction are more likely to occur during the induction phase, as the threshold for shivering is about 35.5 °C, and that of vasoconstriction about 36.5 [38] Thus, shivering is an expected complication of induction which may delay achievement of target temperature [39], especially if SFC is being employed.

Sedation as well as shivering prophylaxis and treatment must be initiated in this phase [2, 37]. Cold-induced diuresis may cause hypokalemia, hypomagnesemia and hypophosphatemia as well as volume depletion which must be monitored and replaced accordingly [16]. Insulin resistance develops and hyperglycemia appears, necessitating monitoring and treatment [2, 16].

Skin counter warming is effective even in SFC [16, 36] as skin mean temperature afferent input accounts for about 20% of the centrally mediated shivering and vasoconstriction response [39]. Given decreased drug clearance observed in TTM, short acting sedatives are preferred. In one study comparing propofol-remifentanil vs midazolam-fentanyl, the former demonstrated earlier awakening and more ventilator free days [40]. Notably the half life of benzodiazepines is known to be prolonged in hypothermia [16].

8.2 Maintenance

Comprises the time between target temperature being reached and the initiation of rewarming.

Patients should be kept at goal temperature for a minimum of 24 h [4, 22], although a longer duration of 48 h has shown a tendency to improved outcomes in post-cardiac arrest [37]. During the maintenance phase, a relatively steady state is reached and focus shifts to maintaining normocapnia, normoxia, normoglycemia, normomagnesemia and normokalemia [4]. Large fluctuations in core temperature are best avoided [22].

8.3 Rewarming

The rewarming phase comprises the end of the maintenance phase and the period required to reach normothermia.
The rewarming phase is critical, as rebound effects may be seen if temperature rises too rapidly, which may hinder benefits derived from TTM. Rapid rewarming may result in severe cerebral hyperthermia [20], systemic vasodilation and hypotension, with subsequent cerebral vasodilation and plateau waves [36] or rebound fever, associated with mortality [1]. Risk for rebound hyperkalemia or increased cerebral metabolic rate or cerebral hypoxia are also pitfalls of rapid rewarming [17,36]. Encountering said phenomena should prompt treatment and slowing or pausing rewarming altogether.

Controlled rewarming is thus recommended at a maximal rate of 0.25–0.5 °C/h if no untoward effects are seen, such as ICP crises [37, 41]. One retrospective study found prolonged rewarming (near 1C/24 h) to be an independent factor for survival and better neurological outcomes in cardiac arrest patients [42]. Rebound fever may also be deleterious, thus maintaining normothermia for 48–72 h after rewarming is also recommendable [2, 17].

Table 2 enlists the common complications encountered with therapeutic hypothermia.

TABLE 2 Commonly complications and caution items encountered in therapeutic hypothermia [2, 10, 11, 20–22, 36, 41, 43]

Condition	Characteristics/treatment
Bleeding diathesis	Concerns for clinically significant hemorrhage caused by ttm are not supported by evidence. Platelet count and function mildly affected below 35 °C, Coagulation factors below 33 °C. Consider platelet or desmopressin administration prior to invasive procedures
Drug metabolism	Hepatic perfusion and enzyme function are diminished in hypothermia, decreasing the clearance of several drugs such as benzodiazepines, opiates, synthetic opiates, paralytics, propofol and phenytoin. This must be taken into account for dosing and neuroprognostication purposes.
Dysrhythmias	A drop in cardiac output is expected and commensurate with decreased metabolic rate. Little risk for severe arrhythmias above 30 °C. Cooling decreases sinus repolarization node hence a degree of bradycardia is to be expected. If hemodynamic instability results, atropine is ineffective and pacing preferable.
Immunosuppression	Cooling impairs inflammation and leukocyte phagocytosis. Rate of infection rises with treatment duration. Pneumonia is the most associated infection, there is no data to support prophylactic antibiotics.

(continued)

TABLE 2 (continued)

Condition	Characteristics/treatment
Hyperglycemia	Hypothermia induces insulin resistance in addition to decreasing it's secretion. Resulting hyperglycemia may necessitate large doses of insulin. Frequent checks and dosing adjustments are especially necessary in the rewarming phase as insulin requirements normalize. Of note, a specific target range conveying benefit has not been elucidated and some authors recommend tolerating hyperlgycmia up to 144 mg/dl.
Electrolyte disturbances	Cooling induces K+ intracellular shift and renal tubular dysfunction, thus hypokalemia. Hypomagnesemia and hypophosphatemia may occur. Frequent blood chemistries and careful correction are warranted, keeping in mind the expected K+ extracellular shift which occurs during rewarming to avoid hyperkalemia. In anuric or severely oliguric patients with renal replacement therapy should be instituted before rewarming
Blood gases	Interpretation of blood gas analysis must account for temperature changes in order to avoid erroneous overestimation of $PaCO_2$ and PaO_2 or overestimation of pH. Metabolic rate falls commesurately with temperature and less CO_2 is generated, and in order to avoid cerebral vasoconstriction, maintaining normocarbia may be reasonable. Thus ventilator settings must be adjusted as with temperature changes, and frequent blood gas analyses are warranted, especially during the induction and rewarming phases

TABLE 2 (continued)

Condition	Characteristics/treatment
Hypovolemia	Increased venous return induced by hypothermia induces release of atrial natriuretic peptide and a decrease in the levels of antidiuretic hormone. This (in combination with other mechanisms such as tubular dysfunction, see later) can lead to a marked increase in diuresis ("cold diuresis")

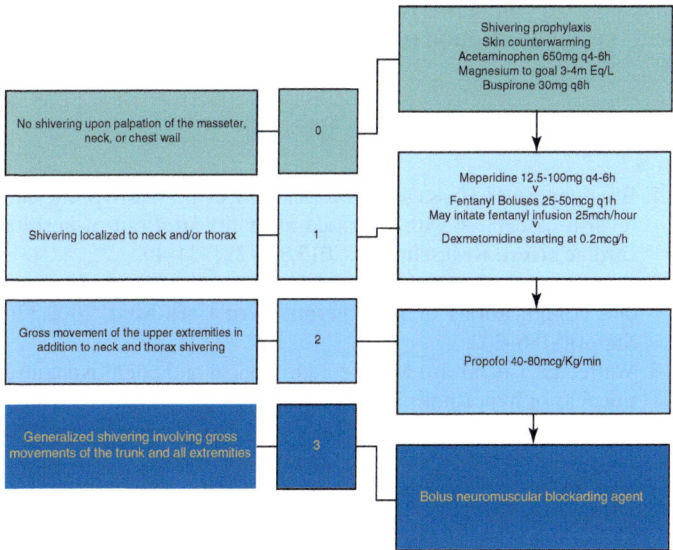

FIGURE 4 Proposed shivering protocol, wherein treatment is tailored to BSAS scores [16, 22, 39, 44, 45]

9 Shivering (Fig. 4)

Shivering is a physiological response to cold temperatures often encountered in the course of TTM which if left rampant may negate any potential benefits [4]. Shivering leads to higher temperature variability and may slow induction [37] as mentioned above. It may also induce a stress response with increased metabolic rate, oxygen consumption, work of breathing, heart rate [2, 4, 36] as well as increased CO_2 production [4]. In awake patients, shivering can increase oxygen consumption by 40–100% [36].

Thus, shivering management must be administered concurrently with TTM initiation and maintained until the rewarming phase is concluded [37]. Several sedatives and hypnotics decrease the shivering threshold [4] and may be be utilized in synergy with non-pharmacological methods such as skin counter-waring with air-circulating blankets or other wam coverings [4, 36]. Shivering management also benefits from a protocolized stepwise approach in order to minimize total dosages and the administration of neuromuscular blockade [45].

References

1. Bro-Jeppesen J, Hassager C, Wanscher M, et al. Post-hypothermia fever is associated with increased mortality after out-of-hospital cardiac arrest. Resuscitation. 2013;84(12):1734–40.
2. Polderman KH. Mechanisms of action, physiological effects, and complications of hypothermia. Crit Care Med. 2009;37(7 Suppl):S186–202.
3. Walter EJ, Carraretto M. The neurological and cognitive consequences of hyperthermia. Crit Care. 2016;20(1):199.
4. Madden LK, Hill M, May TL, et al. The implementation of targeted temperature management: an evidence-based guideline from the Neurocritical Care Society. Neurocrit Care. 2017;27:468–87. https://doi.org/10.1007/s12028-017-0469-5.
5. Greer DM, Funk SE, Reaven NL, Ouzounelli M, Uman GC. Impact of fever on outcome in patients with stroke and neurologic injury: a comprehensive meta-analysis. Stroke. 2008;39(11):3029–35.
6. Walleck CA. Preventing secondary brain injury. AACN Clin Issues Crit Care Nurs. 1992;3(1):19–30.
7. Lazaridis C, Rusin CG, Robertson CS. Secondary brain injury: predicting and preventing insults. Neuropharmacology. 2019;145(Pt B):145–52.
8. Bernard SA, Gray TW, Buist MD, et al. Treatment of comatose survivors of out-of-hospital cardiac arrest with induced hypothermia. N Engl J Med. 2002;346(8):557–63.

9. Andrews PJD, Verma V, Healy M, Lavinio A, Curtis C, Reddy U, et al. Targeted temperature management in patients with intracerebral haemorrhage, subarachnoid haemorrhage, or acute ischaemic stroke: consensus recommendations [Internet]. Br J Anaesth. Elsevier. 2018;121(4):768–75.
10. Cariou A, Payen J, Asehnoune K, Gerard A, Botte A, Brissaud O, Debaty G, Deltour S, Deye N, Engrand N, Francony G, Legreiel S, Levy B, Meyer P, Orban J, Renolleau S, Vigue B, de Saint Blanquat L, Mathien C, Velly L. Targeted temperature management in the ICU: guidelines from a French expert panel. Anaesth Crit Care Pain Med. 2018;37:481–91.
11. Panchal AR, Bartos JA, Cabañas JG. Part 3: Adult basic and advanced life support: 2020 American Heart Association guidelines for cardiopulmonary resuscitation and emergency cardiovascular care. Circulation. 2020;142:S366–468. https://www.ahajournals.org/doi/epub/10.1161/CIR.0000000000000916
12. Hypothermia after Cardiac Arrest Study Group. Mild therapeutic hypothermia to improve the neurologic outcome after cardiac arrest. N Engl J Med. 2002;346(8):549–56.
13. Lascarrou JB, Merdji H, Le Gouge A, et al. Targeted temperature management for cardiac arrest with nonshockable rhythm. N Engl J Med. 2019;381(24):2327–37.
14. Polderman KH. Keeping a cool head: how to induce and maintain hypothermia. Crit Care Med. 2004;32:2558–60.
15. Polderman KH. Induced hypothermia and fever control for prevention and treatment of neurological injuries. Lancet. 2008;371(9628):1955–69.
16. Livesay S, Elmer J, Kirschen M, Peacock S. Emergency neurological life support: resuscitation following cardiac arrest. Neurocrit Care. 2017;27(Suppl 1):134–43. https://doi.org/10.1007/s12028-019-00817-1.
17. Seder DB, Van der Kloot TE. Methods of cooling: practical aspects of therapeutic temperature management. Crit Care Med. 2009;37:S211–22.
18. Fazio CD, Skrifvars MB, Søreide E, Creteur J, Grejs AM, Kjærgaard J, Laitio T, Nee J, Kirkegaard H, Taccone FS. Intravascular versus surface cooling for targeted temperature management after out-of-hospital cardiac arrest: an analysis of the TTH48 trial. Crit Care. 2019;23(1):61. https://doi.org/10.1186/s13054-019-2335-7.
19. Kliegel A, Janata A, Wandaller C, et al. Cold infusions alone are effective for induction of therapeutic hypothermia but

do not keep patients cool after cardiac arrest. Resuscitation. 2007;73:46–53.
20. Polderman KH, Herold I. Therapeutic hypothermia and controlled normothermia in the intensive care unit: Practical considerations, side effects, and cooling methods*. Crit Care Med. 2009;37(3):1101–20.
21. Medi-Therm® III Hyper/Hypothermia Machine MTA6900 Series. https://techweb.stryker.com/Gaymar/TMP/Medi-Term/MTA6900/100974000.pdf.
22. Jain A, Gray M, Slisz S, Haymore J, Badjatia N, Kulstad E. Shivering treatments for targeted temperature management: a review. J Neurosci Nurs. 2018;50(2):63–7. https://doi.org/10.1097/JNN.0000000000000340.
23. IVTM intravascular temperature management catheter specifications. http://www.zoll.com/uploadedFiles/Public_Site/Products/Catheters/Catheters_spec_sheet.pdf.Â.
24. Tømte Ø, Drægni T, Mangschau A, et al. A comparison of intravascular and surface cooling techniques in comatose cardiac arrest survivors. Crit Care Med. 2011;39:443–9. https://doi.org/10.1097/CCM.0b013e318206b80f.
25. Hoedemaekers C, Ezzahti M, Gerritsen A. Comparison of cooling methods to induce and maintain normo-and hypothermia in intensive care unit patients: a prospective intervention study. Crit Care. 2007;11:R91. https://doi.org/10.1186/cc6104.
26. Jun GS, Kim JG, Choi HY, Kang GH, Kim W, Jang YS, Kim HT. A comparison of intravascular and surface cooling devices for targeted temperature management after out-of-hospital cardiac arrest. Medicine. 2019;98(30):e16549. https://doi.org/10.1097/md.0000000000016549.
27. Vaity C, Al-Subaie N, Cecconi M. Cooling techniques for targeted temperature management post-cardiac arrest. Crit Care. 2015;19(1):103. https://doi.org/10.1186/s13054-015-0804-1.
28. Bartlett ES, Valenzuela T, Idris A, Deye N, Glover G, Gillies MA, Taccone FS, Sunde K, Flint AC, Thiele H, Arrich J, Hemphill C, Holzer M, Skrifvars MB, Pittl U, Polderman KH, Ong MEH, Kim KH, Oh SH, Do Shin S, Kirkegaard H, Nichol G. Systematic review and meta-analysis of intravascular temperature management vs. surface cooling in comatose patients resuscitated from cardiac arrest. Resuscitation. 2020;146:82–95. ISSN 0300–9572, https://doi.org/10.1016/j.resuscitation.2019.10.035.
29. Soga T, Nagao K, Kikushima K, et al. Mild therapeutic hypothermia using extracorporeal cooling method in comatose survivors

after out-of-hospital cardiac arrest. Circulation. 2006;114:II_1190. https://www.ahajournals.org/doi/abs/10.1161/circ.114.suppl_18.II_1190-c
30. Ma YJ, Ning B, Cao WH, Liu T, Liu L. Good neurologic recovery after cardiac arrest using hypothermia through continuous renal replacement therapy. Am J Emerg Med. 2013;31(12):1720.e1–3.
31. Bhatti F, Naiman M, Tsarev A, Kulstad E. Esophageal temperature management in patients suffering from traumatic brain injury. Ther Hypothermia Temp Manag. 2019;9(4):238–42.
32. Rhinochill Advantage. http://www.benechill.com/wp/rhinochill-trade/ems-use/.
33. de Waard MC, Biermann H, Brinckman SL, et al. Automated peritoneal lavage: an extremely rapid and safe way to induce hypothermia in post-resuscitation patients. Crit Care. 2013;17:R31. https://doi.org/10.1186/cc12518.
34. Perman SM, Goyal M, Neumar RW, Topjian AA, Gaieski DF. Clinical applications of targeted temperature management. Chest. 2014;145(2):386–93. https://doi.org/10.1378/chest.12-3025.
35. Nielsen N, Wetterslev J, Cronberg T, et al. Targeted temperature management at 33 degrees C versus 36 degrees C after cardiac arrest. N Engl J Med. 2013;369(23):2197–206.
36. Badjatia N. Therapeutic hypothermia protocols. Crit Care Neurol Part II. 2017;141:619–32. https://doi.org/10.1016/b978-0-444-63599-0.00033-8.
37. Taccone FS, Picetti E, Vincent J. High quality Targeted Temperature Management (TTM) after cardiac arrest. Crit Care. 2020;24:6. https://doi.org/10.1186/s13054-019-2721-1.
38. Lopez M, Sessler DI, Walter K, Emerick T, Ozaki M. Rate and gender dependence of the sweating, vasoconstriction, and shivering thresholds in humans. Anesthesiology. 1994;80:780–78.
39. Sessler DI. Defeating normal thermoregulatory defenses. Stroke. 2009;40:e614–21. https://doi.org/10.1161/STROKEAHA.108.520858.
40. Paul M, Bougouin W, Dumas F, Geri G, Champigneulle B, Guillemet L, Salem OBH, et al. Comparison of two sedation regimens during targeted temperature management after cardiac arrest. Resuscitation. 2018;128:204–10, ISSN 0300-9572, https://doi.org/10.1016/j.resuscitation.2018.03.025.
41. Kim SJ, Lee JK, Kim DK, et al. Effect of antibiotic prophylaxis on early-onset pneumonia in cardiac arrest patients treated with therapeutic hypothermia. Korean J Crit Care Med. 2016;31(1):17–24. https://doi.org/10.4266/kjccm.2016.31.1.17.

42. Hifumi T, Inoue A, Kokubu N, et al. Association between rewarming duration and neurological outcome in out-of-hospital cardiac arrest patients receiving therapeutic hypothermia. Resuscitation. 2020;146:170–7. https://doi.org/10.1016/j.resuscitation.2019.07.029.
43. Anderson KB, Poloyac SM, Kochanek PM, Empey PE. Effect of hypothermia and targeted temperature management on drug disposition and response following cardiac arrest: a comprehensive review of preclinical and clinical investigations. Ther Hypothermia Temp Manag. 2016;6(4):169–79. https://doi.org/10.1089/ther.2016.0003.
44. Wang CX, Stroink A, Casto JM, Kattner K. Hyperthermia exacerbates ischaemic brain injury. Int J Stroke. 2009;4(4):274–84.
45. Human T, Tesoro E, Peacock S. Pharmacotherapy pearls for emergency neurological life support. Neurocrit Care. 2017;27(1):51–73. https://doi.org/10.1007/s12028-019-00830-4.

Original Bibliography

Arctic Sun™ Temperature Management System. https://www.crbard.com/Medical/en-US/Products/Arctic-Sun-Temperature-Management-System.

Donnino MW, Andersen LW, Berg KM, Reynolds JC, Nolan JP, Morley PT, Lang E, Cocchi MN, Xanthos T, Callaway CW, Soar J, the ILCOR ALS Task Force, Aibiki M, Böttiger BW, Brooks SC, Deakin CD, Drajer S, Kloeck W, Morrison LJ, Neumar RW, Nicholson TC, O'Neil BJ, Paiva EF, Parr M, Wang T-L, Witt J. Temperature management after cardiac arrest. Circulation. 2015;132(25):2448.

https://www.braincool.se/en/products/rhinochill_en/.

https://www.longdom.org/open-access/untoward-effects-in-the-practice-of-therapeutic-hypothermia-aliterature-update-2329-6925-1000356.pdf.

Merchant RM, Abella BS, Peberdy MA, et al. Therapeutic hypothermia after cardiac arrest: Unintentional overcooling is common using ice packs and conventional cooling blankets. Crit Care Med. 2006;34:S490–4. https://doi.org/10.1097/01.CCM.0000246016.28679.36.

Mechanical Ventilation and Weaning In ICU

Tijo Thomas, Ephrem Teklemariam, and Chitra Sivasankar

1 Introduction

Initial uses of mechanical ventilation were designed to inflate the lung until a specific set pressure was achieved. Since then, there has been an evolution to include a multitude of variable modes of ventilation to best fit a patient's need based on their specific disease pathophysiology [1].

Patients who are mechanically ventilated in the Neurocritical care unit (NCCU) present with unique challenges. They are intubated either due to respiratory failure, brain injury which can be due to trauma, stroke, encephalitis, meningitis, seizures, or multitude of neuromuscular illness. With decreasing levels of consciousness often tongue can fall back and lead to airway obstruction. Also, many of these patients have impaired cough and gag reflex which can lead

---

T. Thomas · E. Teklemariam
Thomas Jefferson University, Philadelphia, PA, USA
e-mail: tijo.thomas@jefferson.edu;
Ephrem.teklemariam@jefferson.edu

C. Sivasankar (✉)
Division of Anesthesiology/Neurosurgery, Thomas Jefferson University, Philadelphia, PA, USA
e-mail: Chitra.sivasankar@jefferson.edu

© The Author(s), under exclusive license to Springer Nature Switzerland AG 2022
N. Arora (ed.), *Procedures and Protocols in the Neurocritical Care Unit*, https://doi.org/10.1007/978-3-030-90225-4_19

to poor secretion clearance and frequent aspiration. Common indications for intubation are included in Fig. 1. These include either failure to ventilate or oxygenate Neuro intensive care patients may have high intracranial pressure (ICP) especially in cases of cerebral edema, large strokes, cardiac arrest, Intracerebral Hemorrhage (ICH), Traumatic Brain Injury (TBI), and Subarachnoid hemorrhage (SAH). The type of brain injury can also affect respiratory drive and pattern [2].

2 Airway Assessment

It is important to assess the airway of a patient before intubation (Fig. 2). However, this is often difficult in ICU as patients are often altered or obtunded and unable to follow com-

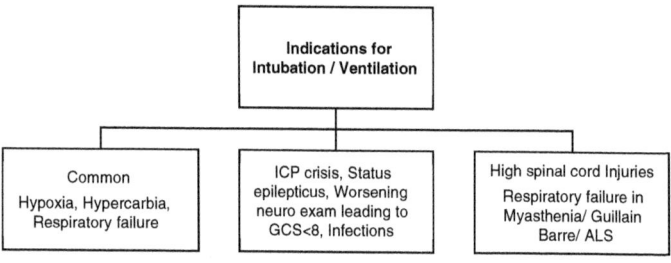

Figure 1 Indications for intubation

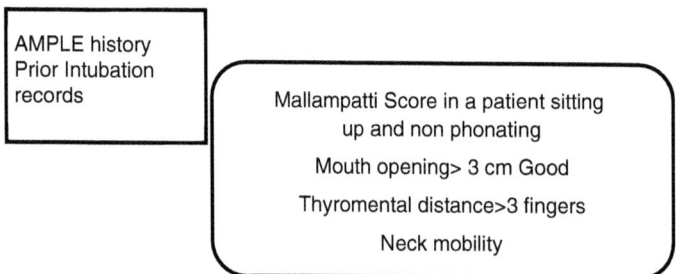

Figure 2 Pre-intubation airway assessment, AMPLE history (allergies, medications, past medical history, last meal, events)

mands. The goal is to identify patients who may have difficult airways and mandating different approaches and help if necessary. Challenges in ICU include significant secretions, hemodynamic instability, increased work of breathing, desaturation as well spinal instability due to trauma, and often inexperienced operators.

The ability to predict a difficult airway is the key to successfully managing it. It is important to have a plan in mind – if plan A does not work you should be able to call for help while trying to do plan B. Patients can be difficult to ventilate or difficult to intubate- there are very few patients who are difficult to ventilate and intubate. In those patients it is important to plan awake fiber optic with either ENT or anesthesia.

There are different mnemonics to quickly remember and learn patients who are difficult to ventilate and intubate See Fig. 3.

3 Predictors of Difficult Ventilation

Bag mask ventilation is the foremost and fundamental skill in airway management. Table 1 Predictors of difficult bag mask include mnemonic- OBESE – BMI >26, Beard or facial hair, Edentulous, Snoring or OSA, Age greater than 55 years. Other factors to look for are limited neck mobility with radiation, fused cervical spine and male sex [5].

4 Predictors of Difficult Intubation – Table 1

Mnemonic used to recognize a patient that is difficult to intubate is LEMON. L for Look. E for Evaluate. M for Mallampati class. O for obstruction and N for neck mobility. Looking externally you are looking at overall patients including head and neck trauma, oral bleeding, obesity, neck circumference, retrognathia, facial hair, stridor, hoarseness of voice. Evaluate the patient using 3-3-2 rule – mouth opening 3 fingerbreadths,

TABLE 1 Difficult mask ventilation and intubation assessment

Difficult mask ventilation	Difficult intubation
Obese – BMI >26	Look Externally
Beard	Evaluate 3-3-2
Edentulous	Mallampatti 3/4
Sleep apnea	Obstruction/Mass
Age >55	Neck Mobility/Circumference >43 cm

TABLE 2 Mallampati scoring (for patient in sitting position)

Class	Description/Difficulty in intubation anticipated
I	Visualization of the soft palate, fauces, uvula and pillars. No anticipated difficulty
II	Visualization of the soft palate, fauces, uvula. No anticipated difficulty.
III	Visualization of the soft palate and base of the uvula. Anticipate moderate difficulty
IV	Soft palate is not visible. Anticipate difficulty.

3 fingerbreadths thyro-mental distance and 2 finger breadths for thyroid-hyoid distance. Mallampati classification (Table 2) can assess the size of the tongue compared to the pharynx based on structures able to be visualized can also help predict difficult intubation. Mallampati class 1 and 2 are considered easier to intubate than 3 and 4. O for anything that might obstruct intubation like an oropharyngeal tumor, foreign body, angioedema. Neck for neck mobility and circumference.

Most of the above mentioned scores are used in the operating room in different subsets of patients. However, one multicenter study evaluated the usefulness of MACOCHA score (Table 3) which can be used in intensive care units (ICU) to predict difficult intubation. Score <3 low risk intubation, higher numbers indicate difficult intubation.

Medications used during intubation are listed below in Table 4. These include pre-induction medications, sedatives, paralytics as well as reversal agents. Each has a specific

Table 3 MACHOCHA variables (Coded from 0 to 12: 0: easy intubation; 12: very difficult intubation)

MACOCHA variables		
Patient related	**M**allampati score III or IV	5
	Apnea syndrome (**O**SA)	2
	Decreased **C** spine Mobility	1
	Limited Mouth **O**pening <3 cm	1
Pathology	GCS <8/**C**oma	1
	Hypoxemia	1
Operator	**N**on anesthesiologist	1
Total		12

limitation and indication. Although first line agents are indicated below, the selection of each agent is dependent on minimizing the possible harmful side effect of each medication. For example, although succinylcholine can helpful in securing airway quickly during intubation, it is typically not used in the NCCU as it can lead to increase in ICP, hyperkalemia especially in patients with history of stroke, TBI, disuse atrophy and neuromuscular disease. Intubation can be done under rapid sequence with the use of paralytics as well as sedative or in some cases with sedation but no paralytics. In the NCCU when there is an emergency intubation, typically would have rapid sequence intubation which can minimize aspiration events [3].

5 Modes of Ventilation

- **Considerations for modes of ventilation**

The ventilator mode describes the characteristics of how the breath is delivered to the patient. The two general approaches consist of either setting volume/flow or pressure as the control variable. The mode of ventilation is at the clinician's discretion. Both volume/flow and pressure targeted modes of ventilation have more in common and can achieve similar goals and minute ventilation goals. Pressure targeted

TABLE 4 Commonly used medications for intubation

Frequently used medications in intubation

Drug	Common Dose ranges	Time to onset	Duration	Indication	Clinical considerations
Induction agents					
Etomidate	0.1–0.3 mg/kg	30 s	3–5 min	Hypotension Increased ICP	Decrease seizure threshold/myoclonus Decrease cortisol synthesis
Propofol	1–2 mg/kg	9–50 s	3–10 min	Increased ICP Seizure disorder	Hypotension Myocardial depression
Ketamine	2 mg/kg IV	1–2 min	5–15 min	Analgesia Asthma/COPD Can be used in hypotension	ICP increase IOP rise

Neuromuscular Blocking Agents				
Succinylcholine	1.5 mg/kg IV	30–60 s	5–15 min	RSI	Hyperkalemia Malignant hyperthermia Myopathy Stroke/denervation >3 d Crush injury >3 days Severe burns >24 h
Rocuronium	0.6–1 mg/kg IV	45–60 s	45–70 min	RSI dose 1 mg/kg	Caution in renal failure Anaphylaxis
Vecuronium	0.1 mg/kg IV	<3 min	45 min		Anaphylaxis
Cisatracurium	0.1–0.2 mg/kg IV	2–3 min	35–45 min	For renal failure and liver failure patients	Hoffman elimination
Reversal Agent				
Sugammedex	16 mg/kg 4 mg/kg 2 mg/kg	2–3min	15 min	For rocuronium reversal	Renal failure Prolonged coags Bradycardia

modes of ventilation will prioritize minimization of barotrauma when compared to volume/flow modes of ventilation which will guarantee a certain minute ventilation.

- **Goals of Mechanical Ventilation in Neurologically injured patients**

  In critically ill patients, goals of mechanical ventilation include oxygenation, ventilation and minimizing ventilator induced lung injury (VALI). In neurologically injured patients, we must also prevent secondary brain injury by preventing hypoxia, prolonged periods of hypocapnia or hypercapnia and elevated ICP. TBI adds a significant layer of complexity since they are excluded from many clinical trials. Permissive hypercapnia and high PEEP can lead to secondary brain injury in these patients. Hypoxemia will decrease cerebral oxygenation resulting in cerebral vasoconstriction and raising ICP. Hypoxia should be avoided at all cost and ARDS net targets (SpO2 >88% and PaO2 >55) are too low.

- **Controlled vs Assisted Breaths.**

  In assist control modes of ventilation, patients can either take controlled breaths or assisted breaths. Clinicians will set the target tidal volume or pressure for a set respiratory rate. If the patient triggers the ventilator, they will receive the set target for every breath and will be able to take more breaths then the set respiratory breaths. The ventilator is assisting the patient by doing most of the work of breathing when the patient triggers the breath, if the patient does not attempt to trigger the mechanical ventilator, they will receive the set target (volume of pressure) for the set respiratory breath.

  In spontaneous breaths, diaphragmatic movement will decrease pleural pressures which will increase venous return. A fully controlled breath must overcome both lung and chest wall resistance to inflate the lung. In patients with significant respiratory demand should be switched to fully controlled ventilation to decrease oxygen consumption.

- **Pressure Regulated Volume Control (PRVC)**

  This is a dual control mode of ventilation which takes components of ACVC and ACPC and combines them. It is a pressure targeted, time cycled breath with decelerating flow. Clinician will set a tidal volume. The ventilator will give the patient a "test breath" and will calculate the compliance and adjust the pressure delivered needed to achieve the volume set by the clinician. The pressure needed to achieve the set tidal volume can change from breath to breath depending on the respiratory compliance of the patient at any given time.

- **Airway Pressure Release Ventilation (APRV)**

This is a time triggered, pressure targeted, time cycled mode of ventilation that extends the I: E ratio which will allow maintenance of mean airway pressure with very quick deflations to maintain ventilation. Pressure high (P high) is the baseline airway pressure that is maintained for time high (T high). Pressure low (P low) is the release pressure usually set to 0 for a certain amount of time termed Time low (T low).

The advantages of APRV include maintenance of high mean airway pressure which lead to consistent alveolar recruitment. This can lead to better V/Q ratio and oxygenation, decreased use of sedation and neuromuscular blockade. Patients will also be able to generate spontaneous breath throughout the ventilatory cycle (Table 5).

- **Noninvasive Positive Pressure ventilation (NIPPV):**

NIPPV provides ventilatory ventilation without the need for invasive artificial airway. It can be delivered with either a face mask that is fitted to the face or a nasal mask and connected to either a small noninvasive mechanical device or mechanical ventilator via tubing. It comes in two forms: (1) Continuous positive pressure ventilation (CPAP) or (2) bilevel positive pressure ventilation (BIPAP) [8].

Both modes of ventilation will increase airway pressure by introducing PEEP. CPAP is equivalent to PEEP. Patients will need to spontaneously breathe with a set continuous PEEP. BIPAP will have set inspiratory pressure and end expiratory pressure. It will be patient triggered, and the volume delivered will be determined by the patient effort. CPAP is commonly used for type one respiratory failure to address hypoxia while BIPAP is used for when hypercapnia and ventilation are the primary concerns.

TABLE 5 Modes of ventilation

Mode	Description	Advantages	Cons	Settings	Monitor
Volume Control (AC-VC)	Every delivered breath is the same tidal volume	Most common mode Achieve minimum minute ventilation Good for lung protective ventilation	Must monitor pressure to avoid barotrauma	Respiratory rate, tidal volume, PEEP, FIO2	Peak and plateau pressure
Pressure Control (AC-PC)	Delivered breaths is a set pressure (IP) for set time (T_i)	Might be more comfortable Able to limit pressure	Frequent monitoring of tidal volume as compliance changes	Respiratory rate, Inspiratory pressure (IP), Inspiratory time (T_i), PEEP, FiO2	Tidal volume, Minute ventilation
Pressure Support (PS)	All breaths initiated by the patient. MV determined by patient	Common mode for weaning (SBT). comfortable	No guaranteed MV.	Pressure support, PEEP, FiO2	Tidal volume, minute ventilation

(continued)

Table 5 (continued)

Mode	Description	Advantages	Cons	Settings	Monitor
Synchronous Intermittent Mandatory Ventilation (SIMV)	Delivers mandatory breaths with fixed TV but allows spontaneous breaths in between mandatory breaths	May improve patient comfort Limit dynamic hyperinflation	Not effective for SBT Not helpful during acute respiratory failure	Respiratory failure, tidal volume, PEEP, FiO2	Peak and plateau pressure
Airway Pressure Release Ventilation (APRV)	Inverse ratio ventilation (I time > E time) & allows patient to breath spont	Improves oxygenation in ARDS spontaneous breath & improve comfort	Risk of VILI Very complex	T_{HIGH}, T_{Lower}, P_{High}, P_{Low}, FiO2	Volume and ventilation (PaCo2)

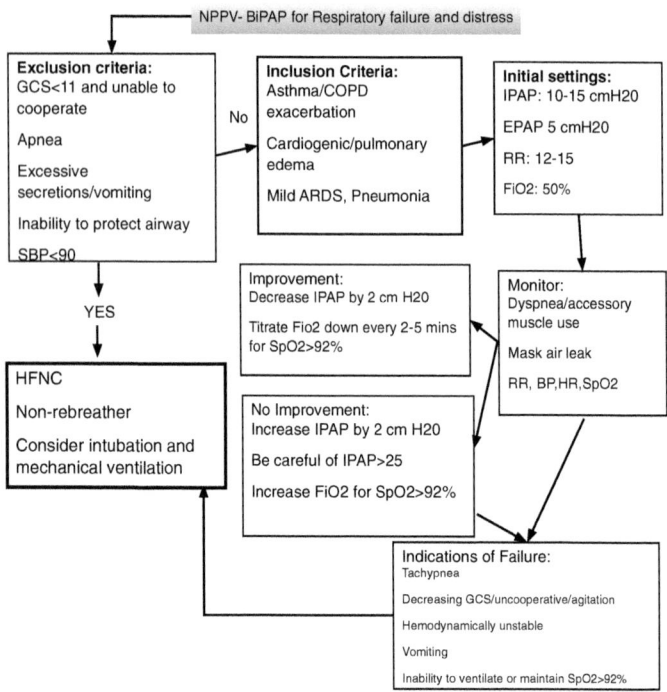

FIGURE 3 NPPV non-invasive positive-pressure ventilation

Patient selection is the most important determinant for the use of NIPPV. Patients with reversible hypoxia from type one respiratory failure (hypertensive pulmonary edema or congestive heart failure) will benefit. Patients with type II respiratory failure (ex. COPD) will experience reduced dyspnea, decrease in intubation rates and improve mortality. NIPPV can also be used post extubation and improve weaning success [6, 7]. Inclusion, exclusion criteria for NIPPV and technique is attached above (Fig. 3).

- **Weaning Protocol**

Assessment of ventilator liberation readiness are traditionally done with respiratory rate, tidal volume, rapid shal-

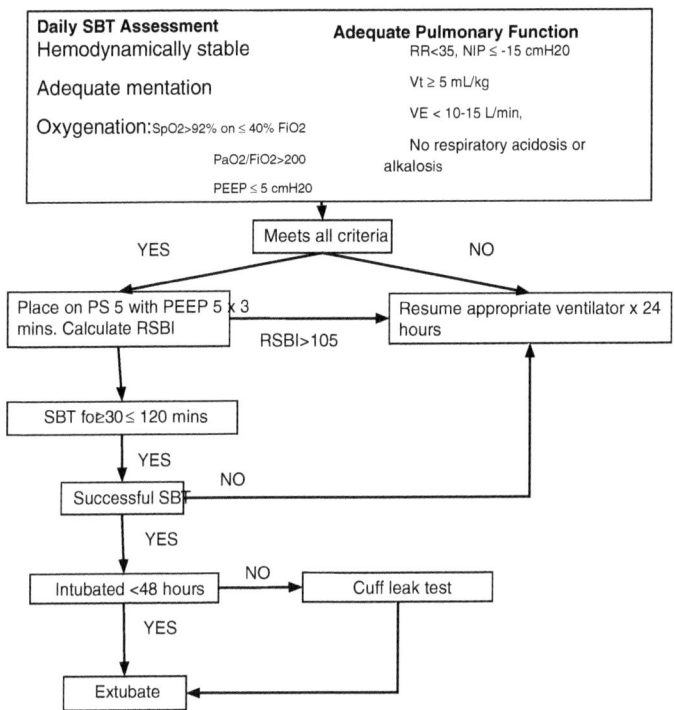

FIGURE 4 Ventilator weaning protocol towards extubation

low breathing index (RSBI), and PaO2 to FiO2 ratio [1]. Features of successful spontaneous breathing trials (SBT) include tidal volume of 4–6 mL/kg, RR 30–38, and RSBI 60–105/L [1]. However, these parameters do not necessarily always predict likelihood of successful extubation [3]. Figure 4 describes ventilator weaning protocols leading to successful extubation.

Multicenter study was done to assess extubation success in patients with severe brain injury [9]. 437 patients were included in the study of which 338 (77%) were successfully extubated. Authors of the study concluded four factors were important – GCS >10, visual pursuit, age >40 and swallow trials.

Table 6 Predictive factors after successful extubation in Brain injury [4, 9]

VISAGE score	Other successful factors
Age <40 years	Negative fluid balance
Extubation day GCS >10	Positive cough reflex
Swallow trials	Positive gag reflex
Visual pursuit	

Table 6 describes historical and exam features found especially in NCCU patients that have shown to predict high likelihood of successful extubation.

References

1. Marino PL. The ICU book. 3rd ed. Lippincott Williams and Wilkins; 2007.
2. Chang W-TW, Nyquist PA. Strategies for the use of mechanical ventilation in the neurologic intensive care unit. Neurosurg Clin. 2013;24:407–16.
3. Lee K. The neuro ICU book. The McGraw-Hill Companies; 2012.
4. Raphael Cinotti MB, Asehnoune K. Management and weaning from mechanical ventilation in neurologic patients. Ann Transl Med. 2018;6(19):381.
5. Saghaei M, Shetabi H, Golparvar M. Predicting efficiency of post-induction mask ventilation based on demographic and anatomical factors. Adv Biomed Res. 2012;1:10.
6. Kraynek B, Best J. What are the clinical indications for non-invasive positive pressure ventilation? The Hospitalist. Dec 2011. Retrieved 26 Sept 2014 from www.the-hospitalist.org/details/article/1409003/What_Are_the_Clinical_Indications_for_Noninvasive_Positive_Pressure_Ventilation.html.
7. Hess DR. Noninvasive ventilation for acute respiratory failure. Respir Care. 2013;58(6):950–72.

8. McNeill GBS, Glossop AJ. Clinical applications of non-invasive ventilation in critical care. Cont Educ Anaesthesia Crit Care Pain. 2012;12(1):3.
9. Asehnoune K, et al. Extubation success prediction in a multicentric cohort of patients with severe brain injury. Anesthesiology. 2017;127(2):338–46.3–37.

Tracheostomy Care

Mohammed Alnijoumi and Troy Whitacre

1 Introduction

Tracheostomy placement is an important step for ventilator weaning in those with prolonged mechanical ventilation needs. Like other invasive procedures and chronic tubes, care must be taken to ensure delivery of the intended benefits and to guard against complications from such a chronic foreign body. The presence of the tracheostomy assists weaning from the mechanical ventilator and potentially allows those who need life-long mechanical ventilation to live at home. However, the chronicity of the foreign tube could lead to stomal injury, tracheal stenosis, hemoptysis, and tracheal infections.

In this chapter, we discuss the care of the tracheostomy tube in the immediate post-placement period, weaning,

---

M. Alnijoumi (✉)
Department of Medicine, University of Missouri, Columbia, MO, USA
e-mail: alnijoumim@health.missouri.edu

T. Whitacre
Respiratory Care Services, MU Health Care, Columbia, MO, USA
e-mail: whitacret@health.missouri.edu

© The Author(s), under exclusive license to Springer Nature Switzerland AG 2022
N. Arora (ed.), *Procedures and Protocols in the Neurocritical Care Unit*, https://doi.org/10.1007/978-3-030-90225-4_20

speaking valve placement, capping trials, decannulation, and chronic long-term care of the tracheostomy tube for those who are dependent on one.

2 Tracheostomy Care

The procedure for insertion of a tracheostomy tube is discussed in detail in chapter Airway Access.

It is worth noting that tracheostomy tubes have different characteristics (Table 1). They are available in assorted sizes, based on either the International Standard Organization

TABLE 1 Characteristics and features of tracheostomy tube

Size:
    International Standard Organization (ISO):
        6, 7, 8, 9, 10
    Jackson:
        4, 6, 8, 10

Length:
    Standard
    Extended Length (XLT):
        Proximal i.e., Vertical
        Distal i.e., Horizontal

Type:
    Single Cannula
    Dual Cannula

Fenestration:
    Present
    Absent

TABLE I (continued)

Shaft:
  Curved
  Angled
Cuff:
  Absent
  Present
    Air-filled
    Water-filled
    Low-pressure, High-volume
    High-volume, Low-pressure, i.e., Tight-to-shaft
    Foam
Material
  Metal:
    Stainless Steel
    Sterling Silver
  Non-metal
    Silicone
    Polyvinyl Chloride (PVC)
    Polyurethane

(ISO) or Jackson sizing. Each size has a different internal diameter (ID) and outer diameter (OD) with varying lengths (specific lengths and diameters of the same size may also differ from company to company). It is very important to familiarize one's self with the products available to him or her, given the difference in measurements between manufacturers. A tracheostomy tube could come as a single- or dual-cannula tube depending on the presence of the inner cannula (Fig. 1). Most tracheostomy tubes come with a dual cannula

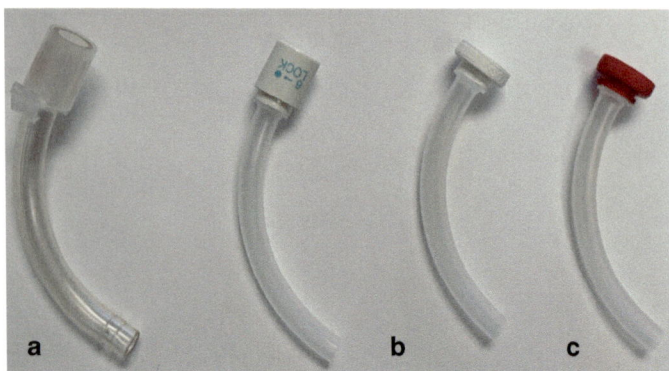

FIGURE 1 (**a**) Disposable inner cannula (size 8); (**b**) Non-disposable inner cannula (size 6); (**c**): Non-disposable inner cannula with integrated decannulating plug

which allows for seamless cleaning and care of the tube. This minimizes tube clogging by allowing the removal of the inner cannula when needed. Tracheostomy tubes made from silicone often come as a single cannula tube given the inherent resistance of silicone to microbial growth. The tracheostomy tube shaft could be angled or curved as it enters the airway. The curvature should allow for minimal pressure to be placed on the posterior wall of the trachea. Most tracheostomy tubes used are non-fenestrated. The presence of a single, or multiple openings along the shaft's angulation or curvature makes the tube a fenestrated tube. Fenestrated tracheostomy tubes are designed to channel more airflow to the larynx and vocal cords and hasten phonation when the cuff is deflated and a speaking valve is present. However, given the location of the fenestrations, they are often occluded by the posterior wall of the trachea and could lead to granulation tissue formation and the potential for tracheal stenosis. The tracheostomy tube comes in standard lengths. However, an extended length (XLT) tracheostomy tube is also commercially available. The extended length portion of the tube could either be proximal (i.e., horizontal) or distal (i.e., vertical). The proximal XLT tracheostomy tubes are often useful in obese patients since they take into consideration increased soft tissue mass at the neck. The distal XLT may be helpful in patients when the distal end of the tracheostomy tube is rocking against the tracheal wall as it angles into the airway. The distal extra-length tube also allows it to be parallel to the tracheal lumen and minimizes obstruction. Additionally, custom-made tracheostomy tubes are an option offered by most manufacturers for those who require specific sizes and/or lengths.

The presence of a 'balloon' cuff differentiates a cuffed tracheostomy tube from a cuffless one. Cuffless tubes traditionally have a better profile and are preferred for patients who are no longer dependent on ventilatory support and have progressed to a speaking valve or capping trial. The balloon cuff is often filled with air, although some manufacturers recommend water. The most frequent type of cuff is a high-volume, low-pressure cuff. This allows it to conform to the airway diameter without significant transluminal pressure; thus, mitigating the risk of tracheal mucosal ischemia and injury. However, low-volume, high-pressure cuffs are also available, known as tight-to-shaft cuffed tubes. The slim profile, without the significant ridges associated with traditional tracheostomy cuffs when deflated, encourages the passage of air around the tracheostomy tube. This provides an enhanced opportunity for phonation and is intended for patients who require infrequent cuff inflation and mechanical ventilatory support. Foam cuffed tracheostomy tubes are also marketed. Made of polyurethane foam covered with a silicone sheath, they have a high residual volume and hence tend to conform to the airway better. The pilot balloon (cuff) is deflated during insertion then opened to ambient air once it is placed into the airway. The balloon expands and contracts with the respiratory cycle which promotes a favorable seal to the tracheal wall. It is important to place the correct-sized foam-cuffed tracheostomy tube as too small of the tube may not provide an adequate seal.

Tracheostomy tubes are manufactured from a variety of materials including stainless steel, sterling silver, silicone, polyvinyl chloride (PVC), and polyurethane. Metal tracheostomy tubes have a slim profile and are resistant to microbial growth. They are also easy to clean and sterilize if needed. However, they lack a balloon cuff and the 15-mm connector to attach to the mechanical ventilator. Non-metal tracheostomy tubes are softer and tend to better conform to the patient's anatomy. However, despite the resistance to biofilm formation, their presence in the trachea leads to surface changes and degradation of the polymeric chain.

The obturator (Fig. 2), which accompanies all types of tracheostomy tubes, facilitates insertion. They should be used

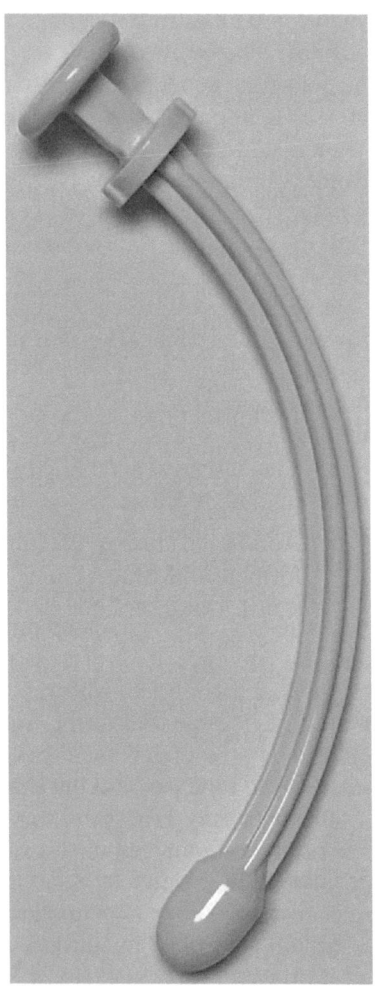

FIGURE 2 Tracheostomy obturator

during tracheostomy changes and be readily accessible-preferably at the head of the bed in hospitalized patients.

3 Post-placement Care

Immediately after tracheostomy placement, the cuff should be inflated, and mechanical ventilation continued. The tracheostomy tube is secured with commercially available tracheostomy ties, most of which are made of cushioned material and fastened to each side of the tracheostomy flange with Velcro. Suturing the tracheostomy to the skin is optional in the author's experience. To guard against pressure injury or ulceration, padded foam is routinely placed between the tracheostomy flange and the sternal notch. A pressure injury is most likely encountered at that location. Pre-cut drain sponges suffice in patients with longer neck anatomy. However, a heavier padded barrier might be helpful with obese patients and those with shorter necks.

The tracheostomy tube size and type should be documented, and the tubes kept clean. Dual- cannula tubes come with an inner cannula that allows for cleaning and ensures the patency of the artificial airway. Inner cannulas may be either disposable or non-disposable. Routine daily changing of the disposable cannula is standard. For non-disposable cannulas, two inner cannulas work better than one. The usable non-disposable cannula is removed and replaced with the second, pre-cleaned non-disposable cannula. This process allows for easy cleaning of the recently removed equipment in preparation for the next change.

For tracheostomy tubes without inner cannulas, care must be taken to educate personnel on removing and replacing the entire tracheostomy tube in case of obstruction. Regardless of the presence or absence of an inner cannula, a replacement tracheostomy tube of the same brand and size, and possibly one sized smaller, should be available for immediate use.

Skin in the peristomal area should be kept dry and clean to decrease the risk of maceration and infection. The peristomal site should be evaluated for signs of redness, tenderness, and firmness. It is equally important to evaluate for signs of pressure injury, especially under the flange. Adequate lighting is an important prerequisite when providing tracheostomy tube care.

If the tracheostomy tube is cuffed, pressure in the pilot balloon should be evaluated when the patient is receiving mechanical ventilation. Cuff pressure should be kept between 20–25 mmHg when inflated to guard against tracheal mucosal ischemia and injury. Pressures over 30 mmHg should be documented and reported to the team. High cuff pressure requirements to maintain a seal may indicate a less than adequate tracheostomy tube size and the tube should be considered for an exchange. For patients with cuffed tracheostomy tubes undergoing speaking valve or capping trials, the importance of fully deflating the cuff before these trials can't be overstated as significant morbidity and even death have been reported. When a cuffed tube is no longer required changing to a cuffless one should be considered.

Adequate humidification of the tracheostomy tube and the distal airway is also essential. Since air flows in and out of the tracheostomy tube, normal anatomic structures that provide heat and humidity are bypassed. Thick, tenacious secretions may slowly accumulate that increase the risk of clogging the tube with inspissated respiratory secretions. Heated (32–34 °C) and humidified (100% relative humidity) air or oxygen-enriched gas can be delivered using a heated humidifier (Fig. 3a, b) or a disposable heat moisture exchanger (Fig. 4), ensuring adequate secretion management and patient comfort.

The tracheostomy tube is designed to be suctioned as needed although scheduled suctioning is usually unnecessary. Suction catheters should be advanced to the tip of the tracheostomy tube before applying suction. Deeper suctioning practices are associated with mucosal injury of the trachea and distal bronchi. Some reports showed that repeated suctioning was found to decrease the rate of tube clogging in

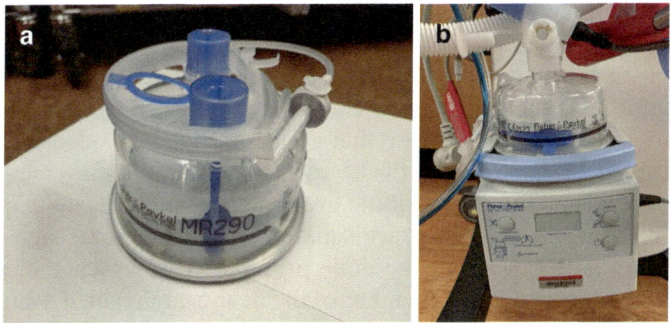

FIGURE 3 (**a**) Heated passive humidifier. (**b**) Heated passive humidifier

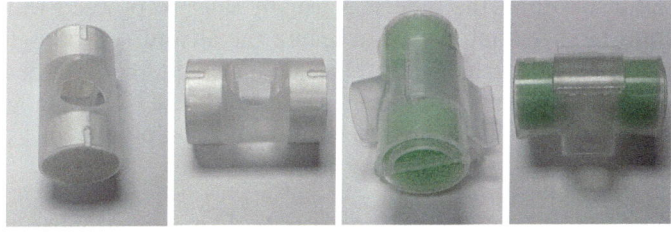

FIGURE 4 Disposable Heat-Moisture Exchanger (HME)

the general ward. Despite this, there is a body of evidence showing repeated suctioning or deep suctioning may lead to tracheitis. Additionally, the routine use of saline bullets to aid in thinning respiratory secretions may lead to hypoxia and could dislodge secretions and microbes from the tracheostomy tube and displace them into the lower respiratory tract.

Protocolized tracheostomy care and specialized healthcare teams to manage inpatient tracheostomy patients are imperative. Studies evaluating the implementation of protocolized care sets have shown a decrease in median time to evaluation by occupational, physical, and speech therapy, and a decrease in tracheostomy days and length of stay. Minimizing the time to decannulation also resulted in shorter hospital stays.

Multidisciplinary teams led to fewer tracheostomy-related complications and higher use of speaking valves. One could postulate that combining those two strategies is essential for improving patient outcomes.

The team must beware that accidental tube dislodgement can occur at any point of the care continuum. Management depends on the timing of the event and the maturity state of the stomal tract. If the tract is mature, replacing the tracheostomy tube can usually be done promptly. The presence of a second provider or a member of the healthcare team, if available, is favored. In the case of a less mature tract, replacement of the dislodged tracheostomy may still be attempted. However, if this step proves difficult or there are questions regarding proper tube placement and the resting position of the distal tip of the tube, it is usually safer to proceed with trans laryngeal intubation to secure the airway. A thorough, investigative evaluation of the stoma could then be performed. Colorimetric capnometry and end-tidal CO_2 capnography are helpful adjuncts to ensure adequate placement.

4 Tracheostomy Weaning to Decannulation

4.1 Downsizing

If the patient is successfully weaned from the mechanical ventilator and no longer requires ventilatory support, the determination to continue care with a life-long tracheostomy tube becomes the providers' decision. This ultimately depends on the patient's condition, underlying clinical diagnosis, and whether the clinical indication for placing the tracheostomy tube still exists.

If it is determined that the tracheostomy tube is not going to be needed for the ongoing treatment of the patient, and the patient has successfully been liberated from the ventilator, consideration to 'downsize' the tracheostomy tube is a strategy that is routinely employed. Downsizing is commonly the first step in the process of weaning from the tracheostomy tube and is performed before decannulation. For downsizing, it is customary to decrease the size of the airway, one step at a time, e.g. if the patient has a size 8.0 tracheostomy tube, downsizing to a 6.0 would be considered standard. Whether it is necessary to downsize further before decannulation is another decision made by the provider. If it is determined that further downsizing is appropriate, the final step would customarily be to change to a 4.0 tracheostomy tube. The 4.0 is generally considered to be the smallest adult-sized airway (in the author's experience, the decision to downsize to a #4.0 tracheostomy tube is mostly unnecessary, and decannulation can be considered when a patient is tolerating a size 6.0 tracheostomy tube). After successful downsizing, speaking valve and/or capping trials are often helpful in determining whether decannulation is likely to be successful.

4.2 Passy-Muir Valve or Speaking Valve

David Muir is the inventor of the Passy-Muir speaking valve (Fig. 5). As a muscular dystrophy patient with quadriplegia, David suffered a respiratory arrest and endured a prolonged course before he eventually underwent a tracheostomy placement procedure. His frustration with the inability to communicate after the tracheostomy prompted him to invent the one-way 'speaking' valve. The Passy-Muir (P-M) valve is a device attached to the 15-mm connector on the protruding end of the tracheostomy tube. During inspiration, the valve opens and air (or oxygen-enriched gas if needed) enters through the tracheostomy tube into the tracheobronchial tree. During exhalation, however, the valve closes, and the exhaled air exits through the larynx, oropharynx, and nasopharynx. The movement of exhaled air is what allows phonation to take place. Added benefits of the P-M valve include the potential to increase end-expiratory pressure and improve swallowing and the sense of smell. But more importantly, it aids with weaning while allowing for phonation and may hasten decannulation.

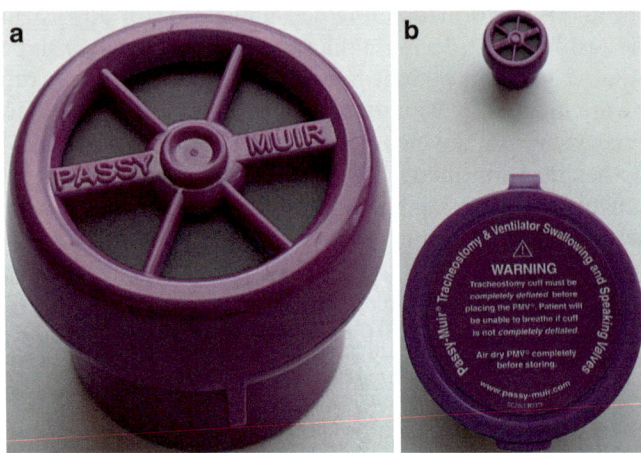

FIGURE 5 (**a**) Passy Muir valve. (**b**) Warning on the PMV box to ensure the balloon cuff is fully deflated

The use of a P-M valve is recommended and encouraged after being liberated from mechanical ventilation. Speaking valve trials are customarily performed under supervision, especially with the initial placement. This can be done by the speech and language pathologist and/or by a respiratory therapist. Certain criteria should be met before this process is left to nursing staff to supervise. When first attempted, the patient must be awake. Patient position is not necessarily important-whether laying down or sitting up-however, in the author's opinion, the head of the bed should be elevated at least 30° for the initial trials. Communicating with the patient on what to expect once the P-M valve is applied helps alleviate the anxiety that often accompanies its' placement since the initial sensation is often overwhelming. Once the valve is applied, the patient's condition is monitored for signs of respiratory distress. It is our practice to ensure that the patient is awake and following commands and can personally remove the speaking valve or call for assistance if respiratory distress develops before placement trials are transitioned to nursing staff supervision only.

The duration of the initial speaking valve trials depends on multiple factors, usually related to the patient, e.g., lack of active respiratory infections and/or the presence of manageable secretions, length of mechanical respiratory support, and the ability to move the upper extremities without limitations (patient overall strength).

As part of the weaning process to eventual decannulation, tolerating the P-M valve trials is essential.

4.3 Capping Trials

An alternative to a P-M valve, capping the tracheostomy also simulates decannulation. The device used is called a tracheostomy cap or a tracheostomy plug and is usually packaged along with the cuffless tracheostomy tube (Fig. 6). However, unlike a P-M valve, capping the tube directs air movement in and out of the respiratory tract during both inhalation and expiration exclusively through the normal anatomical pathway. As such, the patient is less dependent on the tracheostomy, but with a higher imposed work of breathing due to the increase in resistance encountered by the presence of the tracheostomy tube within the lumen of the airway.

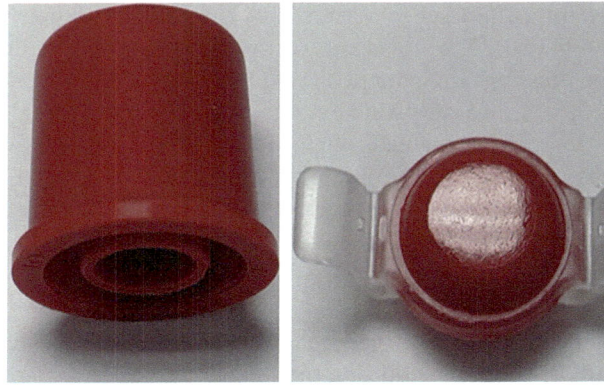

FIGURE 6 Tracheostomy cap/plug

Ideally, if the patient is tolerating the smallest desired tracheostomy tube, capping trials would be initiated after successful use of a P-M valve. However, at institutions without access to a P-M valve, capping trials can begin in the place of the valve. The duration of capping trials depends on patient tolerance. As with the P-M valve, successful capping trials depend on patient strength, manageable secretions, and the absence of uncontrolled respiratory infections. If the patient is tolerant of the initial trial, a full day of capping could be attempted.

Once the patient tolerates a 48-hour continuous capping trial, the patient is considered eligible for decannulation in the author's practice and experience.

4.4 Decannulation

Decannulation, the process of removing the tracheostomy tube, is a rather simple procedure and may be performed in the inpatient or outpatient setting.

At the time of decannulation, the patient is placed in the semi-recumbent position, with the head of the bed elevated to at least 30°. The neck is kept slightly hyperextended. Occasionally, a sitting position with neck hyperextension is preferred. The tracheostomy tube is then removed completely (for cuffed tubes, ensure the cuff is fully deflated before removal). The stoma site is covered with gauze and a pressure dressing. The patient should be instructed to finger-occlude the stoma site whenever she or he phonates. This minimizes air movement through the stoma. The stoma will normally close within 5–7 days of decannulation. If it fails to close within 10–14 days, surgical approximation and closure may be necessary.

Long-term Care

There are patients, who will require a tracheostomy tube indefinitely. Those patients and their caregivers often experience a great deal of anxiety regarding the presence of a tracheostomy tube and its care. Adequate education before discharge from the hospital is crucial to alleviate any associated distress. To ascertain adequate learning of the required steps in tracheostomy care, patients or their caregivers should be taught about the device and then be able to demonstrate proper care, cleaning, and changing of the tracheostomy tube. Repeated evaluation and demonstration of their technique at set intervals ensures adequate retention and solidifies their competence. Formal education for family and caregivers has led to a decrease in the anxiety associated with tracheostomy care as well as the rate of hospital readmissions.

Tracheostomy tubes should be changed as per manufacturer recommendations and not be kept in place longer than suggested. Scanning electron microscopy images of some silicone, PVC, and polyurethane tracheostomy tubes demonstrate evidence of surface changes and degradation of the polymeric chains in as early as 30 days. The risk of infection also increases at 3 months.

Guidelines

Helpful consensus statements and guidelines are published from two, well-recognized professional organizations: The American Academy of Otolaryngology – Head and Neck Surgery and The American Association for Respiratory Care.

We encourage providers taking care of tracheostomy patients to review those regularly.

- Clinical Consensus Statement: Tracheostomy Care.
- AARC Clinical Practice Guidelines: Management of Adult Patients with Tracheostomy in the Acute Care Setting.

Bibliography

1. Perry A, Mallah MD, Cunningham KW, Christmas AB, Marrero JJ, Gombar MA, et al. PATHway to success: Implementation of a multiprofessional acute trauma health care team decreased length of stay and cost in patients with neurological injury requiring tracheostomy. J Trauma Acute Care Surg. 2020;88(1):176–9.

2. Masood MM, Farquhar DR, Biancaniello C, Hackman TG. Association of standardized tracheostomy care protocol implementation and reinforcement with the prevention of life-threatening respiratory events. JAMA Otolaryngol Head Neck Surg. 2018;144(6):527–32.
3. Jung YJ, Kim Y, Kyoung K, Keum M, Kim T, Ma DS, et al. The effect of systematic approach to tracheostomy care in patients transferred from the surgical intensive care unit to general ward. Acute Crit Care. 2018;33(4):252–9.
4. O'Toole TR, Jacobs N, Hondorp B, Crawford L, Boudreau LR, Jeffe J, et al. Prevention of tracheostomy-related hospital-acquired pressure ulcers. Otolaryngol Head Neck Surg. 2017;156(4):642–51.
5. Mah JW, Staff II, Fisher SR, Butler KL. Improving decannulation and swallowing function: a comprehensive, multidisciplinary approach to post-tracheostomy care. Respir Care. 2017;62(2):137–43.
6. Sutt AL, Caruana LR, Dunster KR, Cornwell PL, Anstey CM, Fraser JF. Speaking valves in tracheostomised ICU patients weaning off mechanical ventilation--do they facilitate lung recruitment? Crit Care. 2016;20:91.
7. Colandrea M, Eckardt P. Improving tracheostomy care delivery: instituting clinical care pathways and nursing education to improve patient outcomes. ORL Head Neck Nurs. 2016;34(1):7–16.
8. Sutt AL, Cornwell P, Mullany D, Kinneally T, Fraser JF. The use of tracheostomy speaking valves in mechanically ventilated patients results in improved communication and does not prolong ventilation time in cardiothoracic intensive care unit patients. J Crit Care. 2015;30(3):491–4.
9. Schreiber ML. Tracheostomy: site care, suctioning, and readiness. Medsurg Nurs. 2015;24(2):121–4.
10. Morris LL, McIntosh E, Whitmer A. The importance of tracheostomy progression in the intensive care unit. Crit Care Nurse. 2014;34(1):40–8; quiz 50.
11. Hess DR, Altobelli NP. Tracheostomy tubes. Respir Care. 2014;59(6):956–71; discussion 71-3.
12. Morris LL, Whitmer A, McIntosh E. Tracheostomy care and complications in the intensive care unit. Crit Care Nurse. 2013;33(5):18–30.
13. Mitchell RB, Hussey HM, Setzen G, Jacobs IN, Nussenbaum B, Dawson C, et al. Clinical consensus statement: tracheostomy care. Otolaryngol Head Neck Surg. 2013;148(1):6–20.

14. de Mestral C, Iqbal S, Fong N, LeBlanc J, Fata P, Razek T, et al. Impact of a specialized multidisciplinary tracheostomy team on tracheostomy care in critically ill patients. Can J Surg. 2011;54(3):167–72.
15. Cetto R, Arora A, Hettige R, Nel M, Benjamin L, Gomez CM, et al. Improving tracheostomy care: a prospective study of the multidisciplinary approach. Clin Otolaryngol. 2011;36(5):482–8.
16. Paul F. Tracheostomy care and management in general wards and community settings: literature review. Nurs Crit Care. 2010;15(2):76–85.
17. Parker V, Giles M, Shylan G, Austin N, Smith K, Morison J, et al. Tracheostomy management in acute care facilities–a matter of teamwork. J Clin Nurs. 2010;19(9–10):1275–83.
18. Garrubba M, Turner T, Grieveson C. Multidisciplinary care for tracheostomy patients: a systematic review. Crit Care. 2009;13(6):R177.
19. Backman S, Bjorling G, Johansson UB, Lysdahl M, Markstrom A, Schedin U, et al. Material wear of polymeric tracheostomy tubes: a six-month study. Laryngoscope. 2009;119(4):657–64.
20. Dennis-Rouse MD, Davidson JE. An evidence-based evaluation of tracheostomy care practices. Crit Care Nurs Q. 2008;31(2):150–60.
21. Arora A, Hettige R, Ifeacho S, Narula A. Driving standards in tracheostomy care: a preliminary communication of the St Mary's ENT-led multi disciplinary team approach. Clin Otolaryngol. 2008;33(6):596–9.
22. Bjorling G, Axelsson S, Johansson UB, Lysdahl M, Markstrom A, Schedin U, et al. Clinical use and material wear of polymeric tracheostomy tubes. Laryngoscope. 2007;117(9):1552–9.
23. Eber E, Oberwaldner B. Tracheostomy care in the hospital. Paediatr Respir Rev. 2006;7(3):175–84.
24. Dhand R, Johnson JC. Care of the chronic tracheostomy. Respir Care. 2006;51(9):984–1001; discussion 2–4.
25. Ackerman MH, Mick DJ. Instillation of normal saline before suctioning in patients with pulmonary infections: a prospective randomized controlled trial. Am J Crit Care. 1998;7(4):261–6.
26. Hagler DA, Traver GA. Endotracheal saline and suction catheters: sources of lower airway contamination. Am J Crit Care. 1994;3(6):444–7.
27. Kleiber C, Krutzfield N, Rose EF. Acute histologic changes in the tracheobronchial tree associated with different suction catheter insertion techniques. Heart Lung. 1988;17(1):10–4.

28. Martin KA, Cole TDK, Percha CM, Asanuma N, Mattare K, Hager DN, et al. Standard versus accelerated speaking valve placement after percutaneous tracheostomy: a randomized-controlled feasibility study. Ann Am Thorac Soc. 2021;18(10):1693.
29. Heimer J, Eggert S, Fliss B, Meixner E. Fatal bilateral pneumothorax and generalized emphysema following contraindicated speaking-valve application. Forensic Sci Med Pathol. 2019;15(2):239–42.
30. Barraza GY, Fernandez C, Halaby C, Ambrosio S, Simpser EF, Pirzada MB, et al. The safety of tracheostomy speaking valve use during sleep in children: a pilot study. Am J Otolaryngol. 2014;35(5):636–40.
31. Selleng S, Antal M, Hansen T, Meissner K, Usichenko TI. Pneumothorax and cardiac arrest caused by speaking valve mistaken as moisture exchanger: an incident report. Br J Anaesth. 2013;111(2):297–8.
32. Elpern EH, Borkgren Okonek M, Bacon M, Gerstung C, Skrzynski M. Effect of the Passy-Muir tracheostomy speaking valve on pulmonary aspiration in adults. Heart Lung. 2000;29(4):287–93.
33. Leder SB. Effect of a one-way tracheotomy speaking valve on the incidence of aspiration in previously aspirating patients with tracheotomy. Dysphagia. 1999;14(2):73–7.
34. Lichtman SW, Birnbaum IL, Sanfilippo MR, Pellicone JT, Damon WJ, King ML. Effect of a tracheostomy speaking valve on secretions, arterial oxygenation, and olfaction: a quantitative evaluation. J Speech Hear Res. 1995;38(3):549–55.
35. Passy V, Baydur A, Prentice W, Darnell-Neal R. Passy-Muir tracheostomy speaking valve on ventilator-dependent patients. Laryngoscope. 1993;103(6):653–8.
36. Lewarski JS. Long-term care of the patient with a tracheostomy. Respir Care. 2005;50(4):534–7.

Hemodynamic Monitoring

Kia Ghiassi, Premkumar Nattanmai, and Niraj Arora

1 Introduction

The approach to hemodynamic assessment in the critical care setting has undergone numerous revisions. One of the reasons for this is because of the dynamic nature of hemodynamics within the critically ill demographic, where a wide range of diseases are encountered. Optimal assessment of hemodynamics is limited by invasiveness of the method and perceived accuracy.

Often, when one considers hemodynamic evaluation, intravascular volume status assessment is quite important to consider. Resuscitating a patient with appropriate fluid balance is often challenging. The goal of resuscitation is to optimize preload and thereby increase stroke volume and cardiac

K. Ghiassi (✉) · P. Nattanmai
Department of Neurology, University of Missouri,
Columbia, MO, USA
e-mail: Kgr8v@health.missouri.edu;
nattanmaip@health.missouri.edu

N. Arora
Department of Neurology- Neurocriticalcare unit, University of Missouri, Columbia, MO, USA
e-mail: arorana@health.missouri.edu

output (CO). There is abundant literature mentioning that patients are under-resuscitated or fail to achieve the intended effect of increasing CO with a fluid bolus during the critical phase of hemodynamic instability. Also, it is essential to avoid over-resuscitation as hypervolemia is harmful in itself and causes fluid extravasation, endothelial injury and tissue edema. Alternative to fluids is the use of vasopressors, colloids or blood transfusion products. One should have a clear idea in order to justify the use of one over the other so that fluid resuscitation measures are undertaken promptly and for appropriate duration.

This chapter focuses on different clinical and instrument based parameter approaches which could guide the treating clinician to perform appropriate hemodynamic assessments.

The initial part of the chapter will focus on description of the principles of volume responsiveness along with the techniques and instruments used. In the later part of the chapter, we will discuss the use of ultrasonographic based techniques for fluid responsiveness.

2 Basic Principles of Fluid Resuscitation

In the simplest sense, one can classify cardiovascular function based on arterial and venous synchrony and pairing with the cardiac pump, also referred to as vascular-cardiac pump coupling, dysfunction of the ventricle, and the systemic vessels [65]. The arterial system is a high resistance circuit or series of circuits, through which a given stroke volume is ejected from the left ventricle. Stroke Volume = EDV − ESV, where EDV is end-diastolic volume and ESV is end-systolic volume. As this stroke volume is ejected during systole, potential energy is stored within the aorta and major arteries due to their elastic nature. The capacitance of the aorta and major arteries is low and inversely related to the pressure contained within. Because the ventricular pressure drops below that of the systemic arterial pressure, the aortic valve closes. This is denoted by the dicrotic notch seen on the arterial waveform. During diastole, the blood within the arterial system is driven by the potential energy stored by the vessels' elasticity and overcomes the pressure in the resistance vessels. The elastic recoil of the aorta and major arteries allows for propagation of flow and perfusion of the capillaries. There is release of pressure from the stored energy within the arterial bed throughout systole as well. Blood pressure then decreases till the process is repeated, whereby the left ventricle is filled. Its filling is dependent on the volume-pressure curve of the ventricle and the volume of blood received by the atria through their contraction. This interaction between the stroke volume, elastic recoil of the vessels mentioned, and the resistance of the small arterioles is labeled the Windkessel effect [66].

This explains the relationship between cardiac output and systemic vascular resistance: Mean Arterial Pressure (MAP) = Cardiac Output (CO) x Systemic Vascular Resistance (SVR). The difference between the systolic and diastolic pressures is the pulse pressure and is related to the stroke volume by a constant that reflects the capacitance of the aorta, major arteries, and also the arterial bed. Assuming a constant capacitance, variation in pulse pressure means that stroke volume is changing.

2.1 Frank-Starling Curve

The relationship between length and tension in cardiac muscle is represented by the Frank-Starling Curve which is the relationship between left-ventricular end diastolic pressure and stroke volume for myofibrils. At lower pressures, there is a more dramatic rise in stroke volume for a small change in pressure. The length of this curve is meant to describe cardiac performance and proposes that there is an optimal length between sarcomeres, where tension is maximum. This will lead to the greatest force of contraction. At lengths below or greater than this, contractility will be compromised. Therefore preload can be increased up to a certain point, beyond which, stroke volume, is not increased. With increase in contractility, the curve is shifted upwards, whereby there is less of an increase in left ventricular end diastolic pressure necessary for the same increase in stroke volume. Heart failure would be the inverse of this graphically. Increases in contractility are due to positive inotropes. Decreases in contractility are due to loss of cardiac function (e.g. from myocardial infarction or dilated cardiomyopathy). Increases and decreases in afterload cause downward and upward shifts of the curve, respectively.

Some factors that affect the usefulness of the Frank-Starling Curve are impaired cardiac contractility, increased left ventricular afterload, and a reduction in left ventricular end-diastolic volume due to ventricular hypertrophy.

2.2 Diastolic Volume-Pressure Curve (Fig. 1)

In this figure, the red curve represents normal diastolic function and the yellow curve represents a patient with an acute myocardial infarction. The pressure difference between the

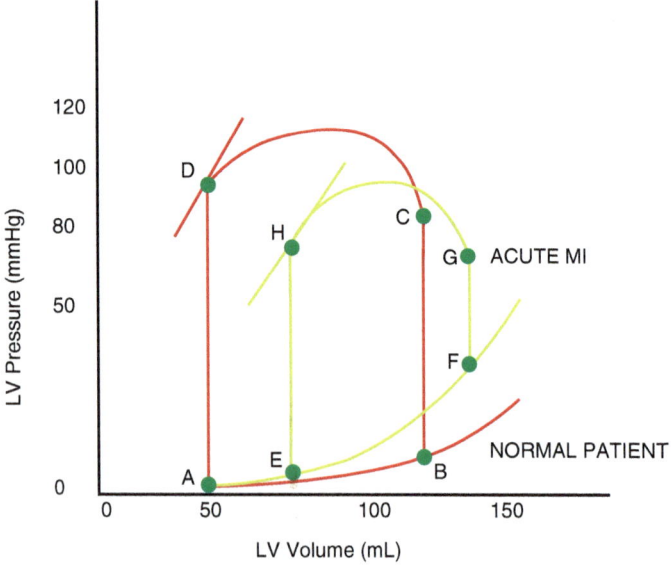

FIGURE 1 Diastolic volume-pressure curve. (Modified from: Wijdicks et al. [68])

juxtacardiac pressure and the intraventricular pressure is the transmural pressure. Here we illustrate this on the y-axis. In a patient with normal myocardial compliance, at a minimum of 50 mL of left ventricular volume is when the transmural pressure rises above zero. This is referred to as the unstressed volume. The addition of volume beyond this point is the stressed volume. In a healthy patient, adding more volume to the left ventricle allows for a rise in left ventricular transmural pressure from point A to B. There is a sharp rise in left ventricular transmural pressure after this point without an increase in volume. This is because the pericardium becomes increasingly stiff with the rise in left ventricular end-diastolic volume. There is a certain amount of volume that the left ventricle must contain before the pericardium significantly stiffens. That volume is generally over 100 mL in a healthy patient. In a patient with a myocardial infarction, the curve can be seen to shift upward and leftward. This means that a higher pressure is required for the same change in left ventricular end-diastolic volume. With more volume in the pericardium, venous return (VR) is impaired due to a rise in right atrial pressure (RAP). This results in a drop in left ventricular end-diastolic volume and hence, CO. By equivalent mechanisms, intra-abdominal hypertension, tension pneumothorax, high positive end-expiratory pressure via mechanical ventilation and large pleural effusions affect the CO. If these pressures are high enough, this results in a lower transmural pressure. Left ventricular preload will decrease, as will left ventricular afterload, however, the net effect is a decrease in stroke volume. Other causes of decreased left ventricular end-diastolic volume include impaired myocardial compliance due to either infiltrative diseases, ischemic heart disease, or hypertrophic cardiomyopathy. Ventricular filling defects, arrhythmias, valvulopathies, and ventricular interdependence from a variety of causes are implicated.

2.3 Contractility (Fig. 1)

Isovolumetric contraction starts at point B, after which the sudden rise in transmural pressure is seen without a concomitant change in volume. The pressure within the left ventricle overcomes the aortic valve and systole occurs. As can be seen, at about 100 mmHg and a volume of 120 mL, there is isovolumetric contraction in the normal heart, until the pressure rises to 80 mmHg (point B to point C). Then the aortic valve opens. The pressure then falls from 120 to 90 mmHg, at which point only 50 mL of blood is inside the left ventricle (point C in point D). In patients with acute myocardial infarction, there is a depressed cardiac function curve.

As in a patient with a myocardial infarction, due to the compromised ejection, end-systolic volume remains at 90 mL with a lower pressure of 75 mmHg (point H). This upward and leftward shift is due to impaired diastolic function. To allow for VR, the left ventricular end-diastolic volume increases to 130 mL. The increase is 20 mmHg. Even with a rise in heart rate, at 110 beats per minute, the stroke volume and the CO as a result are diminished. The increase in systemic vascular resistance could not compensate for the decrease in stroke volume.

Isovolumetric contraction occurs when there is already a left ventricular end-diastolic pressure of approximately 30 mmHg (point F to point G) in patients with acute myocardial infarction. This is because of impaired left ventricular relaxation, which results in reduced ejection fractions. Note that the reduction in left ventricular volume with systole from point C to point D in the healthy patient versus point G to H in the patient with impaired contractility is significantly more. Hence, we have a reduced stroke volume in the patient with an acute myocardial infarction since there is a smaller difference between end-diastolic and end-systolic volume. Isovolumetric relaxation still leaves the empty ventricle at a higher end-diastolic pressure (point E) than in the healthy patient.

In thinking about CO and VR, and CO, one must consider the systemic vessels' capacitance and resistance. Capacitance is the ability to accommodate volume and is the analog of compliance. It is the difference in volume per amount of pressure. Resistance can simply be expressed as the pressure gradient per amount of CO.

2.4 Mean Systemic Filling Pressure (P_{ms})

When there is no active flow in the circulatory system (a very brief moment in time), this represents the mean systemic filling pressure. It is typically at least 10 mmHg. and less than the systemic arterial pressure. Blood moves from the low-volume and high-pressure arterial system into the venous system. The right ventricle pumps blood forward allowing for a drop in right atrial pressure relative to the mean systemic pressure. This creates a suction effect allowing for the blood from the venous system to enter the right atrium. With each stroke volume ejection, the arterial pressure rises and the venous pressure drops both relative to the mean systemic pressure. As per our description above, resistance through a vessel is a function of the pressure gradient divided by flow. Therefore being that the arterial system is a high-pressure system, it has high resistance. The differences in the pressure gradients between these three circulatory systems allow for blood to be driven forward. The mechanisms as described include pressure gradients and intra-chamber suction. Mean systemic pressure varies minimally from the time there is no flow to when there is steady flow. This assumes that the compliance of the circulatory system is constant. When the capacitance of the arterial and venous vessels change, the driving pressure is altered.

In order to maintain appropriate forward flow, the mean systemic pressure must be greater than the right atrial pressure. To augment this, intravascular volume can be increased or capacitance of the venous system decreased. Decreasing the capacitance of the venous system will achieve the same effect as decreasing the unstressed volume. The unstressed volume is the amount of blood needed to fill the vascular bed so that any additional volume will start to affect the stretch on the walls of the vessels. One way to reduce this threshold volume is to use vasoconstricting agents, increase contractility, or reduce afterload. A passive leg raise also shifts blood volume into the stressed volume by transferring volume from the central abdominal vasculature. With less volume required for the unstressed volume, a greater force is exerted on the vessel walls leading to an increase in mean systemic pressure greater to the point that is greater than the venous system pressure. Right atrial pressure decreases and venous return increases.

2.5 Venous Return

The right atrial pressure on the x-axis decreases from 12 to 0 mmHg as it travels from A to B leading to an increase in venous return (Fig. 18). No area to the left of point B on the venous return curve will lead to an increase in venous return. Therefore a right atrial pressure of zero is what will allow for the maximum acceptance difference in mean systemic pressure and right atrial pressure. Any lower and the flow is impaired because of the pressures in the superior vena cava and inferior vena cava decreases below their surrounding pressure. This represents the driving pressure for venous return.

The slope of the relationship between venous return and mean systemic pressure represents the resistance to venous return.

$$RVR = (P_{ms} - RAP)$$

RVR: Resistance to venous return, P_{ms}: Mean systemic pressure, and RAP: Right atrial pressure

Left ventricular function regulates right atrial pressure if no right heart dysfunction is present. Figure 2 illustrates that cardiac output decreases and venous return increases with

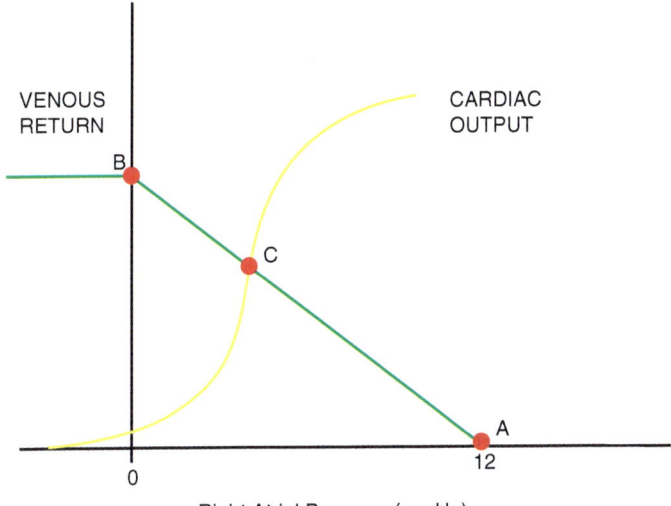

FIGURE 2 Normal relationship between venous return and cardiac output. (Modified from: Wijdicks et al. [68])

decreases in right atrial pressure. Venous return and cardiac output intersect at a given right atrial pressure. VR can be augmented to improve CO by increasing Pms. An upward translation of the curve is shown in Fig. 3. VR and CO curves intersect at a greater CO.

With contractility increased or afterload reduced, the CO curve (red) shifts left. Along either CO curve, the point of intersection between the CO and both VR curves demonstrates that with a higher VR, the CO increases as RAP increases. In hypovolemic patients, improvement in contractility will barely improve cardiac output as noted between the difference in points C and B.

Figure 4 shows that in compromised cardiac function, VR decreases from A to B as the RAP increases. When vasoconstriction takes place, unstressed volume decreases and venous return increases. Therefore, for a higher RAP, there is less of an increase in CO along with signs such as pulmonary and peripheral edema.

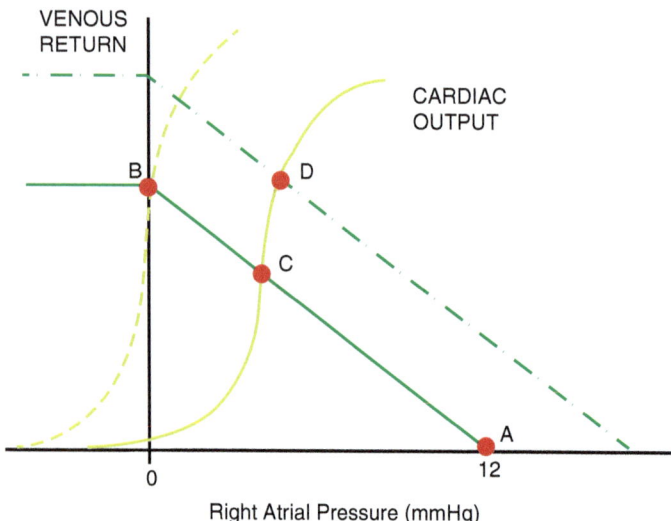

FIGURE 3 Effect of upward shift of venous return curve and improvement in cardiac output in relation to right atrial pressure. (Modified from: Wijdicks et al. [68])

RVR is the resistance to venous return and it is less in states of vasodilatation such as distributive shock, however CO would increase in this state. The opposite is true for vasoconstriction in which the RVR would increase and CO decreases.

Additionally, juxta-cardiac pressures increase the RAP and diminish VR. Examples are positive pressure ventilation and pneumothorax. Pms will have to increase to account for the increase in resistance to venous return. High levels of PEEP do not cause as much of a drop in CO in euvolemic or hypervolemic patients because the baroreceptor reflexiveness is more active than in hypovolemic patients. This explains why intubation in the hypovolemic patient can be extremely detrimental to CO.

It should be noted that fluid responsiveness and the effective arterial volume are not equivalent. Two patients with two different left ventricular functions can both have the same preload but respond differently to the same fluid bolus.

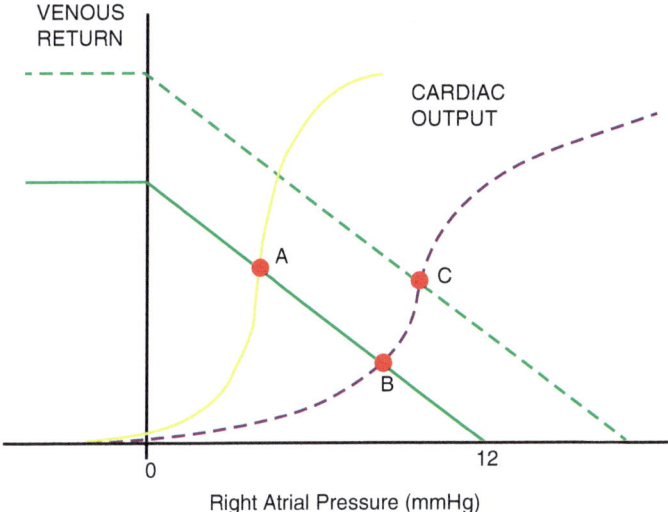

FIGURE 4 Effect of upward shift of venous return curve and diminished cardiac output in relation to right atrial pressure. (Modified from: Wijdicks et al. [68])

3 Hemodynamic Profiles of Shock

Distinguishing between the different types of shock at the basic level involves characterizing its features, specifically the Pulmonary Capillary Wedge Pressure (PCWP), Pulmonary Artery Pressure, Cardiac Output (CO) and subsequently Cardiac Index (CI, a body surface area adjusted form of cardiac output), Systemic Vascular Resistance (SVR), and Right Atrial Systolic and Diastolic pressures.

As illustrated in Fig. 5, **Septic Shock**, which is a form of distributive shock is marked by a preserved CI, at least early on before the possibility of sepsis induced cardiomyopathy. It features a low SVR and PCWP reflecting the low vasomotor tone and the body's attempt to compensate by increasing CI. With regards to the PCWP in Septic Shock, this is low, however it is due to capillary leak. Though some fluids may need to be administered to achieve an appropriate unstressed volume, too much fluid can drive the effective arterial volume

-	PCWP	CI	SVR	RAP	PASP
Normal Parameters	<6–12 mmHg	2.5-4.0	800–1600 (dynes × s)/(cm^5)	<6 mmHg	<25 mmHg
Hypovolemic Shock	↓	↓	↑	↓	↓
Distributive Shock	↓	↑	↓	↓	↓
Cardiogenic Shock	↓←→	↓	↑←→	↑←→	↑←→
Tamponade	↑←→	↓	↑←→	↑	↑←→

FIGURE 5 Hemodynamic profiles of shock. PCWP pulmonary capillary wedge pressure, CI cardiac index, SVR systemic vascular resistance, RAP right atrial pressure, PASP pulmonary artery systolic pressure. (Modified from: https://thoracickey.com/cardiogenic-shock-and-pulmonary-edema/)

into the interstitial space [64]. **Distributive Shock** also entails shock from fulminant hepatic failure, drug overdose, anaphylaxis, and neurogenic etiologies.

Cardiogenic Shock is divided into left ventricular (LV) and right ventricular (RV) failure. It includes patients with arrhythmias and valvulopathies causing compromised CI. Though acute mitral regurgitation has its own hemodynamic profile, it is essentially the same as Cardiogenic Shock due to LV failure. Both have elevated Pulmonary Artery Diastolic Pressures and PCWP due to the associated increase in afterload and increased pressure gradient that the Pulmonary Artery Systolic Pressure has to overcome.

Of note, these are rough guidelines for distinguishing shock types because the early and late hemodynamic profiles of shock can change and there can be mixed shock types as well.

Additionally, through the combination of lactate, central venous oxygen saturation, and assessment of venoarterial dif-

Hemodynamic Monitoring 457

ference in PCO2, shock can be classified into macro-circulatory versus micro-circulatory dysfunction (Fig. 6).

Figure 7 categorizes hemodynamic monitoring tools by invasive and non-invasive means and further details the tools necessary to utilize each.

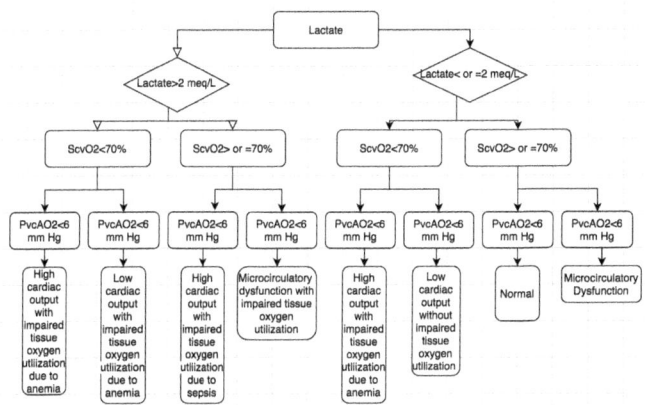

FIGURE 6 Shock states characterization. ScvO2 (central venous oxygen saturation), and PvcAO2 (venous to arterial carbon dioxide pressure difference)

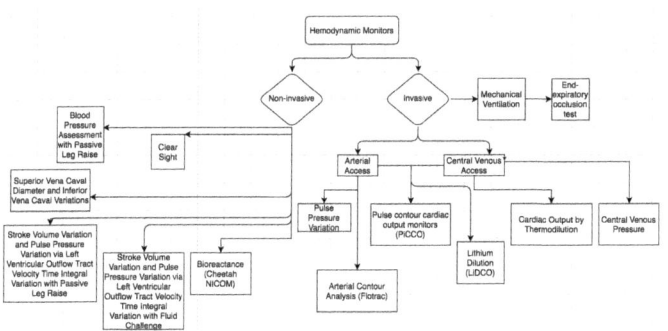

FIGURE 7 Flowchart categorizing hemodynamic monitoring tools

3.1 Methods of Assessment

Static methods: 1. Central Venous Pressure (CVP), 2. Pulmonary Artery Occlusion Pressure (PAOP), 3. Inferior Vena Cava(IVC) diameter collapsibility and distensibility, 4. End-Diastolic Volume (EDV), and correct flow time. They do not predict fluid responsiveness well.

Dynamic methods: 1. Pulse Pressure Variation (PPV), 2. Stroke Volume Variation (SVV), 3. Plethysmographic Variability Index(PVI). Dynamic methods take respirophasic changes in intrathoracic pressure into account, while static methods do not.

Central venous pressure has not been considered dependable as it is a static hemodynamic measure and has not correlated well with echocardiographic measures. It has traditionally been measured at the end of expiration to limit the influence of intrathoracic pressure as best as possible. A 2016 systematic review of 51 studies evaluating 982 critically ill patients showed that prediction of fluid responsiveness was low across all patient subgroups with no positive or negative predictive value over 66% for any central venous pressure from 0 to 20 mmHg [7].

Pulse Pressure Variation (PPV) has been frequently referenced. PPV with a threshold of 15% increase in determining cardiac output was found to be inferior to pulmonary artery occlusion pressure in a 2006 study involving 21 critically ill patients spontaneously breathing while receiving mechanical ventilation or face mask before and after fluid challenge [6]. Both pulse pressure variation and stroke volume variation are less reliable in conditions of spontaneous breathing, arrhythmias, low lung compliance, open chest, increased intra-abdominal pressure, tachypnea, and heart failure [13].

Thermodilution by use of Swan-Ganz catheters had been considered an accurate measure of cardiac output, however it is invasive and not indicated in most patients, especially in the neurocritical care unit. 20 mL of cold saline is injected through the central venous catheter and a thermodilution curve is plotted from the temperatures recorded at the thermistor tip based on the change in temperature from start to the thermistor tip. Additionally Swan-Ganz catheter placement has a number of risks and is not recommended for use in patients with suspected septic shock. It is also contraindicated in patients with coagulopathies, right sided endocarditis, mechanical tricuspid or pulmonic valves. Swan-Ganz catheters and the multitude of assessments that can be made with them have not been demonstrated to reduce mortality or hospital stay [8].

Thermodilution by cardiac output also requires insertion of a Swan-Ganz catheter and thus is invasive and not indicated in most neurocritical care patients. Via injection of a bolus of fluid into the right atrium, the rate of temperature change is plotted as described above.

Pulmonary artery occlusion pressure is an indirect measurement of left ventricular end-diastolic pressure (LVEDP). Limitations include need for precise placement of catheter tip, overestimation of LVEDP in patients with mitral stenosis, and overestimation of LVEDP in those with aortic regurgitation [1].

Additionally, **transpulmonary devices** can estimate cardiac output by analysis of arterial waveforms. These include lithium dilution and ultrasound dilution devices [10]. The lithium dilution device measures injected lithium chloride with an electrode and was found to have cardiac output measurements that were within 15.6% of pulmonary artery catheters [11]. Transpulmonary systems are not reliable in estimating volume responsiveness in several subsets of patients: those with significant arrhythmias, aortic regurgitation, intra-aortic balloon pumps, or spontaneously breathing patients or ventilated patients on less than 8 cc/kg of ideal body weight.

One system that utilizes transpulmonary thermodilution and pulse contour analysis together is **pulse contour cardiac output monitors (PiCCO)**. Fluid management in 350 patients with septic shock and acute respiratory distress syndrome were randomized to PiCCO and central venous pressure monitoring. Target mean arterial pressure was >60 mmHg. This study found no significant difference in mortality, ventilator-free days, or days free of continuous renal replacement therapy [12].

Flotrac is a device that utilizes arterial pressure waveform analysis, which it uses to calculate a cardiac output, stroke volume, stroke volume variation, and systemic vascular resistance. A Flotrac sensor attached to an arterial line monitors changes in vascular tone every 20 s. A database of previously collected patient values are used for comparison. The arterial pressure waveform is continuously analyzed to calculate the mentioned values. It's algorithm is based on Cardiac output = heart rate x stroke volume. The pulse rate is substituted for heart rate. The upslope of the waveform is used to detect pulse. Stroke Volume is calculated as the standard deviation of arterial blood pressure multiplied by a varying coefficient that accounts for changes in vascular resistance and compliance of the vessels between a variety of patient data [3]. There are several requirements, which include patients who are mechanically ventilated at 8 cc/kg (ideal body weight), not taking breaths spontaneously, and who are in sinus rhythm [2]. Most of the literature supporting the use of Flotrac as a hemodynamic monitoring tool is in the surgical population.

There has been demonstrable acceptable agreement in comparing Flotrac to Pulmonary Artery Catheters in cardiac surgery patients [43, 44]. The percentage error was 20%. When evaluating patients with hyperdynamic cardiac status, there was less agreement than when evaluating normal or hypodynamic cardiac status [45]. Flotrac has been shown to be inaccurate when used in patients with low systemic vascular resistance, namely distributive shock [46]. Even after further update of software, to the latest rendition of Flotrac, measurement of cardiac output was still not of acceptable agreement between Flotrac and transesophageal echocardiography during abdominal aortic aneurysm surgery [47].

ClearSight is a continuous non-invasive cardiac output monitoring system. Using a novel pulse contour method and continuous blood pressure monitoring, ClearSight measures cardiac output. With a finger cuff that wraps around the middle phalanx of multiple fingers inflating and deflating, the diameters of the arteries in the fingers are detected via LED. There is a brachial pressure reconstruction that is imputed from the finger pressure waveform. Based on the interactions between systolic and diastolic pressures and arterial impedance, the total arterial compliance is calculated [48]. The ease of use and lack of invasiveness make this a versatile modality. However because of the volume clamping of the fingers, the applied fingers must be changed every 8 h. Limitations include edematous fingers, aortic regurgitation, proximal aortic aneurysms, and severe vasoconstriction. There has been good agreement with pulmonary artery catheters in patients with heart failure [49]. There was good concordance when compared to PiCCO as well [50]. There was however, up to 50% error in the critically ill [51]. Comparison with transesophageal doppler was also poor [52].

And yet with all these options, many of us still rely on a fluid challenge, which can be appropriate, depending on the clinical context. However it is likely overutilized and studies have shown the effects of a fluid bolus on blood pressure measurements are typically transient, lasting approximately 15 min, even in patients deemed to be "fluid responsive". As examined in a meta-analysis, perceived fluid responsiveness in of itself is influenced by the rate of infusion, whereby faster infusions lead to a positive response, defined by an increase in cardiac index by at least 15% [9].

The technical application of many of these hemodynamic monitoring tools is discussed in Table 1. In total, there are limitations to every method of hemodynamic assessment (Table 2), each with varying degrees of validity.

Table 1 Technical application of hemodynamic monitoring tools

Method of monitoring	Application
Central venous pressure (CVP) [54]	With a central venous catheter inserted into the internal jugular vein or subclavian vein, the tip of the catheter should ideally be in the cavoatrial junction Using either a manometer or digital transducer, the transducer is "zeroed" at the level of the right atrium The 3-way stopcock is zeroed when it is closed to the patient. It is then turned to be closed to room air but open to the patient and the transducer. Usually this at the level of the fourth intercostal space in the mid-axillary line (the phlebostatic axis) While supine, the central venous pressure is measured at end-expiration A normal venous pressure is between 8 and 12 mmHg Supposed to represent right atrial pressure

Pulse pressure variation (PPV) [55]	Requires the patient to be in sinus rhythm, mechanically ventilated on 8 cc/kg of ideal body weight tidal volume, and have no significant alterations to chest wall compliance
Ideally, the patient should not be breathing spontaneously, to limit influence from intrathoracic pressure changes
Beat to beat monitoring is necessary: Arterial lines can be used. Additionally, there are non-invasive monitors as well like Nexfin and CNAP-500
Tubing is connected from the arterial line to a transducer which is aligned with the phlebostatic axis, as above
The arterial waveform is condensed to 6.25 mm/s on the monitor through adjusting "speed"
Identify the maximum and minimum waveforms: Maximum waveform should be during inspiration and minimum waveform should be during expiration
Use the cursor to mark the systolic and diastolic values for each waveform
The pulse pressure variation percentage is = $((PP_{max} - PP_{min})/\text{Mean of 2 PP}) \times 100$, where PP is pulse pressure
Pulse Pressure Variations of >12% have been associated with volume responsiveness

(continued)

TABLE 1 (continued)

Method of monitoring	Application
Thermodilution [56]	A Swan-Ganz catheter is inserted with its thermistor tip in the pulmonary artery 5–10 mL of cold saline is injected into the right atrium from the proximal catheter port Saline contacts blood when it travels through the ventricles into the pulmonary artery The temperature of the blood cools and is measured by the thermistor tip in the pulmonary artery The computer detect the change in temperature and uses it impute flow, which represent cardiac output from the right ventricle This is based on the temperature and volume of the cold saline injected Flow is inversely proportional to the change in temperature over time This is repeated three times and the average is taken In order to minimize influence of intrathoracic pressure, perform this at the end of expiration each time
Pulse contour cardiac output monitors (PiCCO) [57]	Both central venous access and arterial access are required A central venous line via the internal jugular veins or subclavian veins should be placed Any arterial access site is acceptable Similar to the procedure for Thermodilution Once calibration is complete, perform three separate injections of 15–30 mL of 0.9% saline that is <8 °C The monitor calculates a number of parameters including Cardiac Output, Extravascular Lung Water, Global End-Diastolic Volume, Intrathoracic Blood Volume, Cardiac Function Index, Global Ejection Fraction, Pulmonary Vascular Permeability Index, Stroke Volume, Stroke Volume Variation, Systemic Vascular Resistance, Pulse Pressure Variation, Left Ventricular Contractility Index, and Central Venous Oxygen Saturation

Lithium dilution (LiDCO) [58]	With the same setup as the PiCCO system, lithium chloride is injected instead of normal saline As opposed to measuring temperature, the sensor measures lithium content It detects this past the site of the arterial line Based on the same principles as Thermodilution, the area under the curve that records lithium concentration over time from site of insertion to site of detection, cardiac output is calculated from this dilution Compared to Thermodilution, it is not affected by the patient's core temperature and additional infusing fluids
IVC collapsibility (IVCCI) [59]	IVCCI is used for spontaneously breathing patients While in B-mode with the phased array probe in the longitudinal subxiphoid view, the last section of the vein, 0.5–3 cm right from the atrium, is located Transition to M-mode, then measure the IVC at maximum diameter (in expiratory phase) and also at minimum diameter (in inspiratory phase) The minimum diameter is subtracted from the maximum diameter and divided by the maximum diameter and multiplied by 100 When the patient is asked to sniff, an index >50% is supposed to correspond to a right atrial pressure of 3 mmHg if the IVC diameter is less than or equal to 2.1 cm On its own, IVCCI <20% is supposed to correspond to high right atrial pressures while <80% is supposed to correspond to low atrial pressures

(continued)

TABLE 1 (continued)

Method of monitoring	Application
IVC distensibility (IVCDI) [60]	The IVCDI is calculated in mechanically ventilated patients. It is the difference between maximum and minimum IVC diameters divided by the minimum diameter × 100 An index >18% suggests that volume expansion is unlikely to be effective in mechanically ventilated patients
Arterial contour analysis (Flotrac) [61]	An arterial line is placed, which is connected to a blood flow sensor Once connected to a monitor and calibrated, the patient's Cardiac Output, Stroke Volume, Stroke Volume Variation, and Systemic Vascular Resistance are calculated
ClearSight [62]	Through the application of the principle of vascular unloading, also known as the volume clamp method, finger cuffs are used to measure arterial pressures by estimation of diameters of arteries within the fingers with reconstruction of brachial arterial pressures
Bioreactance (Cheetah NICOM) [63]	Sensors are attached to the patient's body and then connected to the cable according to corresponding color This can then be used in conjunction with either passive leg raise or a fluid bolus For a passive leg raise, place the patient in semi-recumbent position for 3 min for calibration Then as instructed on the monitor, perform the passive leg raise to 45° for 3 min A stroke volume index >10% is intended to mean that the patient's blood pressure will increase with fluid administration
Passive leg raise	This is a very versatile technique that can be used in conjunction with Bioreactance, Arterial Contour Analysis, and Stroke Volume calculation on bedside ultrasound

Table 2 Summary of methods predicting preload responsiveness with diagnostic threshold and limitations

Method	Threshold	Main limitations
Central venous pressure	8–12 mmHg	Static parameter that has no direct correlation with blood volume. Should especially use in patients with heart transplants, right ventricular dysfunction, in particular
Pulse pressure/stroke volume variations [15]	12%	Cannot be used in case of spontaneous breathing, cardiac arrhythmias, low tidal volume/lung compliance
Inferior vena cava diameter variations [36]	12%	Cannot be used in case of spontaneous breathing, low tidal volume/lung compliance
Superior vena caval diameter variations [36]	36%	Requires performing transesophageal Doppler. Cannot be used in case of spontaneous breathing, low tidal volume/lung compliance
Passive leg raising [46]	10%	Requires a direct measurement of cardiac output
End-expiratory occlusion test [64]	5%	Cannot be used in non-intubated patients. Cannot be used in patients who interrupt a 15-s respiratory hold
"Mini"-fluid challenge (100 mL) [64]	6%	Requires a precise technique for measuring cardiac output
"Conventional" fluid challenge (500 mL) [64]	15%	Requires a direct measurement of cardiac output. Induces fluid overload if repeated

From: Monnet et al. [4]

4 Role of Ultrasound in Hemodynamic Assessment

Increasingly ultrasound has become a popular option both because of its ability to be easily employed as a point of care tool and in being able to take the dynamics of the cardiopulmonary system into account.

Within the arsenal of echocardiography, inferior vena cava diameter, collapsibility index (IVCCI), and distensibility index (IVCDI) are being used more frequently. IVCCI is used for spontaneously breathing patients.

4.1 Method

1. While in B-mode with the phased array probe in the longitudinal subxiphoid view, the last section of the vein, 0.5–3 cm right from the atrium, is located.
2. Transition to M-mode, then measure the IVC at maximum diameter (in expiratory phase) and also at minimum diameter (in inspiratory phase).
3. The minimum diameter is subtracted from the maximum diameter and divided by the maximum diameter and multiplied by 100.
4. When the patient is asked to sniff, an index >50% is supposed to correspond to a CO of 3 mmHg if the IVC diameter is less than or equal to 2.1 cm.

On its own, IVCCI <20% is supposed to correspond to high right atrial pressures while <80% is supposed to correspond to low atrial pressures. However these measures have been not proven to be useful in spontaneously breathing patients [59]. Nine studies have been performed involving spontaneously breathing patients. Three of these studies were negative, two had borderline results, and two involved children in the neurosurgical operating room, and women with pre-eclampsia. One of the positive studies involved patients who were alert enough to follow commands and make a quantitative respiratory effort and the other was criticized for late enrollment of patients after an average of four liters intravenous fluids received. Because of the lack of reproducibility in spontaneously breathing patients, it is not preferred [5].

The IVCDI is calculated in mechanically ventilated patients. It is the difference between maximum and minimum IVC diameters divided by the minimum diameter x 100. An index >18% suggests that volume expansion is unlikely to be effective in mechanically ventilated patients.

Many of these methods are both invasive and unnecessary in the vast majority of neuro-critical care patients to answer the question of what the effective arterial volume is in the patient and also if the patient is fluid responsive with respect to stressed volume. Furthermore, although point of care echocardiography of the patient is now becoming the standard of care for determining the above, it is not an easily applicable skill and requires significant practice under supervision to ensure the clinician is not under or overestimating their measurements, obtains appropriate views that avoid foreshortening, and that the measurements are made within the appropriate clinical context.

The objective of assessing preload and fluid responsiveness of patients in the neuro-intensive care unit is to avoid the morbidity and mortality associated with excess intravenous fluid administration [14]. Fluid overload is an independent predictor for all-cause mortality [16–18]. In a cohort of patients with end-stage renal disease receiving hemodialysis, bedside nuclear magnetic resonance found that the first sign of fluid overload was expansion of the extracellular fluid space of muscle [15]. Beside this very early sign, which would be difficult to detect in most patients, pulmonary edema is another relatively early sign of fluid overload. Other manifestations are heart failure, impaired digestion, and impaired healing.

Beyond maintaining volume status with an appropriate range to optimize cardiac output and thereby optimize oxygen delivery to the heart and other essential organs, the clinician in the neuro-intensive care is concerned with cerebral blood flow (CBF) in particular and cerebral blood volume (CBV). Intracranial pressure (ICP) is a function of intracranial volume and craniospinal compliance. Assuming cerebral auto-regulation is not impaired, ICP is slightly greater than cerebral venous pressure. With an unchanged mean arterial pressure, as ICP increases, cerebral perfusion pressure (CPP) decreases as denoted by the relationship:

CPP = MAP − ICP. Figure 8 shows the relationship between cerebral blood flow and cerebral perfusion pressure. There is a similar relationship between cerebral blood flow and mean arterial pressure shown in Fig. 9.

When CPP falls below 50 mmHg, autoregulation fails and CBF declines. Hypotension, whether it is due to hypovolemia or any other cause, causes vasodilation, which can raise ICP. Because of the increased susceptibility to ischemic secondary injury in the injured brain, maintaining euvolemia is of utmost importance. As per the relationship above, a compensatory increase in MAP for the same elevation in ICP would maintain a constant CPP and it is vital to maintain

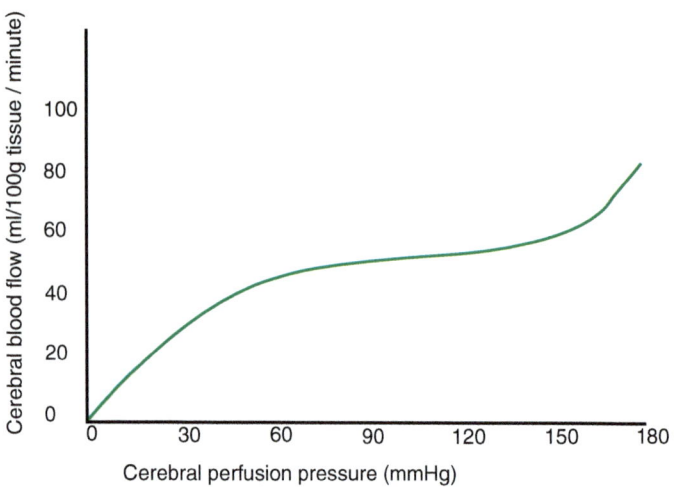

FIGURE 8 Relationship between cerebral blood flow and cerebral perfusion pressure

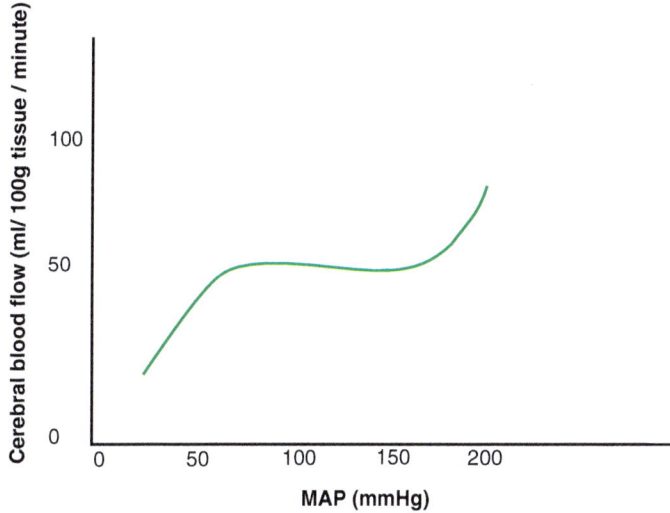

FIGURE 9 Relationship between mean arterial pressure and cerebral blood flow

euvolemia for this. Expansion of plasma volume not only causes autoregulatory vasoconstriction, but it reduces blood viscosity, and improves microvascular blood flow [12].

For this reason, an approach that seeks to minimize the adverse effects of fluid overload is more important than attempting to determine fluid responsiveness and preload in the neurocritical care unit specifically. As mentioned above, pulmonary edema is an early marker of fluid overload, particularly extravascular lung water (EVLW).

Extravascular lung water is the water in the alveoli and interstitium and is quantified through transpulmonary thermodilution. It is of equal significance in cardiogenic and non-cardiogenic pulmonary edema. A normal reference range is 7.3 ± 2.8 mL/kg and values >10 mL/kg are considered the cutoff value for pulmonary edema. Values >15 mL/kg signify severe pulmonary edema. This comes from autopsies in Japan which showed that EVLW >9.8 mL/kg were at the optimal discrimination threshold for pulmonary edema and numbers of 14.6 mL/kg having a positive predictive value of 99% [24].

There have already been efforts made to assess EVLW in critically ill patients with heart failure [20]. One found a positive correlation with a r value of 0.745 between lung ultrasound that demonstrated pulmonary edema and EVLW [21]. Through comparison of the PiCCO system and pulmonary capillary wedge pressure, chest ultrasound had a strong association with EVLW [23]. It is calculated with transpulmonary thermodilution by the method described above along with calculation of the mean transit time of the fluid. This is a surrogate for intrathoracic thermal volume. Global end diastolic volume (GEDV) is calculated as the difference between intrathoracic thermal volume and pulmonary thermal volume. EVLW is determined from its relationship with GEDV. When EVLW has been indexed to height, there has been a strong association with PaO2/FiO2 ratios (AUC: 0.729) and even stronger association with Oxygenation Index (AUC: 0.778) [22]. Furthermore, the decrease in EVLW in the first 48 h of measurement is associated with 28-day survival in ARDS [25]. The advantage of lung ultrasound is that the parameters to be evaluated are easier to learn and apply then echocardiographic skills. There is a much smaller chance of inter-operator variability as well [41]. It still provides the same ease of use because it is a point of care tool. Anesthesia residents were taught to detect pneumothoraces online in 5 min [42]. In addition, lung ultrasound has demonstrated itself a superior tool to chest x-ray in identifying patients with pulmonary edema earlier. There can be a delay of 12 h after patients have developed signs and symptoms of volume overload before corresponding signs are seen on chest x-ray. By the same token, there can be up to a 4 day delay in correlating the resolution of pulmonary edema and x-ray [67].

In addition, when it comes to the diagnosis of pleural effusion, lung ultrasound is superior to chest x-ray in diagnosing and quantifying pleural effusions [33]. Per two systematic reviews of 8 cohort studies with 1048 patients in total, with

CT as a reference, lung ultrasound had a 90.9% pooled sensitivity compared to 50.2% with chest x-ray in detecting pneumothorax [34].

4.2 Basic Principles of Lung Ultrasound and Image Acquisition

The high frequency linear probe, sometimes referred to as the vascular probe, will give better resolution of the pleura than the phased-array probe, being that the depth required is less than for echocardiography. Though the phased-array probe can still be used, especially for identifying deeper structures. The linear probe operates at higher frequencies (8–15 MHz) and typically is meant for superficial distances (1–4 cm). The field of view is linear and is meant for evaluating blood vessels, breast, thyroid, and tendons [53]. The phased array probe has a trapezoidal field of view. At the surface of the probe, the field of view is narrow, but it widens the deeper the waves penetrate. It optimally detects structures between 4 and 8 cm. It operates at lower frequencies (2–6 MHz) and thus higher wavelengths. It is ideally suited for cardiac echocardiography and abdominal exams.

4.3 Method

1. Seat the patient upright. Elevate the head of the bed and use wedges. Expose the thorax completely.
2. Cover the surface of the probe with gel so that an interface can form that excludes any air.
3. Set the ultrasound to 2D Mode (also known as B-mode). Select the lung preset, if available.
4. To evaluate the pleural line, a depth of 3–4 cm will typically be sufficient, otherwise to further evaluate deeper structures, increase the depth to 7 cm. Adjust the gain accordingly. Note the direction of the dot on the top of the screen, which corresponds to the probe marker.

5. There are several protocols that denote the number of regions to examine. The Bedside Lung Ultrasound in Emergency (BLUE protocol) identifies three points for each lung, while there is a 12 point examination for critical care patients. The three point method can be used in each lung.
6. Make sure to keep the probe perpendicular with the skin. With the probe marker pointed in the cranial direction, use two hands.
7. Standing on the right side of the patient, place the hypothenar eminence of your left hand against the clavicle and with your thumbs overlapping place your right hand next to it. The upper BLUE point is at the middle of the hand on the left. The lower BLUE point is at the middle of the hand on the right. The same is done on the other side, standing to the left of the patient. The posterolateral alveolar and pleural syndrome point (PLAPS) is directly behind the patient at the same level of the lower BLUE point. Some use the intersection of the posterior axillary line with the horizontal axis of the lower BLUE point to represent this region (Fig. 10).

Findings of ultrasound can be divided into real images and artifacts.

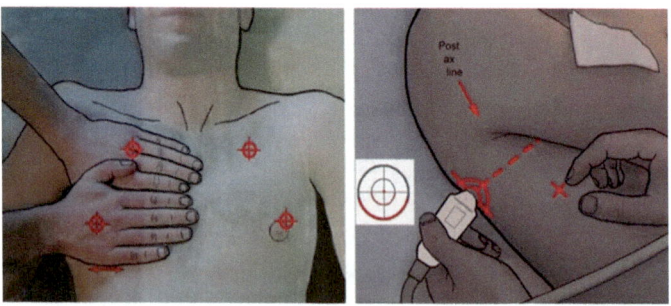

Figure 10 BLUE (left) and PLAPS (right) points shown. (Reprinted from: Lichtenstein [69] (Open Access))

5 Artifacts

The parietal pleura tends to be more easily visualized than the visceral pleura. They lie approximately 0.5 cm below the skin surface, as can be measured by the scale. The transmission of ultrasound waves to the pleura can lead to ultrasounds reverberating, which result in A-lines. A-lines are hyperechoic (bright) and layered in a horizontal orientation below the pleura. This is often a result of a high ratio of gas to volume under the parietal pleura can be present in pneumothorax, hyperinflation, or even normal lung [26]. Predominant A-lines in sequence (A-profile) suggest non-parenchymal disease in patients with respiratory failure suggest COPD, asthma, or pulmonary embolism. In the presence of lobar consolidation it can be associated with pneumonia or ARDS. When there is no lung sliding it is referred to as an A′-profile.

Lung sliding is an artifact that manifests as a horizontal translation of a hyperechoic line at the level of the pleura and represents the parietal and visceral pleura against each other. The lung sliding artifact is created when the visceral pleura slides past the parietal pleura. M-mode allows a thin cut of tissues along the axis of a line to be visualized moving through time. When applied to lung pleura, the presence of lung sliding is commonly referred to as the seashore sign (Fig. 11). Absence of lung sliding can be concerning and indicative of pneumothorax, though is not indicative of it on its own. On M-Mode, the stratosphere sign appears (Fig. 12). When there is no lung sliding, a lung pulse can be seen, in which the visceral pleura only moves with the heart beating. The interface between collapsed lung and pleura is the lung point and can be another sign of pneumothorax, specifically showing where it starts.

B-lines or comet tails are vertical hyperechoic lines that originate from pleural lines and will usually stretch to 5–7 cm in depth (Figs. 13 and 14). They correspond to the number of interlobular septa [39]. Key characteristics are that they obliterate A-lines and usually move with lung sliding when in a group of 3 or more (B profile). If lung sliding is absent, it is a

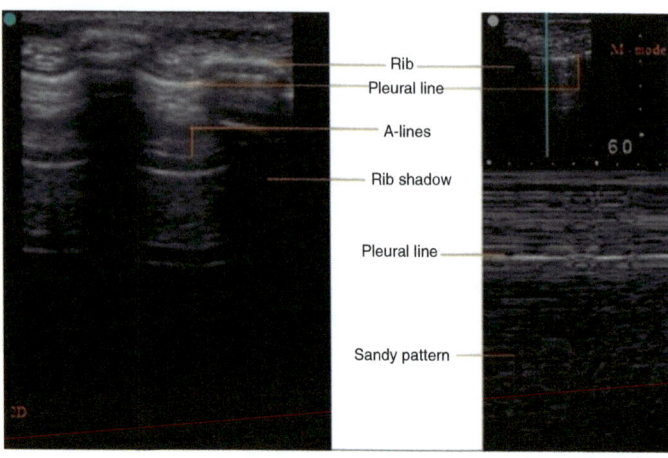

FIGURE 11 Seashore sign on right. (Reprinted from: Saraogi [70] (Open Access))

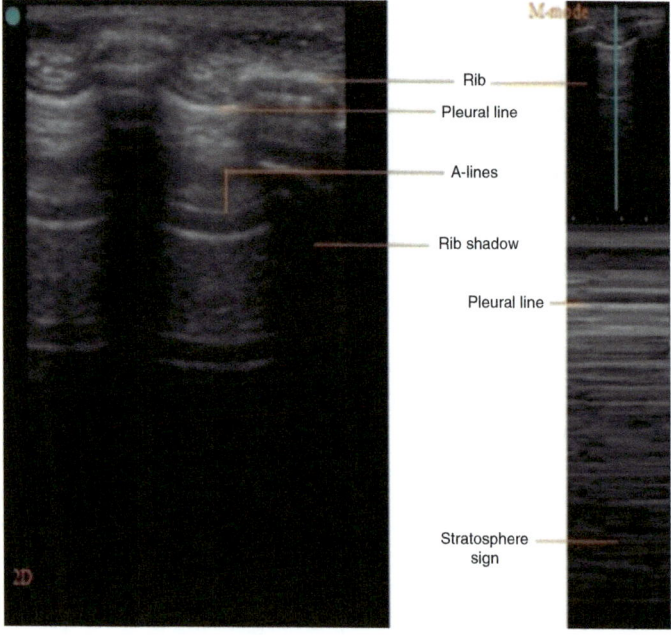

FIGURE 12 Stratosphere sign. (From: Saraogi [70] (Open Access))

Hemodynamic Monitoring 477

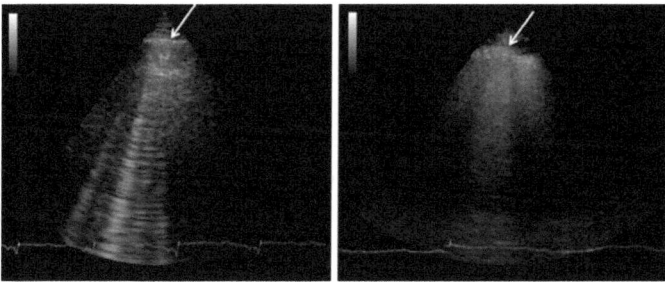

FIGURE 13 Left: B-profile in a patient with pulmonary edema. Arrow represents the pleural line. Right: Different distribution of B-lines creating a B profile that was due to pulmonary fibrosis. Arrow here shows an irregular and more coarse pleural line. (Reprinted from: Gargani and Volpicelli [71] (Open Access))

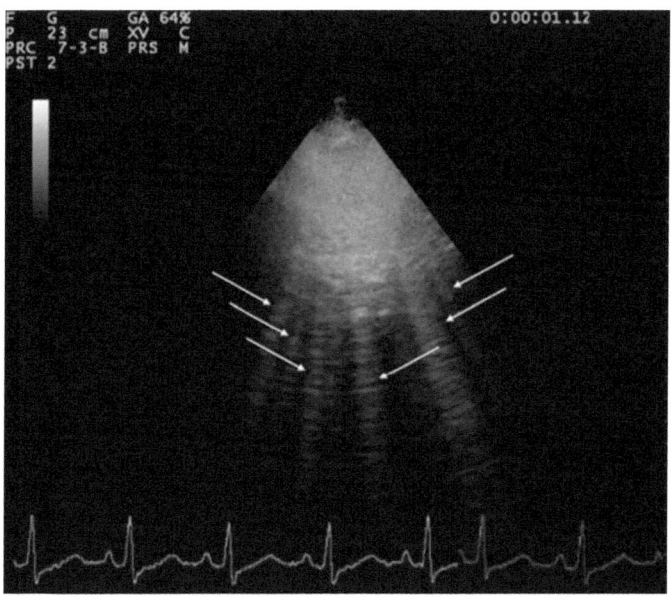

FIGURE 14 B-lines appear as hyperechoic lines originating from the pleural line that extend at least 5 cm. Here they are denoted by arrows. (Reprinted from: Gargani and Volpicelli [71] (Open Access))

B′-profile. Edema engorges interlobular septa allowing ultrasound penetration. An impedance gradient between gas and fluids traps the ultrasound. This forms the B-line, which comes in and out of view. When there is a single B-line it may be normal. When more than two are seen, they are sometimes called lung rockets and are due to pulmonary edema or pulmonary fibrosis. Three or four B-lines in a single view are effects of thickened interlobular septa. Five or more correlate with a severe interstitial syndrome [27].

More recently, efforts to characterize pulmonary edema as cardiogenic vs noncardiogenic have been made. The greater the amount of EVLW, the more B-lines are seen in a group and the closer they are to each other. When severe, they appear as white lung (Fig. 15). With cardiogenic pulmonary edema, B-lines tend to be uniform and lung sliding is normal. They are more often associated with bilateral pleural effusions, which can be detected with ultrasound. In noncardiogenic pulmonary edema, non-uniform B-lines, more

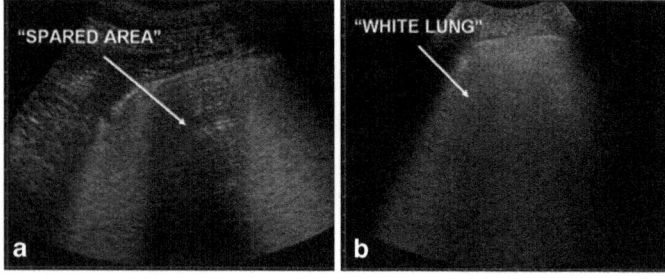

FIGURE 15 Comparison of cardiogenic and non-cardiogenic pulmonary edema in lung ultrasound. (**a**) Non-cardiogenic pulmonary edema, ARDS in this case, showcasing non-homogeneous distribution. (**b**) Cardiogenic pulmonary edema with more evenly distributed alveolar-interstitial pattern. Bottom Left: Jagged, uneven, and thickened pleural line, seen in ARDS. Bottom Right: Thin and even pleural line in cardiogenic pulmonary edema. (Reprinted from: Copetti et al. [72] (Open Access))

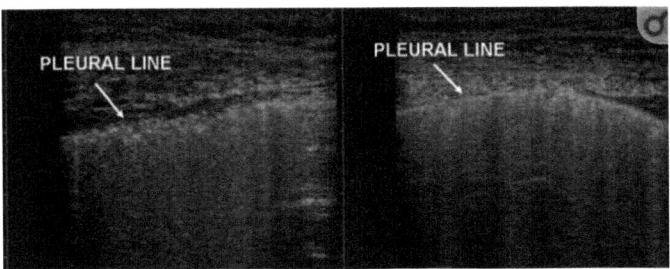

FIGURE 15 (continued)

frequent, with jagged, thickened (>2 mm) non-uniform pleura and uneven tissue patterns (consolidations and spared areas). Lung sliding may be imperceptible, though lung pulse will be present. Air bronchograms are sometimes seen as well. Isolated air bronchograms are shown in Figs. 16 and 17. Linear air bronchograms can also appear in ventilator associated pneumonia (Fig. 18). If the B-lines are 7 mm or more apart, it is more likely due to an interstitial syndrome, whereas distances 3 mm or less are more consistent with pulmonary edema. If the B-lines are irregularly spaced, pneumonia is more likely [32]. Unilateral B-lines are not consistent with pulmonary edema. It will usually be seen within 2 regions per each lung.

C-profiles are simply anterior lung consolidations. This appears as lung tissue and the image may contain an irregular pleural line. C-profiles are sometimes referred to as A/B--profiles as well.

Z-lines are confused with B-lines but are rather shorter vertical comet tails. They arise from the pleural line but tend not to span more than 4 cm at the most, do not obliterate A-lines. The pattern of movement B-lines possess with lung sliding is not present with Z-lines.

Table 3 describes some of these artifacts and more in detail.

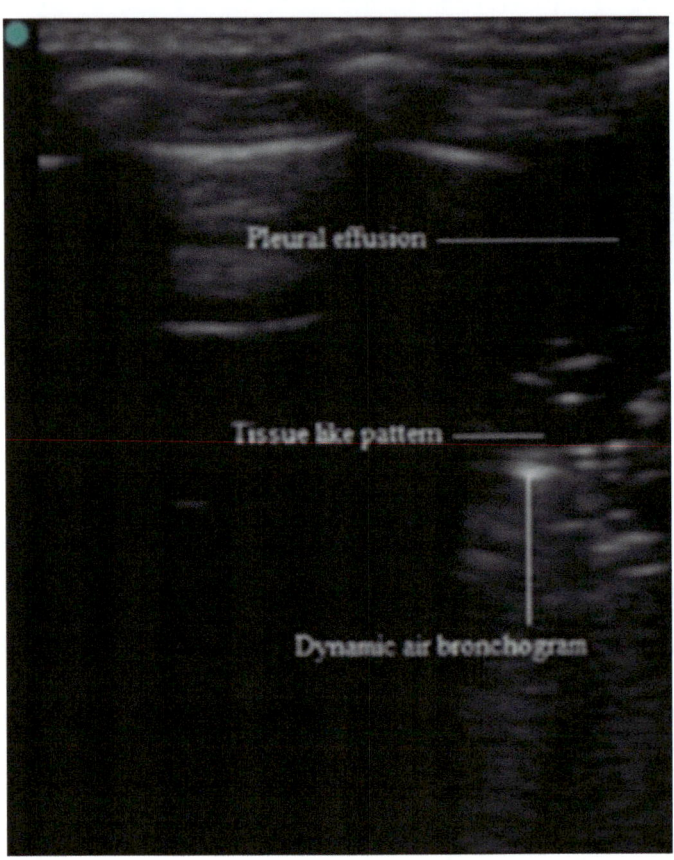

FIGURE 16 Dynamic air bronchogram. (From: Saraogi [70] (Open Access))

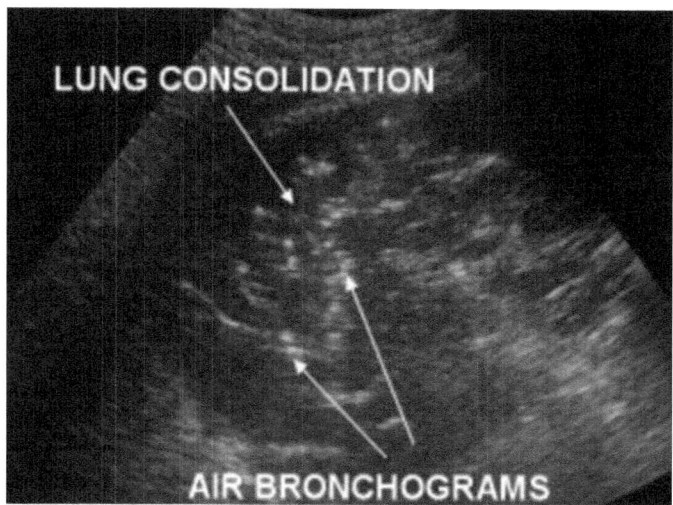

FIGURE 17 Dynamic air bronchograms indicated by arrows. (Reprinted from: Copetti et al. [72] (Open Access))

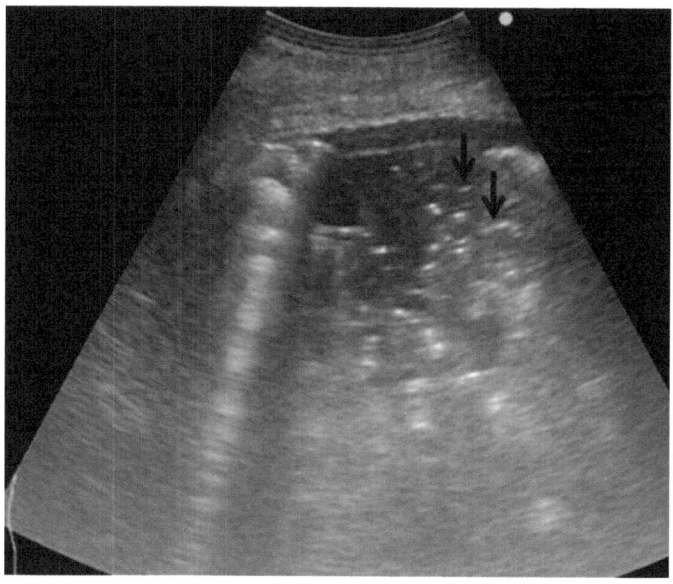

FIGURE 18 Linear air bronchogram. Arrows pointing to the highlighted area. (Reprinted from: Keng and Lee [73] (Open Access))

TABLE 3 Pertinent lung findings

Bat sign	Hyperechoic line visualized within 0.5 cm below the rib and used to identify the pleura (Fig. 19)
Seashore sign	These appear as straight lines above the pleura and coarse more dense echotexture below the line Confirms normal movement of the pleural line with ventilation
Lung pulse	In the setting of no lung sliding, the visceral pleura only moves with the heartbeat
Shred sign	Also known as non-translobar consolidations Hypoechoic regions below the pleura that are ill defined Seen in: Diffuse parenchymal lung disease Ventilator associated pneumonia Less commonly in pulmonary subpleural infarcts
Tissue sign	Homogeneous echotexture Seen in loss of aeration due to pneumonia
Air bronchogram	Static Dynamic Linear Can be seen in ventilator associated pneumonia Punctiform Non-specific

Modified from: Mojoli et al. [75]

6 Real Images

Pulmonary consolidations either go through the lobe or do not. Non-translobar consolidations appear as hypoechoic densities beneath the pleura and translobar consolidations can appear as a deformity within tissue.

Air bronchograms are hyperechoic as compared to consolidations and are within the parenchyma. The dynamic variant is hyperechoic and may shimmer with each respiratory cycle and indicates pneumonia or pulmonary abscess. Static air bronchograms more likely mean the patient has resorptive

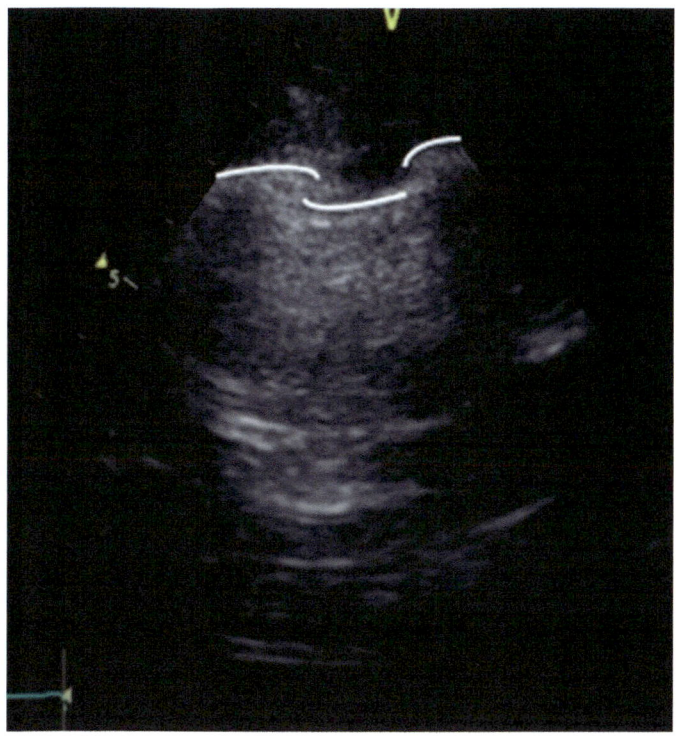

Figure 19 Bat sign. (Reprinted from: Gargani and Volpicelli [71] (Open Access))

atelectasis but can less frequently be seen with pneumonia, as well [28].

Pleural effusions are identified by four features on imaging (Fig. 20):

1. Anechoic space
   (a) Appears black and empty through each respiratory cycle
   (b) There can be variations where it is hypoechoic, complex with pleural effusions, or contains septations
2. Chest Wall

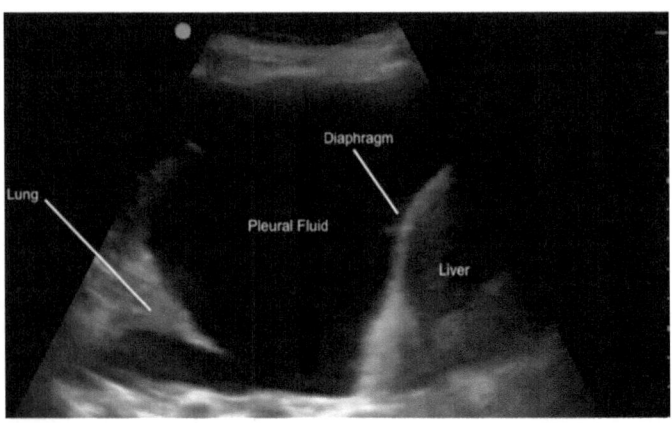

FIGURE 20 Anatomic sonographic characteristics of pleural effusions. (Atkinson et al. [74] (Open Access))

(a) Defined by skin, muscle and rib above the pleura

3. Diaphragm

   (a) Appears as a convexity above the liver or the spleen. There should be contraction and therefore downward movement during inspiration. Make sure to avoid the hepatorenal and splenorenal abscess, which look similar, but are often less echogenic.

4. Lung

   (a) An area under the pleura and above the diaphragm with differing level of echotexture

6.1 Utility in Neuro-Science Intensive Care Unit

Our goal in the neuro-critical care unit is to identify changes consistent with increased EVLW and titrate fluids accordingly. This approach is not wholly independent of knowing the patient's systolic and diastolic functional status, potential valvulopathies, and new versus old regional wall motion abnormalities. Of course modalities such as echocardiography are important. However, for the neuro-intensivist, ordering a formal echocardiogram to establish a baseline of cardiac function in a patient's whose hemodynamic status and preload assessment is unclear would make more sense than attempting to garner an incomprehensive assessment of cardiac function in relation to respiratory function. As mentioned above, factoring in whether the patient is on the ventilator or not, how he/she is synchronizing with it, and the ventilator settings does complicate hemodynamic assessment to more than simply evaluating the IVC.

Using the tools above, a systematic approach has been created to characterize the findings, known as the BLUE Protocol [29], referenced above, designed to diagnose the cause of respiratory failure. This was validated in several studies. In a study of 260 patients with respiratory failure assessed with ultrasound, pulmonary edema, identified as predominant anterior B-lines, had 87% PPV and 99% NPV when compared to the diagnosis by the ICU team [31]. As compared to non-contrast chest CT and clinical outcome, lung ultrasound compared well in diagnosing pulmonary edema [35]. This was with an inter-observer variability of only 4.9% for 295 patients' scans. A simplified lung edema scoring system (SLESS) based off of the BLUE protocol ultrasound points categorized four aeration patterns in septic patients [38]. Scores ranged from 6 (normal aeration) to 24 (bilateral total lung consolidation). This study found that there was good correlation with the MED and SAPS3 scores for sepsis ($r = 0.53$ and 0.55, respectively). It also had a negative correlation with PaO2/FiO2 ratio ($r = -0.62$). One cohort of 37 patients with acute respiratory failure defined as respiratory rate ≥ 30 breaths/minute, $PaO_2 \leq 60$ mmHg, oxygen saturation by pulse oximetry $\leq 90\%$, or $PCO_2 \geq 45$ mm Hg with arterial pH ≤ 7.35 compared chest x-ray findings with the BLUE Protocol, with the reference standard being the final diagnosis made by the critical care team. There was a 90% positive predictive value (PPV) and non-predictive value (NPV) of 91% for pulmonary edema. For pneumonia, PPV was 88% and NPV was 90% [30]. Another study with 308 patients with

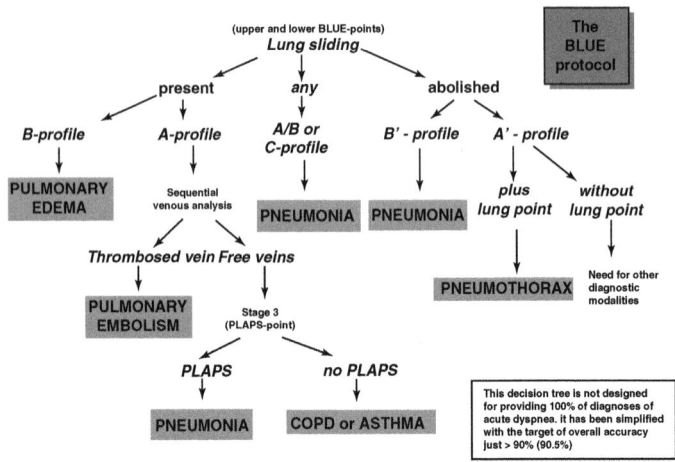

FIGURE 21 BLUE protocol. (From: Lichtenstein [29] (Open Access))

dyspnea comparing the BLUE protocol with the final diagnosis made by the critical care team found that the PPV and NPV for pulmonary edema were 87% and 89%, respectively [31]. There has also been good comparison with pulmonary occlusion pressures [36, 37] and measurement of EVLW in particular [36].

There are more advanced techniques involving evaluating 12 regions in total, which also directly correlate with EVLW, but for our purposes the BLUE protocol will suffice. Within the BLUE protocol (Fig. 21), we are primarily concerned with findings of pulmonary edema. Initially, a shallow view should be taken to examine the pleura for lung sliding. M-Mode can be used to better distinguish the two. The seashore sign is consistent with lung sliding, while the stratosphere sign is not. It is important to check the pleura starting at the upper BLUE point first to see the pleura. If there is not any lung sliding, next check for presence for A-lines. If present, are there several layers of A-lines? This would indicate an A'-profile. If a lung point is detected, by scanning along the periphery of the lung, this can be a pneumothorax. In the absence of lung sliding, a B'-profile could be seen with pneumonia. If lung sliding is present and there are B-profiles bilaterally (3 or more B-lines as defined above), this is usually consistent with pneumonia. Use descriptors mentioned above to distinguish between this and pneumonia. A-profiles with lung sliding present can be pneumonia, pulmonary embolism, COPD, or asthma and distinguishing these is beyond the scope of this chapter. C profiles are typically due to pneumonia. The important take-away from the BLUE protocol is being able to identify immediate abnormalities that suggest the patient has pulmonary edema.

7 Future Directions

There have been an increasing number of applications of lung ultrasound recently. To further elucidate the degree of pulmonary edema, ultrasound rating systems have been created to try to quantify the amount of non-aerated lung tissue [40]. As is, there is a strong correlation between aeration scores and tissue density assessment on CT. Further refinement of the aeration score will hopefully help distinguish the level of aeration within a single lung field. Ideally, with further validation of this method, there can be replacement of frequent chest x-rays in the ICU, which would both minimize radiation exposure and limit costs.

8 Application

In the mechanically ventilated patient, an approach involving the use of Flotrac can be used to assess effective arterial volume. Though it has its limitations, it has been shown to be useful in determining hemodynamic parameters in patients who are known not to be in overt cardiogenic shock. Outside of a formal transthoracic echocardiogram, bedside point of care echocardiography can easily reveal this through E-point septal separation, stroke volume and therefore cardiac output and index calculation through Left Ventricular Outflow Tract

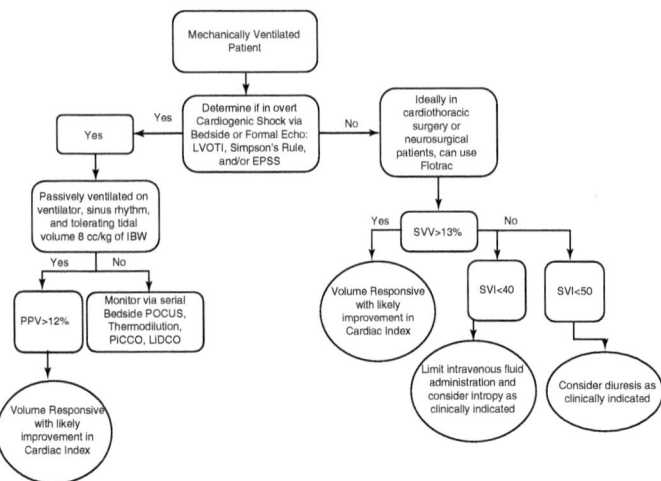

FIGURE 22 Determination of volume status as a function of cardiac output in mechanically ventilated patients

Velocity Time Integral (outside the scope of this chapter). Its use is ideal in the perioperative cardiac patient and also has evidence of utility in neurosurgical patients. As demonstrated in the Algorithm illustrated in Fig. 22, if the patient meets the criteria, Flotrac is an appropriate option. When connected to an arterial catheter, a Stroke Volume Variation (SVV) can be calculated as $SV_{max} - SV_{min}/SV_{mean}$, where SV_{max} is the maximum stroke volume detected in a given amount of time and SV_{min} is the minimum stroke volume detected in the same time period. SV_{mean} is the average of the two values mentioned. If the SVV is greater than 13%, this could indicate that the patient's cardiac output is expected to improve with fluid administration.

References

1. Power P, Bone A, Simpson N, Yap CH, Gower S, Bailey M. Comparison of pulmonary artery catheter, echocardiography, and arterial waveform analysis monitoring in predicting the

hemodynamic state during and after cardiac surgery. Int J Crit Ill Inj Sci. 2017;7:156–62.
2. Krige A, Bland M, Fanshawe T. Fluid responsiveness prediction using Vigileo FloTrac measured cardiac output changes during passive leg raise test. J Intensive Care. 2016;4:63. Published 2016 Oct 6.
3. Biais M, Vidil L, Sarrabay P, Cottenceau V, Revel P, Sztark F. Changes in stroke volume induced by passive leg raising in spontaneously breathing patients: comparison between echocardiography and Vigileo/FloTrac device. Crit Care. 2009;13(6):R195.
4. Monnet X, Marik PE, Teboul JL. Prediction of fluid responsiveness: an update. Ann Intensive Care. 2016;6(1):111. https://doi.org/10.1186/s13613-016-0216-7.
5. Li Y, Yin W, Kang Y. Is ultrasound assessment of the inferior vena cava for fluid responsiveness unlikely to be helpful, or is it just too early to say? Can J Anaesth. 2020;67(6):783–4.
6. Heenen S, De Backer D, Vincent JL. How can the response to volume expansion in patients with spontaneous respiratory movements be predicted? Crit Care. 2006;10(4):R102.
7. Eskesen TG, Wetterslev M, Perner A. Systematic review including re-analyses of 1148 individual data sets of central venous pressure as a predictor of fluid responsiveness. Intensive Care Med. 2016;42(3):324–32.
8. Rajaram SS, Desai NK, Kalra A, et al. Pulmonary artery catheters for adult patients in intensive care. Cochrane Database Syst Rev. 2013;2013(2):CD003408.
9. Toscani L, Aya HD, Antonakaki D, et al. What is the impact of the fluid challenge technique on diagnosis of fluid responsiveness? A systematic review and meta-analysis. Crit Care. 2017;21(1):207.
10. Cecconi M, De Backer D, Antonelli M, et al. Consensus on circulatory shock and hemodynamic monitoring. Task force of the European Society of Intensive Care Medicine. Intensive Care Med. 2014;40(12):1795–815.
11. Costa MG, Della Rocca G, Chiarandini P, et al. Continuous and intermittent cardiac output measurement in hyperdynamic conditions: pulmonary artery catheter vs. lithium dilution technique. Intensive Care Med. 2008;34(2):257–63.
12. Zhang Z, Ni H, Qian Z. Effectiveness of treatment based on PiCCO parameters in critically ill patients with septic shock and/

or acute respiratory distress syndrome: a randomized controlled trial. Intensive Care Med. 2015;41(3):444–51.
13. Monnet X, Marik PE, Teboul JL. Prediction of fluid responsiveness: an update. Ann Intensive Care. 2016;6(1):111.
14. Claure-Del Granado R, Mehta RL. Fluid overload in the ICU: evaluation and management. BMC Nephrol. 2016;17(1):109. Published 2016 Aug 2.
15. Mohammad WH, Elden AB, Abdelghany MF. Chest ultrasound as a new tool for assessment of volume status in hemodialysis patients. Saudi J Kidney Dis Transpl. 2020;31(4):805–13.
16. Agarwal R. Volume overload in dialysis: the elephant in the room, no one can see. Am J Nephrol. 2013;38:75–7.
17. Kalantar-Zadeh K, Regidor DL, Kovesdy CP, Van Wyck D, Bunnapradist S, Horwich TB, et al. Fluid retention is associated with cardio- vascular mortality in patients undergoing longterm hemodialysis. Circulation. 2009;119:671–9.
18. Wizemann V, Wabel P, Chamney P, et al. The mortality risk of overhydration in haemodialysis patients. Nephrol Dial Transplant. 2009;24:1574–9.
19. Perez-Barcena J, Llompart-Pou JA, O'Phelan KH. Intracranial pressure monitoring and management of intracranial hypertension. Crit Care Clin. 2014;30(4):735–50.
20. Picano E, Gargani L, Gheorghiade M. Why, when, and how to assess pulmonary congestion in heart failure: pathophysiological, clinical, and methodological implications. Heart Fail Rev. 2010 Jan;15(1):63–72.
21. Zhang L, Yu W, Zhou C, Chen G. Zhonghua Wei Zhong Bing Ji Jiu Yi Xue. 2020;32(5):585–9.
22. Huber W, Höllthaler J, Schuster T, et al. Association between different indexations of extravascular lung water (EVLW) and PaO2/FiO2: a two-center study in 231 patients. PLoS One. 2014;9(8):e103854.
23. Enghard P, Rademacher S, Nee J, Hasper D, Engert U, Jörres A, et al. Simplified lung ultrasound protocol shows excellent prediction of extravascular lung water in ventilated intensive care patients. Crit Care. 2015;19:36.
24. Tagami T, Sawabe M, Kushimoto S, Marik PE, Mieno MN, Kawaguchi T, Kusakabe T, Tosa R, Yokota H, Fukuda Y. Quantitative diagnosis of diffuse alveolar damage using extravascular lung water. Crit Care Med. 2013;41(9):2144–50.
25. Tagami T, Nakamura T, Kushimoto S, Tosa R, Watanabe A, Kaneko T, Fukushima H, Rinka H, Kudo D, Uzu H, Murai A,

Takatori M, Izumino H, Kase Y, Seo R, Takahashi H, Kitazawa Y, Yamaguchi J, Sugita M, Takahashi H, Kuroki Y, Kanemura T, Morisawa K, Saito N, Irahara T, Yokota H. Early-phase changes of extravascular lung water index as a prognostic indicator in acute respiratory distress syndrome patients. Ann Intensive Care. 2014;4:27.
26. Koenig S, Mayo P, Volipcelli G, Millington SJ. Lung ultrasound for respiratory failure in acutely ill patients: a review [published online ahead of print, 2020 Aug 21]. Chest. 2020;S0012-3692(20)34273-2.
27. Lichtenstein D, Mézière G, Biderman P, Gepner A, Barré O. The comet-tail artifact: an ultrasound sign of alveolar-interstitial syndrome. Am J Respir Crit Care Med. 1997;156:1640–6.
28. Lichtenstein D, Mezière G, Seitz J. The dynamic air bronchogram. A lung ultrasound sign of alveolar consolidation ruling out atelectasis. Chest. 2009;135(6):1421–5.
29. Lichtenstein DA. BLUE-protocol and FALLS-protocol: two applications of lung ultrasound in the critically ill. Chest. 2015 Jun;147(6):1659–70.
30. Dexheimer Neto FL, Andrade JM, Raupp AC, et al. Diagnostic accuracy of the Bedside Lung Ultrasound in Emergency protocol for the diagnosis of acute respiratory failure in spontaneously breathing patients. J Bras Pneumol. 2015;41(1):58–64.
31. Lichtenstein DA, Mezière GA. Relevance of lung ultrasound in the diagnosis of acute respiratory failure: the BLUE protocol [published correction appears in Chest. 2013 Aug;144(2):721]. Chest. 2008;134(1):117–25.
32. Frankel HL, Kirkpatrick AW, Elbarbary M, et al. Guidelines for the appropriate use of bedside general and cardiac ultrasonography in the evaluation of critically ill patients-part I: general ultrasonography. Crit Care Med. 2015;43(11):2479–502.
33. Hooper C, Lee YC, Maskell N, BTS Pleural Guideline Group. Investigation of a unilateral pleural effusion in adults: British Thoracic Society Pleural Disease Guideline 2010. Thorax. 2010;65(Suppl 2):ii4–ii17.
34. Alrajhi K, Woo MY, Vaillancourt C. Test characteristics of ultrasonography for the detection of pneumothorax: a systematic review and meta-analysis. Chest. 2012;141(3):703–8.
35. Volpicelli G, Mussa A, Garofalo G, et al. Bedside lung ultrasound in the assessment of alveolar-interstitial syndrome. Am J Emerg Med. 2006;24(6):689–96.

36. Agricola E, Bove T, Oppizzi M, et al. "Ultrasound comet-tail images": A marker of pulmonary edema: a comparative study with wedge pressure and extravascular lung water. Chest. 2005;127:1690–5.
37. Agricola E, Picano E, Oppizzi M, et al. Assessment of stress-induced pulmonary interstitial edema by chest ultrasound during exercise echocar- diography and its correlation with left ventricular function. J Am Soc Echocardiogr. 2006;19:457–63.
38. Santos TM, Franci D, Coutinho CM, et al. A simplified ultrasound-based edema score to assess lung injury and clinical severity in septic patients. Am J Emerg Med. 2013;31:1656–60.
39. Lichtenstein DA. BLUE-protocol and FALLS-protocol: two applications of lung ultrasound in the critically ill. Chest. 2015;147(6):1659–70.
40. Soummer A, Perbet S, Brisson H, Arbelot C, Constantin JM, Lu Q, et al. Lung Ultrasound Study Group. Ultrasound assessment of lung aeration loss during a successful weaning trial predicts postextubation distress. Crit Care Med. 2012;40:2064–72.
41. Soummer A, Perbet S, Brisson H, Arbelot C, Constantin JM, Lu Q, et al. Lung Ultrasound Study Group. Ultrasound assessment of lung aeration loss during a successful weaning trial predicts postextubation distress. Crit Care Med. 2012;40:2064–72.
42. Krishnan S, Kuhl T, Ahmed W, Togashi K, Ueda K. Efficacy of an online education program for ultrasound diagnosis of pneumothorax. Anesthesiology. 2013;118:715–21.
43. De Backer D, Ospina-Tascon G, Salgado D, Favory R, Creteur J, Vincent JL. Monitoring the microcirculation in the critically ill patient: current methods and future approaches. Intensive Care Med. 2010;36(11):1813–25.
44. Vasdev S, Chauhan S, Choudhury M, Hote MP, Malik M, Kiran U. Arterial pressure waveform derived cardiac output FloTrac/Vigileo system (third generation software): comparison of two monitoring sites with the thermodilution cardiac output. J Clin Monit Comput. 2012;26:115–20.
45. Slagt C, Malagon I, Groeneveld AB. Systematic review of uncalibrated arterial pressure waveform analysis to determine cardiac output and stroke volume variation. Br J Anaesth. 2014;112(4):626–37.
46. Marqué S, Gros A, Chimot L, Gacouin A, Lavoué S, Camus C, Le Tulzo Y. Cardiac output monitoring in septic shock: evaluation of the third-generation Flotrac-Vigileo. J Clin Monit Comput. 2013;27(3):273–9.

47. Kusaka Y, Yoshitani K, Irie T, Inatomi Y, Shinzawa M, Ohnishi Y. Clinical comparison of an echocardiograph derived versus pulse counter derived cardiac output measurement in abdominal aortic aneurysm surgery. J Cardiothorac Vasc Anesth. 2012;26(2):223–6.
48. Perel A, Settels JJ. Totally non-invasive continuous cardiac output measurement with the Nexfin CO-Trek. Ann Update Intensive Care Emerg Med. 2011;1:434–42.
49. Sokolski M, Rydlewska A, Krakowiak B, Biegus J, Zymlinski R, Banasiak W, Jankowska EA, Ponikowski P. Comparison of invasive and non-invasive measurements of haemodynamic parameters in patients with advanced heart failure. J Cardiovasc Med (Hagerstown). 2011;12(11):773–8.
50. Ameloot K, Van De Vijver K, Broch O, Van Regenmortel N, De Laet I, Schoonheydt K, Dits H, Bein B, Malbrain ML. Nexfin noninvasive continuous hemodynamic monitoring: validation against continuous pulse contour and intermittent transpulmonary thermodilution derived cardiac output in critically ill patients. Sci World J. 2013;2013:519080.
51. Stover JF, Stocker R, Lenherr R, Neff TA, Cottini SR, Zoller B, Béchir M. Noninvasive cardiac output and blood pressure monitoring cannot replace an invasive monitoring system in clinically ill patients. BMC Anesthesiol. 2009;12(9):6.
52. American College of Obstetricians and Gynecologists. Invasive hemodynamic monitoring in obstetrics and gynecology: ACOG technical bulletin no. 175. Int J Gynaecol Obstet. 1993;42:199–205.
53. https://lbnmedical.com/ultrasound-transducer-types/. Accessed 12 Oct 2020.
54. https://www.anaesthesia.hku.hk/LearNet/measure.htm. Accessed 12 Oct 2020.
55. Marik PE. Techniques for assessment of intravascular volume in critically ill patients. J Intensive Care Med. 2009;24(5):329–37.
56. Gawlinski A. Measuring cardiac output: intermittent bolus thermodilution method. Crit Care Nurse. 2004;24:74–8.
57. Litton E, Morgan M. The PiCCO monitor: a review. Anaesth Intensive Care. 2012;40(3):393–409. https://doi.org/10.1177/0310057X1204000304.
58. http://www.lidco.com/archives/LiDCOplus_brochure_1914.pdf. Accessed 18 Oct 2020.
59. Kaçar CK, Uzundere O, Yektaş A. A two parameters for the evaluation of hypovolemia in patients with septic shock: Inferior

Vena Cava Collapsibility Index (IVCCI), delta cardiac output. Med Sci Monit. 2019;25:8105–11.
60. Yao B, Liu JY, Sun YB, Zhao YX, Li LD. The value of the inferior vena cava area distensibility index and its diameter ratio for predicting fluid responsiveness in mechanically ventilated patients. Shock. 2019;52(1):37–42.
61. Sangkum L, Liu GL, Yu L, Yan H, Kaye AD, Liu H. Minimally invasive or noninvasive cardiac output measurement: an update. J Anesth. 2016;30(3):461–80.
62. Rogge DE, Nicklas JY, Schön G, et al. Continuous noninvasive arterial pressure monitoring in obese patients during bariatric surgery: an evaluation of the vascular unloading technique (Clearsight system). Anesth Analg. 2019;128(3):477–83.
63. http://cheetah-medical.com/wp-content/uploads/2016/12/Starling-v5.2-Cheat-Sheet-Final.pdf. Accessed 23 Oct 2020.
64. Hariyanto H, Yahya CQ, Widiastuti M, Wibowo P, Tampubolon OE. Fluids and sepsis: changing the paradigm of fluid therapy: a case report. J Med Case Rep. 2017;11(1):30. Published 2017 Feb 4.
65. Wijdicks E, Freedman D, Findlay J, Sen A. Mayo clinic critical care and neurocritical care board review. Cardiovascular system in the critically ill patient. Chapter 4. Oxford University Press; 2019.
66. Safar ME, Lévy BI. Chapter 13: resistance vessels in hypertension. Comprehensive hypertension; 2007. p. 145–50.
67. Kostuk W, Barr JW, Simon AL, et al. Correlations between the chest film and hemodynamics in acute myocardial infarction. Circulation. 1973;48:624–32.
68. Ripoll Sanz JG, Jiramethee N, Diaz-Gomez JL. Cardiovascular system in the critically ill patient. In: Wijdicks E, Freedman D, Findlay J, Sen A, editors. Mayo Clinic critical care and neurocritical care board review. New York: Oxford University Press; 2019.
69. Lichtenstein DA. Lung ultrasound in the critically ill. Ann Intensive Care. 2014;4:1. https://doi.org/10.1186/2110-5820-4-1.
70. Saraogi A. Lung ultrasound: present and future. Lung India. 2015;32(3):250–7. https://doi.org/10.4103/0970-2113.156245.
71. Gargani L, Volpicelli G. How I do it: lung ultrasound. Cardiovasc Ultrasound. 2014;12:25.
72. Copetti R, Soldati G, Copetti P. Chest sonography: a useful tool to differentiate acute cardiogenic pulmonary edema from acute respiratory distress syndrome. Cardiovasc Ultrasound. 2008;6:16. Published 2008 Apr 29. https://doi.org/10.1186/1476-7120-6-16.

73. Keng LT, Lee CF. Ultrasound-guided transthoracic needle aspiration to diagnose invasive pulmonary aspergillosis. Am J Respir Crit Care Med. 2020;201(11):1451–2. https://doi.org/10.1164/rccm.202001-0008LE. PMID: 32078784; PMCID: PMC7258635.
74. Atkinson P, Milne J, Loubani O, Verheul G. The V-line: a sonographic aid for the confirmation of pleural fluid. Crit Ultrasound J. 2012;4(1):19. Published 2012 Aug 24. https://doi.org/10.1186/2036-7902-4-19.
75. Mojoli F, Bouhemad B, Mongodi S, Lichtenstein D. Lung Ultrasound for critically ill patients. Am J Respir Crit Care Med. 2019;199(6):701–14. https://doi.org/10.1164/rccm.201802-0236CI.

Endotracheal Intubation via Direct Laryngoscopy

Jonathan F. Ang and Blaine Michael Winterton

1 Introduction

Endotracheal Intubation (ETI) via direct laryngoscopy (DL) is an important, and often a lifesaving skill for critical care physicians. This chapter will discuss the indications, contraindications, medications, anatomy, preparation, laryngoscope, technique, and confirming proper placement needed for a critical care practitioner to safely conduct an ETI procedure.

2 Indications and Contraindications

Common indications for ETI in the intensive care setting include insufficient oxygenation or ventilation, acute respiratory failure, airway protection in a patient with depressed

---

J. F. Ang (✉)
Division of Pulmonary, Critical Care and Environmental Medicine, University of Missouri, Columbia, MO, USA
e-mail: angj@health.missouri.edu

B. M. Winterton
Department of Medicine, University of Missouri, Columbia, MO, USA
e-mail: bmwhkb@health.missouri.edu

© The Author(s), under exclusive license to Springer Nature Switzerland AG 2022
N. Arora (ed.), *Procedures and Protocols in the Neurocritical Care Unit*, https://doi.org/10.1007/978-3-030-90225-4_22

mental status, for short-term hyperventilation to manage increased intracranial pressure, or to manage copious secretions or bleeding from the airway [1, 2]. When the clinical picture is unclear on the need to intubate, the evaluation of three basic questions can assist the practitioner in determining patients that are requiring intubation versus those who can still be observed [3]. A confirmed answer to one of these three questions identifies the need for intubation in the critical care setting:

1. Is patency or protection of the airway at risk?
2. Is oxygenation or ventilation failing?
3. Is a need for intubation anticipated (what is the expected clinical course)?

Absolute contraindications include supraglottic or glottic pathology that inhibits the placement of an endotracheal tube (ETT) through the glottis or that can be exacerbated by placement of the ETT or maneuvering of the laryngoscope. Such pathology includes blunt trauma to the larynx and penetrating trauma of the upper airway such as hematoma or partial transection of the airway [4]. Furthermore, severe laryngeal or supralaryngeal edema as a consequence of bacterial infection, burns, or anaphylaxis may lead to the impossibility to visualize the laryngeal inlet during laryngoscopy [5].

Relative contraindications to ETI primarily revolve around the potential difficulties of conducting the procedure. These difficulties are often related to the skill set of the clinician, physiologic status of the patient, injuries of the patient, and unique anatomic features of the patient. Under these circumstances, consideration of non-invasive methods of airway support to avoid creating a life-threatening scenario of "cannot intubate-cannot ventilate".

3 Medications

Placement of an endotracheal tube can cause a physiologic stress response (eg, hypertension, tachycardia, cough). The goals of induction agents are to limit these physiological responses. Induction agents are used to achieve unconsciousness and apnea. Examples include propofol, ketamine, and etomidate. In many instances, a combination of these induction agents are used so that less of each individual agent is required. Adjunctive medications are used to supplement the effects of the primary anesthetic induction agent. The most common are opioids and midazolam [6]. Neuromuscular blocking agents are for Rapid Sequence Intubation to achieve optimal intubating conditions and to prevent further physiologic response reflexes (eg, coughing, gagging, straining, and vomiting) that can be seen with airway manipulation. Medications that are often used as neuromuscular blocking agents are succinylcholine and defasciculating agents such as rocuronium [6] (Table 1).

4 Choosing the Medications for ETI in a Neurocritical Patient

ETI can be performed in a neurologically injured patient either just by using sedative medications with or without any neuromuscular blockade. The choice of medication use depends on the intensivist preference and experience, hemodynamic condition of the patient, underlying injury which led to intubation and some underlying conditions which could lead to contraindication for certain medications. Use of propofol in a patient who is already hypotensive should be avoided. Use of neuromuscular blocking agents can be avoided if the patient is already comatose and adequate induction is achieved with other agents. Succinylcholine has very short onset and duration of action, however it is known to cause hyperkalemia, myalgias and rarely malignant hyperthermia. So its use should be avoided in patients with known muscular disorders, immobilised patients (due to stroke, paralysis or traumatic brain injury as there is upregulation of acetylcholine receptors which leads to more potassium efflux and higher chances of hyperkalemia) or genetic predisposition. Ketamine is very appealing for use in induction as it

TABLE 1 Common medications used for induction, suggested dose, advantages and adverse effects [7]

Drug/MOA	Suggested intravenous dose	Advantages	Potential adverse effects
Propofol (GABA agonist)	1–2.5 mg/kg Hypovolemia or hemodynamic compromise: <1 mg/kg	Rapid onset and offset Bronchodilation Anticonvulsant properties	Dose-dependent hypotension and respiratory depression.
Etomidate (GABA agonist)	0.15–0.3 mg/kg Profound hypotension: 0.1–0.15 mg/kg	Rapid onset and offset Hemodynamic stability with no changes in BP, HR, or CO Anticonvulsant properties	Involuntary myoclonic movements Absence of analgesic effects Can cause acute adrenocortical insufficiency
Ketamine (noncompetitive NMDA and glutamate receptor antagonist)	1–2 mg/kg Profound hypotension: 0.5–1 mg/kg	Rapid onset Increases BP, HR, and CO Profound analgesic properties Bronchodilation Preserves airway reflexes and respiratory drive	Increases ICP Increases myocardial oxygen demand Increases pulmonary arterial pressure Psychomimetic effects
Rocuronium (non-depolarising neuromuscular blocker)	0.60–1.00 mg/kg 1.20 mg/kg with RSI	No contraindications Easily reversible by Sugammadex	30–50 min to 25% recovery.

Succinylcholine (depolarising neuromuscular blocker)	0.60–1.50 mg/kg	5–10 min to 25% recovery time Fastest onset Most reliable for rapid tracheal intubation	Contraindicated in High K, muscular dystrophy, pseudocholinesterase deficiency. Myalgia, brady cardia
Fentanyl (Opioid analgesic)	0.5–1 mcg/kg Reduce dose in older adults and if hemodynamic instability	Suppresses airway reflexes during intubation Supplements sedation and reduces dose requirement of IV induction agent	Dose-dependent respiratory depression; possible apnea Pruritus Can cause "rigid chest" syndrome
Midazolam (GABA agonist)	0.5–2 mg Greater than 70 years old: 0.5 mg increments up to 2 mg	Reduces anxiety and produces amnesia Supplements sedation and reduces dose requirement of induction agent Anticonvulsant	Mild systemic vasodilation and decrease in CO Dose-dependent respiratory depression.
Lidocaine (Sodium channel blocker)	1.5 mg/kg	Blunts ICP rise by decreasing MAP and CPP	Use in elevated ICPs is controversial. Decreases seizure threshold Hypotension, potential ventricular tachyarrhythmias

ICP Intracranial Pressure, *MAP* Mean arterial pressure, *CPP* Cerebral perfusion pressure

does not cause hypotension or vasodilation. Ketamine when used alone can cause raised ICP due to increased cardiac contractility but with adequate sedation it can lead to improved cerebral perfusion pressure(CPP) despite elevated ICP. Etomidate is the most hemodynamically inert agent with no significant effect on ICP but preserving the CPP. Its use should be avoided in septic patients when there is a concern of adrenocortical insufficiency due to observation of increased mortality rate in such a population.

In our experience, a combination of fentanyl, midazolam and etomidate has been very effective in most patients with acute brain injuries.

5 Anatomy

The pharynx lies just posterior to the oral cavity and is a passageway for both food and respiratory gases. It extends from the base of the skull to the level of the cricoid cartilage anteriorly and the inferior border of the sixth cervical vertebra posteriorly. The widest level occurs at the hyoid bone (5 cm) vs the narrowest at the level of the esophagus (1.5 cm). Just caudal to the pharynx, the larynx lies opposite the third through sixth cervical vertebrae. This is the crossroads between the food and air passages and consists of cartilages forming the skeletal framework, ligaments, membranes, and muscles. The arytenoid cartilages (cuneiform and corniculate) make up the posterior aspect of the laryngeal inlet. These posterior cartilages are important landmarks as they are the first structures visualized as the epiglottis is lifted during laryngoscopy and possibly the only structure visualized in some patients. The true vocal cords originate below the epiglottic tubercle anteriorly and connect with the arytenoids posteriorly. The vocal cords cover the entrance to the trachea. An optimal laryngoscopic view will allow visualization of the entire length of both vocal cords [8] (See Fig. 1).

Assessment of anatomy can be done by various scoring mechanisms. The Modified Mallampati Test has been deter-

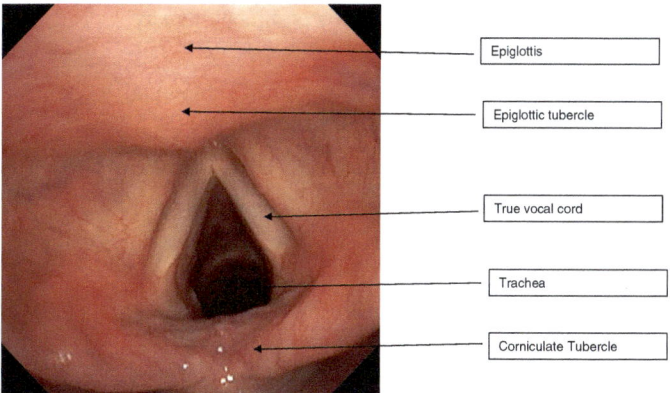

Figure 1 Laryngeal inlet anatomy

mined to have the highest sensitivity of predicting a difficult ETI [9]. The modified Mallampati classification is a simple scoring system that assesses how much the mouth can open to the size of the tongue, estimating the space available for an ETI. A class I is present when the soft palate, uvula, and pillars are visible; class II when the soft palate and the uvula are visible; class III when only the soft palate and base of the uvula are visible; and class IV when only the hard palate is visible [10].

6 Preparation

Proper and careful preparation is imperative for a successful intubation. Being prepared and having a "back-up" plan for when the airway proves to be difficult would increase the odds of a successful intubation.

1. Assess the patient's airway and anatomy, looking for signs of potential difficult airways (Table 2).
2. Preoxygenate the patient to increase oxygen reserve, which allows more time to secure the airway when intubating.

Table 2 Predictors of a difficult airway	History of difficult airway intubation
	Non-compliant sub-mental compliance
	Large neck circumference of >40 cm
	Mallampati Score class 3 or 4
	Thyromental distance <6 cm
	Interincisor gap <4 cm
	Sternomental distance <12 cm
	Head extension <30° from neutral position
	Inability to protrude mandible

3. Prepare and check laryngoscopes. Check that the light source is working.
4. Arrange all tools needed for intubation:
    (a) Laryngoscope, blades
    (b) Endotracheal tubes with different sizes, check for cuff leaks
    (c) Stylet
    (d) Lubricant
    (e) Oral or nasal airway
    (f) End-tidal carbon dioxide monitor or esophageal detector
5. Ensure there is a functioning intravenous access. Preferably two.
6. Attach monitors to the patient: blood pressure, pulse oximetry, cardiac monitoring.
7. Ensure there is a working suction device and bag-valve mask that is connected to oxygen supply.
8. Prepare all medications needed prior to beginning the process of endotracheal intubation.

9. It is imperative to have a backup or alternative approach to secure the airway (i.e. laryngeal mask airway, bougie, cricothyrotomy) and have a secondary plan in case intubation proves difficult.
10. Ensure that the patient has no dentures or loose teeth.

7 Technique

1. Position the patient (sniffing position: head hyperextended, atlanto-occipital extension with head elevation 3 to 7 cm) and induce anesthesia ± neuromuscular blockade.
2. Perform manual ventilation with bag mask ventilation and oropharyngeal airway.
3. Hold the laryngoscope with the left hand.
4. Insert the blade along the right side of the tongue then sweep the tongue towards the left.
5. Advance the tip of the blade in the midline till the laryngeal inlet is visualized

    (a) If using a curved blade, the tip of the blade is positioned above the epiglottis. Fitting into the vallecula to lift the epiglottis indirectly.
    (b) If using a straight blade, the tip of the blade goes below the epiglottis and then lifts directly to visualize the vocal cords.

6. External laryngeal manipulation or bimanual laryngoscopy – during insertion of the blade, the right hand of the laryngoscopist uses the thumb and forefinger to exert pressure externally on the thyroid cartilage, allowing for a better view of the glottis. An assistant then places their finger in the same spot on the thyroid cartilage and the laryngoscopist can proceed with the intubation [11].
7. Pull upward and along the line of the handle to the laryngoscope taking care not to pivot and exert pressure on the teeth.

8. Lift the epiglottis upward to visualize the cords.
9. Inserted pre-lubricated ETT through the vocal cords, stop advancing when the cuff is about 2–3 cm beyond the vocal cords.
10. Remove the stylet, inflate the ETT cuff, and then connect to the bag valve system to ventilate the patient.
11. Confirm placement using End tidal CO2 monitor or esophageal detector and listening to bilateral breath sounds.

8 Confirming Proper Placement of Endotracheal Tube

1. End-tidal carbon dioxide determination using quantitative capnography or colorimetric is an accurate means of confirming ETT in the trachea in a non-cardiac arrest patient. At least five exhalations with a consistent CO2 level before one can assume the ETT is in the trachea [12–14].
2. Clinical findings like bilateral breath sounds on auscultation, misting or fogging of the ETT may help support the likelihood that the ETT is in the trachea. Clinical findings alone should not be used to confirm placement.
3. Esophageal detector device – suction is applied using a syringe or bulb, if ETT is in the airway, air should flow freely. If the ETT is in the collapsible esophagus, there would be little to no airflow. Air flow is evidenced by expansion of suction bulb or aspiration of air in the syringe [14].
4. Chest radiograph – a single view AP chest radiograph determines depth of the ETT, but cannot reliably exclude esophageal intubation.
5. Bronchoscopy – direct visualization with a bronchoscope to visualize tracheal rings is the gold standard to confirm placement of an ETT.

9 Protocol for ETI (Fig. 2)

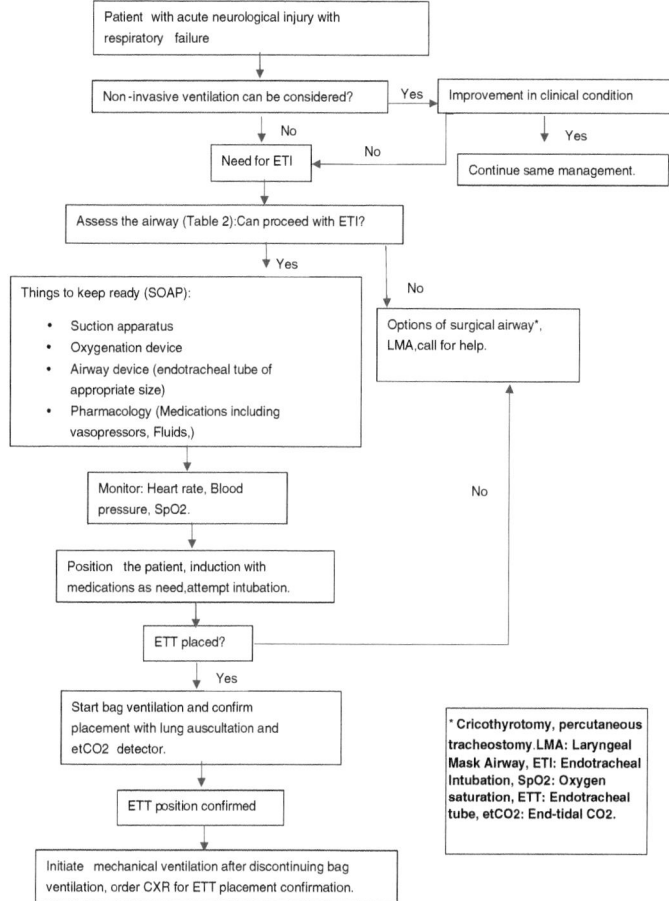

FIGURE 2 Endotracheal intubation protocol

References

1. Ezri TW. Indications for tracheal intubation. In: Hagberg CA, editor. Benumof's airway management: principles and practice. 2nd ed. Philadelphia: Mosby; 2007. p. 371.
2. Eisenkraft JB, et al. Anesthesia for thoracic surgery. In: Clinical anesthesia. 4th ed. Philadelphia: Lippincott Williams and Wilkins; 2001.
3. Brown CA 3rd, et al. The decision to intubate. In: The walls manual of emergency airway management. 5th ed. Philadelphia: Lippincott Williams & Wilkins; 2018. p. 3.
4. Kendall JL, Anglin D, Demetriades D. Penetrating neck trauma. Emerg Med Clin N Am. 1998;16(1):85. Berkow L, Hagberg CA, Crowley M. 2020.
5. Verghese ST, Hannallah RS. Pediatric otolaryngologic emergencies. Anesthesiol Clin North Am. 2001;19(2):237–56.
6. Berkow L, Hagberg CA, Crowley M. Rapid sequence induction and intubation for anesthesia. 7 Sept 2020. Retrieved from UpToDate: uptodate.com/rapid-sequence-induction-and-intubation-rsii-for-anesthesia.
7. King A. Genral anesthesia: intravenous induction agents. 7 Sept 2020. Retrieved from UpToDate: uptodate.com/contents/general-anesthesia-intravenous-induction-agents.
8. Hagber CA, Artime CA, Aziz MF. Hagberg and Benumof's airway management. Philadelphia: Elsevier Inc.; 2018.
9. Khatiwada S, et al. Prediction of difficult airway among patients requiring endotracheal intubation in a tertiary care hospital in Eastern Nepal. JNMA J Nepal Med Assoc. 2017;56(207):314–8.
10. Samsoon GL, Young JR. Difficult tracheal intubation: a retrospective study. Anaesthesia. 1987;42:487.
11. Levitam RM, Mickler T, Hollander JE. Bimanual laryngoscopy: a videographic study of external manipulation by novice intubators. Ann Emerg Med. 2002;40(1):30.
12. Grmec S. Comparison of three different methods to confirm tracheal tube placement in emergency situation. Intensive Care Med. 2002;28(6):701.
13. MacLeod BA, Heller MB, Gerard K, Yealy DM, Menegazzi JJ. Verification of endotracheal tube placement with colotimetric end-tidal CO_2 detection. Ann Emerg Med. 1991;20(3):267.
14. Bozeman WP, Hexter D, Liang HK, Kelen GD. Esophageal detector device versus detection of end-tidal carbon dioxide level in emergency intubation. Ann Emerg Med. 1996;27:595–9.

Vasospasm

Chandra Shekar Pingili and Niraj Arora

1 Introduction

1.1 Incidence and Pathophysiology

Intracranial vasospasm is a highly debated clinical entity. Vasospasm is not always deleterious on the brain. Iatrogenic vasospasm is created by permissive hypocapnia as a transient measure to decrease intracranial Pressure [1–3]. The exact mechanism of vasospasm is yet to be understood. Intracranial bleed with its chemical cascade is speculated to be the reason behind vasospasm leading to delayed cerebral ischemia and anoxic neuropathy. Oxyhaemoglobin, arachidonic acid metabolites, endothelin damage, Nitric oxide scavenging pathway, free radical damage, and perivascular nerve damage are all the postulated mechanisms behind the vasospasm [4]. The incidence of vasospasm varies from 30% to 60% depend-

C. S. Pingili (✉)
Department of Neurocritical Care, University of Missouri, Columbia, MO, USA
e-mail: cpygd@health.missouri.edu

N. Arora
Department of Neurology- Neurocriticalcare unit, University of Missouri, Columbia, MO, USA

ing on the nature of the bleed, the extent of the bleed, and in the case of aSAH, the MFS [5]. Vasospasm is equally seen in aSAH and non-aneurysmal bleeds. In 15% of the cases of SAH, the exact source of bleed is unknown despite CTA and Repeat DSA [6]. However non aSAH carries an overall better prognosis compared to the aneurysmal SAH. MFS was designed to predict the incidence of vasospasm in aneurysmal SAH [7, 8].

Based on Table 1, it is evident that the severity of the bleed and the extent of bleed decides the risk of vasospasm and DCI. Nonaneurysmal PSAH (NPSAH) has a better acute prognosis compared to the aSAH in terms of rebleeding, risk of hydrocephalus, and no decrease in the quality of life. However, the overall prognosis is the same otherwise [10]. Post-traumatic vasospasm was seen in patients with TBI even without brain bleed [5]. Patients with lower Glasgow Coma Scores (GCS) at admission were more likely to develop hemodynamically significant vasospasm, regardless of the presence of traumatic SAH [5]. Only a portion of aSAH patients with radiological vasospasm develop symptomatic vasospasm; 30–70% of aSAH patients show radiological vasospasm on angiography on day 7 post ictus while only

TABLE 1 Showing mFS, risk of DCI from vasospasm and CT scan findings [9]

Modified fisher score (mFS)	Risk of DCI from vasospasm	CT scan findings
0	0	No bleed
1	24%	Minimal/thin SAH/no IVH
2	33%	Minimal/thin SAH/bilateral IVH
3	33%	Dense SAH/no IVH
4	40%	Dense SAH/bilateral IVH

DCI delayed cerebral ischemia, *SAH* subarachnoid hemorrhage, *IVH* intraventricular hemorrhage

20–30% of aSAH patients develop symptomatic vasospasm, and anatomic vasospasm occurs frequently without any signs of ischemia. aSAH vasospasm usually starts after day 4 and can occur at any time until the end of the first 3 weeks. TBI patients tend to develop vasospasm as early as the second day and generally do not last beyond the first 2 weeks. Post-traumatic vasospasm in the absence of tSAH, generally, has an even briefer duration [8]. The incidence of TCD diagnosed vasospasm, angiography-diagnosed vasospasm and the development of clinical vasospasm among those with radiographic vasospasm are significantly higher in a SAH group of patients compared to the tSAH group [11].

Following TBI, the incidence of radiographic vasospasm as measured by TCD and DSA is reported to range between 19–68% and 18.6–41%, respectively. In comparison, the incidence of aSAH-induced vasospasm was noted by TCD to be approximately 38–45% and by DSA to be 43.2%, on average. **Younger age, lower admission GCS, and quantity of cisternal or intracerebral hemorrhage are the risk factors for vasospasm.** Clinical manifestations of DCI are usually that of end-organ damage from anoxic neuropathy [8, 12, 13].

1.2 Diagnostic Modalities

Cerebral vasospasm is a reversible narrowing of the cerebral blood vessels, generally involving the proximal arteries that form the Circle of Willis. Clinical vasospasm is the narrowing of the cerebral artery causing cerebral ischemia with neurological symptoms. Angiographic vasospasm is the narrowing of arteries seen on vascular imaging. DSA has 100% sensitivity and specificity, CTA has a sensitivity of 80% and specificity of 93%. The former is invasive and both risk contrast exposure and are expensive [14].

1. **Transcranial Doppler (TCD)**
   TCD is a cheaper, non-invasive, and bedside procedure with no risk for contrast or radiation exposure. Also, this can be repeated at any time of the day if needed. TCD has

Table 2 TCD sensitivity and specificity [15]

Vessel insonated	Sensitivity (%)	Specificity (%)
MCA	67	99
ACA	42	76
PCA	48	69
Basilar artery	76.9	77
Vertebral artery	43.8	88

MCA Middle Cerebral Artery, *ACA* Anterior Cerebral Artery, *PCA* Posterior Cerebral Artery

Table 3 MCA vasospasm degree [15]

Degree of spasm	Mean flow velocity (cm/s)	Lindegaard ratio
Mild	120–149	3–6
Moderate	150–199	3–6
Severe	>200	>6

a positive predictive value (PPV) of 97%, negative predictive value (NPV) of 78% [15]. Table 2 details the diagnostic usefulness of the TCD based on the vessel insonated. Here we use a 2 Hz probe to delve into the deeper vessels. Table 3 on the other hand details the mean velocities recorded and the risk of vasospasm based on TCD. TCD numbers, combined with the clinical exam will guide the intensivist about the evolution of the vasospasm, prompting them to start medical and or interventional strategies to bring down the spasm.

Based on radiological images, vasospasm is classified depending on the vessel diameter. Severe vasospasm if the reduction in vessel caliber is >50%, moderate if it is between 25–50% and mild if the reduction is <25% [15]. Vasospasm increases the resistance to the blood flow. Mild vasospasm does not affect the blood flow. If the systolic blood pressure (SBP) is maintained above the lower limit of autoregulation, then moderate vasospasm will not have any deleterious consequences. In these two situations, a constant flow is achieved, and the cerebral blood flow velocity (CBFV) will increase with decreasing diameter and the angiographic spasm can be captured on the TCD. Severe spasm on the other hand is beyond the autoregulatory mechanism. A TCD flow velocity below 120 cm/s is normal and spasm is moderate to severe if the velocity is above 200 cm/s in the MCA if the patient is not hyperemic and symptomatic. Iatrogenic SBP augmentation is common in the SAH group of patients and this will increase the flow velocities above 200 cm/second [16]. This should not count as a spastic vessel in the absence of symptoms. TCD should be done daily in the intensive care unit since it is good at predicting the vasospasm [4]. 15% of patients will not have a good temporal window bringing down the usefulness of a bedside TCD. TCD has a better diagnostic yield in the anterior vs posterior circulation and proximal vs distal circulation.

The extracranial component of the internal carotid artery (eICA) is not influenced by the intracranial spasm and the change in velocity has a linear relation to the flow. A ratio of the MCA and ipsilateral e ICA velocities is called the Lindegaard index (LI) and the normal value is 1.7 +/− 4. A day to day trend is a more reliable marker of vasospasm. Values more than 3 suggest a significant spasm and more than 6 is called a severe spasm. Sviri ratio is the basilar artery counterpart of the LI

TABLE 4 Basilar artery vasospasm degree [5, 17]

MFV (cm/s)	BA/vertebral MFV (Sviri ratio)	Inference
>70	>2	Mild vasospasm
>85	>2.5	Moderate to severe spasm
>85	>3	Severe spasm

MFV mean flow velocity, *BA* basilar artery

(Table 4). It is calculated by the ratio of basilar artery mean flow velocity divided by an average of the time-averaged maximum MFV of both the extracranial vertebral arteries.

2. **CT Angiography (CTA)**

    CTA is a relatively cheap and rapid test that can help us in diagnosing the vasospasm. The latest multidetector CTA is fast, uses lesser contrast load, and helps us with 3-dimensional images. The sensitivity and specificity of the CTA is around 80% and 93% respectively. However CTA images are influenced by operator dexterity, beam hardening artifacts like clips and coils, and the time-lapse between contrast infusion and image acquisition. The major limiting factor with the CTA is that it is very sensitive for the proximal vessels only compared to the middle and distal vessels unless there is severe vasospasm. In the latter case, CTA is shown to be as efficacious as the DSA in diagnosing vasospasm. The real application of CT perfusion in the prediction of DCI is still debated and needs further studies [18]. A negative CTA in a patient with high suspicion of vasospasm should prompt further investigation [14, 19].

3. **Time of Flight-MR Angiography (TOF-MRA)**

    TOF-MRA is time of flight Magnetic resonance angiography. This is a noninvasive test and does not involve any contrast boluses. The technique is just an exploitation of the excitation tendency of the flowing blood with resultant signal transmission and high-resolution image capturing. However, this test is 100% sensitive only in the ACA and less than 50% sensitive in the MCA and ICA. MRA is also influenced by the presence of artifacts and signal dissipation is often seen in sites of turbulent flow. Here vasospasm is overestimated. MRA is inferior to the DSA. Since the imaging is T1 dependent, a black-blood MRA (technique that suppress signal from flowing blood while maintaining high signal in the surrounding stationary tissues, thus rendering the vessels black) is suggested to be superior to the TOF-MRA in evaluating the vasospasm [14, 20, 21].

4. **Positron Emission Tomography Scan (PET Scan)**

    PET-scan images offer multipurpose information. These images not only provide us with the diagnosis of vasospasm but also furnish the functional complications of spasm like decreased perfusion, decreased oxygen delivery, tissue metabolism rate, oxygen extraction, mean transit time and cerebral blood volume, etc. However, the overall process is too intricate to apply this modality on a day-to-day basis [14, 22–25].

5. **Digital Subtraction Angiography (DSA)**

    DSA is the gold standard in the diagnosis of vasospasm and also offers room for therapeutic intervention with either balloon angioplasty or intra-arterial vasodilators as detailed below. DSA will also help with quantifying the transit time and the interval between different phases of the circulation. 3-Dimensional (3D) angiography is achieved by reconstruction of the vessel images and this generally offers better information and visualization. However, the 3-DSA is less specific and sensitive compared to the convention DSA because of the pseudo spastic vessel segments. 3-dimensional DSA involves computational reconstruction and processing. In this process, the Clinically relevant information is lost at the expense of achieving a cosmetically appealing image and this is responsible for the diminished clinical returns on the 3-DSA.

    Angioplasty of course carries the risk of thromboembolic complications and recurrence of vasospasm [26, 27]. There is a risk of vessel dissection, brain tissue staining with subsequent non-hemorrhagic ischemia, bleeding from the puncture site with a risk of retroperitoneal bleeds, distal embolism with limb ischemia −0.5% to 2%. The risk of allergic reactions from contrast is around 2% and also contrast carries the risk of nephrotoxicity. The procedure needs an experienced interventionist and there is the risk of radiation exposure too. DSA doesn't offer any insight into cerebral perfusion and ischemia [14, 24, 28].

6. **Single-photon emission computed tomography (SPECT)** **SPECT** is a nuclear study that uses Technetium-99 ions uptake by the tissues after an infusion. The uptake is impaired in patients with vasospasm. The sensitivity and specificity of this study are 89% and 75%. However, this is a nuclear technique that needs Tc-99 to be coupled with a lipophilic substance. The low-resolution imaging with the granular appearance and high acquisition times is another limitation [29, 30]. Also, the abnormal images are compared to the normal part of the brain tissue. In patients with diffuse vasospasm or otherwise with a generalized pathology this study is difficult to consider [14, 24, 31–33].
7. **Xenon (Xe)-133 clearance** is another nuclear imaging modality as above except that inhaled or intravenous Xe-133 is used instead. Despite being a low-cost imaging technique with a lower dose of radiation, the overall image quality is poor, practically making this test not useful [14, 34].
8. **Xenon enhanced computed tomography** is a kind of CTA, where the patient is made to inhale 72% oxygen and 28% xenon and CT images are captured. The poor quality images seen on the routine Xe-133 scans are now overcome with this technique. Along with the anatomical details, this study also helps in estimating the blood flow. The risk of radiation exposure is high here and also there is a risk of elevated ICP [29, 35–38].
9. **Dynamic CT perfusion scan** is now a routine imaging modality in any patient with suspected CVA. This is a functional study that helps us to compute CBV, CBF, MTT, and Tmax. This is a rapid test with a sensitivity and specificity of 74% and 93% respectively. However, the patient is exposed to high doses of iodinated contrast, posterior cerebral artery (PCA) is not imaged on this scan. Patients with marked cardiovascular disease burden and disrupted blood-brain barrier doesn't qualify for this test. All perfusion scans only produce relative flow charts and not absolute flow charts [29, 39–44].

10. **Diffusion-weighted and perfusion-weighted imaging (DWI/PWI)** images the entire brain tissue compared to the CT perfusion studies. Vasospasm causes distal ischemia with subsequent tissue edema. This is seen as a hyperintense lesion on the DWI scan. PWI on the other hand exploits the dynamic susceptibility contrast imaging technique. Gadolinium is the contrast used here compared to the CT study. PWI allows for infusion of the gadolinium followed by measurement of the concentration changes related to the first- pass bolus. The T-2 relaxation changes will be proportional to the degree of perfusion. The sensitivity of this test is as high as 100% at times. However, the study is fraught with limitations like cost, equipment availability, time, metal and meth hemoglobin artifacts [45–48]
11. **Electroencephalogram (EEG):**
Electroencephalography (EEG) can provide a real time, continuous recording with prediction of responses to ischemia. EEG might be representing an early asymptomatic response to ischemia before it clinically manifests. Role of cortical spreading depolarizations (CSD) has been proposed. This is seen on EEG as transient electrographic suppressions associated with local transient brain tissue hypoxia. When the depolarizations happen in clusters and repeat itself, it results in infarction in the setting of hypotension and vasospasm. Some of the small studies proposed the criteria to predict DCI based on decreasing alpha-to-delta power ratio (ADR) or relative alpha power variability (RAV). Epileptiform discharges, rhythmic and periodic ictal–interictal continuum patterns and isolated alpha suppression can all be seen during ischemia. A recent prospective study performed in patients with clinical suspicion of vasospasm who had cEEG done shows that it can accurately predict DCI following SAH. The measures like ADR, RAV, focal slowing, epileptiform discharges or rhythmic or periodic patterns have excellent sensitivity and high specificity. Across baseline risk levels. The number of

patients needed to monitor to predict one additional case of DCI prior to clinical symptoms was between 3 and 7.

2 Prevention of Vasospasm

As a treating intensivist, one is intrigued with the idea of preventing clinical deterioration in a aSAH patient. The temporal course of the vasospasm and its high incidence makes the prevention an attractive strategy. However, in spite of best medical management in terms of prevention, patients might require a myriad of therapies and the prevention of the vasospasm could be difficult.

Prevention of worsening vasospasm can be done with blood pressure augmentation with fluids or intravenous pressors, maintaining euvolemia, avoiding anemia with blood transfusion with target hemoglobin more than 7. Several drugs and strategies have been tried in preventing vasospasm.

1. **Calcium Channel Blockers:** This has more neuroprotective effects than preventing vasospasm. The beneficial effect is hypothesized due to (a) effect on blood rheology by increasing red blood cell deformability, (b) anti-platelet aggregating effect, (c) dilation of collateral leptomeningeal arteries, (d) prevention of calcium entry into ischemic cells which cause cerebral infarction. Several agents are available which are discussed below:

    - **Nimodipine:** It is a calcium-channel blocker (CCB) with preferential central nervous system (CNS) penetration. Blocks dihydropyridine-sensitive L-type calcium channels. Use of nimodipine is a mandated practice in the prevention of aSAH induced vasospasm. This is based on British aneurysm nimodipine trial (BRANT) in 1989 which showed that patients receiving nimodipine had clinically & statistically significant reduction in poor outcome (NNT 8), mainly

driven by a reduction in cerebral infarct (NNT 12). Nimodipine does not alter radiographic vasospasm and has no significant difference in mortality. This is a lipophilic calcium channel blocker that causes vasodilation [49]. Usual dosing is 60 mg orally or via naso-gastric tube every 4 h given within 96 h of symptoms of SAH for 21 day or until the patient is discharged home in good neurological condition, whichever comes first. If a patient gets hypotensive with this regimen, the dose is reduced to 30 mg every 2 h.
- **Nicardipine:** It is shown in a randomized trial that continuous intravenous infusion of high-dose nicardipine (0.15 mg/kg/h) significantly decreases the incidence of symptomatic, angiographic and TCD vasospasm. However, no difference in overall outcome was found and the efficacy has been limited by side effects including prolonged hypotension, pulmonary edema and renal dysfunction, A subsequent randomized trial showed that low-dose nicardipine (0.075 mg/kg/h) treatment is associated with a virtually equivalent benefit in terms of vasospasm prevention but with fewer side effects [68].
- **Nifedipine, diltiazem, verapamil:** These CCBs are less widely used for vasospasm after SAH in the U.S. since the approval of nimodipine [50]. Diltiazem was found to be safe but it has no effect on vasospasm. In a series of 123 SAH patients treated with oral diltiazem instead of nimodipine, 19.5% incidence of delayed ischemic neurological deficit (DID) was noted while favorable outcome with Glasgow Outcome Scale of 4 or 5 was achieved in 75% of patients.

2. **Fasudil:** It is a protein kinase inhibitor but is not available in the United States. In a randomized trial comparing fasudil with nimodipine, no serious adverse events in the fasudil group were reported and the drug was found to be safe and efficient agent for suppressing cerebral vaso-

spasm after subarachnoid hemorrhage surgery for ruptured cerebral aneurysm.
3. **Dantrolene:** Dantrolene is a skeletal muscle relaxant used in the management of malignant hyperthermia, Neuroleptic malignant syndrome and skeletal muscle spasm. This drug works by decreasing the release of calcium ion from the sarcoplasmic reticulum. While the drug is not tested for use in the management of vasospasm like nimodipine, it's often used as an intra arterial bolus when vasospasm is seen during DSA. CNS depression and liver failure are the major side effects of this drug when used in doses above 800 mg per day.
4. **Papaverine** is a potent arterial dilator. However its use as an intra arterial agent in the DSA is now abandoned because of the cardiac and CNS side effects. Also, despite an improvement in the vasospasm with this drug, there's no overall improvement in the neurological outcome.
5. **Estrogens and Erythropoietin** are two humoral agents with proven vasodilatory effects. They both work through the Nitric Oxide mechanism. However to date there are no large trials to support their overall benefit on mortality or morbidity.
6. **Statins** are proven endothelial protective drugs. However they have no role in the prevention of vasospasm [61].
7. **Nitric Oxide (NO)** is a potent vasodilator. It's a proven fact that there is decreased endogenous Nitric oxide in patients with SAH. However to date there are no large randomized controlled studies to support external supplementation of the NO in the management of vasospasm. In Fact some case reports suggest poor outcomes from NO supplementation because of peripheral hypotension from NO, indirectly worsening the spasm.
8. **Cilostazol** is a phosphodiesterase 3 inhibitor. This drug given orally has proven beneficial in the management of vasospasm.

9. **Clazosentan** is an endothelin −1 receptor antagonist. This drug efficiently reverses vasospasm at 3–24 h after administration but there's no overall benefit on the neurological outcomes.
10. **Heparin** is a potent anti inflammatory drug. Several small studies have shown heparin to be effectively counteract the vasospasm in SAH. However there are no large scale studies todate and the drug inherently carries a risk of bleeding in patients already admitted with SAH.
11. **Lumbar drainage of CSF**: Considering blood as an irritant product causing vasospasm, use of lumbar drainage of CSFafter aSAH reduced the prevalence of DID and improved early clinical outcome but failed to improve outcome at 6 months (LUMAS trial).
12. **Intracisternal thrombolysis** (tissue plasminogen activator or urokinase) is still to be validated in large randomized clinical trials however, based on a meta-analysis, the beneficial effect was noted to be clinically and statistically significant.
13. **Cisternal irrigation with tissue plasminogen activator combined with continuous postoperative cisternal drainage** was associated with a low incidence of vasospasm
14. Prophylactic transluminal balloon angioplasty: This has shown no benefit in vasospasm prevention but increased deaths (4%) from vessel rupture which is at higher incidence than the 1.1% reported in the literature.

3   Treatment of Vasospasm (Table 5)

It is pivotal to initiate the treatment of vasospasm sooner rather than later. The threshold to initiate treatment with different interventions has a significant variability. Institutional policies also vary widely and there is no one standard approach to the treatment. If vasospasm is manifesting as a clinical event, prompt action should be taken to treat the symptoms. Sonographic evidence of vasospasm or radiographic evidence of vasospasm needs definite confirmation

TABLE 5 Treatment strategies for vasospasm (medical and interventional) [49–64]

1. Pharmacological

  A. Arterial dilation: CCB
  B. Dantrolene
  C. Fasudil
  D. Magnesium
  E. Statins
  F. Hormones (EPO, estrogen)
  G. Phosphodiesterase inhibitors (Milrinone, papaverine, cilostazol)
  H. Endothelin receptor antagonists (ET_A (clazosentan) and $ET_{A/B}$
  I. Nitric oxide
  J. Heparin
  K. Fibrinolysis

2. Endovascular therapy

  A. Intra-arterial vasodilators as in above
  B. Balloon Angioplasty
  C. Cisternal drainage along with thrombolytics
  D. Combination of A, B, C

with more invasive testing like cerebral angiogram. Any evidence of vasospasm needs vigilance and administration of therapies to prevent DID. The goal of treatment is to improve CBF, prevent DID and have a favourable outcome.

4 Pharmacological Treatment

Intravenous Milrinone infusion (Montreal protocol) is also used for the treatment of vasospasm [54–56]. Milrinone is a phosphodiesterase II inhibitor that selectively inhibits cyclic adenosine monophosphate (cAMP) with an inotropic and vasodilatory effect with a very high affinity for the intracranial vessel receptors compared to the cardiac and peripheral receptors. Cardiac arrhythmias and hypotension are the major side effects of this drug. Milrinone is usually bloused as 0.1–

0.2 mg/kg followed by an infusion at 0.75 mcg/kg/min. The maximum dose on the infusion is 1.25 mcg/kg/min. This drug is renally dosed. The usual recommendation is to keep the MAP >90 mmHg.

For resistant cases of vasospasm, the patient is taken for DSA and repeat DSA if necessary, with intraarterial diltiazem, Milrinone, and Baclofen infusions based on the practitioner's preferences [54, 57–60]. The role of nicardipine and verapamil as oral agents is highly debated with confounding results to date. IV magnesium is used in the management of migraine attacks but has no role in the treatment of SAH vasospasm. Statins also have no role in the management of the vasospasm [61].

Fasudil is a Rho-kinase inhibitor. This is approved for the treatment of vasospasm and DCI in china but not in the United States [62, 63]. Intraarterial papaverine is not used anymore because of its significant neurotoxicity [64]. Cilostazol, an antiplatelet drug has shown to reduce vasospasm and decrease morbidity but not mortality. This however needs further studies [65]. The role of endothelin −1 antagonist clazosentan, heparin are all still debated and need further studies [66, 67].

5 Endovascular Therapy

Pharmacological management is usually the first step in management of vasospasm. However, when the medical therapy fails or the patient develops side effects related to treatment, endovascular therapy is the preferred option available. The options of therapy are mentioned in the table.

A. **Intra-arterial (IA) vasodilators (**Table 6**):** Various agents have been used for vasodilation. The advantage of the IA administration is more distal penetration, better safety with less side effects. Main disadvantage is the need for multiple arterial punctures in cases of recurrent vasospasm, The drugs can be injected in larger or moderate

TABLE 6 Intra arterial vasodilators during DSA [58–60]

Drug	Intra-arterial dose[a]	Comments
Verapamil (CCB)	5–10 mg injected over 2 min	Watch for hypotension, not selective to cerebral vasculature
Nicardipine (CCB)	10–40 mg	Watch for hypotension
Nimodipine (CCB)	5 mg per artery	Not commonly used
Milrinone (PDEi)	5–10 mg per artery	Monitor hypotension, hypokalemia, tachycardia.
Fasudil (Rho kinase inhibitor)	15–45 mg per artery	Not available in the U.S. Good outcome in small studies. Does not lower blood pressure.
Papaverine (Opioid alkaloid)	200–300 mg over 30 min	Paradoxical vasospasm, thrombocytopenia, raised ICP. Now abandoned and not in use.

[a]Doses of medications are based on case-studies

size arteries. Hypotension and raised ICP are potential side effects to be considered.

B. Transluminal Balloon Angioplasty (TBA)

This specialized procedure is effective treatment in case of vasospasm of proximal vessels (more than 2–3 mm diameter) like supraclinoid internal carotid artery, M1 and M2 segments of MCA, A1 segment of ACA, P1 segment of PCA and the basilar artery. TBA causes structural and functional changes in the vessel. There is stretching and disruption of both the degenerative muscle and the proliferative non-muscle components, mainly in the media of the vasospastic arteries. It carries the risk of arterial rupture, embolism, reperfusion injury, occlusion, displacement of aneurysm clip, arterial dissection. Clinical improvement has been noted in about 60–80% cases. This modality should be performed earlier in refractory vasospasm. Best results are obtained if the procedure is performed within 2 h of clinical symptom onset.

C. **Cisternal Drainage along with thrombolytics**

This can be performed at the time of surgery (Clipping) or through cisternal catheters. It has shown to reduce the incidence of vasospasm.

6 Protocol for Vasospasm Management

Figure 1 shows a simplified flowchart for the management of aSAH. Even though the therapy is tailored according to the individual patient requirements, the flowchart could serve as a practical guide for the treating physicians.

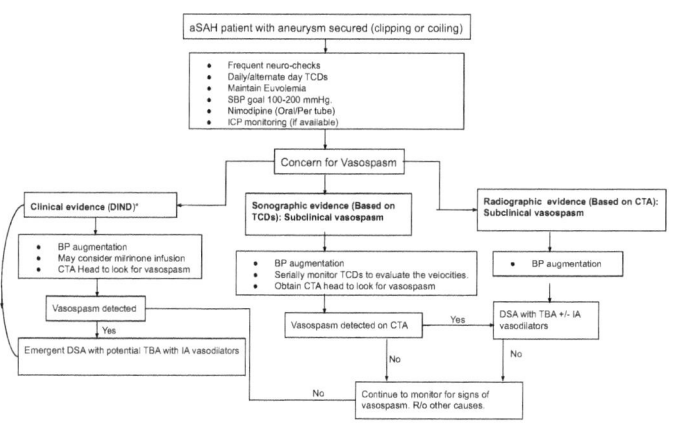

FIGURE 1 Management Protocol for Vasospasm in aSAH

7 Future Directions

The chapter cannot be completed without discussion of the future research and newer developments. The challenges of deciphering the best therapy for prevention and treatment of vasospasm still exist in spite of multiple drugs tried in the past. However, because of constant research in this area there are some novel approaches which might be helpful for the vasospasm.

Haptoglobin is one such protein which has been found to be useful. Hemoglobin disrupts the NO signalling and by its ability to bind to hemoglobin, NO action can function normally to cause vasodilation. Injecting haptoglobin in the CSF of a SAH patient could possibly prevent vasospasm. In animal studies, the results were promising and this would need further clinical trials to validate in humans.

The use of multilevel modality monitoring consisting of PbtO2 monitor, cerebral microdialysis (CMD), and/or EEG each of which provides information on a different aspect of brain physiology might lead to precise diagnosis and treatment. There is some evidence of its use in vasospasm when ICP and CPP monitoring is not helpful. However, since it is an invasive technique it has its own limitations of use and more information based on clinical trials is required before its widespread applicability in clinical practice.

There is a potential role of identifying biomarkers in CSF for detection of vasospasm. Various biomarkers including micro-RNA (mRNA), fibrin degradation product, soluble receptor, and calcium binding protein have been studied. Among those, sphingosine-1-phosphate receptor 4 (S1PR4) mRNA level was found to be elevated in patients developing vasospasm following SAH. Another study identified miR3117-3p as a potential biomarker for in SAH patients with the risk of vasospasm. Certain proteins like D-dimer in CSF and soluble receptor for advanced glycation end products (RAGE) in blood were also elevated in patients who developed cerebral vasospasm. Nevertheless, the role of biomarkers still needs to be validated in larger clinical trials.

References

1. Chapter 142: Hypocarbia and hypercarbia. https://accessanesthesiology.mhmedical.com/content.aspx?bookid=974&sectionid=61590019.
2. Hassler W, Chioffi F. CO_2 reactivity of cerebral vasospasm after aneurysmal subarachnoid haemorrhage. Acta Neurochir. 1989;98(3–4):167–75. https://doi.org/10.1007/BF01407344.
3. Zhou Q, et al. Effects of permissive hypercapnia on transient global cerebral ischemia–reperfusion injury in rats. Anesthesiology. 2010;112(2):288–97. https://doi.org/10.1097/ALN.0b013e3181ca8257.
4. Psychogios K, Tsivgoulis G. Subarachnoid hemorrhage, vasospasm, and delayed cerebral ischemia prevention, effective monitoring, and early detection are the keys to successful management after subarachnoid hemorrhage. Pract Neurol. 2019 Practical Neurology.
5. Nassar HGE, Ghali AA, Bahnasy WS, Elawady MM. Vasospasm following aneurysmal subarachnoid hemorrhage: prediction, detection, and intervention. Egypt J Neurol Psychiatry Neurosurg. 2019;55(1):3. https://doi.org/10.1186/s41983-018-0050-y.
6. Xu L, et al. Management of spontaneous subarachnoid hemorrhage patients with negative initial digital subtraction angiogram findings: conservative or aggressive? Biomed Res Int. 2017;2017:1–10. https://doi.org/10.1155/2017/2486859.
7. Fang Y, et al. New risk score of the early period after spontaneous subarachnoid hemorrhage: for the prediction of delayed cerebral ischemia. CNS Neurosci Ther. 2019;25(10):1173–81. https://doi.org/10.1111/cns.13202.
8. Brown RJ, Kumar A, Dhar R, Sampson TR, Diringer MN. The relationship between delayed infarcts and angiographic vasospasm after aneurysmal subarachnoid hemorrhage. Neurosurgery. 2013;72(5):702–8. https://doi.org/10.1227/NEU.0b013e318285c3db.
9. Frontera JA, et al. Prediction of symptomatic vasospasmafter subarachnoid hemorrhage: the modified fisher scale. Neurosurgery. 2006;59(1):21–7. https://doi.org/10.1227/01.NEU.0000218821.34014.1B.
10. Fu F-W, et al. Perimesencephalic nonaneurysmal subarachnoid hemorrhage caused by transverse sinus thrombosis: a case report

and review of literature. Medicine. 2017;96(33):e7374. https://doi.org/10.1097/MD.0000000000007374.
11. Bauer AM, Rasmussen PA. Treatment of intracranial vasospasm following subarachnoid hemorrhage. Front Neurol. 2014;5:72. https://doi.org/10.3389/fneur.2014.00072.
12. Budohoski KP, et al. Impairment of cerebral autoregulation predicts delayed cerebral ischemia after subarachnoid hemorrhage: a prospective observational study. Stroke. 2012;43(12):3230–7. https://doi.org/10.1161/STROKEAHA.112.669788.
13. Ryttlefors M, Enblad P, Ronne-Engström E, Persson L, Ilodigwe D, Macdonald RL. Patient age and vasospasm after subarachnoid hemorrhage. Neurosurgery. 2010;67(4):911–7. https://doi.org/10.1227/NEU.0b013e3181ed11ab.
14. Mills JN, Mehta V, Russin J, Amar AP, Rajamohan A, Mack WJ. Advanced imaging modalities in the detection of cerebral vasospasm. Neurol Res Int. 2013;2013:1–15. https://doi.org/10.1155/2013/415960.
15. Samagh N, Bhagat H, Jangra K. Monitoring cerebral vasospasm: how much can we rely on transcranial Doppler. J Anaesthesiol Clin Pharmacol. 2019;35(1):12–8. https://doi.org/10.4103/joacp.JOACP_192_17.
16. Kiser TH. Cerebral vasospasm in critically III patients with aneurysmal subarachnoid hemorrhage: does the evidence support the ever-growing list of potential pharmacotherapy interventions? Hosp Pharm. 2014;49(10):923–41. https://doi.org/10.1310/hpj4910-923.
17. Kumar G, Alexandrov AV. Vasospasm surveillance with transcranial Doppler sonography in subarachnoid hemorrhage. J Ultrasound Med. 2015;34(8):1345–50. https://doi.org/10.7863/ultra.34.8.1345.
18. Fragata I, et al. Computed tomography perfusion as a predictor of delayed cerebral ischemia and functional outcome in spontaneous subarachnoid hemorrhage: a single center experience. Neuroradiol J. 2019;32(3):179–88. https://doi.org/10.1177/1971400919829048.
19. Anderson GB, Ashforth R, Steinke DE, Findlay JM. CT angiography for the detection of cerebral vasospasm in patients with acute subarachnoid hemorrhage. AJNR Am J Neuroradiol. 2000;21(6):1011–5.
20. Takano K, Hida K, Iwaasa M, Inoue T, Yoshimitsu K. Three-dimensional spin-echo-based black-blood MRA in the detection

of vasospasm following subarachnoid hemorrhage. J Magn Reson Imaging. 2019;49(3):800–7. https://doi.org/10.1002/jmri.26231.
21. Heiserman JE. MR angiography for the diagnosis of vasospasm after subarachnoid hemorrhage. Is it accurate? Is it safe? Am J Neuroradiol. 2000;21(9):1571–2.
22. Grubb RL, Raichle ME, Eichling JO, Gado MH. Effects of subarachnoid hemorrhage on cerebral blood volume, blood flow, and oxygen utilization in humans. J Neurosurg. 1977;46(4):446–53. https://doi.org/10.3171/jns.1977.46.4.0446.
23. Sarrafzadeh AS, Nagel A, Czabanka M, Denecke T, Vajkoczy P, Plotkin M. Imaging of hypoxic–ischemic penumbra with 18F-fluoromisonidazole PET/CT and measurement of related cerebral metabolism in aneurysmal subarachnoid hemorrhage. J Cereb Blood Flow Metab. 2010;30(1):36–45. https://doi.org/10.1038/jcbfm.2009.199.
24. Carlson AP, Yonas H. Radiographic assessment of vasospasm after aneurysmal subarachnoid hemorrhage: the physiological perspective. Neurol Res. 2009;31(6):593–604. https://doi.org/10.1179/174313209X455754.
25. Sarrafzadeh AS, Haux D, Lüdemann L, Amthauer H, Plotkin M, Küchler I, Unterberg AW. Cerebral ischemia in aneurysmal subarachnoid hemorrhage: a correlative microdialysis-PET study. Stroke. 2004;35(3):638–43. [PubMed] [Ref list].
26. Terry A, et al. Safety and technical efficacy of over-the-wire balloons for the treatment of subarachnoid hemorrhage–induced cerebral vasospasm. FOC. 2006;21(3):1–7. https://doi.org/10.3171/foc.2006.21.3.14.
27. Choi BJ, Lee TH, Lee JI, Ko JK, Park HS, Choi CH. Safety and efficacy of transluminal balloon angioplasty using a compliant balloon for severe cerebral vasospasm after an aneurysmal subarachnoid hemorrhage. J Korean Neurosurg Soc. 2011;49(3):157. https://doi.org/10.3340/jkns.2011.49.3.157.
28. Yao G-E, et al. Vasospasm after subarachnoid hemorrhage: a 3D rotational angiography study. In: Early brain injury or cerebral vasospasm. Vienna: Springer; 2011. p. 221–5. https://doi.org/10.1007/978-3-7091-0356-2_40.
29. Lad SP, Guzman R, Kelly ME, Li G, Lim M, Lovbald K, Steinberg GK. Cerebral perfusion imaging in vasospasm. Neurosurg Focus. 2006;21(3):E7.
30. Yonas H, Pindzola RR, Meltzer CC, Sasser H. Qualitative versus quantitative assessment of cerebrovascular reserves. Neurosurgery. 1998;42(5):1005–10; discussion 1011-2.

31. Rajendran JG, Lewis DH, Newell DW, Winn HR. Brain SPECT used to evaluate vasospasm after subarachnoid hemorrhage: correlation with angiography and transcranial Doppler. Clin Nucl Med. 2001;26(2):125–30.
32. Rawluk D, Smith FW, Deans HE, Gemmell HG, MacDonald AF. Technetium 99m HMPAO scanning in patients with subarachnoid haemorrhage: a preliminary study. Br J Radiol. 1988;61(721):26–9. https://doi.org/10.1259/0007-1285-61-721-26.
33. Lewis DH, Eskridge JM, Newell DW, Grady MS, Cohen WA, Dalley RW, Loyd D, Grothaus-King A, Young P, Winn HR. Brain SPECT and the effect of cerebral angioplasty in delayed ischemia due to vasospasm. J Nucl Med. 1992;33(10):1789–96.
34. Mickey B, Vorstrup S, Voldby B, Lindewald H, Harmsen A, Lassen NA. Serial measurement of regional cerebral blood flow in patients with SAH using 133Xe inhalation and emission computerized tomography. J Neurosurg. 1984;60(5):916–22.
35. Mills JN, Mehta V, Russin J, Amar AP, Rajamohan A, Mack WJ. Advanced imaging modalities in the detection of cerebral vasospasm. Neurol Res Int. 2013;2013:415960. https://doi.org/10.1155/2013/415960.
36. Drayer BP, Wolfson SK, Reinmuth OM, Dujovny M, Boehnke M, Cook EE. Xenon enhanced CT for analysis of cerebral integrity, perfusion, and blood flow. Stroke. 1978;9(2):123–30.
37. Plougmann J, Astrup J, Pedersen J, Gyldensted C. Effect of stable xenon inhalation on intracranial pressure during measurement of cerebral blood flow in head injury. J Neurosurg. 1994;81(6):822–8. https://doi.org/10.3171/jns.1994.81.6.0822.
38. Knuckey NW, Fox RA, Surveyor I, Stokes BA. Early cerebral blood flow and computerized tomography in predicting ischemia after cerebral aneurysm rupture. J Neurosurg. 1985;62(6):850–5. [PubMed] [Ref list].
39. Lindegaard K-F, Nornes H, Bakke SJ, Sorteberg W, Nakstad P. Cerebral vasospasm diagnosis by means of angiography and blood velocity measurements. Acta Neurochir. 1989;100(1–2):12–24. https://doi.org/10.1007/BF01405268.
40. Murphy A, et al. Changes in cerebral perfusion with induced hypertension in aneurysmal subarachnoid hemorrhage: a pilot and feasibility study. Neurocrit Care. 2017;27(1):3–10. https://doi.org/10.1007/s12028-017-0379-6.
41. Harrigan MR, Magnano CR, Guterman LR, Hopkins LN. Computed tomographic perfusion in the management of aneurysmal subarachnoid hemorrhage: new application of an

existent technique. Neurosurgery. 2005;56(2):304–17; discussion 304–317. https://doi.org/10.1227/01.neu.0000148902.61943.df.
42. Aralasmak A, Akyuz M, Ozkaynak C, Sindel T, Tuncer R. CT angiography and perfusion imaging in patients with subarachnoid hemorrhage: correlation of vasospasm to perfusion abnormality. Neuroradiology. 2009;51(2):85–93. https://doi.org/10.1007/s00234-008-0466-7.
43. Hoeffner EG, et al. Cerebral perfusion CT: technique and clinical applications. Radiology. 2004;231(3):632–44. https://doi.org/10.1148/radiol.2313021488.
44. Dankbaar JW, Rijsdijk M, van der Schaaf IC, Velthuis BK, Wermer MJH, Rinkel GJE. Relationship between vasospasm, cerebral perfusion, and delayed cerebral ischemia after aneurysmal subarachnoid hemorrhage. Neuroradiology. 2009;51(12):813–9. https://doi.org/10.1007/s00234-009-0575-y.
45. Sorensen AG, et al. Hyperacute stroke: evaluation with combined multisection diffusion-weighted and hemodynamically weighted echo-planar MR imaging. Radiology. 1996;199(2):391–401. https://doi.org/10.1148/radiology.199.2.8668784.
46. Rordorf G, et al. Diffusion- and perfusion-weighted imaging in vasospasm AFTER subarachnoid hemorrhage. Stroke. 1999;30(3):599–605. https://doi.org/10.1161/01.STR.30.3.599.
47. Wani AA, Phadke R, Behari S, Sahu R, Jaiswal A, Jain V. Role of diffusion-weighted MRG in predicting outcome in subarachnoid hemorrhage due to anterior communicating artery aneurysms. Turk Neurosurg. 2008;18(1):10–6.
48. Hattingen E, et al. Perfusion-weighted MRI to evaluate cerebral autoregulation in aneurysmal subarachnoid haemorrhage. Neuroradiology. 2008;50(11):929–38. https://doi.org/10.1007/s00234-008-0424-4.
49. Das JM, Zito PM. Nimodipine. In: StatPearls [Internet]. Treasure Island: StatPearls Publishing; 2021.
50. Dorhout Mees S, et al. Calcium antagonists for aneurysmal subarachnoid haemorrhage. Cochrane Database Syst Rev. 2007;2007(3):CD000277. https://doi.org/10.1002/14651858.CD000277.pub3.
51. Stippler M, et al. Magnesium infusion for vasospasm prophylaxis after subarachnoid hemorrhage. J Neurosurg. 2006;105(5):723–9. https://doi.org/10.3171/jns.2006.105.5.723.
52. Wong GKC, Poon WS. Magnsium and vasospasm. J Neurosurg. 2007;106(5):938–9; author reply 939-940. https://doi.org/10.3171/jns.2007.106.5.938.

53. Suarez JI, Participants in the International Multidisciplinary Consensus Conference on the Critical Care Management of Subarachnoid Hemorrhage. Magnesium sulfate administration in subarachnoid hemorrhage. Neurocrit Care. 2011;15(2):302–7. https://doi.org/10.1007/s12028-011-9603-y.
54. Durrant JC, Hinson HE. Rescue therapy for refractory vasospasm after subarachnoid hemorrhage. Curr Neurol Neurosci Rep. 2015;15(2):521. https://doi.org/10.1007/s11910-014-0521-1.
55. Nishiguchi M, Ono S, Iseda K, Manabe H, Hishikawa T, Date I. Effect of vasodilation by milrinone, a phosphodiesterase III inhibitor, on vasospastic arteries after a subarachnoid hemorrhage in vitro and in vivo: effectiveness of cisternal injection of milrinone. Neurosurgery. 2010;66(1):158–64; discussion 164. https://doi.org/10.1227/01.NEU.0000363153.62579.FF.
56. Fraticelli AT, Cholley BP, Losser M-R, Saint Maurice J-P, Payen D. Milrinone for the treatment of cerebral vasospasm after aneurysmal subarachnoid hemorrhage. Stroke. 2008;39(3):893–8. https://doi.org/10.1161/STROKEAHA.107.492447.
57. Kieninger M, et al. Side effects of long-term continuous intraarterial nimodipine infusion in patients with severe refractory cerebral vasospasm after subarachnoid hemorrhage. Neurocrit Care. 2018;28(1):65–76. https://doi.org/10.1007/s12028-017-0428-1.
58. Duman E, Karakoç F, Pinar HU, Dogan R, Fırat A, Yıldırım E. Higher dose intra-arterial milrinone and intra-arterial combined milrinone-nimodipine infusion as a rescue therapy for refractory cerebral vasospasm. Interv Neuroradiol. 2017;23(6):636–43. https://doi.org/10.1177/1591019917732288.
59. Keuskamp J, Murali R, Chao KH. High-dose intraarterial verapamil in the treatment of cerebral vasospasm after aneurysmal subarachnoid hemorrhage. JNS. 2008;108(3):458–63. https://doi.org/10.3171/JNS/2008/108/3/0458.
60. Feng L, et al. Intraarterially administered verapamil as adjunct therapy for cerebral vasospasm: safety and 2-year experience. AJNR Am J Neuroradiol. 2002;23(8):1284–90.
61. Liu J, Chen Q. Effect of statins treatment for patients with aneurysmal subarachnoid hemorrhage: a systematic review and meta-analysis of observational studies and randomized controlled trials. Int J Clin Exp Med. 2015;8(5):7198–208.

62. Dee RA, Mangum KD, Bai X, Mack CP, Taylor JM. Druggable targets in the Rho pathway and their promise for therapeutic control of blood pressure. Pharmacol Ther. 2019;193:121–34. https://doi.org/10.1016/j.pharmthera.2018.09.001.
63. Huang Y, Wu J, Su T, Zhang S, Lin X. Fasudil, a Rho-Kinase inhibitor, exerts cardioprotective function in animal models of myocardial ischemia/reperfusion injury: a meta-analysis and review of preclinical evidence and possible mechanisms. Front Pharmacol. 2018;9:1083. https://doi.org/10.3389/fphar.2018.01083.
64. Liu Yf, Qiu HC, Su J. et al. Drug treatment of cerebral vasospasm after subarachnoid hemorrhage following aneurysms. Chin Neurosurg Jl 2, 4 (2016). https://doi.org/10.1186/s41016-016-0023-x.
65. Qureshi AI, et al. Therapeutic benefit of cilostazol in patients with aneurysmal subarachnoid hemorrhage: a meta-analysis of randomized and nonrandomized studies. J Vasc Interv Neurol. 2018;10(2):33–40.
66. Macdonald RL. Endothelin antagonists in subarachnoid hemorrhage: what next? Crit Care. 2012;16(6):171. https://doi.org/10.1186/cc11822.
67. Ma J, Huang S, Ma L, Liu Y, Li H, You C. Endothelin-receptor antagonists for aneurysmal subarachnoid hemorrhage: an updated meta-analysis of randomized controlled trials. Crit Care. 2012;16(5):R198. https://doi.org/10.1186/cc11686.
68. Haley EC Jr, Kassell NF, Torner JC. A randomized trial of nicardipine in subarachnoid hemorrhage: angiographic and transcranial Doppler ultrasound results – a report of the Cooperative Aneurysm Study. J Neurosurg. 1993;78:548–53.

Phenobarbital for Alcohol Withdrawal Syndrome

Carly M. Guay and Kathryn E. Qualls

1 Introduction

Alcohol use disorder is associated with significant morbidity and mortality, with approximately three million deaths attributable to the harmful use of alcohol globally in 2016 [1]. Ethanol is a central nervous system (CNS) depressant that exerts its effects via inhibition of glutamate, an excitatory neurotransmitter, and potentiation of gamma-aminobutyric acid (GABA), an inhibitory neurotransmitter [2]. Upon cessation of alcohol intake or a significant reduction in the amount consumed, patients physically dependent on alcohol may experience alcohol withdrawal syndrome (AWS) as a result of CNS hyperactivity. Signs and symptoms of alcohol withdrawal can vary in severity and include anxiety, insomnia, headache, hallucinations, nausea, diaphoresis, tachycardia, hypertension, hyperthermia, and hyperactive reflexes [3]. In the most severe cases, seizures, delirium, and death may also occur [3]. Although variable from one patient to another, signs and symptoms of withdrawal are most likely to reach peak intensity approximately 48–72 h after a last drink [4].

C. M. Guay (✉) · K. E. Qualls
Pharmacy Department, University of Missouri Health Care, Columbia, MO, USA
e-mail: cmgvbw@health.missouri.edu

© The Author(s), under exclusive license to Springer Nature Switzerland AG 2022
N. Arora (ed.), *Procedures and Protocols in the Neurocritical Care Unit*, https://doi.org/10.1007/978-3-030-90225-4_24

2 Management of Alcohol Withdrawal

According to the American Society of Addiction Medicine (ASAM), the first step in the assessment of alcohol withdrawal is determining whether a patient is at risk of developing severe and/or complicated alcohol withdrawal [3]. Factors associated with increased patient risk for complicated withdrawal include history of alcohol withdrawal delirium or alcohol withdrawal seizure, numerous prior withdrawal episodes, comorbid medical or surgical illness (especially traumatic brain injury), increased age, long duration of heavy and regular alcohol consumption, seizure(s) during the current withdrawal episode, marked autonomic hyperactivity on presentation, and physiological dependence on benzodiazepines or barbiturates [3].

During withdrawal management, severity of alcohol withdrawal should be monitored using a validated assessment scale, such as the Clinical Institute Withdrawal Assessment, Revised (CIWA-Ar) tool [3]. ASAM recommends that the severity of alcohol withdrawal be used to guide initial therapy; patients with mild withdrawal may be managed with pharmacotherapy or supportive care alone, while those with moderate or severe symptoms should receive pharmacotherapy [3].

3 Pharmacotherapy

Regardless of the severity of alcohol withdrawal, ASAM recommends benzodiazepines as first-line treatment due to their known efficacy in preventing seizures and delirium [3]. Benzodiazepines act as positive allosteric modulators on the GABA-A receptor, consequently reducing the autonomic hyperactivity that occurs in the setting of alcohol withdrawal [5]. In patients experiencing resistant alcohol withdrawal, however, severe or complicated withdrawal may occur despite high doses of benzodiazepines. In such instances, ASAM recommends the addition of adjunctive medications such as phenobarbital [3]. Whereas benzodiazepines increase the *frequency* of chloride channel opening caused by GABA-A receptor activation, phenobarbital increases the *duration* of channel opening [6]. Additionally, phenobarbital may provide added beneficial effect via its antagonizing activity on stimulatory N-methyl-D-aspartate (NMDA) receptors, which helps to explain its place in the treatment of benzodiazepine-refractory alcohol withdrawal [7]. ASAM also recommends the use of phenobarbital as monotherapy for patients experiencing any severity of alcohol withdrawal with a contraindication for benzodiazepine use [3]. However, ASAM includes the caveat that "phenobarbital should only be used by clinicians experienced with its use" due to the risk of respiratory depression and over-sedation [3].

When considering patients in the neurocritical care setting, it is important that treatment of AWS does not negatively impact the neurologic exam. While the CNS depressant effects of benzodiazepines can influence neurological assessment, it is theorized that the risk of this occurring with phenobarbital may be lower. However, phenobarbital has a narrow therapeutic index and is a strong inducer of the cytochrome P450 enzyme system, so judicious use and close monitoring are warranted [8].

4 Literature Review

Although there are no studies evaluating phenobarbital for alcohol withdrawal in the neurocritical care setting, there is growing evidence to support its use in patients without neurological injury (Table 1). Rosenson and colleagues [6] conducted a prospective, randomized, double-blind trial comparing a single intravenous dose of phenobarbital (10 mg/kg) to placebo for patients with AWS in the emergency department. All patients received symptom-guided lorazepam, but the addition of a one-time phenobarbital dose resulted in fewer admissions to the intensive care unit (ICU) (8% vs. 25%, difference 17%, 95% confidence interval (CI)

TABLE 1 Summary of primary literature

Author, year	Study design	Setting	Interventions	Outcome measures	Results
Hendey et al., 2011 [4]	Prospective, randomized, double-blind	ED	IV PB (260 mg initial dose, 130 mg subsequent doses) followed by PO placebo [n = 25] IV LZ (2 mg) followed by PO CD [n = 19]	Primary: change in CIWA score from baseline to ED discharge Secondary: ED LOS, hospital admission rates, CIWA score at 48-h reassessment	Primary: PB and LZ significantly decreased the CIWA score from baseline to ED discharge (15.0 to 5.4 and 16.8 to 4.2, P < 0.0001) Secondary: no difference in ED LOS, hospital admission rates, or CIWA scores at discharge and 48-h reassessment
Rosenson et al., 2013 [6]	Prospective, randomized, double-blind	ED	IV PB (10 mg/kg) followed by symptom-guided LZ-based AW protocol [n = 51] Placebo followed by symptom-guided LZ-based AW protocol [n = 51]	Primary: initial level of hospital admission Secondary: use of continuous LZ infusion, hospital LOS, total LZ required per patient, adverse events	Primary: PB resulted in fewer ICU admissions (8% vs. 25%, 95% CI 4–32) Secondary: no difference in hospital LOS or adverse events; PB resulted in decreased use of continuous LZ infusion (4% vs. 31%, 95% CI 14–41) and decreased total LZ required (26 vs. 49 mg, 95% CI 7–40)

Tidwell et al., 2018 [7]	Retrospective cohort	Medical ICU	Tapered PB protocol (starting dose and route of administration dependent on assessment of risk factors) plus as-needed LZ if deemed necessary by provider [n = 60] CIWA-Ar protocol [n = 60]	Primary: ICU LOS Secondary: hospital LOS, use of mechanical ventilation, use of adjunctive pharmacotherapy	Primary: PB protocol resulted in shorter ICU LOS (2.4 vs. 4.4 days, P < 0.001) Secondary: lower incidence of mechanical ventilation (1 vs. 14 patients, P < 0.001) and use of adjunctive agents for symptom control (4 vs. 17 patients, P = 0.002) in PB protocol group; PB protocol resulted in shorter hospital LOS (4.3 vs. 6.9 days, P = 0.004)

(continued)

TABLE 1 (continued)

Author, year	Study design	Setting	Interventions	Outcome measures	Results
Nelson et al., 2019 [12]	Retrospective cohort	ED	IV DZ monotherapy [n = 100] IV LZ plus IV PB [n = 100] IV PB monotherapy [n = 100]	Primary: rate of ICU admission Secondary: rate of mechanical ventilation, admission rate, non-ICU LOS, ICU LOS, total LOS	Primary: no difference in rate of ICU admission among groups (DZ 22%, LZ plus PB 23%, PB 24%, $P = 0.99$) Secondary: no difference in rate of mechanical ventilation, ICU LOS, or non-ICU LOS; total LOS was lowest for patients treated with LZ plus PB ($P = 0.04$); admission rate was highest in the PB monotherapy group (DZ 35, LZ plus PB 47, PB 54, $P = 0.024$)

Nisavic et al., 2019 [9]	Retrospective cohort	Inpatient	BZD-based protocol [n = 419] PB-based protocol [n = 143]	Primary: AW-related complications (seizures, alcoholic hallucinosis, and/or delirium) Secondary: hospital LOS, ICU LOS, discharges AMA, mortality, adverse events	Primary: no difference in AW-related seizures or hallucinosis between groups; higher rates of delirium in BZD group (7% vs. 4%, P = 0.28) Secondary: no difference in hospital LOS, ICU LOS, discharges AMA, or adverse events; one patient death in the BZD group compared to none in the PB group
Nguyen et al., 2020 [10]	Retrospective cohort	ICU	LZ-based AW protocol [n = 36] PB-adjunct (LZ-based AW protocol plus adjunctive PB) [n = 36]	Primary: total treatment duration Secondary: ICU LOS, change in CIWA-Ar score at 24 h	Primary: longer duration of treatment in LZ group, but not statistically significant (3.1 vs. 2.7 days, P = 0.573) Secondary: no difference in ICU LOS; larger change in CIWA-Ar score at 24 h in the LZ group compared to the PB-adjunct group (6.5 ± 8.5 vs. 1.8 ± 9.0 points, P = 0.0275)

(continued)

TABLE 1 (continued)

Author, year	Study design	Setting	Interventions	Outcome measures	Results
Oks et al., 2020 [11]	Retrospective cohort	Medical ICU	IV PB (130 mg every 15 min until RASS 0 to −1) [n = 86]	Primary: rate of mechanical ventilation Secondary: PB treatment duration	Primary: 17 patients (19.8%) required mechanical ventilation, but no patient was intubated due to PB use alone Secondary: mean PB treatment duration was 5.2 ± 2.9 days
Nejad et al., 2020 [13]	Retrospective cohort	Inpatient, ICU, ED	BZD-based protocol [n = 52] PB-based protocol [n = 33]	Primary: development of AW-related complications Secondary: hospital LOS, mortality, adverse events	Primary: 25 patients (48.2%) developed AWD and 38 (73.1%) developed uncomplicated AWS in the BZD group compared to 0 patients in the PB group ($P = 0.0001$) Secondary: hospital LOS was longer in the PB group (12.5 vs. 10.9 days); no difference in mortality; 10 patients (19.2%) developed adverse events in the BZD group compared to 0 patients in the PB group

Abbreviations: *AMA* against medical advice, *AW* alcohol withdrawal, *AWD* alcohol withdrawal delirium, *AWS* alcohol withdrawal syndrome, *BZD* benzodiazepine, *CD* chlordiazepoxide, *CI* confidence interval, *CIWA-Ar* Clinical Institute Withdrawal Assessment for Alcohol, revised, *DZ* diazepam, *ED* emergency department, *ICU* intensive care unit, *IV* intravenous, *LOS* length of stay, *LZ* lorazepam, *mg* milligrams, *PB* phenobarbital, *PO* per os (by mouth), *RASS* Richmond Agitation Sedation Scale

4–32%) [6]. There was no difference in hospital length of stay (LOS) or adverse events between groups [6].

In the medical ICU setting, Tidwell and colleagues [7] conducted a retrospective cohort study comparing a tapered phenobarbital protocol with as-needed lorazepam to a symptom-guided, lorazepam-based alcohol withdrawal protocol. In the phenobarbital group, the starting dose and route of administration was determined based the presence of risk factors for delirium tremens (DT). The investigators found that use of the phenobarbital protocol resulted in shorter ICU and hospital LOS, a lower incidence of mechanical ventilation, and decreased use of adjunctive pharmacologic agents for symptom control [7].

In another retrospective cohort study, Nisavic and colleagues [9] compared a benzodiazepine-based protocol to a phenobarbital-based protocol for inpatients with AWS. While the investigators found no difference in alcohol withdrawal-related seizures or hallucinosis between groups, higher rates of delirium were observed in the benzodiazepine group (7% vs. 4%, P = 0.28) [9]. There was no difference in hospital LOS, ICU LOS, or adverse events between treatment groups [9].

Nguyen and colleagues [10] retrospectively evaluated the use of adjunctive phenobarbital in the ICU setting for patients on a lorazepam-based alcohol withdrawal protocol. Although not statistically significant, the use of adjunctive phenobarbital resulted in a slightly shorter treatment duration (2.7 vs. 3.1 days, P = 0.573) [10]. However, more patients in the phenobarbital-adjunct arm required mechanical ventilation than in the lorazepam arm (3 vs. 0, P = 0.239) [10]. This suggests that there may be an increased risk of respiratory depression with the combined use of phenobarbital and lorazepam.

In the most recent retrospective cohort evaluation, Oks and colleagues [11] assessed 86 patients in the medical ICU setting who received intravenous phenobarbital for symptoms of alcohol withdrawal. In this study, patients were administered 130 mg of phenobarbital every 15 min until a Richmond Agitation Sedation Scale (RASS) score of 0 to −1 was achieved. Overall, 17 patients (19.8%) required mechanical ventilation, but no patient was intubated due to phenobarbital use alone [11]. The mean duration of phenobarbital treatment was 5.2 ± 2.9 days [11].

As a whole, the literature for phenobarbital in AWS is conflicting and does not elucidate a clear role for the agent. Scenarios where the utilization of phenobarbital may be beneficial include the treatment of patients with refractory alcohol withdrawal or patients in whom avoidance of large benzodiazepine doses is preferred, such as those with neurologic injuries (Fig. 1). A randomized controlled trial compar-

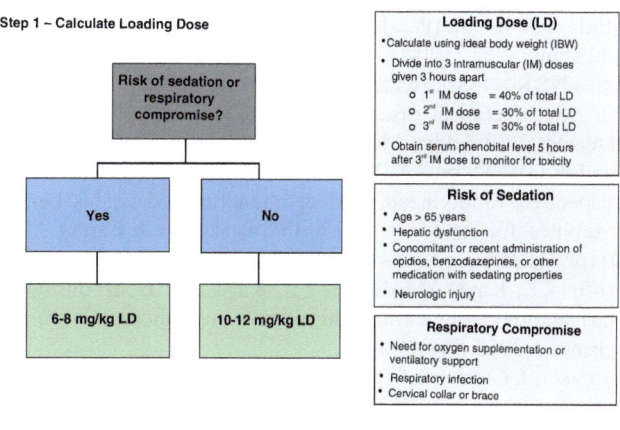

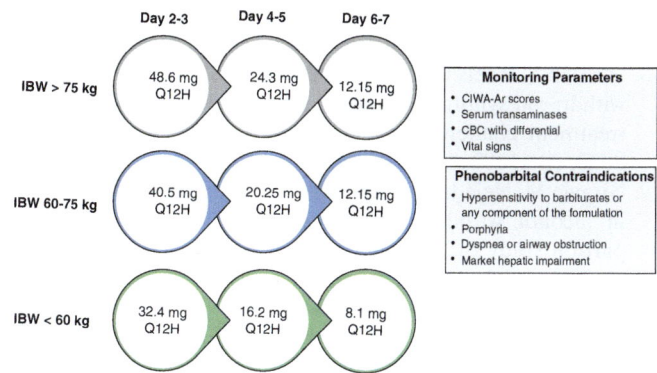

FIGURE 1 Phenobarbital-based alcohol withdrawal protocol [9, 13]

ing phenobarbital monotherapy to benzodiazepine monotherapy in the neurocritical care unit is warranted to clarify the role of barbiturates for alcohol withdrawal in this unique patient population.

References

1. WHO. Global status report on alcohol and health 2018. Geneva: World Health Organization; 2018.
2. Newman RK, Stobart Gallagher MA, Gomez AE. Alcohol withdrawal. In: StatPearls [Internet]. Treasure Island: StatPearls Publishing LLC; 2020. URL: https://www.ncbi.nlm.nih.gov/books/NBK441882/. Accessed December 15, 2020.
3. The ASAM clinical practice guideline on alcohol withdrawal management. J Addict Med. 2020;14(3S Suppl 1):1–72.
4. Hendey GW, Dery RA, Barnes RL, Snowden B, Mentler P. A prospective, randomized, trial of phenobarbital versus benzodiazepines for acute alcohol withdrawal. Am J Emerg Med. 2011;29(4):382–5.
5. Griffin CE, Kaye AM, Bueno FR, Kaye AD. Benzodiazepine pharmacology and central nervous system-mediated effects. Ochsner J. 2013;13(2):214–23.
6. Rosenson J, Clements C, Simon B, et al. Phenobarbital for acute alcohol withdrawal: a prospective randomized double-blind placebo-controlled study. J Emerg Med. 2013;44(3):592–8.
7. Tidwell WP, Thomas TL, Pouliot JD, Canonico AE, Webber AJ. Treatment of alcohol withdrawal syndrome: phenobarbital vs CIWA-Ar protocol. Am J Crit Care. 2018;27(6):454–60.
8. Farrokh S, Roels C, Owusu KA, Nelson SE, Cook AM. Alcohol withdrawal syndrome in neurocritical care unit: assessment and treatment challenges. Neurocrit Care. 2021;34:593–607. https://doi.org/10.1007/s12028-020-01061-8.
9. Nisavic M, Nejad SH, Isenberg BM, et al. Use of phenobarbital in alcohol withdrawal management – a retrospective comparison study of phenobarbital and benzodiazepines for acute alcohol withdrawal management in general medicine patients. Psychosomatics. 2019;60(5):458–67.
10. Nguyen TA, Lam SW. Phenobarbital and symptom-triggered lorazepam versus lorazepam alone for severe alcohol withdrawal in the intensive care unit. Alcohol. 2020;82:23–7.

11. Oks M, Cleven KL, Healy L, et al. The safety and utility of phenobarbital use for the treatment of severe alcohol withdrawal syndrome in the medical intensive care unit. J Intensive Care Med. 2020;35(9):844–50.
12. Nelson AC, Kehoe J, Sankoff J, Mintzer D, Taub J, Kaucher KA. Benzodiazepines vs barbiturates for alcohol withdrawal: analysis of 3 different treatment protocols. Am J Emerg Med. 2019;37(4):733–6.
13. Nejad S, Nisavic M, Larentzakis A, et al. Phenobarbital for acute alcohol withdrawal management in surgical trauma patients – a retrospective comparison study. Psychosomatics. 2020;61(4):327–35.

Diabetic Ketoacidosis and Hyperglycemia

Muhammad Waqar Salam and John Liu

1 Introduction

Among the patient population sufficiently ill to warrant hospital admission, hyperglycemia is exceptionally common, with incidence estimated at about a third of patients. This is significantly more than the prevalence of diabetes mellitus, which is estimated at roughly 10% of the general population [28]. Not only are patients with baseline diabetes at higher risk for inpatient admissions, the various physiologic stresses associated with hospital and ICU care provide additional risk factors for stress hyperglycemia. While common, hyperglycemia is not a benign finding in hospitalized and critically ill patients. Among the population of critically ill patients, multiple studies have suggested that hyperglycemia is associated with a significantly increased risk for mortality and that the effect increases as the degree of hyperglycemia worsens [1, 2]. Unfortunately, management of hyperglycemia is limited by the possibility of treatment-related hypoglycemia, which has similarly negative effects on both length of hospital stay and patient mortality [26].

M. W. Salam (✉) · J. Liu
Division of Endocrinology, Diabetes and Metabolism, Department of Internal Medicine, University of Missouri, Columbia, MO, USA
e-mail: salamm@health.missouri.edu; liujohn@health.missouri.edu

© The Author(s), under exclusive license to Springer Nature Switzerland AG 2022
N. Arora (ed.), *Procedures and Protocols in the Neurocritical Care Unit*, https://doi.org/10.1007/978-3-030-90225-4_25

The patient requiring treatment in the neurocritical care setting poses additional unique challenges due to the potentially more serious effects of hypoglycemia on the central nervous system (CNS) as well as additional factors predisposing patients to hyperglycemia. In this chapter we present an overview of glycemic management in patients with central nervous system injury particularly in the critical care setting beginning with a review of the physiology of glucose homeostasis in the CNS, continuing with the discussion of the risk factors predisposing this unique set of patients to hyperglycemia and hypoglycemia, and concluding with an overview of management considerations and strategies.

2 Glucose Homeostasis in the Brain

Glucose is the essential energy resource of the human central nervous system, which consumes an estimated 100 grams of glucose per day, or about 20% of total glucose in the body, to maintain normal brain function. While a majority (approximately 70%) of the produced adenosine triphosphate (ATP) is used to maintain membrane potential and other aspects of neuronal signaling, the remainder is necessary for basic tasks of cellular upkeep and maintenance [8]. As a result, the central nervous system is very susceptible to the effects of hypoglycemia.

Glucose homeostasis and metabolism in the brain is mediated by glucose transporters (GLUT), which are a family of fourteen transmembrane proteins acting as bidirectional, sodium and ATP independent facilitative transporters of glucose and similar simple carbohydrate molecules [9]. Specifically, GLUT1 and GLUT3 have central roles in maintaining glucose homeostasis in the CNS. GLUT1 is expressed in both the luminal and abluminal surfaces of the blood brain barrier and provides facilitative transportation of glucose from systemic circulation into the central nervous system, driven by the differential in glucose concentration between the two systems. The concentration gradient is maintained by the catabolism of glucose in the central nervous system to meet energy demands. Glucose concentration in the interstitial fluid of the central nervous system is generally 1–2 mmol/L (18–36 mg/dL), or approximately one third that of the plasma. GLUT1 has high affinity for glucose with a Michaelis constant (Km) of 1.5–3 mmol/L (27–54 mg/dL) as compared to typical plasma glucose concentration of 5 mmol/L (90 mg/dL), therefore providing constant glucose transportation under physiologic conditions [10]. GLUT1 is also expressed in astrocytes, providing access to interstitial glucose. GLUT3 is expressed on the surface on neurons and has comparatively higher affinity and capacity in comparison to GLUT1, providing neurons with preferential access to glucose when the glucose concentration is low in the interstitial fluid (maximal affinity at glucose concentration of 2.8 mmol/L or 50 mg/dL) [11]. Intracellular glucose is subject to phosphorylation to glucose-6-phosphate by Hexokinase, an irreversible process that enters the molecule into glycolysis.

Clinically, patients with central nervous system injury exist in hyper-metabolic states with increased consumption of glucose by the brain [12]. Therefore, interruptions in glucose supply due to decline in serum glucose to below the affinity of GLUT1 transportation would have more immediate and severe consequences. Indeed, studies in animal models have demonstrated that expression of GLUT receptors in the brain is significantly up-regulated after induced ischemic events [16, 17]. This likely represents a protective response to meet the increased metabolic demands of the injured brain and emphasizes the importance of maintaining steady glucose supply in the context of a CNS insult.

Additionally, patients with pre-existing diabetes may have adaptations that serve to moderate the degree of hyperglycemia in the central nervous system, potentially by decreasing the transcription or activity of glucose transporters in the brain to decrease movement of glucose into central nervous system cells [13, 14]. While this may be adaptive and helpful in the baseline hyperglycemic state, it could predispose these patients to exaggerated responses to hypoglycemia due to diminished glucose transport capacity. However, the degree and importance of this effect is controversial, with other studies showing conflicting results and no significant effect of hyperglycemia on transcription and activity [15]. Regardless, it is well-recognized clinically that patients with higher baseline blood sugars demonstrate neuroglycopenic symptoms at a significantly higher level of plasma glucose compared to euglycemic patients although the mechanisms and clinical significance of this observation remain uncertain [18, 19].

3 Hyperglycemia and Hypoglycemia in the Neurocritical Care Unit (NCCU)

Patients who are critically ill, either for neurological reasons or otherwise, are at increased risk for hyperglycemia. There are multiple contributing factors, the primary one being the increased levels of stress-related hormones, either released endogenously or given exogenously as part of treatment. Cortisol, one of the most well known stress hormones, acts on its nuclear receptor in target tissues, leading to hyperglycemia through a variety of mechanisms, including increased gluconeogenesis, impaired insulin release, and impaired glucose uptake in peripheral tissues. In patients without sufficient pancreatic reserve to maintain normal plasma glucose, a primarily postprandial hyperglycemia occurs [23]. Dexamethasone, a pharmacologic glucocorticoid commonly used in the neurosurgical setting, is significantly more potent than cortisol and can contribute to dramatic and long-lasting episodes of hyperglycemia due to its longer half-life of approximately 2 days.

Catecholamines, released by the adrenal medulla in response to acute stress, can also lead to hyperglycemia through their actions on the alpha and beta adrenergic receptors. This is primarily mediated by activation of the beta-2 adrenergic receptor, which leads to both increased insulin and glucagon secretion by direct stimulation of pancreatic beta cells and increased hepatic glycogenolysis and gluconeogenesis [24]. The net effect of beta-2 adrenergic receptor stimulation is generally hyperglycemia. Alpha-1 adrenergic receptors are also thought to play a role in promoting hyperglycemia by increasing gluconeogenesis [25]. In addition to endogenously secreted epinephrine and norepinephrine, pharmacologic vasopressors particularly norepinephrine used to support blood pressure in the critical care setting result in similar effects by these mechanisms.

Patients in the NCCU have several additional clinical factors that predispose to hyperglycemia. For instance, patients who are ventilator-dependent or having dysphagia following a neurologic insult, frequently require tube feeding which appears to be an independent risk factor for development of hyperglycemia. Although there is lack of data regarding etiology and frequency, patients receiving enteral nutrition appear to be at an increased risk for hyperglycemia. For instance, one study comparing insulin Glargine and sliding scale insulin in treating fifty patients on enteral nutrition noted that over half of the patients did not have pre-existing diabetes on presentation [20]. While the precise etiology for this high prevalence of hyperglycemia remains unclear, it may include the high carbohydrate load of enteral nutrition products. Moreover, continuous tube feeding has been associated with decreased levels of endogenous insulin and Incretin secretion and increased insulin resistance in animal models [22].

Due to the frequently unpredictable clinical course of critically ill patients, hypoglycemia is as serious a concern as hyperglycemia. As with hyperglycemia, hypoglycemic episodes in hospitalized patients are associated with increased length of stay and increased mortality rates [26]. The primary risk factor for hypoglycemia in hospitalized patients appears to be the difference in oral intake. Not only are critically ill patients more prone to interruptions in oral intake due to procedural or diagnostic testing requirements, they may have significantly higher caloric intake at baseline. Although, in theory, basal insulin should be dosed based on basal insulin requirement, in practice many patients have excessively high doses of basal insulin providing at least partial meal time coverage. This disproportion in the basal and bolus insulins, can lead to hypoglycemic episodes upon withdrawal of baseline oral nutrition. This is a special consideration in patients with type 1 diabetes as the autoimmune destruction of the pancreas leads to a deficiency in glucagon as well as insulin within 5 years of diagnosis [27], impairing the counter-regulatory response to hypoglycemia.

Patients requiring higher doses of insulin to manage their hyperglycemia due to any of the previously discussed factors (stress hormones, glucocorticoid and vasopressor therapy, enteral feeding) are also prone to hypoglycemia as their condition and the underlying risk factors improve or resolve. This may occur gradually over the course of days, such as with glucocorticoid therapy, or may occur very rapidly over the course of hours, such as with withdrawal of enteral feeds or vasopressor therapy. Overall, the high degree of unpredictability and rapidly changing clinical circumstances requires a flexible and rapidly titratable method of insulin delivery to minimize the risk of hypoglycemia to the particularly vulnerable human brain following an acute insult.

4 Management of Hyperglycemia in the NCCU

The exact goals of glycemic control in inpatients have been the subject of numerous studies and professional society guidelines. The landmark 2009 NICE-SUGAR trial compared critically ill patients randomized to target ranges of 81 to 108 mg/dL (categorized as Intensive Insulin Therapy) compared to target glucose under 180 mg/dL (conventional therapy). The study showed that patients in the IIT group had a significantly higher risk for hypoglycemia and had a higher mortality rate [3]. This effect has been replicated in other smaller studies [4] and has led to the recommendation of a less aggressive glycemic target for critically ill patients ranging from 140–180 mg/dL according to the American Heart Association/American Stroke association (AHA), American

Diabetes Association (ADA) and 150–180 according to the Society of Critical Care Medicine SCCM [6–8].

In the neuro-critical care patient population, the glycemic targets remain an area of debate though there are several meta-analyses on the subject looking at different targets and their association with various outcomes. A 2012 meta-analysis of sixteen randomized control trials involving 1248 neuro-critical care patients compared target ranges of 70–140 mg/dL with a glucose target of 144–300 mg/dL and noted that the group with lower glucose target had increased risk of hypoglycemia though it did not affect morality. The study additionally noted worse outcomes, especially with neurological recovery, among patients with glucose >200 mg/dL and suggested an intermediate target range [31]. A separate meta-analysis of nine studies including 1459 critically ill neurosurgical or neurological patients comparing tight glycemic control (defined individually per study, generally 80–120 mg/dL) compared to conventional glycemic control noted decreased rates of infection and improved neurological outcomes among the tight glycemic control group but also increased rates of hypoglycemia and no impact on mortality [32]. While the precise glucose target range for neuro-critical care patients remains debatable, a target of 140 or 150 to 180 appears reasonable in general to limit both hypoglycemia and risk for infection and poor neurological outcomes associated with hyperglycemia.

Hyperglycemia in the critical care setting is best treated with insulin monotherapy and outpatient non-insulin diabetes medications, in general, are discontinued on admission due to various reasons. Specifically, metformin can be associated with increased risk of lactic acidosis in patients with acute renal injury, sulfonylureas can contribute to hypoglycemia with unpredictable dose responses, SGLT-2 inhibitors can contribute to DKA and urinary tract infections, and GLP-1 agonists can lead to nausea and vomiting with decrease in the caloric intake. Insulin, therefore, remains the mainstay for treatment of hyperglycemia in the neuro-critical care setting. Insulin also offers the advantage of rapid titration, frequent dosing if needed and a more predictable dose response curve.

Insulin can be delivered by two main routes: subcutaneous injection of short and long acting insulin analogues and intravenous infusion of regular insulin. In general, insulin infusion remains the preferred method for glycemic control in the neuro-critical care patient population [5]. Intravenous insulin infusion has a number of advantages over multiple daily injections, primarily including more flexible dose titration due to the short half-life of intravenous insulin (blood glucose begins to recover approximately 15 min after infusion is held [29]) and the frequent monitoring of glucose values to guide dosing. Additionally, the intravenous route bypasses differences in insulin absorption rate, which may be affected in patients with poor peripheral perfusion and variable absorption of the subcutaneous insulin. Lastly, intravenous insulin infusion achieves target glucose much more rapidly compared to subcutaneous insulin due to rapid dose titration and should be considered for patients who have significant hyperglycemia on admission to the intensive care unit.

These advantages are especially desirable in neuro-critical care patients due to the plethora of risk factors for hyperglycemia and hypoglycemia previously discussed. For instance, patients with significant acute medical stress or patients on vasopressors may have transiently elevated insulin requirements that could rapidly reverse upon resolution of stress or discontinuation of vasopressors. These patients may also exhibit impaired perfusion of subcutaneous tissues due to hypotension or vasoconstriction, rendering subcutaneous insulin absorption unreliable. Critically ill patients may also have persistently poor or absent oral caloric intake, increasing the risk for hypoglycemia with a long acting subcutaneous basal insulin such as insulin Glargine or Determir.

There are a variety of intravenous insulin protocols available, which differ by institution. These may include dose titration tables or conventional calculations. In general, the desirable characteristics of an acceptable insulin infusion protocol include

(i) appropriate glycemic targets
(ii) instructions regarding glucose monitoring and dose titration
(iii) determination of dose titration based on glucose reading and the rate of change of glucose (calculated by comparing with the previous glucose reading)
(iv) appropriate measures for prevention and treatment of hypoglycemia
(v) demonstration to be clinically safe and effective [30].

Generally, glucose is monitored every 1 h in patients on intravenous insulin to guide dose titration. This has traditionally been done by use of glucometer though the use of continuous glucose monitoring systems (CGMS) is being studied as a safer and more effective alternative. Once target glucose has been achieved and maintained for few hours, monitoring can be switched to every 2 h depending on the protocol. If enteral/tube feeding is initiated, an increase in the infusion rate is to be expected though the infusion rate tends to stabilize once goal tube feeds have been achieved for several hours [21]. Continuous tube feeding as opposed to bolus feeding is the preferred method of feeding and leads to more predictable insulin dose titration. If tube feeds are interrupted for any reason such as diagnostic testing or procedural reasons, down titration of the infusion rate is usually in order to minimize the risk of hypoglycemia.

For patients with pre-existing type 1 diabetes mellitus, basal insulin coverage is of paramount importance to prevent ketoacidosis particularly in the context of superimposed stress of critical illness. This can be achieved with insulin infusion as discussed above though consideration should be given to initiate the insulin infusion at a lower rate given their tendency for higher insulin sensitivity and wider fluctuations in the glucose readings.

Figure 1 gives an overview of our suggested approach to hyperglycemia in the neuro-critical care setting. Adjustments to this general approach and the target glucose range can be made as deemed clinically appropriate for a patient's medical condition.

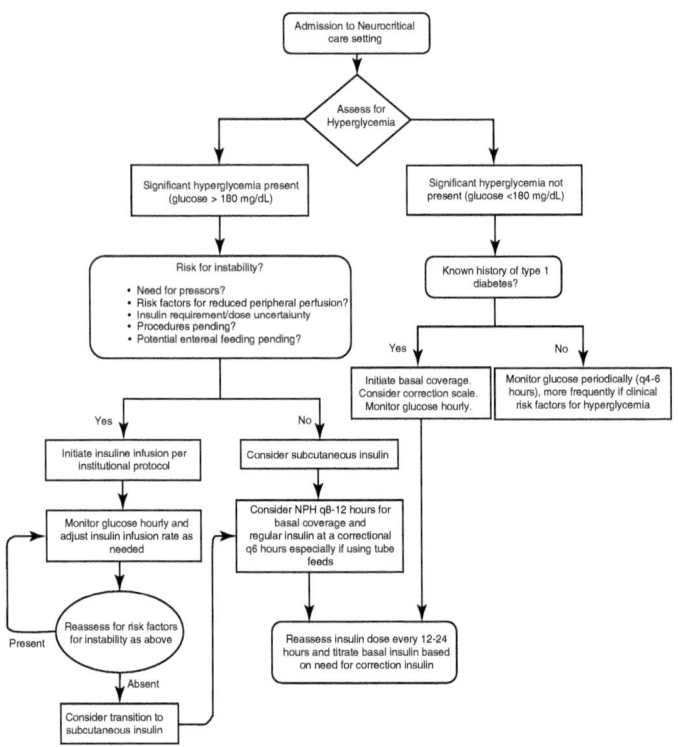

FIGURE 1 Approach to hyperglycemia in the NCCU

The management principles for treatment of diabetic ketoacidosis (DKA) in the NCCU is similar to those in the general population with intravenous insulin, fluid resuscitation and electrolyte replacement being the key components. A more liberal glucose target (typically <250 mg/dL) may be initially appropriate until the ketoacidosis is resolved and the anion gap normalizes. It is common practice to switch intravenous fluids to dextrose containing fluids (e.g. D5/0.45% NS) once blood glucose reaches 200–250 mg/dL. This ensures delivery of adequate amounts of insulin to help normalize the anion gap while minimizing the risk of hypoglycemia. Potassium level should be monitored closely (every 2–4 h) and replaced as necessary. Once anion gap is closed, hyperglycemia and hypovolemia corrected, a switch to the more commonly employed critical care glucose target of 140–180 can be made.

Subcutaneous insulin is the major option for glycemic control in hyperglycemic patients with relatively stable insulin requirements and with good subcutaneous absorption. Dosing of subcutaneous insulin can be determined by a variety of methods. For patients on insulin infusion, a calculation for the total daily dose can be made from the insulin infusion. Typically, 80% of the total daily dose of intravenous insulin is used as the total daily dose of subcutaneous insulin. This can be subdivided into basal and bolus insulin. For subcutaneous insulin, use of short or intermediate acting insulin analogues such as Aspart, Lispro or Neutral Protamine Hagedorn (NPH) is preferred over use of long acting insulin analogs such as Glargine, Determir or Degludec. For patients with pre-existing diabetes on insulin therapy, outpatient doses can be used to estimate total daily insulin requirements, although many patients have decreased oral intake and improved insulin adherence in the hospital setting compared to baseline and dose should be reduced by approximately 25–30% to minimize the risk of hypoglycemia. For patients requiring insulin therapy who were not on insulin therapy at baseline or have not been treated with insulin infusion, total daily dose can be estimated by using an approximation of 0.3 to 0.5 units per kilogram of body weight, depending on degree of estimated insulin resistance. Patients receiving glucocorticoid therapy may require an increased amount of prandial/bolus insulin compared to the basal dose given the mechanism of hyperglycemia as we had previously discussed.

Basal insulin may be initially given in the form of intermediate acting insulin such as NPH at 8–12 h intervals. Many institutions employ NPH insulin every 8–12 h as basal insulin for patients who do not require intravenous insulin but who may experience fluctuating or uncertain basal insulin requirements. The increased frequency of dosing has the benefit of allowing more frequent dose titration to rapidly address

Table 1 Pharmacokinetic characteristics for commonly used types of subcutaneous insulin

Type of insulin	Onset of action	Peak effect	Duration of action
Regular	15–30 min	2–3 h	6–8 h
Lispro, Aspart	5–15 min	60–90 min	3–4 h
NPH	2 h	6–8 h	8–16 h
Glargine	2 h	No peak	20–24 h
Degludec	2 h	No peak	>40 h

hyperglycemia or hypoglycemia in patients whose exact requirements are unclear or changing rapidly with their clinical condition. If a longer acting insulin analogue (Glargine, Determir, Degludec) is to be used for basal coverage, reduced dosing at 12 h intervals as opposed to once a day dosing may be prudent to minimize risk of hypoglycemia. Table 1 summarizes the pharmacokinetic properties for commonly used types of insulin.

In the case of patients receiving continuous enteral/tube feeds, various methods can be used to address the associated hyperglycemia. In patients being treated with insulin infusion, an increase in the infusion rate is to be anticipated with the initiation of the tube feeds as previously discussed. Once the goal rate of tube feeds is achieved, the infusion rate tends to stabilize at a new higher rate. For patients being treated with subcutaneous insulin, management of hyperglycemia associated with tube feeding may be more challenging. Use of various methods has been advocated in this setting. Basal insulin together with correctional regular insulin dosed every 4 to 6 h has been shown to be effective [32] although this may carry a higher risk for hypoglycemia, especially in the event of withdrawal of enteral nutrition. This, however, can be ameliorated by promptly starting dextrose-containing fluids in the case of interruption in enteral nutrition. A proportion of the additional dose needed on the correctional scale can then be added to the basal insulin dose. Again, use of NPH at 8–12 h intervals may provide a bigger margin of safety when compared with longer acting insulin analogues.

As an alternative method, approximately one third of total daily insulin could be given as basal insulin with the remainder given every 4 to 6 h as scheduled doses of fixed dose regular insulin with additional correction factor [33]. This has the benefit of improved flexibility and potentially decreased risk of hypoglycemia.

References

1. Falciglia M, Freyberg RW, Almenoff PL, D'Alessio DA, Render ML. Hyperglycemia-related mortality in critically ill patients varies with admission diagnosis. Crit Care Med. 2009;37(12):3001–9. https://doi.org/10.1097/CCM.0b013e3181b083f7.
2. Krinsley JS. Association between hyperglycemia and increased hospital mortality in a heterogeneous population of critically ill patients. Mayo Clin Proc. 2003;78(12):1471–8. https://doi.org/10.4065/78.12.1471.
3. NICE-SUGAR Study Investigators, Finfer S, Chittock DR, et al. Intensive versus conventional glucose control in critically ill patients. N Engl J Med. 2009;360(13):1283–97. https://doi.org/10.1056/NEJMoa0810625.
4. Brunkhorst FM, Engel C, Bloos F, et al. Intensive insulin therapy and pentastarch resuscitation in severe sepsis. N Engl J Med. 2008;358(2):125–39. https://doi.org/10.1056/NEJMoa070716.
5. American Diabetes Association. Diabetes care in the hospital: standards of medical care in diabetes—2020. Diabetes Care. 2020;43(Supplement 1):S193–202. https://doi.org/10.2337/dc20-S015.
6. Qaseem A, Chou R, Humphrey LL, Shekelle P, Clinical Guidelines Committee of the American College of Physicians. Inpatient glycemic control: best practice advice from the Clinical Guidelines Committee of the American College of Physicians. Am J Med Qual. 2014;29(2):95–8. https://doi.org/10.1177/1062860613489339.
7. Jacobi J, Bircher N, Krinsley J, et al. Guidelines for the use of an insulin infusion for the management of hyperglycemia in critically ill patients. Crit Care Med. 2012;40(12):3251–76. https://doi.org/10.1097/CCM.0b013e3182653269.

8. Dienel GA. Brain glucose metabolism: integration of energetics with function. Physiol Rev. 2019;99(1):949–1045. https://doi.org/10.1152/physrev.00062.2017.
9. Mueckler M, Thorens B. The SLC2 (GLUT) family of membrane transporters. Mol Asp Med. 2013;34(2–3):121–38. https://doi.org/10.1016/j.mam.2012.07.001.
10. Patching SG. Glucose transporters at the blood-brain barrier: function, regulation and gateways for drug delivery. Mol Neurobiol. 2017;54(2):1046–77. https://doi.org/10.1007/s12035-015-9672-6.
11. Simpson IA, Dwyer D, Malide D, Moley KH, Travis A, Vannucci SJ. The facilitative glucose transporter GLUT3: 20 years of distinction. Am J Physiol Endocrinol Metab. 2008;295(2):E242–53. https://doi.org/10.1152/ajpendo.90388.2008.
12. Bergsneider M, Hovda DA, Shalmon E, et al. Cerebral hyperglycolysis following severe traumatic brain injury in humans: a positron emission tomography study. J Neurosurg. 1997;86(2):241–51. https://doi.org/10.3171/jns.1997.86.2.0241.
13. Hou WK, Xian YX, Zhang L, et al. Influence of blood glucose on the expression of glucose trans-porter proteins 1 and 3 in the brain of diabetic rats. Chin Med J. 2007;120(19):1704–9.
14. Pardridge WM, Triguero D, Farrell CR. Downregulation of blood-brain barrier glucose transporter in experimental diabetes. Diabetes. 1990;39(9):1040–4. https://doi.org/10.2337/diab.39.9.1040.
15. Simpson IA, Appel NM, Hokari M, et al. Blood-brain barrier glucose transporter: effects of hypo- and hyperglycemia revisited. J Neurochem. 1999;72(1):238–47. https://doi.org/10.1046/j.1471-4159.1999.0720238.x.
16. McCall AL, Van Bueren AM, Nipper V, Moholt-Siebert M, Downes H, Lessov N. Forebrain ischemia increases GLUT1 protein in brain microvessels and parenchyma. J Cereb Blood Flow Metab. 1996;16(1):69–76. https://doi.org/10.1097/00004647-199601000-00008.
17. Benarroch EE. Brain glucose transporters: implications for neurologic disease. Neurology. 2014;82(15):1374–9. https://doi.org/10.1212/WNL.0000000000000328.
18. Boyle PJ, Schwartz NS, Shah SD, Clutter WE, Cryer PE. Plasma glucose concentrations at the onset of hypoglycemic symptoms in patients with poorly controlled diabetes and in nondiabetics. N Engl J Med. 1988;318(23):1487–92. https://doi.org/10.1056/NEJM198806093182302.

19. Amiel SA, Sherwin RS, Simonson DC, Tamborlane WV. Effect of intensive insulin therapy on glycemic thresholds for counter-regulatory hormone release. Diabetes. 1988;37(7):901–7. https://doi.org/10.2337/diab.37.7.901.
20. Korytkowski MT, Salata RJ, Koerbel GL, et al. Insulin therapy and glycemic control in hospitalized patients with diabetes during enteral nutrition therapy: a randomized controlled clinical trial. Diabetes Care. 2009;32(4):594–6. https://doi.org/10.2337/dc08-1436.
21. Pancorbo-Hidalgo PL, García-Fernandez FP, Ramírez-Pérez C. Complications associated with enteral nutrition by nasogastric tube in an internal medicine unit. J Clin Nurs. 2001;10(4):482–90. https://doi.org/10.1046/j.1365-2702.2001.00498.x.
22. Stoll B, Puiman PJ, Cui L, et al. Continuous parenteral and enteral nutrition induces metabolic dysfunction in neonatal pigs. JPEN J Parenter Enteral Nutr. 2012;36(5):538–50. https://doi.org/10.1177/0148607112444756.
23. Scaroni C, Zilio M, Foti M, Boscaro M. Glucose metabolism abnormalities in Cushing syndrome: from molecular basis to clinical management. Endocr Rev. 2017;38(3):189–219. https://doi.org/10.1210/er.2016-1105.
24. Philipson LH. beta-Agonists and metabolism. J Allergy Clin Immunol. 2002;110(6 Suppl):S313–7. https://doi.org/10.1067/mai.2002.129702.
25. Barth E, Albuszies G, Baumgart K, et al. Glucose metabolism and catecholamines. Crit Care Med. 2007;35(9 Suppl):S508–18. https://doi.org/10.1097/01.CCM.0000278047.06965.20.
26. Turchin A, Matheny ME, Shubina M, Scanlon JV, Greenwood B, Pendergrass ML. Hypoglycemia and clinical outcomes in patients with diabetes hospitalized in the general ward. Diabetes Care. 2009;32(7):1153–7. https://doi.org/10.2337/dc08-2127.
27. McCrimmon RJ, Sherwin RS. Hypoglycemia in type 1 diabetes. Diabetes. 2010;59(10):2333–9. https://doi.org/10.2337/db10-0103.
28. Smiley D, Umpierrez GE. Management of hyperglycemia in hospitalized patients. Ann N Y Acad Sci. 2010;1212:1–11. https://doi.org/10.1111/j.1749-6632.2010.05805.x.
29. Skjaervold NK, Lyng O, Spigset O, Aadahl P. Pharmacology of intravenous insulin administration: implications for future closed-loop glycemic control by the intravenous/intravenous route. Diabetes Technol Ther. 2012;14(1):23–9. https://doi.org/10.1089/dia.2011.0118.

30. Kelly JL. Continuous insulin infusion: when, where, and how? Diabetes Spectr. 2014;27(3):218–23. https://doi.org/10.2337/diaspect.27.3.218.
31. Kramer AH, Roberts DJ, Zygun DA. Optimal glycemic control in neurocritical care patients: a systematic review and meta-analysis. Crit Care. 2012;16(5):R203. Published 2012 Oct 22. https://doi.org/10.1186/cc11812.
32. Gosmanov AR, Umpierrez GE. Management of hyperglycemia during enteral and parenteral nutrition therapy. Curr Diab Rep. 2013;13(1):155–62. https://doi.org/10.1007/s11892-012-0335-y.
33. Mabrey ME, Barton AB, Corsino L, et al. Managing hyperglycemia and diabetes in patients receiving enteral feedings: a health system approach [published correction appears in Hosp Pract (1995). 2015;43(5):308]. Hosp Pract (1995). 2015;43(2):74–8. https://doi.org/10.1080/21548331.2015.1022493.

Electrolyte Management

Kathryn E. Qualls and Niraj Arora

1 Introduction

The management of electrolytes remains a cornerstone of care while patients are in the intensive care unit (ICU). Electrolyte derangements may increase morbidity and mortality of these patients [1]. When considering replacement one should consider the following main electrolytes: calcium, magnesium, potassium, phosphorus, and sodium. Reference ranges for the aforementioned electrolytes in adult patients are defined in Table 1. There are many parenteral and enteral products that can be utilized for electrolyte replacement.

K. E. Qualls (✉)
Pharmacy Department, University of Missouri Health Care, Columbia, MO, USA
e-mail: quallske@health.missouri.edu; quallske@umsystem.edu

N. Arora
Department of Neurology- Neurocriticalcare unit, University of Missouri, Columbia, MO, USA
e-mail: arorana@health.missouri.edu

© The Author(s), under exclusive license to Springer Nature Switzerland AG 2022
N. Arora (ed.), *Procedures and Protocols in the Neurocritical Care Unit*, https://doi.org/10.1007/978-3-030-90225-4_26

TABLE 1 Electrolyte reference ranges [2]

Electrolyte	Reference range
Calcium	8.5–10.8 mg/dL (Ionized – 1.1–1.32 mmol/L)
Magnesium	1.5–2.2 mEq/L
Phosphorus	2.6–4.5 mg/dL
Potassium	3.5–5 mEq/L
Sodium	136–145 mEq/L

2 Calcium Management

Aberrations in calcium are common in acutely ill individuals – including hypocalcemia and hypercalcemia. With the severity of disease of these patients variable, the ionized calcium level should be measured for effective evaluation [3]. Normal ionized calcium levels are 1.1 to 1.3 mmol/L. In neurocritical care, the role of calcium cannot be undermined as calcium plays an essential role in the pathophysiology of acute neurological conditions such as stroke, traumatic brain injury and seizures. Hypocalcemia has been associated with coagulopathy leading to intracerebral hemorrhage expansion [4]. The purpose of checking calcium levels in ICU setting is to correct the levels if low levels of calcium are noted as hypocalcemia is a predictor of disease severity and mortality in ICU [5].

Hypocalcemia is defined as an ionized level <1.11 mmol/L. There are two different intravenous products utilized for replacement and they are calcium gluconate and calcium chloride. Calcium chloride is typically utilized in urgent or emergent situations with central venous access secondary to the risk of tissue necrosis [6]. Calcium gluconate is the primary intravenous repletion agent utilized and replacement is shown in Table 2.

Hypercalcemia is defined as an ionized calcium of >1.3 mmol/L. Malignancies and hyperparathyroidism are the cause for most cases of hypercalcemia. Hypercalcemia affects

Table 2 Hypocalcemia management

Serum ionized calcium (mmol/L)	Replacement dose and route	Laboratory evaluation
>1.11	No replacement needed	AM Labs
1.05–1.11	1 gram calcium gluconate IV	AM Labs
0.99–1.04	2 grams calcium gluconate IV	4 h after replacement
0.93–0.98	3 grams calcium gluconate IV	4 h after replacement
<0.93	4 grams calcium gluconate IV	4 h after replacement

many different systems in the body including neuromuscular, gastrointestinal, renal, cardiovascular and skeletal [6]. Treatment to lower calcium should happen if patients are symptomatic. This can be achieved with intravenous fluids, pharmacological agents, and/or hemodialysis. Pharmacological agents for hypercalcemia treatment include calcitonin, pamidronate, zoledronate, and cinacalcet [7, 8].

3 Magnesium Management

Magnesium is utilized throughout the human body, as it is a cofactor in reactions powered by adenosine triphosphate [7]. Normal magnesium levels are 1.5–2.2 mg/dL. Hypomagnesemia occurs in many patients with neurological injuries and can be associated with delayed cerebral ischemia [6]. The treatment for magnesium levels that are outside the normal range should be corrected and maintained throughout hospitalization.

Hypomagnesemia is defined as a serum magnesium level <2 mg/dL. Hypomagnesemia is commonly recognized when patients are also deficient in potassium, calcium and/or phosphorus as many of these present together. Magnesium should

TABLE 3 Hypomagnesemia treatment

Serum magnesium (mg/dL)	Replacement dose and route	Laboratory evaluation
>2	No replacement needed	AM Labs
1.5–2	2 grams IV	4 h after replacement
<1.5	4 grams IV	4 h after replacement

be given in these instances to ensure appropriate response to other electrolyte repletion. Replacement doses are described in Table 3.

Hypermagnesemia is defined as a magnesium level >5 mg/dL. As the magnesium level increases, so does the severity of complications associated with hypermagnesemia; these can include drowsiness, bradycardia, muscle flaccidity, respiratory depression, and QT prolongation [7]. Hypermagnesemia is rare but should be considered in life threatening instances. Common treatments include discontinuing sources of parenteral/enteral magnesium, intravenous fluids, and hemodialysis [6].

4 Phosphorus Management

Phosphorus homeostasis is almost exclusively maintained by the kidneys; while the main use of phosphorus in the body is for the formation of bone and teeth it also serves as a component of adenosine triphosphate (ATP) [2, 7]. Energy storage and metabolism are key functions of ATP and utilized through many different organ systems thus giving rise to why phosphorus is so vital. Normal phosphorus levels are 2.6–4.5 mg/dL and should be evaluated throughout the duration of the hospitalization [2].

Hypophosphatemia is defined as a phosphorus level of <3 mg/dL. Severe hypophosphatemia with a level of <1 mg/

dL gives rise to central nervous signs and symptoms including but not limited to generalized weakness, encephalopathy, seizures and peripheral neuropathy [6, 7]. When deciding on phosphorus replacement, consideration of the degree of potassium replacement should be evaluated as well. Replacement doses are described in Table 4. Phosphorus products available on the market are included in Tables 5 and 6. Most phosphorus products have an additional electrolyte with them whether that be sodium or potassium.

TABLE 4 Hypophosphatemia management

Serum phosphorus (mg/dL)	Replacement dose and route		Laboratory evaluation
>3	No replacement needed		AM Labs
2.7–3	1 tablets/packets oral/per tube		AM Labs
2.1–2.7	2 tablets/packets oral/per tube	15 mmol IV	AM Labs
1.5–2	2 tablets/packets oral/per tube q4h for 2 doses	30 mmol IV	4 h after replacement
<1.5	45 mmol IV		2 h after replacement

TABLE 5 Enteral phosphorus products [9]

Enteral product	Phosphorus content (mmol)	Potassium content (mEq)	Sodium content (mEq)
Phosphorus tablet (KPhos neutral)	8	1.1	12
Phosphate-potassium packet (Phos-NaK powder)	8	7.1	7.1

TABLE 6 Intravenous phosphorus products [10, 11]

Intravenous product	Product content
Potassium phosphorus	For every 3 mmol of Phosphorus, there are 4.4 mEq of Potassium
Sodium phosphorus	For every 3 mmol of Phosphorus, there are 4 mEq of Sodium

Hyperphosphatemia is defined as a phosphorus level of >4.5 mg/dL. The most common cause of hyperphosphatemia is renal insufficiency -- whether this be acute or chronic [6]. Treatment includes phosphate binders, intravenous fluids and renal replacement therapy. Several phosphate binders are currently available for use but are typically not utilized in critically ill patients.

5 Potassium Management

The most common cation in the body is potassium and is stored intracellularly as well as extracellularly [7]. Normal potassium levels are 3.5–5 mEq/L [2]. When looking at the epidemiology of potassium derangements, several etiologies should be considered; these include decreased or increased potassium intake, cellular shifts, and increased or decreased potassium loss [6]. Potassium plays a major role in the resting membrane potential and changes in concentrations can affect cardiac, neural, and muscular tissues [7].

Hypokalemia is defined as potassium of <3.5 mEq/L. The major presenting factor with hypokalemia is a cardiac arrhythmia or abnormality [6]. Other symptoms associated with hypokalemia include fatigue, myalgia, hepatic encephalopathy, and constipation. Table 7 describes replacement options for potassium as well as next steps in laboratory monitoring and evaluation.

Hyperkalemia is commonly defined as a potassium of >5.5 mEq/L and is associated with cardiac abnormalities, muscle weakness or paralysis. Renal dysfunction and failure are the most common etiologies of hyperkalemia [7].

Table 7 Hypokalemia management

Serum potassium (mEq/L)	Replacement dose and route	Laboratory evaluation
>3.9	No replacement needed	AM Labs
3.6–3.9	20 mEq IV or PO	AM Labs
3.2–3.5	40 mEq IV or PO	4 h after replacement
2.8–3.1	60 mEq IV or PO	4 h after replacement
<2.7	80 mEq IV Only	2 h after replacement

Table 8 Hyperkalemia management

Mechanism of action	Prescribed methods for treatment of hyperkalemia
Potassium shift intracellularly	10 units regular insulin IV and 1 amp of D50W 10 mg albuterol nebulizer treatment
Potassium excretion	Furosemide 40 mg IV Hemodialysis Potassium Binders

Table 9 Potassium binders [12–14]

Potassium binder	Dose	Onset of action
Sodium Polystyrene Sulfate	Oral: 15 grams up to four times per day Rectal: 30 grams every 6 h	2–6 h
Patiromer	Oral: 8.4 grams daily	7 h
Sodium Zirconium Cyclosilicate	Oral: 10 grams three times per day for 48 h; maintenance of 10 grams daily	1 h

Treatment options for hyperkalemia are outlined in Tables 8 and 9. One notable electrocardiography change is the peak T waves that can be associated with hyperkalemia [12]. Prior to hyperkalemia treatment, administration of calcium intravenously is recommended to stabilize the myocardium [7].

6 Sodium Management

Sodium for many clinicians is the most important cation when looking at the management of a variety of disease states in the neurocritical care unit (NCCU). Sodium is a vital player in the regulation of volume throughout the body [7] and a great agent to utilize for elevated intracranial pressure management. Hyponatremia and hypernatremia will be discussed further with focus on the neurological injury spectrum.

Hyponatremia is defined as a sodium of <130 mEq/L with a critical level necessitating immediate attention of <120 mEq/L. The two most common etiologies of hyponatremia include cerebral salt wasting syndrome (CSWS) and syndrome of inappropriate antidiuretic hormone (SIADH). Neurological injuries that have the potential to have hyponatremia as side effects include the following: central nervous system infections, stroke, subarachnoid hemorrhage, traumatic brain injury, transsphenoidal pituitary surgery and other intracranial malignancies [6]. The clinical features of CSW and SIADH are described in Table 10.

The calculation for FE_{urate} is shown below [15]:

$$FE_{urate} = \frac{\text{Urine Uric acid} \times \text{Serum creatinine}}{\text{Serum Uric acid} \times \text{Urine creatinine}} \times 100$$

Laboratory testing to consider for diagnosis are described below:

1. Serum sodium: 135–145 mEq/L
2. Urine Osmolality: 50–1200 mOsm/kg (average: 500–850 mOsm/kg water)
3. Plasma osmolarity: 275–290 mOsm/Kg
4. Urine sodium: up to 20 mEq/L (40–220 mEq/day)
5. Serum Glucose: 70–140 mg/dL

TABLE 10 Clinical features of SIADH and CSWS

Clinical feature	SIADH	CSWS
Volume status	Euvolemic/hypervolemic	Hypovolemic
FE_{urate} relation to Serum Na [15]	Correction of hyponatremia normalize FE_{urate} to 4–11%	Correction of hyponatremia leads to persistent elevated FE_{urate}
Treatment	Fluid restriction, hypertonic saline, demeclocycline, furosemide	Normal saline, hypertonic saline, fludrocortisone

It is essential to first identify the triggering factors for hyponatremia and have a systematic approach before considering the treatment (Fig. 1). In most cases in NCCU, treatment with salt tablets, hypertonic saline solution or fludrocortisone can be considered unless dealing with hypervolemic hyponatremia where the treatment of the underlying disorder is a must. Medications are described further in Tables 11, 12, and 13.

Hypernatremia is defined as a sodium of >145 mEq/L. This is typically seen in patients with diabetes insipidus and after the treatment with hypertonic saline in the NCCU [6]. Other etiologies can include medication induced, inappropriate dietary intake, or fluid loss. Diabetes insipidus is defined as a deficiency in plasma antidiuretic hormone and produces the inability to conserve free water.

The treatment of hypernatremia usually necessitates eliciting appropriate history before undergoing treatment. Figure 2 describes an approach to the diagnosis and management of hypernatremia. Diagnosis of diabetes insipidus requires due vigilance in considering history of increased thirst, recording of intake and output, trends of rising sodium before treatment with desmopressin (Table 14) is considered. Though there is no protocolized approach for treatment of diabetes insipidus, these patients usually require intravenous or subcu-

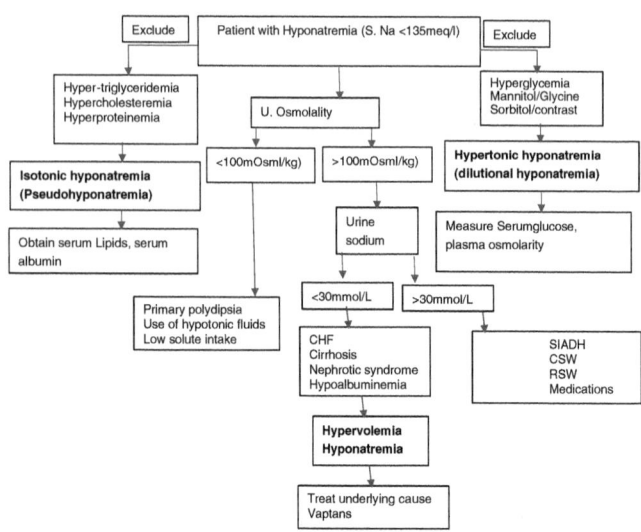

FIGURE 1 Hyponatremia protocol. SIADH Syndrome of inappropriate anti-diuretic hormone, CSW Cerebral salt wasting, RSW Renal salt wasting, CHF Congestive Heart Failure

TABLE 11 Medications for the treatment of SIADH [16, 20]

Medication	Mechanism of action	Dose
Demeclocycline	Inhibition of antidiuretic hormone activity	300 mg every 12 h; max of 1200 mg/day
Salt tablets	Sodium supplementation	1–2 g every 8 h; max of 16 g/day 1 g = 17.1 mEq of sodium

TABLE 12 Medications for the treatment of CSWS [17]

Medication	Mechanism of action	Dose
Fludricortisone	Increased reabsorption of sodium from renal distal tubules	0.1 mg daily; max of 0.4 mg/day

TABLE 13 Sodium chloride concentrations [18]

Hypertonic saline concentration (%)	Osmolality (mOsm/L)
0.9	308
1.5	513
3	1026
23.4	8008

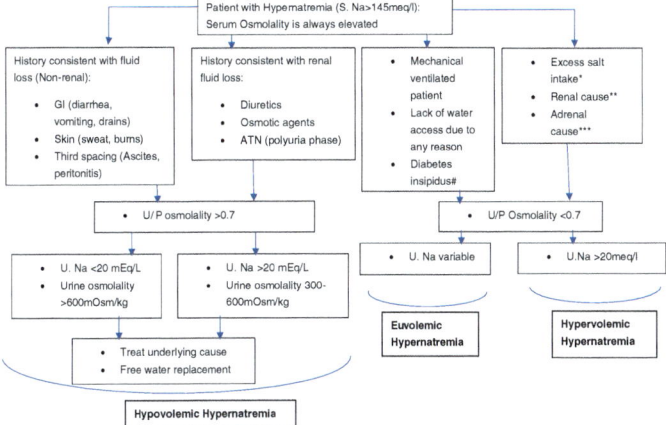

FIGURE 2 Approach to hypernatremia. U Urine, P Plasma, ATN Acute tubular necrosis, * Hypertonic saline infusions, high salt infusions, ** Primary aldosteronism: Look for HTN and hypokalemia, *** Cushing's syndrome, # Central or nephrogenic

TABLE 14 Medications for the treatment of hypernatremia [19, 21]

Medication	Mechanism of action	Dose
Desmopressin	Increases cyclic adenosine monophosphate in renal tubular cells	0.25–1 mcg IV or SC every 12–24 h

taneous desmopressin initially before oral/intranasal desmopressin is considered. In most cases, DI resolves by itself in a few days to weeks and the patient does not require long term medication management.

7 Summary

Electrolyte management in the NCCU is a learned skill and one that providers should understand and implement ways to ensure appropriate management is completed. There are a variety of mechanisms by which to adjust electrolytes to obtain optimal serum levels. While electrolyte management can be tedious, it can be lifesaving in patients admitted to the NCCU.

References

1. Lee JW. Fluid and electrolyte disturbances in critically ill patients. Electrolyte Blood Press. 2010;8(2):72–81.
2. Schmidt J, Wieczorkiewicz J. Interpreting laboratory data: a point-of-care guide. Bethesda: American Society of Health-System Pharmacists; 2012. p. 33, 98, 118, 123, 140, 141.
3. French S, Subauste J, Geraci S. Calcium abnormalities in hospitalized patients. South Med J. 2012;105(4):231–7.
4. Morotti A, Charidimou A, Phuah CL, Jessel MJ, Schwab K, Ayres AM, et al. Association between serum calcium level and extent of bleeding in patients with intracerebral hemorrhage. JAMA Neurol. 2016;73(11):1285–90.
5. Sanaie S, Mahmoodpoor A, Hamishehkar H, Shadvar K, Salimi N, Montazer M, et al. Association between disease severity and calcium concentration in critically ill patients admitted to intensive care unit. Anesth Pain Med. 2018;8(1):e57583.
6. Medenwald B, Halstead M, Suarez JI. Acid-base and electrolyte disturbances. In: Darsie ME, Mohett AM, editors. The Pocket Guide to Neurocritical Care: a concise reference for the evaluation and management of neurologic emergencies. Neurocritical Care Society; 2020. p. 184–203.

7. McEvoy C, Murray PT. Electrolyte disorders in critical care. In: Hall JB, Schmidt GA, Kress JP, editors. Principles of critical care. 4th ed. McGraw-Hill; 2015. Accessed 21 Oct 2020.
8. Maier JD, Levine SN. Hypercalcemia in the intensive care unit: a review of pathophysiology, diagnosis, and modern therapy. J Intensive Care Med. 2015;30(5):235–52.
9. Potassium phosphate and sodium phosphate. In: Specific Lexicomp Online Database [database on the Internet]. Hudson: Lexicomp Inc.; 2021. [updated 29 Dec 2020; cited 15 Feb 2021].
10. Potassium phosphate. In: Specific Lexicomp Online Database [database on the Internet]. Hudson: Lexicomp Inc.; 2021. [updated 13 Dec 2020; cited 15 Feb 2021].
11. Sodium phosphate. In: Specific Lexicomp Online Database [database on the Internet]. Hudson: Lexicomp Inc.; 2021 [updated 26 Feb 2021; cited 28 Feb 2021]. Levis JT. ECG diagnosis: hyperkalemia. Perm J. 2013;17(1):69. https://doi.org/10.7812/TPP/12-088.
12. Sodium polystyrene sulfonate. In: Specific Lexicomp Online Database [database on the Internet]. Hudson: Lexicomp Inc.; 2021 [updated 2 Feb 2021; cited 28 Feb 2021].
13. Patiromer. In: Specific Lexicomp Online Database [database on the Internet]. Hudson: Lexicomp Inc.; 2021 [updated 26 Feb 2021; cited 28 Feb 2021].
14. Sodium Zirconium Cyclosilicate. In: Specific Lexicomp Online Database [database on the Internet]. Hudson: Lexicomp Inc.; 2021 [updated 2 Feb 2021; cited 28 Feb 2021].
15. Maesaka JK, Imbriano LJ, Miyawaki N. Determining fractional urate excretion rates in hyponatremic conditions and improved methods to distinguish cerebral/renal salt wasting from the syndrome of inappropriate secretion of antidiuretic hormone. Front Med (Lausanne). 2018;5:319.
16. Demeclocycline. In: Specific Lexicomp Online Database [database on the Internet]. Hudson: Lexicomp Inc.; 2021 [updated 17 Mar 2021; cited 20 Mar 2021].
17. Fludricortisone. In: Specific Lexicomp Online Database [database on the Internet]. Hudson: Lexicomp Inc.; 2021 [updated 5 Feb 2021; cited 20 Mar 2021].
18. Sodium chloride. In: Specific Lexicomp Online Database [database on the Internet]. Hudson: Lexicomp Inc.; 2021 [updated 26 Mar 2021; cited 26 Mar 2021].

19. Desmopressin. In: Specific Lexicomp Online Database [database on the Internet]. Hudson: Lexicomp Inc.; 2021 [updated 26 Mar 2021; cited 26 Mar 2021].
20. Braun MM, Barstow CH, Pyzocha NJ. Diagnosis and management of sodium disorders: hyponatremia and hypernatremia. Am Fam Physician. 2015;91(5):299–307.
21. Broch Porcar MJ, Rodríguez Cubillo B, Domínguez-Roldán JM, et al. Practical document on the management of hyponatremia in critically ill patients. Med Intensiva (Engl Ed). 2019;43(5):302–16. English, Spanish.

Plasmapheresis

Zeeshan Azeem, Angela Emanuel, and Kunal Malhotra

1 Introduction

Apheresis is derived from the Greek word "Aphairesis"– to take away by force [1]. The term Plasmapheresis was coined by John J. Abel in 1914 in his report, "Plasma removal with return of the corpuscles(plasmapheresis)" wherein he reported that a large amount of plasma could be collected from an animal if the red blood cells were to be returned [2].

Therapeutic plasma exchange (TPE) is defined by the American Society for Apheresis (ASFA) 2019 guidelines as "A therapeutic procedure in which the blood of the patient is passed through a medical device which separates plasma from the other components of blood". TPE involves plasma removal and replacement with a solution such as a colloid solution (e.g., albumin and/or plasma) or a combination of a crystalloid/colloid solution [3].

From remote history, it has been known to mankind that there are potentially toxic substances called "humors" which accumulate in the blood of critically-ill patients and that the removal of these would be beneficial for patients. Dating back

---

Z. Azeem · A. Emanuel · K. Malhotra (✉)
Karl D Nolph Division of Nephrology, University of Missouri, School of Medicine, Columbia, MO, USA
e-mail: malhotrak@health.missouri.edu

© The Author(s), under exclusive license to Springer Nature Switzerland AG 2022
N. Arora (ed.), *Procedures and Protocols in the Neurocritical Care Unit*, https://doi.org/10.1007/978-3-030-90225-4_27

one thousand years B.C, Bloodletting, the practice of draining blood from sick patients, has been around. The practice of bloodletting peaked in the eighteenth century and as we know, it has tremendously evolved in the last 5–6 decades [1].

The technique was first introduced as a possible treatment for Guillain-Barré syndrome (GBS) in 1978 and further research over the next few years found it to be significantly beneficial in treatment of GBS. By late 80s, TPE was extensively used as a first line treatment in the acute management of GBS and myasthenic crisis [4].

TPE has emerged as a powerful therapeutic modality in the treatment of autoimmune mediated neurological disorders [5]. Autoimmune neurological conditions are mediated by autoantibodies that cause cellular injury to various components of the nervous system. Majority of the patients present with focal neurological deficits such as motor weakness, hyporeflexia, altered pain perception, stroke and seizures. Delays in initiating appropriate treatment may result in irreversible neurological injuries and permanent impairment of function [1].

2 Basic Nomenclature

Apheresis – A general term for "taking away" a targeted cell type or substance from blood. Apheresis includes plasmapheresis (plasma) and cytapheresis (blood cells).
The term "pheresis," which is a shortened pronunciation (slang) for apheresis, is not used.

Plasmapheresis – A general term used to denote selective removal of plasma. Plasma can be separated from blood using centrifugation or filtration.
Plasmapheresis is mostly used to collect plasma from a healthy blood donor for transfusion (i.e., plasma donation).

Therapeutic apheresis – A general phrase that denotes replacement of plasma with another fluid such as colloid, crystalloid, or allogeneic plasma.
It also implies removal or replacement of abnormal or excessive cells for the purpose of achieving a clinical benefit.

Therapeutic plasma exchange (TPE) – A phrase that was historically used synonymously with "therapeutic apheresis" because in the past only plasma was used as replacement fluid. However, TPE is now applied specifically to procedures that involve replacement solely with plasma.
TPE is also referred to as plasma exchange or therapeutic plasmapheresis and involves removal of patient plasma and replacement with allogeneic or autologous plasma. Plasma removed during plasma exchange must not be used for transfusion to another individual, according to regulations from the US Food and Drug Administration (FDA).

Therapeutic cytapheresis (hemapheresis) – A term used to denote selective removal of abnormal blood cells (e.g., sickled cells [erythrocytapheresis, red blood cell exchange]) or excessive numbers of cells (eg, platelets [thrombocytapheresis], white blood cells [leukocytapheresis]).

Dialysis – A diffusion-based treatment best suited for the removal of fluid or small molecules (e.g., uremic toxins, some drugs) from the blood using a filter. Fluid is removed by filtration (convection); solutes are removed by diffusion.

Plasma filtration – A technique that separates plasma from cellular components with a highly permeable filter (plasma filter) using a dialysis or hemofiltration machine.

3 Indications of Therapeutic Plasma Exchange (Table 1)

Plasma exchange is increasingly being used in neurological settings for the treatment of numerous clinical conditions [6]. Neurological diseases including myasthenia gravis, Guillain Barre' syndrome (GBS) and chronic inflammatory demyelinating polyneuropathy (CIDP) are among the most frequent indications TPE [7]. TPE is also employed in treatment of connective tissue diseases, hematological, nephrological, endocrinological and metabolic disorders [8]. Table1 presents the common indications of TPE based on the clinical utility as recommended by American society for Apheresis (ASFA) Guideline on the Use of Therapeutic Apheresis in Clinical Practice-Evidence-Based Approach [9].

TABLE I Indications of Therapeutic Plasma exchange (TPE) based on the strength of evidence on its clinical utility- American Society for Apheresis (ASFA), 2010

Category I (Apheresis is accepted as first-line therapy)	Category II Apheresis is accepted as second-line therapy)	Category III Role of apheresis therapy is not established. Decision making is individualized
Acute inflammatory demyelinating polyradiculoneuropathy (GBS) Primary treatment	Myasthenia gravis (Chronic, long-term treatment)	Chronic focal encephalitis (Rasmussen encephalitis)
Myasthenia gravis (Acute, short-term treatment)	Multiple sclerosis	Neuromyelitis optica spectrum disorders (NMOSD)
Acute stroke secondary to sickle cell disease	Neuromyelitis optica spectrum disorders (NMOSD)	Paraneoplastic neurologic syndromes as anti-myelin-associated glycoprotein (MAG) neuropathy and multiple myeloma
Stroke prophylaxis in non-acute Sickle cell disease	Acute disseminated encephalomyelitis (ADEM): Steroid refractory	Sudden sensorineural hearing loss
CIDP	Pediatric Autoimmune Neuropsychiatric Disorders Associated with Streptococcal Infections (PANDAS)	Progressive multifocal leukoencephalopathy (PML) associated with natalizumab
		Sydenham's Chorea-severe

3.1 Principles

TPE involves an extracorporeal blood purification method targeted to remove large molecular weight substances from a patient's plasma. Henceforth, the removal of circulating alloantibodies, autoantibodies, cytokines, immune and other inflammatory mediators is believed to be the principal mechanism of action through which TPE renders its benefit [10].

There is a wide array of neurological conditions where pathological production of auto-antibodies have been implicated, such as:

- the antibodies against nicotinic acetylcholine receptor in MG [11]
- antibodies against P/Q-type voltage-gated calcium channels in Lambert-Eaton syndrome [12]
- Anti-Myelin Oligodendrocyte Glycoprotein (MOG) antibodies in MS [13]

Clinical utility of TPE is based on at least one of the following conditions [6]:

- The substance targeted for removal must have a sufficiently long half-life so that extracorporeal removal is more rapid than endogenous clearance pathways.
- The substance to be removed must be acutely toxic and/or resistant to conventional therapy so that the rapid elimination from the extracellular fluid by therapeutic apheresis is indicated.
- The substance to be removed should be sufficiently large, with a molecular weight greater than 15,000 daltons, so that it cannot be easily removed by less expensive purification techniques such as hemofiltration or high-flux hemodialysis.

3.2 Mechanisms of Action

Therapeutic plasma exchange constitutes an extracorporeal blood purification technique designed to remove large molecular weight particles from plasma. The removal of circulating autoantibodies, immune complexes, cytokines, and other inflammatory mediators is thought to be the principal mechanism of action [10].

Clinical benefit from plasma exchange is primarily observed in diseases with a self-limited course, whereas a long-term effect in chronic disorders is less frequently achieved. Furthermore, the intravascular and extravascular distribution of substances that are desired to be removed by plasma exchange has to be considered. Most large molecular weight substances have considerable concentrations in the extravascular space. After removal of the substance in the intravascular space, there may be a rapid substance redistribution into the intravascular space, which usually requires repeated treatments with plasma exchange [10].

Research has shown plasmapheresis can lead to alteration of cellular networks of T cells, plasma cells and macrophages. TPE can mediate an enhanced production of immune cells [14], immunoglobulins [15], suppressor T-cell function [16] and a deviation of cytokine patterns redressing a disturbed T-helper type 1 and T-helper type 2 balance [17].

The rate of removal of substances during TPE is conventionally expressed as a first-order kinetic due to slow equilibration of large molecular weight molecules between the vascular space and the interstitial space. Because of this, it is estimated that the exchange of a single volume of plasma will lower the level of a specific macromolecule by 50% to 60% and 1.4 plasma volumes exchange will lower the levels of target substances by 75%. This explains why complete removal of pathogenic antibodies is nearly impossible to achieve [6].

4 Technique (Fig. 1)

Therapeutic plasma exchange is based on the separation of plasma from the blood's cellular elements. This can be achieved in the following ways:

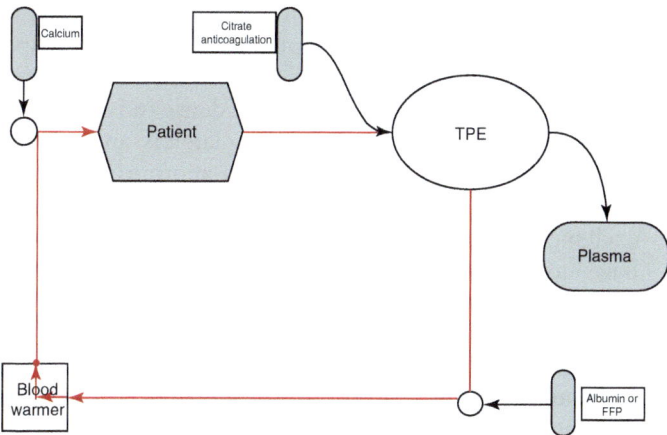

FIGURE 1 Figure presents the simplified circuit of TPE

1. **Membrane Filtration or Membrane plasma separation** (MPS) [18, 19]: Also referred to as mTPE, this technique involves separating blood components based on their particle size. Plasma filter membranes used in TPE typically have pore size of 0.2 μm to 0.5 μm in diameter (which is approximately 30 times the diameter of pores in conventional high-flux hemofilter membranes used in dialysis circuits). This ensures removal of particles up to a molecular weight of 3 million Daltons(D). The size of platelets and red blood cells is between 2 and 3 μm, which corresponds to 10 times the size of a pore. Albumin measures 0.01 μm, which is 30 times smaller than a pore and passes easily through the membrane, as do IgM (0.03 μm) and cryoglobulins (0.1 μm) [19, 20]. Substances that can pass through includes immunoglobulins, immune complexes, complement factors, lipoproteins, and endotoxin [6]. During this process, the patient's plasma leaves the side pores of the membrane filter and is replaced by an appropriate replacement fluid. This requires maintaining an adequate transmembrane pressure to prevent plugging of the pores from cellular components [4]. TPE is also possible using NxStage and Prismaflex continuous renal replacement therapy (CRRT) machines.

2. **Centrifugation:** also referred to as cTPE, this process involves separating blood components based on their specific gravity. The whole blood is pumped into a separation chamber and centrifuged pushing the dense red cells to the periphery, followed by white cells, platelets and plasma. The machine is designed to apply an appropriate *g* force and sensors to detect a state of equilibrium. During this exchange, the patient's plasma is diverted into a collection bag and subsequently replaced with a replacement fluid while other components are returned to the patient [21]. Major differences between the two techniques of TPE are highlighted in Table 2.
3. **Immunoadsorption:** This is a newer modality that allows a more selective removal of circulating antibodies by binding to a ligand resulting in removal of immunoglobulin fractions

TABLE 2 Comparison of the Membrane Filtration and Centrifugation techniques of Therapeutic Plasma Exchange [23]

Characteristic	Membrane Filtration	Centrifugation
Access	Central	Central & peripheral
Blood flow rate(ml/min)	150	10–150
Plasma extraction(ml/min)	30%	Variable
Anticoagulation	Heparin, citrate or none	Citrate
Separation	Size	Specific gravity
Molecular Weight cut off (Dalton: D)	3 million	Not applicable
Replacement Fluid	Fresh Frozen plasma, Albumin	Fresh Frozen plasma, Albumin
Alternative use	Dialysis	Stem cell harvest for possible Bone Marrow transplant

Note: Adapted and modified from Williams and Balogun [23]

[22]. Following adsorption, the plasma and cellular components are combined and reinfused. Adsorption has been utilized in treatment of several neurological disorders, notably Multiple sclerosis (MS) and Myasthenia Gravis (MG) [6].

4.1 Vascular Access for Therapeutic Plasma Exchange

Vascular access is the conduit by which TPE is performed. Blood flow into the device enables the process of centrifugation or membrane filtration to occur. Suboptimal flow may result in a suboptimal procedure, including longer procedural times, decreased efficiency, and the need to abort it before the target plasma volume has been processed [24]. The access options range from a large-bore needle to cannulate the patient's peripheral veins to the use of intravascular or implantable access devices (IVADs), such as arteriovenous (AV) shunts or AV fistulae; central venous catheters (CVCs); and CVCs tunneled with a port (port-CVCs) [24]. Centrifugation based TPE requires blood flow rates that range from 50 to 120 mL/min while membrane-based TPE requires a higher blood flow rate, ranging from 150 to 200 mL/min. Patient's underlying disease and mental status can impact their ability to produce tension, thus enabling blood to enter into the device if peripheral veins are being considered. Vascular anatomy; body habitus; hygiene; hydration; status as an inpatient, outpatient, or critically ill patient; and prior medications also affect the decision. Furthermore, the availability of personnel and resources to obtain vascular access are often important determinants, especially when emergent TPE is needed [24].

Peripheral Veins Peripheral antecubital veins are cannulated using 16- to 18-gauge Teflon or silicone coated dialysis-type steel needles. The maximum blood flow achieved is 80 cc per minute and makes this type of access suitable only for centrifugation techniques [25, 26].

Central Venous Catheters (CVC) Central vein catheters include both nontunneled and tunneled catheters. Nontunneled, semi-rigid catheters are usually made of polyurethane, and are designed for ease of insertion, and have lower thrombogenicity than rigid catheters. They are used for short-term use (usually less that 2 weeks) [27]. Tunneled catheters, which are designed for long-term use (weeks to months), are usually made of silicone and are more biocompatible, flexible and have the least thrombogenicity. Peripherally inserted central catheters (PICC lines) are too small in caliber (4–5 F) to accommodate the negative pressure and blood flow rates required for TPE procedures and should not be used. Catheters should be at least 11.5 F in adults. Catheters are the most common vascular access type used for TPE procedures in North America, South America and Asia [26, 27]. Despite the differences in CVC designs, an advantage of CVCs is that they allow for consistent and adequate flow rates required for apheresis. Complications include catheter occlusion due to thrombosis, infections (localized and systemic), catheter breakage, and embolism [24]. A study evaluating the rate of complications from CVC placement for apheresis procedures in the intensive care unit demonstrated that insertion of CVCs was associated with early and late complications, such as pneumothorax, arterial puncture, and air embolism [26].

AV fistula these are surgically created by direct anastomosis of an artery and a vein and are an appropriate choice for patients who undergo chronic TPE procedures. Common sites for AV fistulae include the radiocephalic or brachiocephalic anastomosis. AV fistulae, which have been used predominantly in hemodialysis (HD), are increasingly being utilized in apheresis. However, according to the WAA and an international registry report, among the different IVADs, AV fistulae were the least commonly used in apheresis, ranging from 2% to 4% of procedures [28, 29]. AV fistulae are often used as the vascular access of choice in patients on HD who also require TPE.

Port-CVCs Ports are tunneled chambers that are implanted under the skin, usually in the subcutaneous tissue of the anterior chest wall, with the distal tip of the attached tubing terminating at the junction of the right atrium and the superior vena cava. This vascular access option should be considered for patients who require long-term TPE procedures. The tubing is made of silicone or polyurethane, and the chamber (cylindrical or funnel-shaped) can be single or double and may be made of titanium, plastic, silicone, or a combination of these materials [24, 30]. The advantages of "ports" are the low rates of infection, potential long-term use, and patient comfort and increased quality of life, because they are able to participate in different types of physical activity, including swimming [24].

4.2 Anticoagulation

To prevent extracorporeal clotting, an anticoagulant is usually added to the patient's blood as it is withdrawn. A buffered dextrose solution containing citrate (acid citrate dextrose [ACD]), which chelates ionized plasma calcium, is the most commonly used anticoagulant for centrifugation apheresis procedures [25]. Unfractionated heparin may also be used, either alone or in combination with ACD. Heparin is the anticoagulant of choice for membrane plasma separation methods. Under special circumstances, a patient may be systemically anticoagulated with heparin, thereby obviating the need for extracorporeal anticoagulation. This latter approach requires careful monitoring and incurs a higher potential risk of bleeding [25]. The half-life of citrate is approximately 30 minutes in patients with normal liver and renal function. Citrate metabolism is severely impaired and plasma ionized calcium levels are significantly reduced in patients with acute hepatic failure undergoing therapeutic plasma exchange [31]. Citrate-induced metabolic alkalosis can develop in patients with renal failure [32]. In contrast to heparin, citrate infusion does not induce an anticoagulant effect in vivo [25]. Symptoms and signs of citrate toxicity include a metallic taste in the mouth, perioral numbness, distal paresthesia, muscle twitching, spasm, nausea, tetany, and prolonged Q-T interval. Hypokalemia and hypomagnesemia may also occur [32, 33]. Albumin replacement fluid does not contain citrate but may lead to hypocalcemia because of avid calcium binding [34]. Therefore, supplemental calcium is often added to albumin return fluid during plasma exchange procedures. Continuous reinfusion of extracorporeal heparin during TPE procedures prolongs the clotting time. Patients at high risk for bleeding or with concerns of heparin sensitivity should undergo apheresis exclusively with ACD. If heparin is required in a patient with a high risk of bleeding, the activated clotting time should be closely monitored. Heparin-induced bleeding may be reversed with protamine [25]. Although the use of anticoagulation in cTPE is essential, mTPE can be performed without the use of anticoagulation. Similar to anticoagulation-free hemodialysis and hemofiltration, the use of saline to prerinse the circuit, higher blood flow rates leading to shorter treatment times and lack of air–blood interface (this being present with the NxStage System One TPE tubing system) can all contribute to simplifying the treatment without the use of anticoagulation [20].

4.3 Replacement Fluids

During TPE, the patient's fluid volume removed must be replaced to prevent marked volume depletion.

While fresh frozen plasma (FFP) is universally used as the RF in thrombotic thrombocytopenic purpura (TTP) as it contains the missing ADAMTS13 enzyme, the von Willebrand factor cleaving enzyme, it carries a small risk for viral transmission and can cause citrate toxicity if used in large volume exchanges. Some patients, who may be pre or post invasive procedures, or with pre-existing coagulopathy, or with current bleeding or increased risk of bleeding due to nonselective removal of coagulation proteins during TPE; may require FFP at the end of procedure to replace coagulation factors and reduce the risk of further blood loss [20].

For most other indications, albumin and/or saline are the replacement fluids of choice. The optimal choice often varies with the clinical setting. Five percent albumin is used for most conditions; saline for hyperviscosity; and some combination of albumin and saline if cost is a consideration. Albumin has no risk of viral transmission and some patients experience pyrogenic reactions but these are rare [35].

5 Prescription of Therapeutic Plasma Exchange

For most conditions in which therapeutic plasma exchange is used, it is considered acceptable to perform 1–1.5 plasma volume exchanges per procedure. Most currently available cell separators can perform one complete volume exchange in 1.5 to 2 hours. The following formula can be used to estimate the plasma volume in an adult [36]:

$$\text{Estimated plasma volume}(\text{in liters}) = 0.07 \times \text{weight}(\text{kg}) \times (1 - \text{hematocrit})$$

The frequency of the procedure depends upon the neurological disease and severity of the condition. Most of the acute neurological conditions require plasma exchange 2–3 times per week till improvement and the frequency is tapered over time depending upon the clinical condition. Average number of procedures required for most acute conditions is 5–7 but varies with the clinical situation [37].

6 Summary of Recommendations for Use of TPE in Neurology Intensive Care

Therapeutic plasma exchange is used in a wide range of acute neurological conditions. Table 3 summarizes the available evidence and ASFA recommendation for use of TPE in acute neurological illnesses.

TABLE 3 Summary of recommendations for therapeutic plasma exchange in neuro-critical care patients

Clinical condition	Evidence	AAN and ASFA Recommendation
GBS/AIDP	A recent Cochrane found moderate quality evidence showing significantly more improvement with plasma exchange than with supportive care alone, without a significant increase in serious adverse events [38].	Plasma exchange in Guillain–Barré syndrome and AIDP as an established and effective treatment with a strong level of evidence [37, 39].
CIDP	Moderate- high quality evidence showing that plasma exchange gave short-term improvement in disability and nerve function. However, plasma exchange may be followed by rapid deterioration, with requiring maintenance plasma exchange [40].	Plasma exchange is effective in CIDP and can be offered as a first line agent, where indicated, with strong level of evidence [37, 39].
MG	Proven efficacy for acute state but insufficient evidence to prove long term efficacy of plasmapheresis in MG [41].	Randomized studies have proven the clinical effectiveness of plasma exchange in moderate-to-severe myasthenia gravis and for pre-thymectomy patients [37, 39].

Table 3 (continued)

Clinical condition	Evidence	AAN and ASFA Recommendation
MS	MS patients with acute fulminating disease and antibodies to MOG responded to plasma exchange [4].	Plasma exchange is probably effective as an adjuvant treatment for severe relapsing forms of multiple sclerosis and in corticosteroid-unresponsive fulminant forms; however, it is unlikely to be effective in progressive forms [37, 39].
NMOSD	First-line therapy with plasma exchange may be superior to high-dose corticosteroid pulse therapy in achieving complete remission in transverse myelitis but not in optic neuritis. Escalation therapy with plasma exchange increases remission [42].	Plasma exchange is probably effective in corticosteroid-refractory acute attacks but probably ineffective as a maintenance therapy [37, 39].
Autoimmune encephalitis	When used in combination with corticosteroids and immunoglobulins may expedite remission [4].	Plasma exchange is probably effective in autoimmune encephalitis as the titers of LGI1 and CASPR2 autoantibodies decrease with plasma exchange and this is associated with clinical improvement [37].

ASFA American Society for Apheresis; *AAN* American Association of Neurologists; *ADEM* acute disseminated encephalomyelitis; *CIDP* chronic inflammatory demyelinating polyneuropathy; *NMOSD* neuromyelitis optica spectrum disorders

7 Complications and Monitoring

Plasma exchange is generally considered a safe procedure. Various studies have suggested the risk of complications as high as 40% but the risk of life threatening complications is quoted as 0.025% to 4.75% [43].

The common complications that can occur during or post-plasma exchange procedure are shown in Table 4.

TABLE 4 Complications of Therapeutic plasma exchange [43, 45]

	Complication	Clinical Features
Vascular access related	Hemorrhage	Hypotension, pallor, tachycardia
	Infection / sepsis	Fever, hypotension, tachycardia
	Pneumothorax	Shortness of breath, pain, hypotension
Anticoagulation related	Citrate induced hypocalcemia	Perioral or distal tingling, paresthesia
	Depletion coagulopathy	
	Thrombocytopenia	
	Anemia	Pallor, dyspnea, weakness
	Thrombosis	
Infection	Depletion of immunoglobulin	
	Viral transmission from replacement fluid	
Reaction to replacement fluids	Anaphylactoid reactions	Fever, rigors, urticaria, wheezing, hypotension, laryngospasm

TABLE 4 (continued)

	Complication	Clinical Features
	Reactions associated with ACE inhibitors	
Electrolyte abnormalities	Hypokalemia	Cramps, arrythmias
	Alkalosis	
	Hypocalcemia and hypercalcemia	
Other	Apneic events	
	Complement mediated membrane bio-incompatibility	Hypotension, dyspnea and chest pain
	Chills and hypothermia due to inadequately warmed replacement fluid	
	Drug removal	
	Cardiac arrythmias	
	Pulmonary edema	
	Transfusion related lung injury	
	Vitamin removal	

Clinical parameters such as vital signs every 15 minutes and signs and symptoms of hypocalcemia (numbness or tingling of the fingers, nose, or tongue) and allergic reaction should be monitored before, during and after the procedure.

Laboratory parameters including complete blood count, comprehensive metabolic panel (potassium and ionized calcium), coagulation studies, disease specific parameters such as antibody levels should be conducted before and after each procedure [44].

8 Contraindications

Therapeutic plasma exchange is a relatively safe procedures, however, it is contraindicated in following conditions [45]:

- Active infection
- Non availability of central line or large bore peripheral lines
- ACE inhibitor treatment in last 24 hours
- Hemodynamic instability
- Allergy to fresh frozen plasma or albumin
- Allergy to heparin, if heparin is the only option for anticoagulation.
- Hypocalcemia- relative contraindication.

9 Conclusion

Therapeutic Plasma exchange is an effective modality for a wide range of acute and chronic neurological diseases mediated by autoantibodies. It is increasingly being used in the clinical conditions where rapid removal of autoantibodies is critical to improve outcome. Further research is needed to strengthen the evidence for its use in a wider range of acute neurological conditions. Programs must consider all available options and have resources to arrange for urgent TPE in ICU setting for safe and effective treatments.

References

1. Nguyen TC, Kiss JE, Goldman JR, Carcillo JA. The role of plasmapheresis in critical illness. Crit Care Clin. 2012;28(3):453–68, vii.
2. Kambic HE, Nosé Y. Historical perspective on plasmapheresis. Ther Apher. 1997;1(1):83–108.
3. Padmanabhan A, Connelly-Smith L, Aqui N, Balogun RA, Klingel R, Meyer E, et al. Guidelines on the use of therapeutic Apheresis in clinical practice - evidence-based approach from the writing Committee of the American Society for Apheresis: the eighth special issue. J Clin Apher. 2019;34(3):171–354.

4. Osman C, Jennings R, El-Ghariani K, Pinto A. Plasma exchange in neurological disease. Pract Neurol. 2020;20(2):92–9.
5. Tombak A, Uçar MA, Akdeniz A, Yilmaz A, Kaleagası H, Sungur MA, et al. Therapeutic plasma exchange in patients with neurologic disorders: review of 63 cases. Indian J Hematol Blood Transfus. 2017;33(1):97–105.
6. Lehmann HC, Hartung HP, Hetzel GR, Stüve O, Kieseier BC. Plasma exchange in neuroimmunological disorders: part 2. Treatment of neuromuscular disorders. Arch Neurol. 2006;63(8):1066–71.
7. Clark WF, Rock GA, Buskard N, Shumak KH, LeBlond P, Anderson D, et al. Therapeutic plasma exchange: an update from the Canadian Apheresis Group. Ann Intern Med. 1999;131(6):453–62.
8. Gwathmey K, Balogun RA, Burns T. Neurologic indications for therapeutic plasma exchange: 2011 update. J Clin Apher. 2012;27(3):138–45.
9. Szczepiorkowski ZM, Winters JL, Bandarenko N, Kim HC, Linenberger ML, Marques MB, et al. Guidelines on the use of therapeutic apheresis in clinical practice--evidence-based approach from the Apheresis Applications Committee of the American Society for Apheresis. J Clin Apher. 2010;25(3):83–177.
10. Lehmann HC, Hartung HP, Hetzel GR, Stüve O, Kieseier BC. Plasma exchange in neuroimmunological disorders: part 1: rationale and treatment of inflammatory central nervous system disorders. Arch Neurol. 2006;63(7):930–5.
11. Drachman DB. Myasthenia gravis. N Engl J Med. 1994;330(25):1797–810.
12. Lennon VA, Kryzer TJ, Griesmann GE, O'Suilleabhain PE, Windebank AJ, Woppmann A, et al. Calcium-channel antibodies in the Lambert-Eaton syndrome and other paraneoplastic syndromes. N Engl J Med. 1995;332(22):1467–74.
13. Berger T, Rubner P, Schautzer F, Egg R, Ulmer H, Mayringer I, et al. Antimyelin antibodies as a predictor of clinically definite multiple sclerosis after a first demyelinating event. N Engl J Med. 2003;349(2):139–45.
14. Dau PC. Increased proliferation of blood mononuclear cells after plasmapheresis treatment of patients with demyelinating disease. J Neuroimmunol. 1990;30(1):15–21.
15. Dau PC. Increased antibody production in peripheral blood mononuclear cells after plasma exchange therapy in multiple sclerosis. J Neuroimmunol. 1995;62(2):197–200.

16. De Luca G, Lugaresi A, Iarlori C, Marzoli F, Di Iorio A, Gambi D, et al. Prednisone and plasma exchange improve suppressor cell function in chronic inflammatory demyelinating polyneuropathy. J Neuroimmunol. 1999;95(1–2):190–4.
17. Goto H, Matsuo H, Nakane S, Izumoto H, Fukudome T, Kambara C, et al. Plasmapheresis affects T helper type-1/T helper type-2 balance of circulating peripheral lymphocytes. Ther Apher. 2001;5(6):494–6.
18. Ahmed S, Kaplan A. Therapeutic plasma exchange using membrane plasma separation. Clin J Am Soc Nephrol. 2020;15(9):1364–70.
19. Redant S, De Bels D, Ismaili K, Honoré PM. Membrane-Based Therapeutic Plasma Exchange in Intensive Care. Blood Purif. 2021;50(3):290–97. https://doi.org/10.1159/000510983. Epub 2020 Oct 22. PMID: 33091920
20. Gashti CN. Membrane-based therapeutic plasma exchange: a new frontier for nephrologists. Semin Dial. 2016;29(5):382–90.
21. Vrielink. LCCa. Principles of Apheresis technology. 2014.
22. Koll RA. Ig-Therasorb immunoadsorption for selective removal of human immunoglobulins in diseases associated with pathogenic antibodies of all classes and IgG subclasses, immune complexes, and fragments of immunoglobulins. Ther Apher. 1998;2(2):147–52.
23. Williams ME, Balogun RA. Principles of separation: indications and therapeutic targets for plasma exchange. Clin J Am Soc Nephrol. 2014;9(1):181–90.
24. Ipe TS, Marques MB. Vascular access for therapeutic plasma exchange. Transfusion. 2018;58(Suppl 1):580–9.
25. Linenberger ML, Price TH. Use of cellular and plasma apheresis in the critically ill patient: part 1: technical and physiological considerations. J Intensive Care Med. 2005;20(1):18–27.
26. Schönermarck U, Bosch T. Vascular access for apheresis in intensive care patients. Ther Apher Dial. 2003;7(2):215–20.
27. Golestaneh L, Mokrzycki MH. Vascular access in therapeutic apheresis: update 2013. J Clin Apher. 2013;28(1):64–72.
28. Stegmayr B, Ptak J, Wikström B, Berlin G, Axelsson CG, Griskevicius A, et al. World apheresis registry 2003-2007 data. Transfus Apher Sci. 2008;39(3):247–54.
29. Malchesky PS, Koo AP, Skibinski CI, Hadsell AT, Rybicki LA. Apheresis technologies and clinical applications: the 2007 International Apheresis Registry. Ther Apher Dial. 2010;14(1):52–73.

30. Walser EM. Venous access ports: indications, implantation technique, follow-up, and complications. Cardiovasc Intervent Radiol. 2012;35(4):751–64.
31. Apsner R, Schwarzenhofer M, Derfler K, Zauner C, Ratheiser K, Kranz A. Impairment of citrate metabolism in acute hepatic failure. Wien Klin Wochenschr. 1997;109(4):123–7.
32. McLeod BC, Sniecinski I, Ciavarella D, Owen H, Price TH, Randels MJ, et al. Frequency of immediate adverse effects associated with therapeutic apheresis. Transfusion. 1999;39(3):282–8.
33. Schlenke P, Frohn C, Steinhardt MM, Kirchner H, Klüter H. Clinically relevant hypokalaemia, hypocalcaemia, and loss of hemoglobin and platelets during stem cell apheresis. J Clin Apher. 2000;15(4):230–5.
34. Weinstein R. Hypocalcemic toxicity and atypical reactions in therapeutic plasma exchange. J Clin Apher. 2001;16(4):210–1.
35. Pool M, McLeod BC. Pyrogen reactions to human serum albumin during plasma exchange. J Clin Apher. 1995;10(2):81–4.
36. Kaplan AA. A simple and accurate method for prescribing plasma exchange. ASAIO Trans. 1990;36(3):M597–9.
37. Schwartz J, Padmanabhan A, Aqui N, Balogun RA, Connelly-Smith L, Delaney M, et al. Guidelines on the use of therapeutic Apheresis in clinical practice-evidence-based approach from the writing Committee of the American Society for Apheresis: the seventh special issue. J Clin Apher. 2016;31(3):149–62.
38. Chevret S, Hughes RA, Annane D. Plasma exchange for Guillain-Barré syndrome. Cochrane Database Syst Rev. 2017;2:CD001798.
39. Cortese I, Chaudhry V, So YT, Cantor F, Cornblath DR, Rae-Grant A. Evidence-based guideline update: plasmapheresis in neurologic disorders: report of the Therapeutics and Technology Assessment Subcommittee of the American Academy of Neurology. Neurology. 2011;76(3):294–300.
40. Mehndiratta MM, Hughes RA, Pritchard J. Plasma exchange for chronic inflammatory demyelinating polyradiculoneuropathy. Cochrane Database Syst Rev. 2015;2015(8):CD003906. https://doi.org/10.1002/14651858.CD003906.pub4. PMID: 26305459; PMCID: PMC6734114.
41. Gajdos P, Chevret S, Toyka KV. Intravenous immunoglobulin for myasthenia gravis. Cochrane Database Syst Rev. 2012;12:CD002277.
42. Kleiter I, Gahlen A, Borisow N, Fischer K, Wernecke KD, Wegner B, et al. Neuromyelitis optica: evaluation of 871 attacks and 1,153 treatment courses. Ann Neurol. 2016;79(2):206–16.

43. Szczeklik W, Wawrzycka K, Włudarczyk A, Sega A, Nowak I, Seczyńska B, et al. Complications in patients treated with plasmapheresis in the intensive care unit. Anaesthesiol Intens Ther. 2013;45(1):7–13.
44. Filipov JJ. Plasma exchange in clinical practice. 2018.
45. Kaplan AA. Therapeutic plasma exchange: core curriculum 2008. Am J Kidney Dis. 2008;52(6):1180–96.

Intravenous Immunoglobulin

Biswajit Banik and Niraj Arora

1 Introduction

History begins in 1981, when Imbach et al. reported that when high-dose IVIG was applied in 4 children with refractory immune thrombocytopenic purpura, patient's symptoms significantly improved and platelet count increased and could be maintained at normal levels with IVIG infusion every 1 to 3 weeks [1]. Subsequently a series of cases treated with IVIG had shown good success [2]. These unique findings facilitated the development of new treatment strategies for other autoimmune diseases. Intravenous immunoglobulin is generally considered a safe treatment option. It has widely been used for treatment of neurological disorders of variable etiology,

B. Banik
Department of Neurology, University of Missouri, Columbia, MO, USA

N. Arora (✉)
Department of Neurology- Neurocriticalcare unit, University of Missouri, Columbia, MO, USA
e-mail: arorana@health.missouri.edu

autoimmune disease, immunodeficiency related disease, autoimmune blood disorders and cancer.

Intravenous immunoglobulin G is a polymeric, highly purified preparation of IgG class that is derived from large pools of plasma donors. Immunoglobulin G is the primary effector molecule for humoral immune response. IVIG is a mixture of normal polyclonal IgG extracted from thousands of healthy humans. It has a broad spectrum of antibody activity, antibody to self and foreign antigen, anti-idiotypic antigen. It plays an immunoregulatory role in autoantibody mediated autoimmune disorders and also systemic inflammatory disease [1].

IVIG has multiple immunomodulatory mechanisms of action. It inhibits complement activation and MAC formation, neutralizes pathogenic cytokines, down regulates antibody production, and most importantly modulates macrophage-mediated phagocytosis through blockade of Fc receptor.

2 Composition

IVIG is similar to IgG subtypes in normal plasma with an average half-life of 3–4 weeks. It contains complete IgG antibodies, small amounts of IgA, IgM, soluble cluster of differentiation (CD)-4, CD8 and human leukocyte antigen molecules. Additionally, IVIG can react with plasma proteins (eg, complement components) and Fcγ receptors on secretory cells because the complete Fc fragment is present. IVIG contains a large number of variable antibody regions with extensive activities directed against external antigens. For autoimmune diseases, IVIG infusions have dual functions: immune related protein substitution and immune system regulation [3, 4].

3 Mechanism of Action

As IVIG preparations are extracted from plasma pooled from thousands of donors, it contains antibodies directed against a broad range of pathogens as well as numerous foreign and self-antigens. Given the heterogeneity of numerous disorders treated with IVIG, most possibly different autoimmune disease pathways mediate the clinical efficacy. It has been difficult to explain a common mechanistic understanding of this medication that is applicable to all neurological diseases [1].

IVIG molecule has two functional domains, two antigen binding fragments F_{ab}, which determines specificity of antibody molecules. And constant Fc region, which is critical for the initiation of effector response.

Below is the proposed mechanism of action of IVIG:

1. **Immune-related protein substitution:**
   Papain hydrolyses IgG molecules into 3 fragments. Two F_{ab} and one F_c fragment. The regulatory effects of F_{ab} are essential in the replacement therapy for immunodeficiency. In primary immune deficiency, this replacement therapy replenishes antibodies that have the intrinsic capacity to recognize foreign antigen or neutral pathogen specific IgG regulation. IgG binds to pathogen specific bacterial or viral protein toxins and helps neutralize them and in the elimination process [5, 6].
2. **Immune system regulation:**
   High dose IVIG is used as immunomodulatory therapy for autoimmune and inflammatory disease. This mechanism is more complex and not completely understood. Proposed mechanism includes modulation of expression and function of Fcγ receptor, inhibition of complement cascade, modulation of immune regulatory cytokines and neutralization of autoantibodies.

   As Receptors for IgG, Fcγ receptors are expressed in all immune cells which mediate a wide and robust range of cellular action. After transfusion IVIG, it significantly increases total IgG level, and blocks the effect of Fcγ receptor because of saturation. In animal model one evidenced mechanism shows, the binding of sialylated IgG Fc to DC-SIGN (Dendritic cell specific intra-cellular adhesion molecule 3 grabbing non integrin) or DC-SIGN related protein 1 result in upregulation of inhibitory FcγR IIb; thus decreases inflammation caused by autoantibodies [5]. Moreover, FcRn, which is expressed in endothelial cells, increases half life in circulation. High dose IVIG blocks the function of FcRn, resulting in increased catabolism of endogenous pathogenic IgG, promoting elimination of pathogenic autoantibodies [7].

High dose IVIG can inhibit the complement cascade by sequestering complement away from deposited autoantibody and modulating antibody complement dependent tissue damage [8]. Sharif et al. reported, in 21 GBS patients, IVIG transfusion reduced circulating TNF-Alpha and IL-1B, thereby alleviating clinical syndrome [9].

IVIG contains anti-idiotypic antibodies. Which can bind to variable regions of autoantibodies acting as neutralizing antibodies and block subsequent epidemic response [10]. Bayry et al. studies the effect of IVIG on DCs, and found that IVIG can inhibit the differentiation and maturation of DCs in vitro, suppresses the secretion of IL-12 by mature DCs, and enhances production of IL-10 at the same time. IVIG-induced down-regulation of costimulatory molecules associated with modulation of cytokine secretion resulted in the inhibition of autoreactive and alloreactive T-cell activation and proliferation. Modulation of DC maturation and function by IVIG is of potential relevance to its immunomodulatory effects in controlling specific immune responses in autoimmune diseases [11].

4 Immunoglobulin in Neurological Diseases

IVIG has been shown to be useful for neurological treatment of new-onset or recurrent immune mediated neurological diseases and also for long term maintenance treatment of chronic neurological diseases. Moreover, IVIG may have applications in the management of intractable autoimmune epilepsy, paraneoplastic syndrome, autoimmune encephalitis, neuromyelitis Optica. Subcutaneous immunoglobulin (SCIg) is newly emerging, and is a potential future alternative.

Though the bioavailability of SCIg is lower in comparison to IVIG, homeostatic level is more stable. Current studies shows both has pharmacological equivalence [3].

4.1 Neurological Dose of IVIG

Current recommended high dose for treatment of acute neurological issues is 2 gm/kg divided over 2–5 days or 0.4 gm/kg/day for 5 days. When clinical improvement is not obvious, some patients may receive a second course of IVIG treatment but further studies are required to demonstrate efficacy. For maintenance of therapy, dosage depends on the characteristics of disease, health condition, and other comorbidities of the patient. Notably, the clinical effect of IVIG therapy is related to dose [3].

4.2 Neurological Disorders Treated with IVIG

1. **Guillain Barre syndrome: (FDA approved)**

GBS is a type of polyradiculoneuropathy. Exact pathogenesis is not knows, but often seen in post infectious diseases, most commonly C. Jejuni, CMV, EBV infection. Recently, COVID related GBS cases are also widely reported. Typically, but now always pt. presents with ascending motor weakness, in severe cases can involve respiratory muscles and autonomic nervous system causing major morbidity or death. CSF typically shows Albumino-cytological dissociation, electrodiagnostic changes evolving within 4 weeks. There are multiple variants of GBS which are beyond scope to discuss here. But no particular variant has shown better or worse response to IVIG or PLEX therapy. Oftentimes, patients require close monitoring and treatment at ICU level care. The mainstay of treatment of such a case is plasmapheresis or IVIG. Plasmapheresis is not available in all hospitals, has more risk and side effects. In comparison, IVIG is relatively safer and easy to administer. Though PLEX has a shorter onset of action, overall both treatments are considered equally effective [12]. Van der Meche and Schmitz found IVIG is as least effective as, or may be superior to PLEX. As he found median time to recovery as shorter, fewer complications were observed in comparison to PLEX. The study found that median time to improvement by one grade was 41 days with plasma exchange and 27 days with immune globulin therapy (P = 0.05). The immune globulin group had significantly fewer complications and less need for artificial ventilation [13]. Combination of both PLEX and IVIG does not provide any additional benefit. Combining IVIG, PLEX with 500 mg IV methylprednisolone produces no incremental response [14].

2. Chronic Inflammatory demyelinating polyneuropathy (CIDP)

CIDP is an inflammatory neuropathy, classically characterized by a slowly progressive onset and symmetrical, sensorimotor involvement. However, there are many phenotypic variants, suggesting that CIDP may not be a discrete disease entity but rather a spectrum of related conditions. While the abiding theory of CIDP pathogenesis is that cell-mediated and humoral mechanisms act together in an aberrant immune response to cause damage to peripheral nerves, the relative contributions of T cell and autoantibody responses remain largely undefined [15]. In most cases there is a relapsing remitting clinical pattern. Treatment includes induction therapy and maintenance therapy. Randomized controlled trials (RCTs) have shown that IVIG, plasma exchange, and corticosteroids are effective treatments for CIDP [16–19]. The efficacy of 2gm/kg induction has been confirmed, some pt. has shown clear reduction in symptoms. One of the largest RCT published by Hughes et al. reported, IVIG slowed short-term and long-term benefits and a good tolerability profile, with prolonged relapse time. Patients received a baseline loading dose of 2 g/kg over 2–4 days and then a maintenance infusion of 1 g/kg over 1–2 days every 3 weeks for up to 24 weeks [20]. An open-label Phase III clinical trial that included 49 patients from different centers, investigated IVIG as maintenance treatment for CIDP. After induction therapy with IVIG 0.4 g/kg/day for 5 days, the patients were given 1 g/kg every 3 weeks for 52 weeks for maintenance treatment. At 28 weeks, 77.6% of patients' clinical symptoms were alleviated; additionally, at 52 weeks, 69.4% of patients had sustained remission [21]. The ICE trial, the largest ever conducted in patients with CIDP, has shown that IVIG is safe and effective not only for the short term but also for the long term, leading to the first FDA-approved indication for a brand of IVIG [20]. In most patients, IVIG only became effective after 6 weeks, necessitating at least two infusions before concluding that the treatment is ineffective [22]. Maintenance IVIG therapy is needed, usually with 1 g/kg every 4–6 weeks, but the exact frequency and dosage should be tailored according to the duration of clinical remission following treatment and degree of efficacy. In up to 20% of patients, the disease becomes chronically stable or inactive, so to avoid unnecessary and costly overtreatment, the usefulness of continuing IVIG therapy should be periodically challenged by skipping one or two doses [1]. It is a challenging decision whether to start a patient on IVIG, PLEX or prednisone as all work. Clinically, patients more likely to respond to IVIG therapy seem to be those with disease duration of less than 1 year, with a relapsing course and electrophysiological signs of demyelination on conduction block [23, 24]. In some patients with CIDP treatment, response to IVIG fades over time, requiring other forms of immunotherapy.

3. Multifocal motor neuropathy (FDA approved for IVIG)

MMN is a rare disease associated with motor nerve damage. Its clinical manifestations include slow, progressive, asymmetric limb weakness, mainly involving the distal end, without sensory nerve involvement. Electrophysiologic

TABLE 1 Other neurological conditions in which IVIG can be used for treatment [29]

Anti MAG demyelinating neuropathy
Myasthenia gravis
Lambert Eaton Myasthenic Syndrome (LEMS)
Inflammatory myopathies
Stiff person syndrome
Multiple sclerosis
Neuromyelitis optica
Autoimmune encephalitis

characteristics include focal motor conduction block, and some patients are positive for ganglioside GM1 antibodies [25]. Unlike GBS and CIDP, IVIG is the only effective therapy, steroid and PLEX showed no clinical response. The current primary treatment option for MMN is IVIG therapy (0.4 g/kg for 5 consecutive days), which is based on a meta-analysis of data from 4 double blind RCTs that included 34 patients with MMN [25–27]. The improvement lasts from 3–6 weeks, requiring reinfusion at almost predictable time periods. As symptoms diminish, the electrophysiological conduction block may resolve but, in some patients, axonal loss or new conduction blocks can manifest during long-term treatment.

Other indications for IVIG are listed in Table 1.

5 Adverse Effect and Management

Use of IVIG is not without adverse effects and risk versus benefits should be taken into consideration before committing the patient to long term IVIG infusion. Table 2 lists the adverse effects of IVIG infusion [28].

TABLE 2 Adverse Effects and clinical manifestations of IVIG[28]

Effects and incidence	Clinical symptoms and signs	Timing	Comments
Immediate adverse effects			
Flu-like symptoms (80%)	flushing, nausea, fatigue, fever, chills, malaise, and lethargy	Develop as early as 30 minutes to 24 hours.	Related to the presence of cytokines such as IL-6, TNF-α in the products. Associated with rapid infusion and can be decreased by slowing the rate of infusion.
Skin reactions (6%)	urticaria, spot papules, eczema, pompholyx, lichenoid dermatitis, and desquamation. Epidermolysis	Usually develop within 2 weeks of infusion.	Exact mechanism is not known but steroids help in treatment. No reported deaths related to skin reactions. Consider switching to another IVIG batch formulation.
Cardiovascular reactions (rare case reports)	Bradycardia, supraventricular tachycardia, bradycardia	Usually during administration of IVIG	Telemetry for early identification of arrhythmias. More common if history of coronary artery disease present.
Pulmonary reactions (rare case reports)	Transfusion related acute lung injury (TRALI)	Within 6 hours of administration of IVIG	Usually a diagnosis of exclusion. Can improve with proper mechanical ventilation but carries a high mortality.

(continued)

TABLE 2 (continued)

Effects and incidence	Clinical symptoms and signs	Timing	Comments
Delayed adverse effects			
Hematologic reactions	Thrombotic events: Stroke, myocardial infarction (1–16%)	Within 24 hours of infusion	Caused due to an increase in plasma viscosity (most important), the activation of procoagulant factors, vasospasm, autoimmune vasculitis, and an increased platelet count. High risk factors: high dose (≥ 35 g/day), oral contraceptive use, advanced age, prior/current thrombosis, pre existing atherosclerotic disease, elevated serum viscosity, a hereditary hypercoagulable state or ITP. Early detection in high risk cases and use of antithrombotics if needed.
	Hemolysis (1.6%): asymptomatic to anemia	12 hours to 10 days after the first infusion of IVIG	Risk factor: Blood group A, B or AB, high dose of IVIG, Supportive management helps in most cases.
	Neutropenia	4 days after infusion	Recovers in 2 weeks. Steroids may help.

TABLE 2 (continued)

Effects and incidence	Clinical symptoms and signs	Timing	Comments
Neurological reactions	Headache (50%)	Starts 6–12 h after an infusion and can last between 24 and 72 h	Mechanism is not known but risk factors include high IVIG dose or migraine history. Pain medications like acetaminophen, aspirin, NSAIDs, migraine medications could help to decrease or prevent headache. Can switch to an alternate brand or lower the rate of infusion. Rule out aseptic meningitis
	Aseptic meningitis (0.5–1%): headache, nausea, fever, meningitis signs.	Within 48 h of infusion.	risk factors include high IVIG dose or migraine history. CSF shows elevated nucleated cells, high protein, and negative cultures.
	PRES (rare): headache, seizure, altered mentation, visual disturbance	During infusion	Resolves when the infusion is stopped. MRI brain findings are characteristic.
	Seizures (rare)	Usually with other clinical manifestations	Could be generalized or focal. Look for other etiologies.
Renal and electrolyte effects	Acute kidney injury	Within 10 days of IVIG. Peak at 5 days.	Suspected due to immune complex deposition in the glomeruli, osmotic nephritis, hemolysis-associated acute tubular obstruction, and transient vascular ischemia due to a reduction in renal perfusion. Risk factors include older age, diabetes, chronic kidney injury, dehydration.

(continued)

TABLE 2 (continued)

Effects and incidence	Clinical symptoms and signs	Timing	Comments
	Hyponatremia, hypomagnesemia	Any time during transfusion of IVIG	Recover spontaneously
Infection risk	Hepatitis C (not reported since 1994)		Not routinely tested
	Hepatitis B antibodies	Passive transfer possible.	Recommended to measure HBV antibodies in high risk cases.

PRES: posterior reversible encephalopathy syndrome

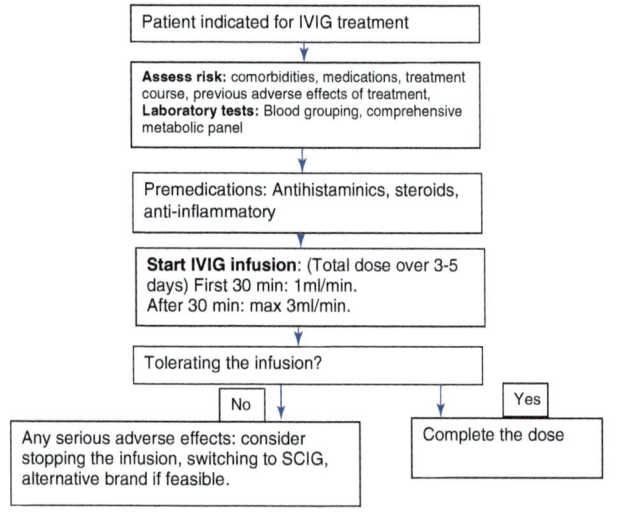

FIGURE 1 Protocol for IVIG infusion [28]

Protocol for IVIG infusion Fig. 1 [28].

6   Conclusion and Future Directions

Even though IVIG has been now used in a variety of neurological as well as non-neurological conditions, there are no controlled trials for the use of this therapy. Understanding the risk-benefit ratio for IVIG is essential before long term use of this therapy is considered. Whether the dosing should be based on ideal body weight or actual body weight also needs to be taken into account during dose calculation. Oral administration of IVIG might attenuate some adverse effects but more research is needed in this regard.

References

1. Lünemann JD, Nimmerjahn F, Dalakas MC. Intravenous immunoglobulin in neurology--mode of action and clinical efficacy. Nat Rev Neurol. 2015;11(2):80–9. https://doi.org/10.1038/nrneurol.2014.253. Epub 2015 Jan 6. PMID: 25561275
2. Schmidt RE, Budde U, Schäfer G, Stroehmann I. High-dose intravenous gammaglobulin for idiopathic thrombocytopenic purpura. Lancet. 1981;2(8244):475–6. https://doi.org/10.1016/s0140-6736(81)90810-2. PMID: 6115233
3. Chen Y, Wang C, Xu F, Ming F, Zhang H. Efficacy and tolerability of intravenous immunoglobulin and subcutaneous immunoglobulin in neurologic diseases. Clin Ther. 2019;41(10):2112–36. https://doi.org/10.1016/j.clinthera.2019.07.009. Epub 2019 Aug 21. PMID: 31445679
4. Chaigne B, Mouthon L. Mechanisms of action of intravenous immunoglobulin. Transfus Apher Sci. 2017;56(1):45–9. https://doi.org/10.1016/j.transci.2016.12.017. Epub 2016 Dec 30. PMID: 28161150
5. Chwab I, Nimmerjahn F. Intravenous immunoglobulin therapy: how does IgG modulate the immune system? Nat Rev Immunol. 2013;13(3):176–89. https://doi.org/10.1038/nri3401. Epub 2013 Feb 15. PMID: 23411799
6. Durandy A, Kaveri SV, Kuijpers TW, Basta M, Miescher S, Ravetch JV, Rieben R. Intravenous immunoglobulins--understanding properties and mechanisms. Clin Exp Immunol. 2009;158 Suppl 1(Suppl 1):2–13. https://doi.org/10.1111/j.1365-2249.2009.04022.x. PMID: 19883419; PMCID: PMC2801035

7. Roopenian DC, Akilesh S. FcRn: the neonatal Fc receptor comes of age. Nat Rev Immunol. 2007;7(9):715–25. https://doi.org/10.1038/nri2155. Epub 2007 Aug 17. PMID: 17703228
8. Basta M, Dalakas MC. High-dose intravenous immunoglobulin exerts its beneficial effect in patients with dermatomyositis by blocking endomysial deposition of activated complement fragments. J Clin Invest. 1994;94(5):1729–35. https://doi.org/10.1172/JCI117520. PMID: 7962520; PMCID: PMC294563
9. Sharief MK, Ingram DA, Swash M, Thompson EJ. I.v. immunoglobulin reduces circulating proinflammatory cytokines in Guillain-Barré syndrome. Neurology. 1999;52(9):1833–8. https://doi.org/10.1212/wnl.52.9.1833. PMID: 10371531
10. Roux KH, Tankersley DL. A view of the human idiotypic repertoire. Electron microscopic and immunologic analyses of spontaneous idiotype-anti-idiotype dimers in pooled human IgG. J Immunol. 1990;144(4):1387–95. PMID: 2303712
11. Bayry J, Lacroix-Desmazes S, Carbonneil C, Misra N, Donkova V, Pashov A, Chevailler A, Mouthon L, Weill B, Bruneval P, Kazatchkine MD, Kaveri SV. Inhibition of maturation and function of dendritic cells by intravenous immunoglobulin. Blood. 2003;101(2):758–65. https://doi.org/10.1182/blood-2002-05-1447. Epub 2002 Aug 29. PMID: 12393386
12. Hughes RA, Swan AV, van Doorn PA. Intravenous immunoglobulin for Guillain-Barré syndrome. Cochrane Database Syst Rev. 2012;(7):CD002063. https://doi.org/10.1002/14651858.CD002063.pub5. Update in: Cochrane Database Syst Rev. 2014;(9):CD002063. PMID: 22786476
13. van der Meché FG, Schmitz PI. A randomized trial comparing intravenous immune globulin and plasma exchange in Guillain-Barré syndrome. Dutch Guillain-Barré Study Group. N Engl J Med. 1992;326(17):1123–9. https://doi.org/10.1056/NEJM199204233261705. PMID: 1552913
14. Randomised trial of plasma exchange, intravenous immunoglobulin, and combined treatments in Guillain-Barré syndrome. Plasma Exchange/Sandoglobulin Guillain-Barré Syndrome Trial Group. Lancet. 1997;349(9047):225–30. PMID: 9014908.
15. Mathey EK, Park SB, Hughes RA, Pollard JD, Armati PJ, Barnett MH, Taylor BV, Dyck PJ, Kiernan MC, Lin CS. Chronic inflammatory demyelinating polyradiculoneuropathy: from pathology to phenotype. J Neurol Neurosurg Psychiatry. 2015;86(9):973–85. https://doi.org/10.1136/jnnp-2014-309697. Epub 2015 Feb 12. PMID: 25677463; PMCID: PMC4552934

16. Mendell JR, Barohn RJ, Freimer ML, Kissel JT, King W, Nagaraja HN, Rice R, Campbell WW, Donofrio PD, Jackson CE, Lewis RA, Shy M, Simpson DM, Parry GJ, Rivner MH, Thornton CA, Bromberg MB, Tandan R, Harati Y, Giuliani MJ. Working Group on Peripheral Neuropathy. Randomized controlled trial of IVIG in untreated chronic inflammatory demyelinating polyradiculoneuropathy. Neurology. 2001;56(4):445–9. https://doi.org/10.1212/wnl.56.4.445. PMID: 11222785
17. Dyck PJ, Litchy WJ, Kratz KM, Suarez GA, Low PA, Pineda AA, Windebank AJ, Karnes JL, O'Brien PC. A plasma exchange versus immune globulin infusion trial in chronic inflammatory demyelinating polyradiculoneuropathy. Ann Neurol. 1994;36(6):838–45. https://doi.org/10.1002/ana.410360607. PMID: 7998769
18. Hughes R, Bensa S, Willison H, Van den Bergh P, Comi G, Illa I, Nobile-Orazio E, van Doorn P, Dalakas M, Bojar M, Swan A. Inflammatory Neuropathy Cause and Treatment (INCAT) Group. Randomized controlled trial of intravenous immunoglobulin versus oral prednisolone in chronic inflammatory demyelinating polyradiculoneuropathy. Ann Neurol. 2001;50(2):195–201. https://doi.org/10.1002/ana.1088. PMID: 11506402
19. Dyck PJ, Daube J, O'Brien P, Pineda A, Low PA, Windebank AJ, Swanson C. Plasma exchange in chronic inflammatory demyelinating polyradiculoneuropathy. N Engl J Med. 1986;314(8):461–5. https://doi.org/10.1056/NEJM198602203140801. PMID: 3511382
20. Hughes RA, Donofrio P, Bril V, Dalakas MC, Deng C, Hanna K, Hartung HP, Latov N, Merkies IS, van Doorn PA; ICE Study Group. Intravenous immune globulin (10% caprylate-chromatography purified) for the treatment of chronic inflammatory demyelinating polyradiculoneuropathy (ICE study): a randomised placebo-controlled trial. Lancet Neurol. 2008;7(2):136–44. https://doi.org/10.1016/S1474-4422(07)70329-0. Erratum in: Lancet Neurol. 2008 Sep;7(9):771. PMID: 18178525.
21. Kuwabara S, Mori M, Misawa S, Suzuki M, Nishiyama K, Mutoh T, Doi S, Kokubun N, Kamijo M, Yoshikawa H, Abe K, Nishida Y, Okada K, Sekiguchi K, Sakamoto K, Kusunoki S, Sobue G, Kaji R, Glovenin-I CIDP Study Group. Intravenous immunoglobulin for maintenance treatment of chronic inflammatory demyelinating polyneuropathy: a multicentre, open-label, 52-week phase III trial. J Neurol Neurosurg Psychiatry. 2017;88(10):832–8. https://doi.org/10.1136/jnnp-2017-316427. Epub 2017 Aug 2. PMID: 28768822; PMCID: PMC5629934

22. Latov N, Deng C, Dalakas MC, Bril V, Donofrio P, Hanna K, Hartung HP, Hughes RA, Merkies IS, van Doorn PA. IGIV-C CIDP Efficacy (ICE) Study Group. Timing and course of clinical response to intravenous immunoglobulin in chronic inflammatory demyelinating polyradiculoneuropathy. Arch Neurol. 2010;67(7):802–7. https://doi.org/10.1001/archneurol.2010.105. Epub 2010 May 10. PMID: 20457948

23. Vermeulen M, van Doorn PA, Brand A, Strengers PF, Jennekens FG, Busch HF. Intravenous immunoglobulin treatment in patients with chronic inflammatory demyelinating polyneuropathy: a double blind, placebo controlled study. J Neurol Neurosurg Psychiatry. 1993;56(1):36–9. https://doi.org/10.1136/jnnp.56.1.36. PMID: 8429321. PMCID: PMC1014761

24. Hahn AF, Bolton CF, Zochodne D, Feasby TE. Intravenous immunoglobulin treatment in chronic inflammatory demyelinating polyneuropathy. A double-blind, placebo-controlled, crossover study. Brain. 1996;119(Pt 4):1067–77. https://doi.org/10.1093/brain/119.4.1067. PMID: 8813271

25. Azulay JP, Blin O, Pouget J, Boucraut J, Billé-Turc F, Carles G, Serratrice G. Intravenous immunoglobulin treatment in patients with motor neuron syndromes associated with anti-GM1 antibodies: a double-blind, placebo-controlled study. Neurology. 1994;44(3 Pt 1):429–32. https://doi.org/10.1212/wnl.44.3_part_1.429. PMID: 8145910

26. Van den Berg LH, Kerkhoff H, Oey PL, Franssen H, Mollee I, Vermeulen M, Jennekens FG, Wokke JH. Treatment of multifocal motor neuropathy with high dose intravenous immunoglobulins: a double blind, placebo controlled study. J Neurol Neurosurg Psychiatry. 1995;59(3):248–52. https://doi.org/10.1136/jnnp.59.3.248. PMID: 7673950; PMCID: PMC486021

27. Federico P, Zochodne DW, Hahn AF, Brown WF, Feasby TE. Multifocal motor neuropathy improved by IVIG: randomized, double-blind, placebo-controlled study. Neurology. 2000;55(9):1256–62. https://doi.org/10.1212/wnl.55.9.1256. PMID: 11087764

28. Guo Y, Tian X, Wang X, Xiao Z. Adverse effects of immunoglobulin therapy. Front Immunol. 2018; https://doi.org/10.3389/fimmu.2018.01299.

29. Lünemann JD, Quast I, Dalakas MC. Efficacy of intravenous immunoglobulin in neurological diseases. Neurotherapeutics. 2016;13(1):34–46.

Brain Death

Kunal Bhatia and Niraj Arora

1 Introduction

Devastating brain injuries are well-recognized causes of irreversible cessation of neurological function [1]. The concept of brain death was first recognized in 1959 by Mollaret and Goulon, who coined the phrase "coma dépassé" (meaning "a state beyond coma") [2]. In 1968 the Ad Hoc Committee of Harvard Medical School to examine the definition of Brain Death, described the first clinical definition of brain death. The committee defined irreversible coma, or brain death, as unresponsiveness and lack of receptivity, the absence of movement and breathing, the absence of brain-stem reflexes, and coma whose cause has been identified [3]. Subsequently, The President's Commission report on "guidelines for the

K. Bhatia
Department of Neurology, Division of Neurocritical Care, Washington University School of Medicine, St. Louis, MO, USA

N. Arora (✉)
Department of Neurology- Neurocriticalcare unit, University of Missouri, Columbia, MO, USA
e-mail: arorana@health.missouri.edu

determination of death" provided a legal definition for brain death in 1981 that led to the Uniform Determination of Death Act (UDDA). As per the UDDA, brain death is defined as "irreversible cessation of all functions of the entire brain, including the brain stem" and equates this concept with the more traditional "irreversible cessation of circulatory and respiratory functions" [4]. However, the UDDA did not describe the clinical methodology or medical standards for determination of brain death. Hence, in 1995 the American Academy of Neurology (AAN) published evidence-based practice parameters providing medical standards for clinical determination of brain death in adults, which were later updated in 2010 [5, 6].

Despite the availability of these well-established parameters, there continues to be a wide variance in the practice of clinical determination of brain death both nationally and worldwide. Some of the common factors observed include variations in prerequisites prior to testing, inconsistencies in the concept, lack of uniformity with regards to the components of the examination, apnea testing technique, requirement for ancillary testing, and discrepancies in documentation [7–11]. This chapter focuses on providing an algorithmic, step-by-step approach to clinical determination of brain death by neurological criteria in adults including the role of ancillary tests, brain death documentation and potential confounding factors.

2 Procedure for Declaration of Death by Neurological Criteria

The three essential findings necessary to confirm "irreversible" cessation of all functions of the entire brain, including the brain stem include: coma (with a known cause), absence of brainstem reflexes, and apnea. The term "irreversible" refers to determining the cause of coma, exclusion of potentially confounding medical conditions and intoxications, and observing the patient for a period of time to exclude the possibility of recovery [6]. Brain death examination can be performed by a qualified physician including neurologists, neurosurgeons, neurointensivists or a critical care physician who is familiar with the clinical criteria and is comfortable performing all aspects of the examination. Alternatively, a neurology consultation could be obtained, with declaration supervised by a neurocritical care trained physician. In addition, physicians should be able to differentiate brain death from other forms of severe brain damage wherein some of the brain functions are preserved with a likelihood of recovery after prolonged periods of time [12–14]. Physicians should also involve the family members throughout the process of brain death declaration, giving ample time to understand the concept of "brain death by neurological criteria" being equivalent to "death", which can eventually help families take important decisions like withdrawal of care, organ donation, and prevent inappropriate use of resources.

The diagnosis of brain death can usually be made clinically at patient bedside. However, several criteria, as described below, must be met prior to initiating declaration of death by neurologic criteria [6]. While only a single complete examination (with apnea testing) is required to declare death based on neurologic criteria, a repeat assessment is advisable in instances wherein there is discordance between the severity of brain injury seen on neuroimaging and clinical examination findings. In such a situation, decision to re-evaluate after a period of interval should be made by the consulting neurologist or neurointensivist and depends on the individual patient characteristics.

1. Step 1: Establishing irreversibility

    The determination of brain death requires the identification of the proximate cause and irreversibility of coma. Etiology should be determined through clinical history, physical examination, neuroimaging, and/or laboratory testing. There must be evidence of an acute devastating central nervous system (CNS) illness that is compatible with the clinical diagnosis of brain death. Traumatic brain injuries [subarachnoid hemorrhage (SAH), epidural hematoma, subdural hematoma, intracerebral hemorrhage (ICH), intraventricular hemorrhage (IVH)], aneurysmal SAH followed by hypertensive ICH are some of the most common events leading to brain death [9, 15]. Other causes that can lead to irreversible loss of brain function include hypoxic-ischemic brain injury, fulminant hepatic failure and ischemic stroke.

2. Step 2: Pre-requisites and Exclusions

   (i) Excluding confounding conditions:

   The physicians should determine and exclude any conditions that may confound the assessment of cortical or brainstem functions and hence interfere with brain death testing. It is recommended that the following confounders, as listed below, should be considered and eliminated in the context of the primary brain injury; if such an injury is severe enough, then these factors may not be important enough to exclude a clinical diagnosis of brain death. If correction of these confounding states is not reasonable, ancillary testing should then be considered [16].

   (a) Severe metabolic, electrolyte, acid-base, and endocrine disturbances that could affect the examination must be corrected.
   (b) Encephalopathy associated with hepatic failure, uremia and hyperosmolar states.
   (c) Pharmacological paralysis with neuro-muscular blocking agents should be excluded with use of train-of-four stimulator. Presence of a twitch or absent twitches on train-of-four with maximal ulnar nerve stimulation signifies continued NM blockade.
   (d) Use of CNS depressing medications, including exposure to toxin agents, should be excluded as it may alter the assessment of neurological function including some of the ancillary tests like electroencephalography (EEG). Calculation of drug clearance using 5 elimination half-lives (assuming

normal hepatic and renal function) should be kept in mind before negating the effects of sedative medications [17]. On the other hand, elimination half-life may be prolonged in presence of organ dysfunction and/or organ dysfunction and should be taken into consideration. If there are concerns for a toxic exposure, drug screen can be ordered or plasma drug levels can be obtained serially, if available.

(e) If alcohol intoxication is suspected or confirmed, the alcohol blood level must be 80 mg/dL or lower [17].

(ii) Normal core body temperature:

A core body temperature of ≥36 °C, as determined by esophageal, bladder, rectal probe, or use of central venous or arterial catheter; should be maintained. Various measures like warming blanket, thermal mattress or automated temperature regulation devices can be used to maintain normal core body temperature. This is important as presence of hypothermia may delay the rise in pCO2 and hence may interfere with results of apnea testing [6]. Furthermore, hypothermia can temporarily blunt brainstem reflexes confounding the results of brain death testing [5, 16].

(iii) Normal systolic blood pressure (SBP):

Systolic blood pressure ≥100 mmHg or a mean arterial pressure (MAP) of at least 60 should be maintained prior to and during brain death testing [17]. Hypotension is often common after devastating brain injury secondary to loss of vascular tone or hypovolemia from diabetes insipidus, and minimum SBP thresholds should be maintained with use of vasopressors and/or fluids if required [18, 19].

(iv) Observation period:

It is recommended that physicians should wait for a minimum of 24 hours after achieving normothermia in patients treated with targeted temperature management (TTM), specifically in post cardiac arrest patients with suspicion for anoxic brain injury [17]. There is no specific time period for other brain injuries and should be determined on a case-case basis by the physician, especially if there is uncertainty about the irreversible nature of the primary brain injury.

3. Step 3: Clinical Neurological examination

   Clinical examination should elicit complete absence of brain function i.e., both cerebral and brainstem function. This can be achieved by an assessment for coma and demonstration of brainstem areflexia.

   (i) Coma – Patients must demonstrate a complete loss of responsiveness to external stimuli. Eye opening or eye movement either spontaneously or to noxious stimuli is absent. There must be no brain-mediated motor responses (including purposeful movements, decorticate or decerebrate posturing, shivering, seizures) to noxious stimuli applied centrally and peripherally. Central pain stimulation can be applied to certain areas such as the supraorbital notch, the ankle of the jaw, upper trapezius, the anterior axillary fold, and the sternum. Response to peripheral pain stimulation can be assessed by applying nail bed pressure. It is important to emphasis that certain reflexive movements originating from the spinal cord or peripheral nerve may occur in brain death. They are common and can occur either spontaneously or after tactile stimulation. Some of the common spinal reflex movements that have been described in literature and are acceptable findings compatible with the diagnosis of brain death include:

   - Undulating toe flexion response - repetitive flexion and extension of toes with passive displacement of foot or plantar tactile stimulation [20, 21].
   - Triple flexion response – characterized by flexion at the hip, knee and ankle upon foot stimulation [20].
   - Unilateral upper extremity pronation extension reflex in response to a cutaneous stimulus or passive anterior neck flexion [20, 22].

- Facial myokymia – undulating, subtle, repetitive contractions of facial muscles due to facial nerve denervation [20].
- Respiratory-like movements - shoulder elevation and adduction, back arching, intercostal expansion without significant tidal volumes [23, 24].
- Lazarus sign - bilateral arm flexion, shoulder adduction, and hand raising to the chest/neck, triggered by passive head flexion and sternal stimulation [20, 23–27].
- Spinal Myoclonus – Multifocal, asymmetric myoclonus involving lower limbs and abdominal muscles [28].
- Truncal movements – asymmetric opisthotonos posturing of the trunk [25].
- Muscle fasciculations of trunk and extremities [20].
- Flexor plantar response – plantar flexion triggered by plantar stimulation [29].
- Eyelid opening – unilateral or bilateral eyelid opening with noxious stimulus to ipsilateral nipple [30].

(ii) Absent brainstem reflexes [6, 31–33]

   (a) Absent pupillary light reflex – The pupils must be fixed in a midsize or dilated position (4–9 mm) with absent pupillary response (direct and consensual) to bright light, as determined with the naked eye, magnifying glass, or a pupilometer. However, pupils can be unequal and of any shape (oval/round/irregular). Severe eye trauma, cataract, prior ophthalmic surgery, exposure to drugs like atropine and scopolamine can influence pupillary reactivity necessitating ancillary testing.

   (b) Absent oculocephalic (OCR) and oculovestibular (OVR) reflexes – There should be absence of any ocular movements (doll's eye) with rotating the head briskly from side to side passively. Cervical spine injury should be ruled out prior to performing oculocephalic testing. Oculovestibular testing is performed by irrigating each ear with ice-cold water. Head is elevated to 30 degree to align the horizontal semicircular canals in the vertical position after the patency of external auditory canal is confirmed. A rupture tympanic membrane should be ruled out as this can lead to increased risk of ear infections. This is followed by irrigating each ear with 50 cc of ice-cold water for at least 60 seconds using a syringe. There should be an interval of 5 mins between testing each ear to allow the endolymph temperature to equilibrate. The eyes should be observed carefully for 1 minute and there should be absence of any extra-ocular movements.

(c) Absent corneal reflex – The cornea should be touched at the external border of iris in both the eyes using a cotton swab or squirts of saline water. No eyelid movement should be seen. In the setting of anophthalmia, severe orbital edema, prior corneal transplantation, or scleral edema or chemosis, appropriate testing of corneal reflexes may be challenging, hence ancillary testing should be used in such instances.

(d) Absence of facial motor responses – Noxious stimulus or deep pressure is applied on the condyles at the level of the temporomandibular joints, supraorbital ridge or sternal notch. There should be absence of grimacing or any facial muscle movements. Severe facial trauma or swelling may preclude evaluation of facial motor response, so ancillary testing should be considered in this setting.

(e) Absence of cough and gag reflexes – The cough reflex can be tested by examining the cough response to deep tracheal suctioning. The suction catheter should be placed deep into the trachea up to the level of carina for appropriate testing. To elicit gag reflex, posterior pharyngeal wall is stimulated bilaterally with the help of a tongue depressor or a suction catheter. In persons with high cervical cord injury, phrenic nerve may be injured which may confound the results of cough reflex and necessitate ancillary testing.

4. Step 4: Apnea testing

    Apnea testing is an essential component of brain death determination in comatose patients. It is a clinical bedside test that assesses the response of respiratory centers in a functional brainstem (medulla) to increased levels of pCO2 (hypercarbia) and decreased pH (respiratory acidosis). In an intact brainstem a rise in pCO2 should decrease central nervous system pH causing stimulation of central chemoreceptors to trigger respiration in adults. The lack of respiratory effort in response to hypercarbia implies destruction of the most caudal part of the brainstem. In patients with intracranial hypertension, a consequence of cerebral edema and compromised CNS autoregulation system, apnea testing may elevate intracranial pressure. Hence, apnea testing should be performed last after completing rest of the clinical evaluation and signs consistent with brain death [6, 17, 31–33]. However, in patients with high cervical cord injury, apnea testing should not be performed due to damage to phrenic nerve and ancillary testing is indicated. Before initiating apnea testing, certain pre-requisites, as detailed below, should be met.

Pre-requisites for apnea testing:

(a) Normothermia – a core body temperature of at least 36 °C or 96.8 °F should be maintained. This can be achieved with use of warming blankets, thermal mattresses, automated temperature regulation systems.

(b) Normotension – SBP ≥ 100 or a MAP of 60, with use of vasopressors, inotropes, and/or fluids as required, should be maintained. It is recommended that an arterial line be placed for continuous BP monitoring and titration of vasopressors accordingly to maintain BP parameters during apnea testing.

(c) Normocarbia – Apnea testing should begin with a normal PaCO2 levels (35–45 mm Hg). It is recommended that hyperventilation should be reversed and minute ventilation be adjusted to achieve normocarbia.
(d) Euvolemia – patients should be evaluated for volume status and cardiovascular stability prior to commencing apnea testing.

Procedure:

(a) Ventilator settings – Patients should be preoxygenated with 100% oxygen for at least 10 minutes with 100% oxygen to a achieve a PaO2 level >200 mm Hg. Ventilation frequency should be kept between 10–12 breaths per minute. Reduce positive end-expiratory pressure (PEEP) to 5 cm H2O as it prevents de-recruitment and decreases the risk of cardiovascular instability. A baseline blood gas (PaO2, PaCO2, pH) should be obtained prior to disconnecting the ventilator.
(b) Disconnect the ventilator and preserve oxygenation by placing an insufflation catheter through the endotracheal tube close to the level of the carina in the trachea. Oxygen is administered at ~6 L/min through the oxygen catheter. Alternatively, T piece system can also be used to provide oxygen via standard corrugated tubing connected to 100% oxygen at a flow of 12 L/min [34]. This allows PaCO2 to rise without producing hypoxia.
(c) Undrape the patient's chest and abdomen and observe for any respiratory movements (chest or abdominal wall excursions) for a minimum of 8–10 minutes.
(d) Obtain a repeat blood gas if there is absence of any respiratory movements after approximately 8–10 minutes.
(e) Apnea is confirmed if blood gas shows PaCO2 ≥ 60 mmHg or a rise in PaCO2 ≥ 20 mmHg above baseline (particularly in patients with chronic CO2 retention like COPD or Obesity hypoventilation syndrome), and supports the diagnosis of brain death.
(f) If results remain inconclusive but patient is hemodynamically stable during the procedure, the test may be repeated

for a longer period of time (i.e., 10–15 minutes) after the patient is again adequately preoxygenated.
(g) Apnea testing should be aborted if [6]:

- Spontaneous respirations are witnessed during apnea testing,
- SBP drops to <90 mm Hg or MAP <60 mm Hg despite titration of fluids, inotropes, and/or vasopressors
- Oxygen saturation drops <85% for >30 seconds.
- Unstable arrhythmia occurs.

(h) If the patient becomes unstable secondary to cardiovascular instability or hypoxia and apnea testing is aborted, a blood gas must be obtained and patient should be hyperventilated with an ambu-bag connected to 100% oxygen until the vital signs are stabilized after which time pre testing ventilation should be resumed. If the PaCO2 goal is achieved, apnea testing can be considered positive. If PaCO2 target is not met, ancillary testing should then be pursued.
(i) If spontaneous respirations were observed during the procedure and apnea testing was aborted, it is recommended to repeat apnea testing after 24 hours if the remaining of the clinical evaluation is consistent with a diagnosis of brain death.

Modifications in Apnea testing:

Declaration of apnea in brain death patients can be harmful due to the various adverse effects such as hypotension, hypoxia, acidosis, arrhythmias, asystole, pneumothorax, and cardiac arrest using conventional methods [34–39]. Due to inherent risks associated with apnea testing, a safe and efficient method should be used to prevent further injury and deleterious effects to the patients. A modified apnea test may be used at the discretion of the performing provider, particularly in patients with hemodynamic instability. The modified apnea test does not involve disconnecting patients from the ventilator and limits infection risk to healthcare providers and staff members from aerosolization of infected droplets in patients with contagious respiratory illness. It is useful in preventing alveolar collapse in patients with acute respiratory distress syndrome due to maintenance of continuous positive airway pressure (CPAP)/positive end expiratory pressure (PEEP), and allows steady and slow increase in PaCO2 levels rather than rapid changes in PaCO2 levels and thus limits hemodynamic instability [35, 39–42].

Procedure for Modified apnea test without disconnecting ventilator:

(a) Similar baseline pre-requisites are met, as with conventional apnea testing, prior to commencing modified apnea test i.e. a normal core body temperature (≥ 36 °C or 96.8 °F), normotension (SBP > 100 mm Hg), euvolemia and no hypoxia.

(b) Pre-oxygenate with 100% O2 for 10 minutes and connect end tidal CO2 monitor (ETCO2). A baseline ABG should be obtained with confirmation of normocarbia (PaCO2 between 35–45 mm Hg).

(c) Commence hypoventilation while still connected to the ventilator by reducing minute ventilation (MV) by at least 50% from stable baseline ventilator settings. Reduce respiratory rate to 2 breaths/min and reduce tidal volume to 50% of current ventilator settings. Apnea alarm should be increased accordingly (45–60 secs) to prevent frequent alarming from prolonged apnea. Maintain initial PEEP level (5 cm H2O) but may be increased or decreased depending on the clinical situation. Attention should be paid to flow sensitivity trigger settings as a low sensitivity can lead to auto cycling and may be misinterpreted as respiratory effort. Similarly, keeping a low-pressure sensitivity for patients on pressure support ventilation may falsely trigger breaths secondary to pressure changes from a hyperdynamic precordium.

(d) After 10 minutes, obtain a blood gas and ABGs should be drawn periodically until PaCO2 levels are ≥ 60 mm Hg or ≥ 20 mm Hg from baseline values.

(e) After reaching a target PaCO2 level, ventilator mode is switched to CPAP to ensure airway maintenance by applying continued PEEP and maximizing the likelihood of adequate alveolar oxygenation.
(f) The patient is observed for signs of respiration for 60 seconds. If no respiratory effort is seen apnea testing is then confirmed. At this time patient should then be returned to previous ventilator settings.
(g) If patient becomes hemodynamically unstable, an ABG should be obtained and the test is aborted, returning the patient to previous ventilator settings.
(h) If the PaCO2 goal is achieved, apnea testing can be considered positive. If PaCO2 target is not met, an ancillary test can be performed as per the provider's discretion.

Modified Apnea test with maintenance of PEEP:
Another modification in modified apnea testing has been used widely and incorporated in the 2010 AAN guidelines for determination of brain death, involves maintenance of PEEP either by delivering CPAP at 10 cm H2O directly via ventilator or through the use of a T-piece tube with a CPAP valve connected at the outflow end [6]. The first approach involves the use of a ventilator and disabling the rescue breaths while maintaining a CPAP of 10 cm H2O [41, 43]. Another approach involves the use of a 10-cm H_2O PEEP valve attached to a T-piece directly attached to the ETT and delivering oxygen at 12 L/min [34]. The remaining parameters for apnea testing remain the same i.e. ABG is obtained at 10 mins and periodically thereafter until PaCO2 ≥ 60 mm Hg or rise in PaCO2 ≥ 20 mm Hg. Apnea is confirmed if there is absence of any respiratory movements in presence of hypercarbia. These techniques can prevent the decruitment of lungs, reduce the risk of hypoxemia, and increase hemodynamic stability by preventing blood pressure fluctuations as compared to the traditional O_2 insufflation method.

Pre-Apnea test recruitment maneuver:
Pre-apnea test recruitment maneuver has also been used recently which prevents alveolar collapse and hypoxemia, particularly in patients with low lung compliance like ARDS. The procedure involves utilizing delivering a PEEP of 5 cm H2O in increments every three breaths to a maximum of 25 cm H2O which is maintained for 2 mins. This is followed by disconnecting the ventilator and providing oxygen at 6 L/min via a tracheal insufflation catheter or connecting a CPAP valve at the end of the endotracheal tube at 20 cm H2O [44]. Blood gas is drawn after 10 mins and a rise in PaCO2 $\geq$ 20 mm Hg above the baseline or PaCO2 $\geq$ 60 mm Hg with absence of respiratory movements confirms apnea.

5. Step 5: Ancillary testing

When the full clinical examination, including the assessment of brain stem reflexes and the apnea test, is conclusively performed, no additional testing is required to determine brain death. However, when uncertainty exists in the clinical evaluation of brain death or when the apnea test cannot be performed, ancillary tests can then be performed [6]. Ancillary tests, also referred to as "confirmatory tests", should be considered in the following situations [45]:

- Severe facial trauma
- Preexisting pupillary abnormalities
- Toxic levels of sedative agents, aminoglycosides, anticholinergic agents, tricyclic antidepressants, antiepileptic drugs, chemotherapeutic agents, or neuromuscular blocking agents
- Severe pulmonary disease resulting in carbon dioxide retention
- uncertainty regarding interpretation of possible spinally mediated movements

Ancillary tests can be discussed under two subcategories: tests to assess cessation of cerebral blood flow (Table 1), and tests to assess electrophysiological function or loss of electrical activity of brain (Table 2) [5, 6, 17]. These tests should be

TABLE 1 Ancillary tests for cerebral blood flow

Ancillary Test	Findings consistent With Brain death	Advantages	Disadvantages	Sensitivity/ Specificity (%)
Conventional 4-vessel Angiography	Absence of intracerebral blood flow at or beyond carotid bifurcation or circle of Willis or of the vertebral arteries above the level of the atlanto-occipital junction [5, 47].	Reference "gold standard" for ancillary tests.	Invasive Requires transport to imaging suite False negative -contrast stasis or delayed filling in intracranial arteries [17, 48].	100/100 [47, 49]
Radionuclide perfusion Scintigraphy	Absent uptake of radio isotope tracer (99mTc-labeled (HMPAO) into the cerebral circulation demonstrates the "hollow skull" or "empty light bulb" sign [5, 17].	Can be performed bedside No exposure to contrast agent	Limited availability Limited evaluation of posterior cerebral circulation flow	88.4/100 [50]

(continued)

TABLE 1 (continued)

Ancillary Test	Findings consistent With Brain death	Advantages	Disadvantages	Sensitivity/ Specificity (%)
Transcranial doppler Ultrasound	Small systolic peaks in early systole without diastolic flow or reverberating flow, suggest very high vascular resistance [5]. Both anterior and posterior circulation should be evaluated	Inexpensive Easily available Can be performed bedside	Operator dependent/ expertise required 10–20% of patients may have no acoustic windows	88–99/98–100 [51]
Computed tomography angiography	Absence of opacification of intracranial circulation and deep cerebral veins [52].	Widely available	Exposure to contrast agent False negatives – stasis filling Not currently validated against above accepted tests	62–99/100 [53]

| Magnetic resonance angiography | Absence of intracranial arterial blood flow [6]. | Not affected by vascular stasis Visualization improved with gadolinium administration | Requires transport to imaging suite Prolonged time during which patient needs to lie flat, not safe for unstable patients Not currently validated against above accepted tests | 93–100/100 [54] |

Table 2 Ancillary tests for electrophysiological function

Ancillary test	Findings consistent With Brain death	Advantages	Disadvantages	Sensitivity/ Specificity (%)
EEG	Electrocerebral silence i.e. no detectable electrical activity (≥2 microvolts) is found during a 30-minute recording at increased sensitivity [5, 55].	Inexpensive Non-invasive Can be performed at bedside	In ICU setting, electrical background noise can produce numerous artifacts/ false readings. Confounded by sedation, hypothermia, toxic states, metabolic disorders	53–80/97 [49, 56]
Somatosensory Evoked Potentials	Bilateral absence of N20-P22 response with median nerve stimulation in the setting of an intact signal in the brachial plexus and spinal cord [5].	Inexpensive Non-invasive Can be performed at bedside Less confounded by sedation as compared to EEG	Confounded by cervical spinal cord injury, metabolic disturbances, hypothermia and brainstem lesions.	100/78 [57]

| Auditory Evoked Potentials | Bilateral absence of brainstem responses to an auditory stimulus (Waves III to V) in the presence of preserved cochlear response (Wave I) [58]. | Inexpensive Non-invasive Can be performed at bedside Less confounded by sedation as compared to EEG | Confounded by hypothermia, isolated cranial nerve 8th injury, brainstem lesions. Not useful as an isolated test. |

interpreted carefully by the provider and in the right context as false positive or false negative results have been reported and are not uncommon [46]. Ancillary testing should never be performed in a patient who does not meet the prerequisites for neurologic determination of death.

Step 6: Brain death certification and Medical Record documentation.

Declaration and time of death have both significant medical (e.g., organ/tissue donation) and nonmedical consequences, such as the initiation of mourning and preparation for burial. After the completion of brain death evaluation, the physician should certify in the patient's medical record whether the patient "meets the neurological criteria for death", and cause of death. As per the AAN practice parameters all phases of the determination of brain death must be documented in the medical record. The medical record must indicate:

- Etiology and irreversibility of coma.
- Absence of cerebral responsiveness.
- Absence of brain stem reflexes.
- Absence of respiration with $PaCO_2 \geq 60$ mm Hg (or ≥ 20 mm Hg increase over baseline normal $PaCO_2$).
- Justification for, and result of, ancillary tests if used.

The time of death that should be documented is the time the $PaCO_2$ reached the target value. In patients with an aborted apnea test, the time of death is when the ancillary test has been officially interpreted.

3 Current Evidence and Guidelines

In the United States, the use of neurological criteria to declare death was first legally defined by the UDDA in 1981 [4]. The UDDA recognized both "death by neurological criteria" and cardiopulmonary criteria in the definition of death and has been adopted by all the 50 states in concept, statutorily or judicially [59]. However, in the United States, most jurisdictions neither specify nor specifically identify the relevant criteria for determination of "brain death by neurological criteria", and instead note that brain death should be determined in accordance with the "currently accepted medical standards." Only two states – Nevada and New Jersey, have laws that mention the medical criteria that should be employed when determining brain death should be in accordance with the guidelines published by American Academy of Neurology in 2010 [6, 60, 61]. The 2010 AAN guidelines for brain death determination is largely derived from the definition of brain death provided by UDDA – "cessation of all functions of the entire brain, including the brain stem." To ensure the "cessation of brain function", physicians should determine the presence of unresponsive coma, absence of brainstem reflexes, and the absence of respiratory drive after a CO_2 challenge. The flowchart depicted in Fig. 1 summarizes the approach to brain death determination by neurological criteria and is based on the "accepted standards" as recommended by the American Academy of Neurology in their 2010 guidelines. Despite the availability of these well established and validated guidelines, there is widespread practice variation observed from institution to institution within the US. Greer et al. reviewed 492 hospital brain death policies across different institutions in the United States and noted significant variability. Approximately, 33.1% of policies required specific expertise in neurology or neurosurgery to diagnose brain death. Most hospitals (65.9%) required 2 separate examinations to determine brain death, and 20.9% required more than 2 examinations. For hospital policies that required more than 1 examination, 54.1% specified a waiting period between examinations; at least 6 hours in 71.1% of the policies. A specific waiting period of at least 24 hours was observed in 5.9% of the hospital policies in patients with cardiac arrest. Regarding pre-requisites for clinical testing, absence of hypotension was required by more than half of the protocols (56.2%) and 79.4% required a core body temperature of at least 36 °C. Most policies required apnea testing (97.4%) but only 83.5% specified a final $PaCO_2$ level

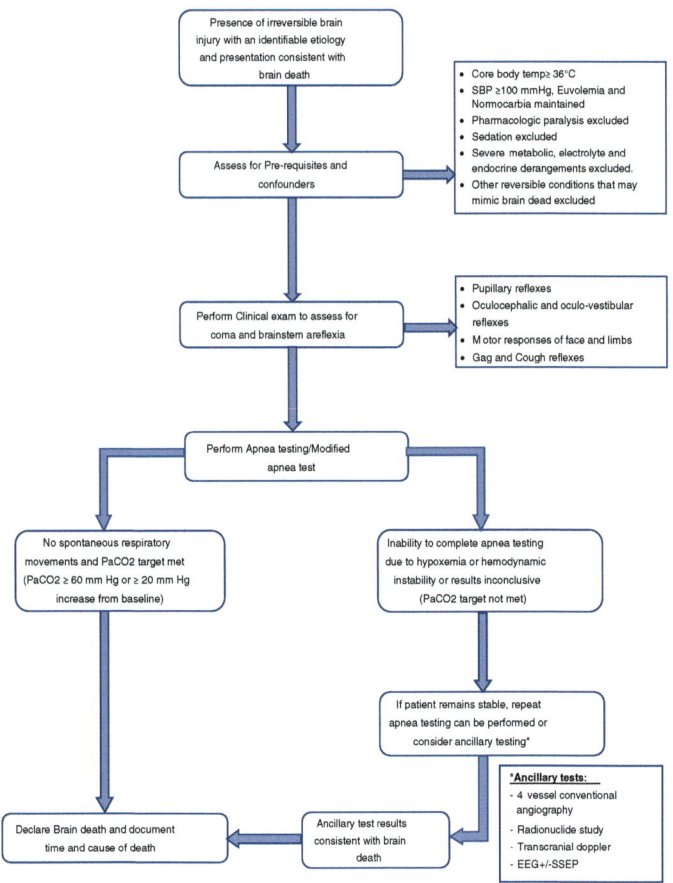

FIGURE 1 Flow Diagram for Determination of Brain Death by Neurologic Criteria

(≥60 mmg Hg). Ancillary testing was observed to be a mandatory requirement in 6.5% of the policies. Of the available options, EEG was listed as an ancillary test in 78.8%, transcranial Doppler ultrasonography in 33.0%, conventional cerebral angiography in 71.3%, and a radionuclide cerebral blood flow study in 72.3% of the policies [10]. This study highlighted ongoing gaps between the hospital policies for determination of brain death and practice parameters updated by AAN in 2010, across different institutions in the United States.

Some variability also exists in the requirements for brain death declaration across different states in the United States. For example, Florida requires two physicians, one of whom is the primary treating physician and the other a board-certified specialist in Neurology, neurosurgery, anesthesiology, internal medicine or surgery [62]. In Georgia and Alaska, a registered nurse has the authority to declare brain death, although a supervising physician is required to certify brain death within 24 hours [63, 64].

Surprisingly, notable differences exist throughout the world in the criteria for diagnosing brain death. For example, United Kingdom adheres to the concept of "brainstem death" rather than "whole brain death" as adopted in the United States. The Code of Practice of the Academy of Royal Medical Colleges defines death as "irreversible loss of the capacity for consciousness, combined with irreversible loss of the capacity to breathe." It further states that "the irreversible cessation of brain stem function (brain stem death) will produce the forementioned clinical state and therefore brain stem death is equivalent to the death of the individual" [65]. The U.K brainstem death criteria (U.K code), as described by Pallis and Harley, emphasizes on three sequential steps while evaluating patients for brainstem death:

- Ensuring that certain preconditions have been met
- Excluding reversible causes of apneic coma
- Clinical examination confirming brainstem areflexia and documenting persistent apnea.
- Functional etiologies of coma such as hypothermia, drug intoxication and metabolic disturbances must be excluded.

The U.K code requires testing of 5 brainstem reflexes: (a) pupillary response to light, (b) corneal reflex, (c) vestibulo-ocular reflex, (d) cranial motor nerve response, and (e) gag or reflex response to tracheal suctioning. As far as apnea testing is confirmed, a rise in $PaCO_2$ level ≥ 50 mm Hg with absence of any respiratory movement is considered consistent with a brainstem death as compared to a level of ≥60 mm Hg in the United States [65]. Another difference is the need for retesting to ensure observer error has not occurred.

The Canadian Neurocritical Care group has established brain death determination guidelines which is comparable to those formulated in the United States, though subtle differences exist. It recommends determination of brain death by physicians with experience in brain death criteria, and in the event of organ procurement, two physicians neither involved in the care of the patient nor part of the organ transplant team, should be engaged in brain death determination [66]. However, the criteria used for apnea testing used ($PaCO_2 \geq 60$ mm Hg) is comparable to that used in the United States.

In Australia and New Zealand, determination of brain death requires "irreversible cessation of all function of the brain", as in the United States. However, the Australia and New Zealand Intensive Care Society (ANZICS) guidelines for brain death require demonstration of absent intracranial flow either by 4 vessel conventional angiography or radionuclide study in conditions where clinical diagnosis cannot be met. A 4-hour observation period is required before the first clinical examination can begin [67].

4 Special Case Scenarios

1. **Therapeutic hypothermia:**
   Given the advances in cardiopulmonary resuscitation and critical care management, the use of targeted temperature management (TTM) in the setting of neurological injury has been expanded to management of patients with traumatic brain injury, ischemic stroke, intracerebral hemorrhage, subarachnoid hemorrhage, and status epilepticus; as compared to out of hospital cardiac arrest patients previously [68]. It can be challenging to identify brain death after treatment with TTM because cooling can temporarily blunt brainstem reflexes [5, 16]. Other factors like use of

sedative drugs prior to, or during the use of TTM, can further confound the results of clinical evaluation due to delayed drug clearance. It is recommended that neuroimaging be obtained after rewarming in patients treated with TTM, if the clinical findings are consistent with brain death. If the neuroimaging findings are consistent with severe cerebral edema, 24 hours after rewarming to at least 36 °C, use of sedative drugs and other confounders should be excluded before determination of brain death. Ideally, clinical examination must be delayed until at least 5 elimination half-lives of the drug administered with the longest half-life has passed before performing an evaluation for brain death. After all the confounders have been addressed, clinical examination for brain death determination can be initiated 24 hours after the patient has been rewarmed to at least 36 °C. A cerebral blood flow study can be considered if results remain inconclusive [17].
2. **Patients requiring Extracorporeal Membrane Oxygenation (ECMO):**

    ECMO can be used to provide respiratory support only (Veno-Venous ECMO) for patients with refractory hypoxemia or to provide both respiratory and circulatory support (Veno-Arterial ECMO) for patients with refractory hypoxemia and severe cardiac and/or hemodynamic failure. Such patients are at increased risk of complications leading to brain injury. Hence, determination of brain death can be challenging especially while circulation is extracorporeally supported. The same fundamentals of brain death determination– etiology, prerequisites, clinical examination including brainstem reflexes, and indications for ancillary testing – should be applied to patients on ECMO. However, there is a lack of consensus or guidance on the appropriate procedure for apnea testing in such patients [69, 70]. The following steps should be used while performing apnea testing in patients on ECMO [17].

    (i) The extracorporeal blood flow should be maintained during the clinical evaluation and apnea test in order to prevent hemodynamic instability and achieve a MAP ≥ 60 mmHg in adults, for patients receiving V-A ECMO.

(ii) Pre-oxygenation should be provided by administering 100% O2 via the mechanical ventilator and increasing the O2 in the membrane lung from the ECMO machine to 100% for 10 minutes.
(iii) Similar to apnea testing in general, 100% oxygen should be delivered while patient is disconnected from ventilator either by using a tracheal cannula, an AMBU bag connected to a PEEP valve, or to the lungs via CPAP on the mechanical ventilator, a resuscitation bag with a functioning PEEP valve, or by maintenance of CPAP/PEEP without disconnecting the ventilator.
(iv) titrating the sweep gas flow rate to 0.5–1.0 L/min while maintaining oxygenation. This ensures minimal CO2 removal and promotes arterial CO2 accumulation.
(v) Observe for any spontaneous respiratory movements with serial measurement of blood gases. Similar criteria i.e. a pH < 7.30 and PaCO2 of at least 60 mmHg, or ≥20 mmHg above the patient's baseline PaCO2 for persons with pre-existing hypercapnia; should be achieved before brain death is confirmed.
(vi) Test should be aborted in case of hemodynamic instability or hypoxemia and patient should be returned to mechanical ventilation and prior ECMO sweep gas flow rate. Ancillary testing can be considered at this point for further evaluation.

5 Future Prospects

Accurate diagnosis of brain death depends on performing a valid clinical evaluation based on the current standards published by AAN, along with maintenance of complete documentation including the time and cause of death, in the medical record. Future prospective studies are required on brain death determination with a focus on examining safe and alternative ways for performing apnea testing, especially in the current COVID-19 pandemic era wherein disconnecting patients from mechanical ventilator can expose the healthcare staff to increased risk of infections. Furthermore, laws should be amended to ensure uniformity in the criteria for brain death declaration across different states within a country. Institutions should adopt and change their respective institutional policies for brain death testing in accordance with the "current accepted medical standards."

References

1. Souter MJ, Blissitt PA, Blosser S, Bonomo J, Greer D, Jichici D, Mahanes D, Marcolini EG, Miller C, Sangha K, Yeager S. Recommendations for the critical care management of devastating brain injury: prognostication, psychosocial, and ethical management : a position statement for healthcare professionals from the Neurocritical Care Society. Neurocrit Care. 2015;23(1):4–13.
2. Mollaret P, Goulon M. Le coma depasse. Rev Neurol (Paris). 1959;101:3–15.
3. A definition of irreversible coma: REPORT of the ad hoc committee of the Harvard Medical School to examine the definition of brain death. JAMA. 1968;205:337–40.
4. Guidelines for the determination of death: report of the medical consultants on the diagnosis of death to the President's commission for the study of ethical problems in medicine and biochemical and behavioral research. JAMA. 1981;246:2184–6.
5. Wijdicks EFM. Determining brain death in adults. Neurology. 1995;45:1003–11.
6. Wijdicks EF, Varelas PN, Gronseth GS, Greer DM. American Academy of Neurology. Evidence-based guideline update: determining brain death in adults: report of the Quality Standards Subcommittee of the American Academy of Neurology. Neurology. 2010;74(23):1911–8.
7. Greer DM, Varelas PN, Haque S, Wijdicks EF. Variability of brain death determination guidelines in leading US neurologic institutions. Neurology. 2008;70(4):284–9.
8. Wijdicks EFM. Brain death worldwide: accepted fact but no global consensus in diagnostic criteria. Neurology. 2002;58:20–5.

9. Wahlster S, Wijdicks EF, Patel PV, Greer DM, Hemphill JC 3rd, Carone M, Mateen FJ. Brain death declaration: practices and perceptions worldwide. Neurology. 2015;84(18):1870–9.
10. Greer DM, Wang HH, Robinson JD, Varelas PN, Henderson GV, Wijdicks EFM. Variability of brain death policies in the United States. JAMA Neurol. 2016;73:213–8.
11. Lewis A, Bakkar A, Kreiger-Benson E, Kumpfbeck A, Liebman J, Shemie SD, Sung G, Torrance S, Greer D. Determination of death by neurologic criteria around the world. Neurology. 2020;95(3):e299–309.
12. Patterson JR, Grabois M. Locked-in syndrome: a review of 139 cases. Stroke. 1986;17:758.
13. Stojkovic T, Verdin M, Hurtevent JF, et al. Guillain-Barré syndrome resembling brainstem death in a patient with brain injury. J Neurol. 2001;248:430.
14. Danzl DF, Pozos RS. Accidental hypothermia. N Engl J Med. 1994;331:1756.
15. Wijdicks EF, Rabinstein AA, Manno EM, Atkinson JD. Pronouncing brain death: contemporary practice and safety of the apnea test. Neurology. 2008;71(16):1240–4.
16. Mathur M, Ashwal S. Pediatric brain death determination. Semin Neurol. 2015;35(2):116–24.
17. Greer DM, Shemie SD, Lewis A, et al. Determination of brain death/death by neurologic criteria: the world brain death project. JAMA. 2020;324(11):1078–97.
18. Smith M. Physiologic changes during brain stem death--lessons for management of the organ donor. J Heart Lung Transplant. 2004;23(9 Suppl):S217–22.
19. Power BM, Van Heerden PV. The physiological changes associated with brain death-current concepts and implications for treatment of the brain-dead organ donor. Anaesth Intensive Care. 1995;23:26–36.
20. Saposnik G, Maurinoj SR, Bueri JA. Undulating toe movements in brain death. Eur J Neurol. 2004;11:723–7.
21. McNair NL, Meador KJ. The undulating toe flexion sign in brain death. Mov Disord. 1992;7:345–7.
22. Jorgensen EO. Spinal man after brain death. Acta Neurochir. 1973;28:259–73.
23. Urasaki E, Tokimura T, Kumai J, Wada S, Yokota A. Preserved spinal dorsal horn potentials in a brain-dead patient with Lazarus' sign. J Neurosurg. 1992;76:710–3.

24. Ropper A. Unusual spontaneous movements in brain-dead patients. Neurology. 1984;34:1089–92.
25. Heytens L, Verlooy J, Gheuens J, Bossaert L. Lazarus sign and extensor posturing in a brain-dead patient. J Neurosurg. 1989;71:449–51.
26. Conci F, Procaccio F, Arosio M, Boselli L. Viscero-somatic and viscero-visceral reflexes in brain death. J Neurol Neurosurg Psychiatry. 1986;49:695–8.
27. de Freitas GR, Lima MASD, Andre C. Complex spinal reflexes during transcranial Doppler ultrasound examination for the confirmation of brain death. Acta Neurol Scand. 2003;108:170–3.
28. Fujimoto K, Yamauchi Y, Yoshida M. Spinal myoclonus in association with brain death. Rinsho Shinkeigaku. 1989;11:1417–9.
29. Ivan L. Spinal reflexes in cerebral death. Neurology. 1973;23:650–2.
30. Friedman A. Sympathetic response and brain death. Arch Neurol. 1984;41:15.
31. Shemie SDHL, Hornby L, Baker A, et al. the International Guidelines for Determination of Death phase 1 participants, in collaboration with the World Health Organization. International guideline development for the determination of death. Intensive Care Med. 2014;40(6):788–97.
32. Academy of Medical Royal Colleges. A code of practice for the diagnosis and confirmation of death; 2008.
33. Australian and New Zealand Intensive Care Society. The ANZICS statement on death and organ donation. ANZICS; 2013.
34. Le'vesque S, Lessard MR, Nicole PC, Langevin S, LeBlanc F, Lauzier F, et al. Efficacy of a T-piece system and a continuous positive airway pressure system for apnea testing in the diagnosis of brain death. Crit Care Med. 2006;34(8):2213–6.
35. Benzel EC, Mashburn JP, Conrad S, Modling D. Apnea testing for the determination of brain death: a modified protocol. J Neurosurg. 1992;76(6):1029–31.
36. Jeret JS, Benjamin JL. Risk of hypotension during apnea testing. Arch Neurol. 1994;51(6):595–9.
37. Goudreau JL, Wijdicks EF, Emery BA. Complications during apnea testing in the determination of brain death: predisposing factors. Neurology. 2000;55(7):1045–8.
38. Saposnik G, Rizzo G, Vega A, Sabbatiello R, Deluca JL. Problems associated with the apnea test in the diagnosis of brain death. Neurol India. 2004;52(3):342–5.

39. Scott JB, Gentile MA, Bennett SN, Couture M, MacIntyre NR. Apnea testing during brain death assessment: a review of clinical practice and published literature. Respir Care. 2013;58(3):532–8.
40. Gutmann D, Marino P. An alternative apnea test for the evaluation of brain death. Ann Neurol. 1991;30(6):852.
41. al Jumah M, McLean DR, al Rajeh S, Crow N. Bulk diffusion apnea test in the diagnosis of brain death. Crit Care Med. 1992;20(11):1564–7.
42. Ahlawat A, Carandang R, Heard SO, Muehlschlegel S. The modified Apnea test during brain death determination: an alternative in patients with hypoxia. J Intensive Care Med. 2016;31(1):66–9.
43. Solek-Pastuszka J, Biernawska J, Iwanczuk W, et al. Comparison of two Apnea test methods, oxygen insufflation and continuous positive airway pressure during diagnosis of brain death: final report. Neurocrit Care. 2019;30:348–54.
44. Hocker S, Whalen F, Wijdicks EF. Apnea testing for brain death in severe acute respiratory distress syndrome: a possible solution. Neurocrit Care. 2014;20:298–300.
45. Webb A, Samuels O. Brain death dilemmas and the use of ancillary testing. Continuum (Minneap Minn). 2012;18(3):659–68.
46. Wijdicks EFM. The case against confirmatory tests for determining brain death in adults. Neurology. 2010;75(1):77Y83.
47. Braum M, Ducrocq X, Huot JC, Audibert G, Anxionnat R, Picard L. Intravenous angiography in brain death: report of 140 patients. Neuroradiology. 1997;39(6):400–5.
48. Flowers WM Jr, Patel BR. Persistence of cerebral blood flow after brain death. South Med J. 2000;93(4):364–70.
49. Paolin A, Manuali A, Di Paola F, et al. Reliability in diagnosis of brain death. Intensive Care Med. 1995;21(8):657–62.
50. Joffe AR, Lequier L, Cave D. Specificity of radionuclide brain blood flow testing in brain death: case report and review. J Intensive Care Med. 2010;25(1):53–64.
51. Chang JJ, Tsivgoulis G, Katsanos AH, Malkoff MD, Alexandrov AV. Diagnostic accuracy of transcranial Doppler for brain death confirmation: systematic review and meta-analysis. AJNR Am J Neuroradiol. 2016;37(3):408–14.
52. Qureshi AI, Kirmani JF, Xavier AR, Siddiqui AM. Computed tomographic angiography for diagnosis of brain death. Neurology. 2004;62(4):652–3.
53. Kramer AH, Roberts DJ. Computed tomography angiography in the diagnosis of brain death: a systematic review and meta-analysis. Neurocrit Care. 2014;21(3):539–50.

54. Matsumura A, Meguro K, Tsurushima H, Komatsu Y, Kikuchi Y, Wada M, Nakata Y, Ohashi N, Nose T. Magnetic resonance imaging of brain death. Neurol Med Chir (Tokyo). 1996;36(3):166–71.
55. Guideline three: minimum technical standards for EEG recording in suspected cerebral death. American Electroencephalographic Society. J Clin Neurophysiol. 1994;11(1):10–3.
56. Grigg MM, Kelly MA, Celesia GG, Ghobrial MW, Ross ER. Electroencephalographic activity after brain death. Arch Neurol. 1987;44(9):948–54.
57. Su Y, Yang Q, Liu G, et al. Diagnosis of brain death: confirmatory tests after clinical test. Chin Med J. 2014;127(7):1272–7.
58. Firsching R, Frowein RA, Wilhelms S, Buchholz F. Brain death: practicability of evoked potentials. Neurosurg Rev. 1992;15(4):249–54.
59. Lewis A, Cahn-Fuller K, Caplan A. Shouldn't dead be dead?: the search for a uniform definition of death. J Law Med Ethics: a journal of the American Society of Law, Medicine & Ethics. 2017;45:112–28.
60. An Act Relating to the Determination of Death, 2017 Nevada Acts ch. 315 (A.B. 424), effective Oct 1, 2017.
61. NJ Admin. Code § 13:35–6A.4.
62. FL Stat. § 382.009 (2013).
63. Ga. Code Ann. § 31–10-16.
64. Ala. Code § 22–31-1.
65. Academy of Medical Royal Colleges. A code of practice for the diagnosis and confirmation of death. Academy of Medical Royal Colleges; 2008.
66. Canadian Neurocritical Care Group. Guidelines for the diagnosis of brain death. Can J Neurol Sci. 1999;26(1):64–6.
67. Australian and New Zealand Intensive Care Society. The ANZICS statement on death and organ donation. 4th ed; 2019.
68. Cariou A, Payen JF, Asehnoune K, et al. Targeted temperature management in the ICU: guidelines from a French expert panel. Ann Intensive Care. 2017;7(1):70.
69. Madden MA, Cho P, Habashi S, N. Successful apnea testing during veno-venous extracorporeal membrane oxygenation (VV-ECMO). Neurocrit Care. 2012;17:S123.
70. Saucha W, Solek-Pastuszka J, Bohatyrewicz R, Knapik P. Apnea test in the determination of brain death in patients treated with extracorporeal membrane oxygenation (ECMO). Anaesthesiol Intensive Ther. 2015;47(4):368–71.

Continuous Renal Replacement Therapy

Zeeshan Azeem, Angela Emanuel, and Kunal Malhotra

This chapter is aimed at describing the following in the subsequent sections:

- The key risk factors for acute kidney injury in the Neuro-ICU patient population
- Diagnosis of AKI
- Principles, indications & modes of RRT
- Different forms of continuous renal replacement (CRRT) modalities
- Types of Dialysis Access
- Dialysis prescription with emphasis on key adjustments warranted in Neuro-ICU
- Principles of anticoagulation
- Strategies for AKI Prevention
- Novel Approaches for improving AKI Care
- Conclusion

Z. Azeem · A. Emanuel · K. Malhotra (✉)
Karl D Nolph Division of Nephrology, University of Missouri, School of Medicine, Columbia, MO, USA
e-mail: malhotrak@health.missouri.edu

© The Author(s), under exclusive license to Springer Nature Switzerland AG 2022
N. Arora (ed.), *Procedures and Protocols in the Neurocritical Care Unit*, https://doi.org/10.1007/978-3-030-90225-4_30

1 Introduction

Neurocritical care encompasses a wide range of neurological conditions and patient populations including those with primary neurological diseases as well as those with neurological sequelae from other medical and surgical conditions. Neurological illness is often associated with a poor clinical outcome. Specialized neurocritical care, as a discipline, evolved from neurosurgical postoperative care and management. Outcome of this patient group is increasingly determined by non-neurological complications rather than the underlying neurologic or neurosurgical diseases. Among these non-neurologic complications, AKI is an independent risk factor for mortality after traumatic brain damage, ischemic stroke, intracerebral and subarachnoid hemorrhage [1–4]. A recent nationwide survey from China found that mortality of AKI patients in the Neurocritical care Unit (NCCU) was around 10% [5]. AKI in the setting of critical illness is considered a significant contributor to poor outcome irrespective of the primary diagnoses or condition that warranted ICU care [6–8].

Patients with chronic kidney disease also constitute a large proportion of Neuro-ICU patients because of higher incidence of neurologic complications such as uremic encephalopathy, higher rates of ischemic and hemorrhagic stroke as well increased frequency of seizures [9].

Moreover, hypertension in patients with kidney disease is a significant risk factor for ischemic and hemorrhagic stroke. The risk of stroke rises further in patients on hemodialysis [10, 11].

2 Risk Factors for Renal Injury in the ICU

There are several risk factors for the development of acute kidney injury in critically ill patients. Among pre-existing conditions, hypertension, diabetes mellitus, coronary artery disease, peripheral arterial disease, cardiovascular disease and chronic kidney disease are significant risk factors. Among neurological conditions, except for ischemic stroke, no underlying disease was significantly associated with AKI. ICU patients in particular are at risk of AKI due to the concomitant infection, use of antibiotic therapy and nephrotoxic medication [1, 12].

3 Diagnosing Acute Kidney Injury in Critically-Ill Patients (Table 1)

AKI in Neurocritical care patients may be present on admission or develop during the hospital course. Early detection of AKI has been a challenge in critically-ill patients, leading to the development of several criteria for diagnosis and staging of AKI. The Acute Kidney Injury Network (AKIN) criteria is the most widely used criteria for the definition of AKI. The AKIN criteria define AKI as an abrupt (within 48 hrs) absolute rise in serum creatinine concentration of >0.3 mg/dl from baseline; >50% increase from baseline or oliguria of <0.5 ml/kg/hour for >6 hours. If the diagnosis of AKI is only based on presence of oliguria, it is crucial to ensure that adequate volume replacement has been attempted and renal tract obstruction excluded [13].

Other criteria that have been used are RIFLE (Risk, Injury, Failure; Loss and End-stage kidney disease) and KIDGO (Kidney Disease: Improving Global Outcomes). The review of available literature shows that all these criteria perform equally well in predicting mortality in critically-ill patients in the diagnosis of AKI [14].

4 Indications of Renal Replacement Therapy (Table 2)

Renal replacement therapy is indicated in a variety of renal and non-renal conditions. The most commonly encountered renal indications in intensive care settings are AKI complicated

TABLE 1 RIFLE/AKIN/KDIGO criteria for diagnosis and staging of AKI [15]

Classification	Definition for AKI	Stage	Serum Creatinine criteria for AKI staging
RIFLE	Increase in Serum Creatinine (SCr) ≥ 50% within 7 days	Risk	To ≥1.5 times baseline
		Injury	To ≥2 times baseline
		Failure	To ≥3 times baseline ≥44 µmol/L increase to at least 354 µmol/L
AKIN	Increase in SCr ≥ 26.5 µmol/L or ≥50% within 48 h	1	Increase in SCr ≥ 26.5 µmol/L or to 1.5–2 times baseline
		2	To 2–3 times baseline
		3	To ≥3 times baseline or ≥26.5 µmol/L or increase to at least 354 µmol/L or initiation of RRT
KDIGO	Increase in SCr ≥ 26.5 µmol/L within 48 h or ≥50% within 7d	1	Increase in SCr ≥ 26.5 µmol/L within 48 hours or to 1.5–2 times baseline
		2	To 2–3 times baseline
			To ≥3 times baseline or increase to at least 354 µmol/L or initiation of RRT

Note. *RIFLE* Renal Injury Failure Loss ESRD, *AKIN* Acute Kidney Injury Network, *KDIGO* Kidney Disease Global Outcomes

TABLE 2 Conventional indications for renal replacement therapy [17]

Fluid overload resistant to diuretic therapy
Metabolic acidosis refractory to medical management
Hyperkalemia refractory to medical management
Uremic symptoms or signs (encephalopathy, pericarditis, and bleeding diathesis)
Poisoning with a dialyzable drug or toxin
Hyperthermia refractory to regular cooling techniques
Life-threatening electrolyte derangements in the setting of acute kidney injury
Progressive azotemia or oliguria unresponsive to medical management

by hemodynamic instability and AKI associated with heart failure, volume overload, hypercatabolic states, liver failure, and brain swelling. Non-renal indications include but are not limited to sepsis, multi-organ failure (MOF), and adult respiratory distress syndrome [16].

5 Timing of RRT- Is Early Initiation of RRT Beneficial?

The most appropriate timing for the initiation of RRT has been a subject of considerable debate especially when acute kidney injury is not accompanied by major metabolic complications (e.g., acidosis, hyperkalemia, uremia) and fluid disturbances [18].

Early or accelerated RRT is the initiation of RRT before the onset of major complications. In standard or delayed RRT, treatment is started once the patient develops one of the following: a serum potassium level of ≥6.0 mmol/liter, a pH of ≤7.20 or a serum bicarbonate level of ≤12 mmol/liter, evidence of severe respiratory failure based on a ratio of the partial pressure of arterial oxygen(P) to the fraction of inspired oxygen(F) of ≤200, clinical perception of volume overload or persistent acute kidney injury for at least 72 hours of admission [19].

There is a consensus that RRT should be initiated as soon as possible in the presence of above parameters, however, in the cases of kidney injury without these complications the benefit of early RRT is uncertain [20]. Patients with AKI especially with fluid overload, who also have poor physiological reserve, may benefit from "early RRT" before the absolute indications develop. A generalized policy of early initiation of RRT may lead to unnecessary intervention in patients who would have recovered without such a treatment [20].

Most available evidence in favor of the early RRT has been derived from observational studies. Data from the Program to Improve Care in Acute Renal Disease (PICARD) trial, a multi-center observational study of AKI, showed that among the patients who required RRT with no previous chronic kidney disease (CKD), RRT initiation at a lower BUN ≤76 mg/dL compared to ≥76 mg/dL was associated with lower 14- and 28-day mortality [21].

The subgroup analysis of Finnish Acute Kidney Injury study (FINNAKI) concluded that initiation of RRT, once an absolute indication had developed (delayed initiation), was associated with higher 90-day mortality compared to early RRT [22].

Standard vs Accelerated Initiation of RRT in Acute Kidney Injury trial (STARRT-AKI) is the most recent RCT comparing accelerated versus standard initiation of RRT in critically ill patients. The results suggest that an accelerated renal-replacement strategy was not associated with a lower risk of death at 90 days [23]. In a recent systematic review and meta-analysis of randomized trials comparing delayed and early RRT strategies in patients with AKI, it was found that timing of RRT initiation does not affect survival in critically ill patients with severe acute kidney injury in the absence of urgent indications for RRT [24]. The authors recommended delaying RRT initiation with close patient monitoring, to reduce the use of RRT, thereby saving health resources. However, hemodialysis is associated with increased intracranial pressure (ICP) in Neuro-ICU patients, and the magnitude of the increase may be related to initial plasma urea levels. This finding might justify early initiation of RRT in neurocritical care unit patients to avoid high urea gradients [25].

In summary, in critically-ill patients the decision to initiate RRT should be individualized based on patients' physiological reserve according to their age, cardiovascular risk factors, pulmonary comorbidities, baseline renal function and the trend of inflammatory and renal injury markers.

6 Renal Replacement Therapies in NCCU

Intermittent or continuous renal replacement therapy (CRRT) remains the mainstay of therapy in treating AKI and refractory volume overload in the ICU. The available literature suggests that CRRT has a survival advantage over intermittent Hemodialysis (IHD) in hemodynamically compromised patients. The choice of renal replacement modality remains controversial due to lack of evidence from randomized controlled trials [26]. Many institutions across the US offer both therapies and have established different criteria in determining which one to use.

7 Types of Renal Replacement Therapy (RRT) (Table 3)

- IHD (Intermittent Hemodialysis)
- CRRT (Continuous Renal Replacement Therapy)
- Hybrid (SLED, Slow Low-Efficiency Dialysis)

IHD and continuous hemodialysis (HD) circuits utilize similar principles. Blood is removed from the patient, pumped through a dialysis filter and returned to the patient following removal of surplus water and waste. Intermittent dialysis pro-

TABLE 3 Comparison of modalities for RRT [27]

	Intermittent RRT	Hybrid RRT	Continuous RRT
Solute transport	Diffusion~Hemodialysis	Diffusion~Hemodialysis Convection~Hemofiltration	Diffusion~Hemodialysis Convection~Hemofiltration
Subtypes	Intermittent Hemodialysis (IHD) Isolated Hemofiltration (IUF)	Extended Dialysis (ED) or Sustained low-efficiency dialysis (SLED) or prolonged intermittent RRT(PIRRT)	Continuous Venovenous hemodialysis (CVVHD) Continuous Venovenous hemofiltration (CVVHF) Hemodialfiltration (CVVHDF) or Slow Continuous ultrafiltration (SCUF)
Duration	4–6 hours	6–16 hours	24 hours or more
Effect	Fast small solute removal+/-Fast fluid removal	Slower fluid & solute removal	Slower fluid & solute removal High total clearance of solutes
Use of standard RRT Machines	Yes	Yes	No

Note. *RRT* renal replacement therapy
Adapted from Schaubroeck et al. [27]. Copyright © 2020 Sage publication

vides renal replacement for brief intervals (3–4 h), usually daily or every 2–3 days. CRRT provides continuous 24-h per day therapy. The major difference between intermittent and continuous therapies is the speed and mechanism by which water and wastes are removed. IHD removes large amounts of water and wastes in a short period of time using principally diffusion compared with CRRT which works at a slower and steady rate using diffusion, convection or a combination of both. IHD allows chronic renal failure patients to limit the amount of time that they receive dialysis, the rapid removal of water and wastes during intermittent treatments may be poorly tolerated in unstable patients in the critically ill patients.

8 CRRT

8.1 Principles of CRRT

CRRT includes continuous hemofiltration, hemodialysis or a combination of the two i.e., hemodiafiltration.

Hemodialysis (HD) involves diffusion of solutes from high concentration compartment to low concentration compartment across the dialysis membrane. The blood and the dialysate move in opposite directions across the membrane to maximize the concentration gradient. Therefore, during HD, urea, creatinine, and potassium move from blood to dialysate, while other solutes, such as calcium and bicarbonate, move from dialysate to blood. The net effect is the desired changes in the plasma concentrations of blood urea nitrogen and plasma creatinine concentration along with an elevation in the plasma calcium and bicarbonate concentrations [16].

Hemofiltration (HF) involves the use of a hydrostatic pressure gradient referred to as transmembrane pressure (TMP) in order to induce the filtration (or convection) of plasma water across the membrane of the hemofilter. The frictional forces between water and solutes (called solvent drag) results in the convective transport of small and middle molecular weight solutes (<5000 Da) in the same direction as water. Different filter membrane properties can produce different ultrafiltration rates at a constant TMP. A filter that is more permeable to water will allow more water to travel across the membrane at a given TMP. A filter with a high permeability to water is called high-flux membrane [16]. To prevent hypovolemia, any water removed during HF is returned to the blood before it reaches the patient. This is called "replacement" fluid or "substitution" fluid. The process of HF itself removes smaller solutes (such as urea and electrolytes) in roughly the same concentration as the plasma resulting in very subtle change in plasma concentration of these solutes compared with HD [16].

8.2 Modes of CRRT

CRRT incorporates several modes of RRT utilizing different mechanisms of clearance, principally diffusive and convective clearance, as described above.

Some of the commonest used modes are [28]:

- Continuous arteriovenous hemofiltration (CAVH)
- Continuous venovenous hemofiltration (CVVH)
- Sustained low efficiency (SLED) or extended daily dialysis (EDD) Dialysis membranes
- Slow continuous ultrafiltration (SCUF)
- Continuous arteriovenous hemodialysis (CAVHD or CAVD)
- Continuous venovenous hemodialysis (CVVHD or CVVD)
- Continuous arteriovenous hemodiafiltration (CAVHDF)
- Continuous venovenous hemodiafiltration (CVVHDF)

As detailed above as to the principles of RRT, each mode uses a unique strategy with some using convective clearance (CVVH) while other modes use diffusive clearance or some combination of convective and diffuse clearance (CVVHDF). This complexity in machine configuration extends further to include options such as pre-filter or post-filter solution replacement in convective modes, to different filter technology in modes that utilize diffusion alone or a combination of diffusion & convection.

The neuro-intensivist is responsible for the majority of the decisions in the care of a critically-ill patient in the Neuro-ICU. This includes adjusting vasopressors, adding new antibiotics, initiating and managing nutritional supplementation, giving fluids or colloids for hemodynamic support or continually monitoring hemodynamic parameters. Therefore, understanding CRRT and its different modalities is extremely important since CRRT affects, among other things, drug clearance and dosing, including antibiotics and vasopressors, and also affects nutritional support. These effects are dependent on CRRT mode, type of clearance, mode configuration, and filter type. The use of anticoagulation for CRRT, in liaison with a nephrologist, is another vital area that needs to be managed and understood by the neuro-intensivist [16].

9 Is CRRT Superior Than Other Modalities?

Current evidence-base suggests that CRRT offers no definite benefits to mortality or preservation of renal function when compared to IHD [17]. IHD, SLED and CRRT are complementary modalities whose use should be individualized based on patient's clinical context and logistics including staff and equipment availability. Multiple modalities can be used on the same patient at different times based on changing clinical needs. IHD is considered the first-line therapy in situations requiring rapid correction of electrolytes (hyperkalemia), urgent fluid removal, and poisoning especially if patients can tolerate it from a hemodynamic standpoint [17].

In summary, CRRT is primarily used in hemodynamically unstable patients in the ICU setting followed by a transition to IHD once vasopressor support is no longer required [17]. Major advantages of CRRT are listed in the Table 4:

TABLE 4 Major advantages of CRRT [16]

Slow and steady removal of solute or fluid removal avoids abrupt changes in body fluid volume and composition (especially beneficial in neurocritical patients)
Superior control of body temperature, fluid, and metabolic profile
Continuous control of azotemia, electrolytes, and acid–base balance
Continuous removal of fluid in volume overload clinical situations
Administration of parenteral nutrition and other fluids without concern for volume excess due to continuous ultrafiltration
Can lower intracranial pressure as opposed to routine IHD which can sometimes raise intracranial pressure
Removal of circulating inflammatory substances including cytokines, activated components of complement, and derivatives of the arachidonic acid

10 CRRT Dosing

CRRT dose represents the volume of blood purified per unit of time and is quantified by effluent rate normalized to body weight (unit: mL/kg/h). In clinical practice, effluent comprises net ultrafiltrate along with replacement fluid and dialysate, depending on the CRRT modality.

The current KDIGO guidelines recommend that patients treated with CRRT should receive an effluent flow rate of 20 to 25 mL/kg/h. In clinical practice, in order to achieve a delivered dose of 20–25 ml/kg/h, it is generally necessary to prescribe a slightly higher dose at 25–30 ml/kg/h, and to account for treatment interruptions in CRRT. The dose should be frequently assessed and adjusted according to the clinical situation [17, 29].

The optimal RRT dosing for AKI has been an area of extensive study in recent times. A large majority of early data came from studies in septic patients with AKI. Initial data suggested survival benefit with relatively higher effluent flow rate (>35 ml/kg/hr). It was understood that high effluent flow rate reduces vasopressor requirements thus improving hemodynamic stability and expedites removal of inflammatory mediators in sepsis. The IVOIRE study, consisting of 137 patients with septic shock- associated AKI, compared an effluent flow rate of 70 ml/kg/hr with 35 ml/kg/hr and found no significant difference in vasopressor requirement and 28-day mortality between the two groups [30].

The two landmark trials, the VA/NIH Acute Renal Failure Trial Network (ATN) study [31] and the Randomized Evaluation of Normal versus Augmented Level (RENAL) Replacement Therapy Study [32] compared HVHF (High Volume Hemofiltration) versus standard therapy found that higher-intensity treatment was not associated with reduced mortality, improved renal recovery or reduced rate of non-renal organ failure when compared with less intensive therapy. Both studies also showed significantly more hypotensive episodes requiring vasopressor support and hypophosphatemia in the high-intensity group.

In conclusion, high effluent flow rates do not affect mortality but are associated with greater electrolyte disturbances, nursing requirements, nutritional demands and difficulty in maintaining therapeutic drug doses [17, 29, 31].

11 Dialysis Access

Two commonest types of access for RRT include:

1. **Arteriovenous (AV):** In patients with pre-existing AV fistula or graft.
   Here the systemic blood pressure drives the blood into the extracorporeal circuit via an arterial needle, which after dialysis is then returned via a venous needle.
2. **Venovenous (VV):**
   Requires one double lumen catheter (occasionally two catheters are used) to be placed in a vein. It requires an extracorporeal blood pump to circulate blood through the dialysis machine.

Traditional RRT circuits removed blood from arterial access sites and returned purified blood via venous catheter, thus utilizing patients' own blood flow A-V gradient and alleviating the need for pump. However, these circuits carry increased risk of aeroembolism, ischemia of limb, hematoma formation, hemorrhage, arterial wall injury and spasm of the artery cannulated [33].

Current CRRT machines have a pump and hence use a veno-venous access. Temporary double-lumen venous dialysis catheters are the most common form of RRT access in the ICU setting. They can be inserted quickly at the bedside and used immediately. This method gives rapid and constant blood flow rate, improved dialyzer performance and decreased circuit and dialyzer clotting [16]. Major access-related complications include aneurysm formation, infections, ischemic steal syndrome, thrombosis, venous hypertension among hemodialysis patients using a fistula, difficult cannulation, bleeding, hematoma, catheter insertion, and endovascular intervention [34].

12 Anticoagulation

Extracorporeal circuit clotting is a major issue with CRRT primarily due to the accumulation of proteins in a process called concentration polarization. Common causes of clotting are listed in Table 5. Significant loss of therapeutic time occurs in replacing clotted hemofilters, which diminishes the efficacy of the treatment.

TABLE 5 The commonest reasons for circuit clotting [35]

1. Suboptimal or inadequate anticoagulation
2. Poor quality vascular access
3. Poor attention to optimal machine operation
4. Sudden changes and patient positioning that can alter catheter function
5. Decreased blood flow
6. Induced clotting due to stasis

Increasing the dose of anticoagulation for all the causes other than the first one can potentially be dangerous. Therefore, every clotting episode ought to be analyzed and addressed accordingly.

13 Types of Anticoagulation for CRRT [17]

It can be divided into four categories:
- Regional Anticoagulation
- Systemic Anticoagulation
- Anticoagulation in Special Situations/Other Agents
- No Anticoagulation

13.1 Regional Anticoagulation (Table 6)

According to the KDIGO guidelines, RCA is the preferred anticoagulation modality in CRRT [29]. As the name implies, this technique keeps the dialysis circuit from clotting (regional) and allows for prolonged filter life without the need for sys-

TABLE 6 Advantages and disadvantages of Regional Citrate Anticoagulation (RCA) [37]

Advantages	Disadvantages
Lower cost	Technically more difficult
Reduced bleeding rates	to perform than systemic
Longer hemo-filter survival	anticoagulation with unfractionated
Similar overall mortality	heparin (UFH)
when compared to systemic	Potential metabolic complications
anticoagulation (heparin-based)	such as hypocalcemia, hypomagnesaemia and hypernatremia
	Metabolic alkalosis (in preserved liver function), and high anion gap metabolic acidosis (in liver dysfunction)
	Relatively contraindicated in acute liver injury and cardiogenic shock with significant lactic acidosis

temic anticoagulation. Therefore, it can safely be used in patients with moderate to high risk of bleeding. The two available options are regional citrate anticoagulation (RCA) and regional heparin anticoagulation (RHA). Principle of RCA is that the citrate binds to calcium (and to some extent, magnesium) thereby impairing function of the calcium-dependent clotting factors. Most of the citrate-calcium complexes are subsequently removed in the effluent and the portion that enters the blood circulation is metabolized in the liver where they are converted to bicarbonate and the calcium is released [36]. Since the post filter blood reentering the circulation has lower ionized calcium due to binding with citrate, calcium needs to be infused via a central line to avoid hypocalcemia. Ionized calcium is monitored frequently at prefilter and post filter level. Based on pre-filter calcium, calcium infusion is titrated to maintain normal ionized calcium in blood and based on post filter calcium, citrate infusion is titrated to ensure adequate lowering of ionized calcium within the dialysis circuit for effective anticoagulation. Since the calcium- citrate complex is broken down by the liver, patients with liver failure can accumulate citrate that can lead to metabolic acidosis.

RHA involves pre-filter infusion of unfractionated heparin (UFH) and neutralization with protamine infusion post-filter. RHA has progressively fallen out of vogue & and carries significant risk of anaphylactoid reaction secondary to protamine. In addition, hypotension, leukopenia and thrombocytopenia have also been reported. RHA has also been associated with a shorter hemofilter survival compared to RCA [38].

13.2 Systemic Anticoagulation (Table 7)

Per KDIGO guidelines, UFH infusion is typically a second-line option (when RCA is contraindicated), with the current evidence suggesting that RCA is superior in terms of bleeding risk and hemofilter survival [29, 37].

Low-molecular heparin (LMWH) carries lower risk for HIT & bleeding when compared to UFH. However, the key issue being limited experience with its use. Serial factor Xa

TABLE 7 Advantages and disadvantages of systemic anticoagulation [39–41]

Advantages	Disadvantages
Established experience of its use Reversibility with protamine Popular due to ease of use	Heparin-induced thrombocytopenia (HIT) is one of the major complications associated with heparin use. It typically develops within five to ten days of heparin use and usually requires immediate discontinuation of heparin. The activated partial thromboplastin time (aPTT) needs to be closely monitored with a goal between 40 and 45 seconds.

monitoring is also required to maintain therapeutic dose. Limited data from RCTs highlights that LMWH has similar rates of bleeding as reported with UFH, however, carries much higher incidence of bleeding when compared to RCA [42]. It has been noted that hemo-filter survival with LMWH anticoagulation may be slightly superior to UFH [43].

14 Special Considerations for CRRT Prescription in Neurocritical Care Patients

Renal replacement therapy may exacerbate brain injury by raising intracranial pressure which reduces the cerebral blood flow and also by ultrafiltration leading to reduced blood supply [44]. Therefore, the prescription of the RRT should be modified accordingly. In addition, some other important considerations are maintaining cardiovascular stability, choice of anticoagulation especially in the patients who have recently suffered intracerebral bleeding and in whom intracranial pressure monitoring is being undertaken [45].

Figure 2 describes the simple protocol which can be considered for CRRT in critical care patients.

1. <u>Maintaining adequate cerebral blood flow in hemodialysis patients:</u>

Maintenance of adequate cerebral blood supply is one of the major considerations in NCCU patients. Healthy non-anemic patients on hemodialysis may have reduced cerebral blood flow as assessed by transcranial Doppler measurements of the middle cerebral artery resulting in reduced cortical oxygen supply [46]. Moreover, during hemodialysis, middle cerebral blood flow falls with increasing ultrafiltration leading to a drop in cerebral oxygen saturation. The regulatory response to changes in arterial carbon dioxide tension remains intact. Patients should be monitored closely and supplemental oxygen provided to avoid cerebral hypoxia. Careful attention should be given to avoid hypotension during dialysis as patients in neurocritical care units may either have or are at risk of cerebral edema leading to increased intracranial pressure and further reduction in cerebral perfusion pressure [10]. Davenport demonstrated the relationship in mean arterial pressure and intracranial pressure during the dialysis session as shown in Fig. 1 (Fig. 2).

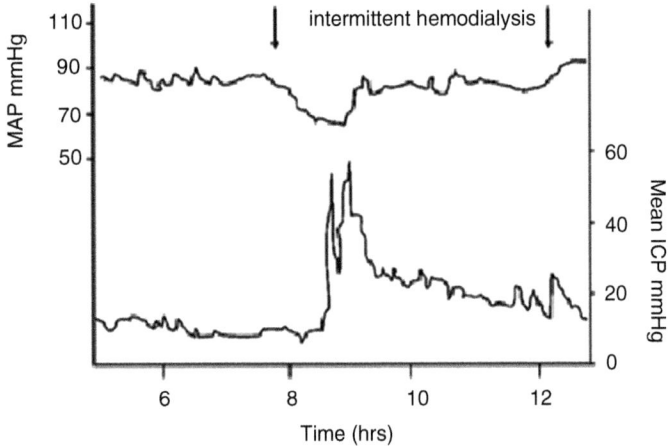

FIGURE 1 Relationship between the MAP and ICP during dialysis in a patient with subdural hemorrhage [47]. Fall in mean arterial blood pressure (MAP) at the start of renal replacement therapy, associated with an increase in intracranial pressure (ICP) and fall in cerebral perfusion pressure (CPP) in a hemodialysis patient post neurosurgical evacuation of subdural hemorrhage

Continuous Renal Replacement Therapy

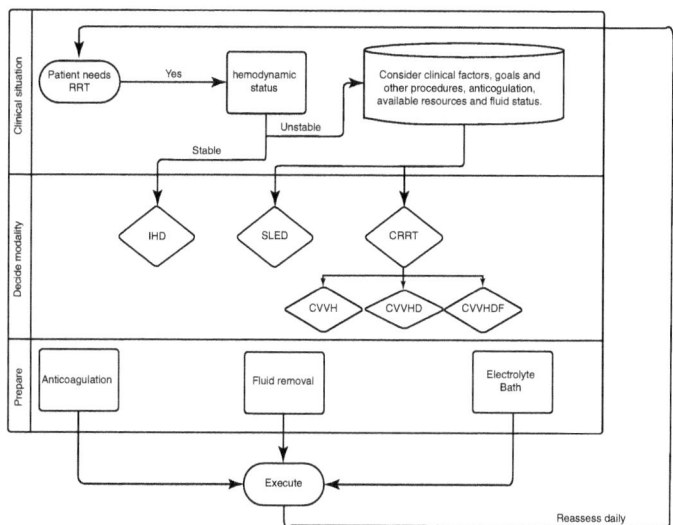

FIGURE 2 Protocol decision for CRRT

Patient survival and favorable outcome require vigilant monitoring and appropriate adjustment of renal replacement therapy [6]. Following modifications in CRRT dosing can ensure hemodynamic stability and this maintains appropriate cerebral blood flow:

(a) Use of greater dialysate sodium, potassium and calcium concentration reduced the risk of reduction in systemic blood pressure and therefore maintained adequate cerebral perfusion [11].
(b) Treatment should be designed to both slow down the rate of change of serum urea and osmolality, and to maintain cardiovascular stability [47].
(c) Hemofiltration techniques, particularly predilutional, will further reduce the rate of urea clearance.
(d) Dialysate with highest potassium concentration should be chosen to reduce the risk of cardiac arrhythmias.
(e) Low serum calcium in patients with kidney disease increases the risk of cardiovascular instability. A dialysate with high calcium concentration can mitigate this effect.

(f) Cooling of dialysate to 35 °C will also reduce the risk of hypotension during dialysis [48].
(g) Cardiovascular stability can be improved by choosing a biocompatible dialyzer, and priming with isotonic bicarbonate to minimize bradykinin generation, preventing hypotension when patients are first connected to the extracorporeal circuit [47].

2. <u>Minimizing cerebral edema:</u>

Elevated ICP may be the consequence of primary neurological condition or as a result of renal replacement therapy. Some degree of cerebral oedema is seen with routine outpatient hemodialysis patients. During hemodialysis, serum urea falls rapidly during the first hour. There is a delay in the transport of urea from the brain cells into the plasma compared to the dialyzer clearance of urea. This leads to a urea gradient which is proportional to fall in plasma osmolality. As water moves at a much faster rate than urea via aquaporin channels, there is a net movement of water down the osmotic gradient from plasma to brain cells resulting in cerebral edema [49].

The renal replacement therapy should be tailored to avoid abrupt reduction in plasma osmolality. Following measures should be taken to achieve this goal:

(a) Intermittent therapy is associated with abrupt changes in hemodynamics and intracranial pressures. Therefore, in the presence of severe neurological illness and unconsciousness, continuous renal replacement or hybrid therapies are preferred. Intermittent therapy can be considered when imaging shows limited cerebral damage with no cerebral edema [11].
(b) Urea clearance depends upon diffusion, therefore, reducing the surface area of the dialyzer, rate of flow of blood and dialysate and decreasing the time of the dialysis session would slow down the process of diffusion. Rate of diffusion is also proportional to initial concentration of urea so increasing the frequency of dialysis will

reduce the pre-dialysis urea levels and absolute fall in urea levels [11].
(c) Sodium is osmotically active solute, so increasing sodium concentration can mitigate the effects of fall in urea. This can be achieved by setting the dialysate sodium concentration 5–10 mEq// higher than serum sodium.
(d) Dialysate fluid contains supraphysiological bicarbonate concentration to correct metabolic acidosis due to renal failure. The bicarbonate reacts with plasma hydrogen ions to form water and carbon dioxide. This carbon dioxide passes into the cell and leads to increased intracellular osmolality and cell swelling. This worsens the cerebral edema in patients with neurological conditions and thus the dialysis prescription should be adjusted to deliver a relatively lower bicarbonate concentration of 30–32 mEq/L [11].

3. Choice of appropriate anticoagulant:

In many patients admitted to neuro-ICU, the blood-brain barrier may be disrupted and there is a potential risk of local hemorrhage into the damaged area. Therefore, excessive systemic anticoagulants should be avoided in patients with recent hemorrhage and those with catheters in situ to monitor ICP. Regional anticoagulation with citrate being infused pre-dialyzer and a calcium free dialysate is preferred as well as CRRT without any anticoagulant. In case of CRRT, predilution is preferred to prevent hemoconcentration in the circuit. In addition, in post dilution mode, the filtration fraction - calculated as effluent rate/plasma flow rate - should be below 20 to 25% [50]. Other regional anticoagulants include prostanoids which can lead to vasodilation and reduced cerebral blood flow [11]. Serine protease inhibitors have been used in patients at high risk of bleeding due to short half-life but the use is limited due to cost and availability [51]. Heparin rinsing of dialyzers, which have been surface modified to adsorb heparin, have been successfully used to dialyze patients without systemic anticoagulation [52].

Theoretically, PD can be considered as an alternative since it does not need any anticoagulation. Concerns on this modality are the efficacy and the effects on intra-abdominal pressure. The intra-abdominal pressure may increase secondary to infusion of PD fluid in the abdominal cavity, which may have diverse effects on intracranial pressure and cerebral perfusion. Increased abdominal pressure may translate into increased intracranial pressure. Further, intra-abdominal hypertension may also decrease systemic preload and increase afterload, leading to lower blood pressure and decreased cerebral perfusion pressure [50, 53, 54].

15 Prevention of AKI

In addition to the early identification & management of critically-ill patients with AKI in the Neuro-ICU, special attention needs to be given to preventive measures for its development. The commonest first step should be to modify interventions or treatments that can potentially cause or precipitate kidney injury. Some of the important strategies include:

- Prevention and treatment of infectious complications lower the incidence of AKI and hereby improve outcome in neurocritical care.
- Maintaining adequate renal perfusion is pivotal in preventing acute kidney injury. Careful yet optimal use of crystalloids or colloid solutions ensure it. Volume expansion combined with the use of vasopressor agents might be required to optimize renal perfusion in septic patients.
- Nephrotoxic substances such as hydroxyethyl starch solutions are best avoided in high-risk patients and those with established AKI.

- Avoid non-steroidal anti-inflammatory drugs (NSAIDs) and nephrotoxic antibiotics especially aminoglycosides; consider using alternative analgesics and antibiotics deemed safe in renal injury.
- For Imaging, avoid CT with contrast, if possible. Use ultrasound, non-contrast computed tomography (CT) or an MRI instead.
- If an intervention using iodinated contrast agent is being planned, adequate hydration should be ensured & medications such as ACE (angiotensin converting enzyme) inhibitors, ARB (angiotensin receptor blocker), NSAIDs may need to be held.

16 Novel Approaches

Early diagnosis and treatment of kidney injury in critically ill patients is of paramount importance for a favorable outcome. There is an increasing interest in the role of biomarkers in early identification of acute kidney injury. Several categories of real time biomarkers are under investigation in an effort to expedite diagnosis and treatment of AKI (Table 8).

Current evidence from clinical studies supports the use of new biomarkers in prevention and management of AKI. Substantial gaps in knowledge remain, and more research is necessary [56].

The combined Tissue Inhibitor of Metalloproteinases-2 (TIMP-2) and Insulin-like Growth Factor-Binding Protein 7 (IGFBP7) (commonly marketed as NephroCheck® by Astute Medical, San Diego, CA – now part of BioMérieux, Inc., Lyon, France) is a commercially available test that has the potential to transform how we detect and treat AKI, however it has poor specificity, limiting clinical utility [57].

TABLE 8 summarizes the findings of several studies investigating modern biomarkers of AKI in a variety of clinical settings for several clinical end points [55]

	Perioperative AKI			Critically ill			Emergency Room	
	Early post-op. AKI	AKI progression	Long-term mortality	Early diagnosis of AKI	Type of AKI (Transient vs intrinsic)	Need for RRT	Early diagnosis of AKI	Type of AKI (Transient vs intrinsic)
Urine NGAL	+	−	+	+	+	+	+	+
Blood NGAL	+	+	?	−	?	−	?	?
Blood CysC	+	−	?	+	+	+	?	?
Urine IL-18	+	+	+	+	+	+	+	+
Urine KIM-1	+	−	+	+	−	−	+	+
Urine LFABP	−	−	+	?	?	−	+	+

TIMP-2 IGFBP-7	?	?	?	+	?	+	?
Urine protein/ Albumin	+	+	+	?	?	?	?

Note. *AKI* Acute kidney Injury; *CysC* Cystatin C; *IGFBP7* Insulin like growth factor binding protein 7; *IL-18* Interleukin 18; *KIM-1* Kidney injury molecule 1; *LFABP* liver fatty acid binding protein; *NGAL* Neutrophil gelatinase associated lipocalin; *op* operative; *RRT* renal replacement therapy; *TIMP-2* Tissue inhibitor of metalloproteinases-2; + Data published displays the ability to detect this aspect of AKI; – Data published does not display ability to detect this aspect of AKI;? No large data published on this biomarker/aspect of AKI

17 Conclusion

- The management of critically ill patients with concomitant neurological and kidney disease is challenging.
- Early recognition of AKI and appropriate intervention can prevent long term disability.
- Careful consideration of the pathophysiology and modification of renal replacement therapy is needed to achieve optimal outcome.

References

1. Büttner S, et al. Incidence, risk factors, and outcome of acute kidney injury in Neurocritical Care. J Intensive Care Med. 2020;35(4):338–46.
2. Wang D, et al. Epidemiology of acute kidney injury in patients with stroke: a retrospective analysis from the neurology ICU. Intern Emerg Med. 2018;13(1):17–25.
3. Qureshi AI, et al. Acute kidney injury in acute ischemic stroke patients in clinical trials. Crit Care Med. 2020;48(9):1334–9.
4. Qureshi AI, et al. Systolic blood pressure reduction and acute kidney injury in intracerebral hemorrhage. Stroke. 2020;51(10):3030–8.
5. Tang X, et al. Acute kidney injury burden in different clinical units: data from nationwide survey in China. PLoS One. 2017;12(2):e0171202.
6. Litmathe J, et al. Predictors and outcome of ICU readmission after cardiac surgery. Thorac Cardiovasc Surg. 2009;57(7):391–4.
7. Andrikos E, et al. Epidemiology of acute renal failure in ICUs: a multi-center prospective study. Blood Purif. 2009;28(3):239–44.
8. Charbonney E, et al. Prognosis of acute kidney injury requiring renal replacement therapy in solid organ transplanted patients. Transpl Int. 2009;22(11):1058.
9. Cislaghi F, Condemi AM, Corona A. Predictors of prolonged mechanical ventilation in a cohort of 5123 cardiac surgical patients. Eur J Anaesthesiol. 2009;26(5):396–403.
10. Hirsch KG, Josephson SA. An update on neurocritical care for the patient with kidney disease. Adv Chronic Kidney Dis. 2013;20(1):39.

11. Davenport A. Changing the hemodialysis prescription for hemodialysis patients with subdural and intracranial hemorrhage. Hemodial Int. 2013;17(Suppl 1):S22–7.
12. Iseki K, O.D.S.G, Fukiyama K. Clinical demographics and long-term prognosis after stroke in patients on chronic haemodialysis. The Okinawa Dialysis Study (OKIDS) Group. Nephrol Dial Transplant. 2000;15(11):1808-13.
13. Mehta RL. Acute Kidney Injury Network: report of an initiative to improve outcomes in acute kidney injury. Crit Care. 2007;11(2):31.
14. Levi TM. Comparison of the RIFLE, AKIN and KDIGO criteria to predict mortality in critically ill patients. Rev Bras Ter Intensiva. 2013;25:290.
15. Li Z, et al. Identification and predicting short-term prognosis of early cardiorenal syndrome type 1: KDIGO is superior to RIFLE or AKIN. PLoS One. 2014;9(12):e114369.
16. Patel P, et al. Continuous renal replacement therapies: a brief primer for the neurointensivist. Neurocrit Care. 2010;13(2):286–94.
17. Ahmed AR, Obilana A, Lappin D. Renal replacement therapy in the critical care setting. Crit Care Res Pract. 2019;2019:6948710.
18. Bouchard J, Cutter G, Mehta R. Timing of initiation of renal-replacement therapy in acute kidney injury. N Engl J Med. 2020;383(18):1796.
19. Bagshaw SM, Darmon M, Ostermann M. Current state of the art for renal replacement therapy in critically ill patients with acute kidney injury. Intensive Care Med. 2017;43:841–54.
20. Gaudry S, Hajage D, Schortgen F. Initiation strategies for renal-replacement therapy in the intensive care unit. N Engl J Med. 2016;375:122–33.
21. Chertow GM, et al. Reasons for non-enrollment in a cohort study of ARF: the Program to Improve Care in Acute Renal Disease (PICARD) experience and implications for a clinical trials network. Am J Kidney Dis. 2003;42:507.
22. Nisula S. Incidence, risk factors and 90-day mortality of patients with acute kidney injury in Finnish intensive care units: the FINNAKI study. Intensive Care Med. 2013;39:420.
23. Bagshaw SM, et al. Timing of initiation of renal-replacement therapy in acute kidney injury. N Engl J Med. 2020;383(3):240–51.
24. Gaudry S, et al. Delayed versus early initiation of renal replacement therapy for severe acute kidney injury: a systematic review

and individual patient data meta-analysis of randomised clinical trials. Lancet. 2020;395(10235):1506–15.
25. Anton L, Damholt MB, Wiis J, Kelsen J, Strange DG, Møller K. Intracranial pressure during hemodialysis in patients with acute brain injury. Acta Anaesthesiol Scand. 2019;63(4):493–9.
26. Wang AY, Bellomo R. Renal replacement therapy in the ICU: intermittent hemodialysis, sustained low-efficiency dialysis or continuous renal replacement therapy? Curr Opin Crit Care. 2018;24(6):437–42.
27. Schaubroeck HA, et al. Acute cardiorenal syndrome in acute heart failure: focus on renal replacement therapy. Eur Heart J Acute Cardiovasc Care. 2020;9(7):802–11.
28. Malhotra K. Dialysis in acute setting. J Acad Hosp Med. 2015;7(4):1.
29. Khwaja A. KDIGO clinical practice guidelines for acute kidney injury. Nephron. 2012;120(4):c179.
30. Joannes-Boyau O, et al. High-volume versus standard-volume haemofiltration for septic shock patients with acute kidney injury (IVOIRE study): a multicentre randomized controlled trial. Intensive Care Med. 2013;39:1535–46.
31. Palevsky PM, et al. Intensity of renal support in critically ill patients with acute kidney injury. N Engl J Med. 2008;359(1):7–20.
32. Bellomo R, et al. Intensity of continuous renal-replacement therapy in critically ill patients. N Engl J Med. 2009;361(17):1627–38.
33. Burchardi H. History and development of continuous renal replacement techniques. Kidney Int Suppl. 1998;66:S120–4.
34. Al-Jaishi AA, et al. Moist clinical epidemiology. Complications of the arteriovenous fistula: a systematic review. JASN. 2017;28:1839.
35. Joannidis M, Straaten HMO-V. Patency of the circuit in continuous renal replacement therapy. Crit Care. 2007;11(4):218.
36. Morabito S, et al. Regional citrate anticoagulation for RRTs in critically ill patients with AKI. Clin J Am Soc Nephrol. 2014;9(12):2173–88.
37. Stucker F, et al. Efficacy and safety of citrate-based anticoagulation compared to heparin in patients with acute kidney injury requiring continuous renal replacement therapy: a randomized controlled trial. Crit Care. 2015;19:91.
38. Gattas DJ, et al. A randomized controlled trial of regional citrate versus regional heparin anticoagulation for continuous renal replacement therapy in critically ill adults. Crit Care Med. 2015;43(8):1622–9.

39. Uchino S, et al. Continuous renal replacement therapy: a worldwide practice survey. The beginning and ending supportive therapy for the kidney (B.E.S.T. kidney) investigators. Intensive Care Med. 2007;33(9):1563–70.
40. Karakala N, Tolwani A. We use heparin as the anticoagulant for CRRT. Semin Dial. 2016;29(4):272–4.
41. van de Wetering J, et al. Heparin use in continuous renal replacement procedures: the struggle between filter coagulation and patient hemorrhage. J Am Soc Nephrol. 1996;7(1):145–50.
42. Oudemans-van Straaten HM, et al. Citrate anticoagulation for continuous venovenous hemofiltration. Crit Care Med. 2009;37(2):545–52.
43. Joannidis M, et al. Enoxaparin vs. unfractionated heparin for anticoagulation during continuous veno-venous hemofiltration: a randomized controlled crossover study. Intensive Care Med. 2007;33(9):1571–9.
44. Davenport A. Intradialytic complications during hemodialysis. Hemodial Int. 2006;10(2):162–7.
45. The Brain Trauma Foundation. The American Association of Neurological Surgeons. The Joint Section on Neurotrauma and Critical Care. Guidelines for cerebral perfusion pressure. J Neurotrauma. 2000;17(6-7):507–11.
46. Findlay MD, et al. Investigating the relationship between cerebral blood flow and cognitive function in hemodialysis patients. J Am Soc Nephrol. 2019;30(1):147–58.
47. Davenport A. Practical guidance for dialyzing a hemodialysis patient following acute brain injury. Hemodial Int. 2008;12(3):307–12.
48. Selby NM, McIntyre CW. A systematic review of the clinical effects of reducing dialysate fluid temperature. Nephrol Dial Transplant. 2006;21(7):1883–98.
49. Trinh-Trang-Tan MM, Cartron JP, Bankir L. Molecular basis for the dialysis disequilibrium syndrome: altered aquaporin and urea transporter expression in the brain. Nephrol Dial Transplant. 2005;20(9):1984–8.
50. Hoste EA, Dhondt A. Clinical review: use of renal replacement therapies in special groups of ICU patients. Crit Care. 2012;16(1):201.
51. Choi JY, et al. Nafamostat Mesilate as an anticoagulant during continuous renal replacement therapy in patients with high bleeding risk: a randomized clinical trial. Medicine (Baltimore). 2015;94(52):e2392.

52. Richtrova P, et al. The AN69 ST haemodialysis membrane under conditions of two different extracorporeal circuit rinse protocols a comparison of thrombogenicity parameters. Nephrol Dial Transplant. 2007;22(10):2978–84.
53. De Laet I, Citerio G, Malbrain ML. The influence of intraabdominal hypertension on the central nervous system: current insights and clinical recommendations, is it all in the head? Acta Clin Belg. 2007;62(Suppl 1):89–97.
54. Hunter JD, Damani Z. Intra-abdominal hypertension and the abdominal compartment syndrome. Anaesthesia. 2004;59(9):899–907.
55. Koyner JL, Parikh CR. Clinical utility of biomarkers of AKI in cardiac surgery and critical illness. CJASN. 2013;8(6):1034–42.
56. Ostermann M, et al. Recommendations on acute kidney injury biomarkers from the acute disease quality initiative consensus conference: a consensus statement. JAMA Netw Open. 2020;3(10):e2019209.
57. El-Khoury JM. Nephrocheck®: checkmate or reality check? Ann Clin Biochem. 2021;58(1):3–5.

Delirium

Arpit Aggarwal and Oluwole Popoola

1 Introduction

Delirium is one of the most commonly encountered complications in patients admitted to neurocritical care units. Several terms have been used to describe this syndrome like altered mental status, encephalopathy, acute confusional state and brain failure. Although these terms are used interchangeably it can create confusion among providers. For the purpose of this chapter, the term delirium will be used. Delirium is multifactorial and develops from complex interactions between risk factors and noxious insults [1].

2 Epidemiology

The prevalence and incidence of delirium varies across care settings, increasing with the complexity of the care setting, with highest rates in postoperative, intensive care units (ICU) and palliative care settings. Delirium is present in 10–23% of hospitalized patients, with an additional 24–31% of these

---

A. Aggarwal (✉) · O. Popoola
Clinical Psychiatry, University of Missouri, Columbia, MO, USA
e-mail: Aggarwalar@health.missouri.edu;
oluwolepopoola@health.missouri.edu

© The Author(s), under exclusive license to Springer Nature Switzerland AG 2022
N. Arora (ed.), *Procedures and Protocols in the Neurocritical Care Unit*, https://doi.org/10.1007/978-3-030-90225-4_31

patients developing delirium during hospitalization [2, 3]. A systematic review of critically ill adults admitted to the ICU estimates that a third of these patients have delirium [4]. Whereas, among neurocritical care unit patients, the prevalence of delirium ranges between 12–46% and the incidence is between 23.6–26.8% [5, 6].

Delirium is more common among the elderly across care settings, with prevalence rates as high as 87% among elderly patients admitted to the ICU [7]. Among neurocritical care unit patients, the median and mean ages of patients with delirium are 62 and 69 years respectively [5, 6]. Hospitalized men are generally more likely to have delirium than women [2, 4, 5] which also holds true for patients in the neurocritical care unit [6].

3 Risk Factors

Risk factors for delirium can be viewed as predisposing and precipitating factors [8]. Delirium results from a complex interplay of predisposing factors, precipitating factors and context of care. Patients with higher vulnerability (more predisposing factors), need only mild precipitating factors to trigger delirium. Whereas, in less vulnerable patients (fewer predisposing factors), delirium is more likely to result from serious precipitating factors. While addressing precipitating factors is essential to the immediate management of delirium, addressing predisposing factors is critical to mitigating future episodes of delirium and the negative outcomes associated with it [8].

Predisposing factors of delirium include [9].

- Advanced age (over 65 years)
- Pre-existing cognitive impairment such as dementia
- Malnutrition and dehydration
- Sensory deprivation such as hearing or visual impairments
- Impaired functional status

- Severe medical diseases such as chronic renal and liver diseases, neurological diseases
- Multiple psychoactive, anticholinergic and sedative medications
- Chronic alcohol use.

General precipitating factors for delirium include [9–11]:

- Sedative-hypnotic and anticholinergic medications
- Polypharmacy
- Metabolic derangements
- Infections such as urinary tract infections and pneumonia
- Hypoxia, shock
- Fever or hypothermia
- Dehydration
- Severe acute illnesses
- Major surgeries such as orthopedic and cardiac surgeries
- Pain and prolonged sleep deprivation
- Recreational substance use and withdrawal

Precipitating factors that are unique to the neurocritical care unit [8, 12] are:

- Non-dominant hemispheric stroke,
- Head trauma
- Intracranial bleeding
- CNS infection (encephalitis, meningitis)
- CNS tumors
- Seizures
- Hypertensive encephalopathy
- Invasive mechanical ventilation.

4 Diagnosis

Delirium is essentially a clinical diagnosis. It is supported by clinical, laboratory, imaging and other diagnostic features of the predisposing, precipitating or etiologic factors. The diagnosis of delirium can thus be conceptualized into two parts: First, identifying delirium; and second, identifying the causes.

1. **Identifying delirium:**

   Identifying delirium relies on a detailed history and mental status examination. History can be obtained from the patient when possible. In most cases, due to cognitive deficits that limits reliability of the history obtainable from the patient, information can be gathered from patient's charts, caregivers, family members and acquaintances. A detailed alcohol and drug use history is particularly important as the approach to management of substance withdrawal delirium is significantly different from delirium due to other etiologies.

4.1 Clinical Presentation

The core symptoms of delirium include disturbances in attention (such as reduced ability to direct, focus, sustain and shift attention), awareness (such as reduced orientation to the environment) and another area of cognition (such as memory, perception, visuospatial ability and language). The timing and course of the development of these symptoms are key features of the history; they tend to have an acute onset and fluctuate in severity during the day [13]. Ancillary symptoms of delirium include disorganized thought process, mood alterations, altered sleep-wake cycle, altered level of consciousness, psychomotor agitation or retardation.

A mental status examination will reveal objective evidence of the cognitive disturbances in delirium. The Folstein Mini-Mental State Examination (MMSE), the Saint Louis University Mental Status (SLUMS) Exam and the Montreal Cognitive Assessment (MoCA) are useful tools that test attention, orientation and other relevant cognitive domains commonly affected in delirium [14–16]. Bedside tests of attention include the digit span; spelling "WORLD" backwards or recitation of the days of the week or months of the year backwards; and alternating alphabet recitation and counting (a verbal form of the Trails B test). If the patient is nonverbal, a handy test is to ask yourself if the patient looks back at you. Visuospatial ability can be assessed at bedside using the clock-drawing test or the intersecting pentagon copying test. Perceptual disturbances include illusions, auditory and visual hallucinations.

Role of Rating Scales

Rating scales serve different purposes in the assessment of delirium. They can be used as aids in the formal diagnosis of delirium or to measure severity and track its course. See Table 1 below for a list of validated delirium rating scales. The Confusion Assessment Method (CAM) is the most widely used delirium rating scale worldwide [17, 18]. It is an algorithm of four core symptoms of delirium, designed for use by nonpsychiatric clinicians to aid in the diagnosis of delirium in high risk settings. The CAM-ICU is an adaptation of the CAM, for use in ICU patients; and has been specifically validated in neurocritical care patients for the diagnosis of delirium. The Intensive Care Delirium Screening Checklist

Table 1 Different rating scales and its utility

Rating Scale	Utility	Patient population
Confusion Assessment Method (CAM)	Diagnostic	General hospital settings
CAM for Intensive Care Unit (CAM-ICU)	Diagnostic	Intensive care units
Intensive Care Delirium Screening Checklist (ICDSC)	Diagnostic	Intensive care units
Delirium Rating Scale (DRS)	Severity rating	General hospital settings
CAM – Severity Scale (CAM-S)	Severity rating and prognostication	General hospital patients and Intensive care units
Memorial Delirium Assessment Scale (MDAS)	Severity rating and monitoring	General hospital patients and intensive care units

(ICDSC) is another rating scale that has been validated for diagnoses of delirium among neurocritical care patients [6, 19, 20]. The Memorial Delirium Assessment scale (MDAS) has also been validated for use among critically ill patients admitted to the ICU. It is a 10- item scale that is administered after diagnosis of delirium is made, to determine severity and monitor its course [21]. Another modification of the CAM, the CAM-S, is useful in monitoring, risk stratification and prognostication of delirium [18].

Role of EEG, Neuroimaging and Biomarkers

The EEG in delirium is almost always abnormal. There are however no pathognomonic EEG patterns in delirium. Most cases of non-alcohol withdrawal delirium show generalized (diffuse) slowing – delta waves – and increased amplitude [22]. Therefore, EEG is helpful when the identification of delirium is obscured by other psychiatric co-morbidities. It could also be useful in identifying causes of delirium. Specific EEG patterns could suggest specific causes of delirium; for example, the presence of triphasic waves suggests underlying metabolic derangements such as hepatic encephalopathy [18].

No consistent neuroimaging correlates have been validated for diagnosing delirium. However, a recent systematic review of neuroimaging in delirium included studies that used MRI, f-MRI, arterial spin labelling MRI, CT, SPECT, diffusion tensor imaging, transcranial doppler, near infrared spectroscopy, proton MRI spectroscopy and 2-fluoro-2-deoxyglucose positron emission tomography. The systemic review found associations with white matter hyperintensities, lower brain volume, atrophy, dysconnectivity, impaired cerebral autoregulation, reduced blood flow and cerebral oxygenation, and glucose hypometabolism [23].

Various biomarkers have been explored in the diagnosis of delirium. Inflammatory biomarkers such as C-reactive proteins and interleukins have particularly been studied due to the central role that inflammation is thought to play in the development of delirium. However, none has yet been validated for diagnoses or monitoring of delirium [18].

2. **Identifying the cause of delirium:**

After delirium has been diagnosed, identification of the cause(s) becomes the principle task. This is sometimes obvious, especially in the neurocritical care patient population. However, a careful clinical evaluation for precipitants of delirium is essential since their correction is critical to effective management of delirium. Modifiable predisposing factors should also be identified as their correction would prevent future episodes of delirium. A thorough history, physical examination, medication review, laboratory tests, imaging studies and other indicated diagnostic studies should be performed.

The history could unravel temporal associations between onset of delirium and potentially related medical conditions such as development of a urinary tract infection, starting a new medication, cessation of alcohol use, etc. A medication review should correlate dosage initiation and changes with behavioral changes.

Physical examination could reveal signs of head trauma such as lacerations or bruises; signs of CNS infection such as fever and nuchal rigidity; signs of metabolic derangements such as asterixis; signs of stroke such as unilateral weakness and hyporeflexia; among others.

Brain imaging and a panel of basic laboratory tests geared at the most common causes of delirium should be ordered in every patient with delirium. More specific testing should be done if the clinical evaluation suggests more specific pathology. Examples include CSF studies, serum heavy metals, antinuclear antibodies, urine porphyrins and HIV.

5 Prevention

It is estimated that 30–40% of delirium cases are preventable [1].

Non pharmacological interventions that target modifiable risk factors of delirium have been shown to reduce the incidence of delirium [24]. Some of the interventions that have been shown to be effective include:

- Frequent reorientation by using clocks, calendars, clearly written daily schedules, windows with outside view and verbal re-orientation.
- Cognitive stimulation – This strategy is more helpful in patients with pre-existing cognitive impairments but at the same time sensory overstimulation should be avoided.
- Hearing and visual aids for patients with impairments, with frequent reinforcements to use them.
- Restoring physiological sleep-wake cycle by reducing ambient noise during night time and use of relaxing music.
- Minimum use of physical restraints and using range of motion exercises to promote early mobilization.
- Maintaining proper hydration and avoiding volume depletion.
- Minimizing use of medications that can precipitate delirium like benzodiazepines, antihistamines, dihydropyridines and opioids [25].
- Pain management: Pain is an important risk factor for delirium and clinicians should consider the risks of using an opioid medication that might worsen delirium, nonopioid medications should be used where possible.

Pharmacological interventions to prevent delirium have been studied using various agents like Cholinesterase inhibitors, antipsychotics, dexmedetomidine, gabapentin and melatonin but have shown mixed results and are not routinely recommended [26–31].

6 Management

Delirium is considered a medical emergency and early identification and treatment of the underlying medical condition is important. Treatment of delirium includes simultaneous management of behavioral disturbances and treatment of underlying medical conditions.

The most common medical conditions causing delirium include:

- Metabolic causes – electrolyte disturbances, infections, organ failures and fluid imbalance.
- Drug induced [32]
- Sedative or alcohol withdrawal
- Wernicke encephalopathy – Thiamine supplementation [33].

Treatment of agitation and behavioral disturbances include pharmacological and non-pharmacological interventions.

- Non pharmacological interventions – Mild cases of delirium may respond well to environment changes that target modifiable risk factors (discussed in the 'prevention' section above). Special units that implemented these changes have been shown to improve the functional outcome in patient who are at high risk for developing delirium [34]. Physical restrains should be reserved for the most severe cased and alternatives like continuous observation by a familiar person or a professional sitter should be used. Multicomponent interventions (e.g. promotion of sleep-wake cycles, meaningful sensory stimulation, preferred music listening, pre-operative patient education, stimulation of cognitive activities, use of orientation devices and effective communication) have been shown to be an effective intervention for delirium [35].
- Antipsychotic medications: There is mixed data regarding the efficacy of using antipsychotic medications to treat delirium. While antipsychotics appear to manage the agitation well, the total duration of delirium does not seem to improve much with their use [36]. No medications are currently approved by the US Food and Drug Administration (FDA) for the treatment of delirium and there is a boxed warning with use of atypical (second-generation) antipsychotics for increased risk of death and cerebrovascular events in patients with dementia [37]. Due to the longer clinical experience with Haloperidol, it remains the standard therapy for managing agitation in this patient population. However, other agents like risperidone, olan-

zapine, quetiapine and ziprasidone have shown similar efficacy in treating delirium [38].
- Benzodiazepines can be effective in cases of delirium due to alcohol and sedative withdrawals but they can worsen confusion and sedation in delirium due to other causes [39]. Other sedative agents like propofol and dexmedetomidine are sometimes used in the critical care settings for management of pain and anxiety in delirium patients.

7 Outcomes

Critically ill patients in the ICU who develop delirium have higher morbidity burden including increased length of ICU stays, longer duration on mechanical ventilation, worsened cognitive function, and increased costs. Delirium in the ICU has been shown to be associated with up to 2-3-fold increase in duration of mechanical ventilation and 2-4-fold increase in time to ICU discharge [40, 41]. In addition, delirium is associated with increased rates of cognitive impairment at time of discharge and up to 12 months after discharge [42, 43]. Higher severity and longer duration of delirium is associated with increased odds of cognitive impairment [9, 10, 42, 43]. Longer delirium duration has also shown an independent association with disability in activities of daily living and worse motor-sensory function [11].

Patient with delirium are more likely to die during hospitalization and up to one year after hospitalization, when compared with those without delirium. The duration of delirium is also associated with mortality. Critically ill patients with delirium in intensive care units are 2 to 3 times more likely to die during hospitalization [4, 12], and 3 times more likely to die 6 months after discharge [4, 44]. Each day of delirium in the ICU is associated with 10% increase in 1-year mortality [42, 45].

While hyperactive and mixed-type delirium are more likely to attract attention and intervention from the care team, hypoactive delirium rates are notably higher among

ICU patients and associated with worse outcomes [46]. Though delirium is generally considered to be acute, signs of delirium can persist for 12 months or longer especially in patients with risk factors like dementia [47].

References

1. Inouye SK, Westendorp RG, Saczynski JS. Delirium in elderly people. Lancet (London, England). 2014;383(9920):911–22.
2. Levkoff SE, Evans DA, Liptzin B, Cleary PD, Lipsitz LA, Wetle TT, et al. Delirium. The occurrence and persistence of symptoms among elderly hospitalized patients. Arch Intern Med. 1992;152(2):334–40.
3. O'Keeffe S, Lavan J. The prognostic significance of delirium in older hospital patients. J Am Geriatr Soc. 1997;45(2):174–8.
4. Salluh JI, Wang H, Schneider EB, Nagaraja N, Yenokyan G, Damluji A, et al. Outcome of delirium in critically ill patients: systematic review and meta-analysis. BMJ. 2015;350:h2538.
5. Patel MB, Bednarik J, Lee P, Shehabi Y, Salluh JI, Slooter AJ, et al. Delirium monitoring in neurocritically ill patients: a systematic review. Crit Care Med. 2018;46(11):1832–41.
6. von Hofen-Hohloch J, Awissus C, Fischer MM, Michalski D, Rumpf JJ, Classen J. Delirium screening in neurocritical care and stroke unit patients: a pilot study on the influence of neurological deficits on CAM-ICU and ICDSC outcome. Neurocrit Care. 2020;33(3):708.
7. Pisani MA, McNicoll L, Inouye SK. Cognitive impairment in the intensive care unit. Clin Chest Med. 2003;24(4):727–37.
8. Inouye SK. Delirium in older persons. N Engl J Med. 2006;354(11):1157–65.
9. Gunther ML, Morandi A, Krauskopf E, Pandharipande P, Girard TD, Jackson JC, et al. The association between brain volumes, delirium duration, and cognitive outcomes in intensive care unit survivors: the VISIONS cohort magnetic resonance imaging study*. Crit Care Med. 2012;40(7):2022–32.
10. Girard TD, Jackson JC, Pandharipande PP, Pun BT, Thompson JL, Shintani AK, et al. Delirium as a predictor of long-term cognitive impairment in survivors of critical illness. Crit Care Med. 2010;38(7):1513–20.

11. Brummel NE, Jackson JC, Pandharipande PP, Thompson JL, Shintani AK, Dittus RS, et al. Delirium in the ICU and subsequent long-term disability among survivors of mechanical ventilation. Crit Care Med. 2014;42(2):369–77.
12. Salluh JI, Soares M, Teles JM, Ceraso D, Raimondi N, Nava VS, et al. Delirium epidemiology in critical care (DECCA): an international study. Crit Care. 2010;14(6):R210.
13. American Psychiatric Association, editor. Diagnostic and statistical manual of mental disorders. 5th ed. Washington, DC: American Psychiatric Association; 2013.
14. Cockrell JR, Folstein MF. Mini-mental state examination (MMSE). Psychopharmacol Bull. 1988;24(4):689–92.
15. Nasreddine ZS, Phillips NA, Bedirian V, Charbonneau S, Whitehead V, Collin I, et al. The Montreal Cognitive Assessment, MoCA: a brief screening tool for mild cognitive impairment. J Am Geriatr Soc. 2005;53(4):695–9.
16. Tariq SH, Tumosa N, Chibnall JT, Perry MH 3rd, Morley JE. Comparison of the Saint Louis University mental status examination and the mini-mental state examination for detecting dementia and mild neurocognitive disorder--a pilot study. Am J Geriatr Psychiatry. 2006;14(11):900–10.
17. Inouye SK, van Dyck CH, Alessi CA, Balkin S, Siegal AP, Horwitz RI. Clarifying confusion: the confusion assessment method. A new method for detection of delirium. Ann Intern Med. 1990;113(12):941–8.
18. Oh ES, Fong TG, Hshieh TT, Inouye SK. Delirium in older persons: advances in diagnosis and treatment. JAMA. 2017;318(12):1161–74.
19. Ely EW, Inouye SK, Bernard GR, Gordon S, Francis J, May L, et al. Delirium in mechanically ventilated patients: validity and reliability of the confusion assessment method for the intensive care unit (CAM-ICU). JAMA. 2001;286(21):2703–10.
20. Gusmao-Flores D, Salluh JI, Chalhub RA, Quarantini LC. The confusion assessment method for the intensive care unit (CAM-ICU) and intensive care delirium screening checklist (ICDSC) for the diagnosis of delirium: a systematic review and meta-analysis of clinical studies. Crit Care. 2012;16(4):R115.
21. Shyamsundar G, Raghuthaman G, Rajkumar AP, Jacob KS. Validation of memorial delirium assessment scale. J Crit Care. 2009;24(4):530–4.
22. Engel GL, Romano J. Delirium, a syndrome of cerebral insufficiency. J Chronic Dis. 1959;9(3):260–77.

23. Nitchingham A, Kumar V, Shenkin S, Ferguson KJ, Caplan GA. A systematic review of neuroimaging in delirium: predictors, correlates and consequences. Int J Geriatr Psychiatry. 2018;33(11):1458–78.
24. Hshieh TT, Yue J, Oh E, Puelle M, Dowal S, Travison T, et al. Effectiveness of multicomponent nonpharmacological Delirium interventions: a meta-analysis. JAMA Intern Med. 2015;175(4):512–20.
25. Clegg A, Young JB. Which medications to avoid in people at risk of delirium: a systematic review. Age Ageing. 2011;40(1):23–9.
26. Gamberini M, Bolliger D, Lurati Buse GA, Burkhart CS, Grapow M, Gagneux A, et al. Rivastigmine for the prevention of postoperative delirium in elderly patients undergoing elective cardiac surgery--a randomized controlled trial. Crit Care Med. 2009;37(5):1762–8.
27. Hirota T, Kishi T. Prophylactic antipsychotic use for postoperative delirium: a systematic review and meta-analysis. J Clin Psychiatry. 2013;74(12):e1136–44.
28. Li X, Yang J, Nie XL, Zhang Y, Li XY, Li LH, et al. Impact of dexmedetomidine on the incidence of delirium in elderly patients after cardiac surgery: a randomized controlled trial. PLoS One. 2017;12(2):e0170757.
29. Cheng H, Li Z, Young N, Boyd D, Atkins Z, Ji F, et al. The effect of Dexmedetomidine on outcomes of cardiac surgery in elderly patients. J Cardiothorac Vasc Anesth. 2016;30(6):1502–8.
30. Sultan SS. Assessment of role of perioperative melatonin in prevention and treatment of postoperative delirium after hip arthroplasty under spinal anesthesia in the elderly. Saudi J Anaesth. 2010;4(3):169–73.
31. de Jonghe A, van Munster BC, Goslings JC, Kloen P, van Rees C, Wolvius R, et al. Effect of melatonin on incidence of delirium among patients with hip fracture: a multicentre, double-blind randomized controlled trial. CMAJ. 2014;186(14):E547–56.
32. Carter GL, Dawson AH, Lopert R. Drug-induced delirium. Incidence, management and prevention. Drug Saf. 1996;15(4):291–301.
33. Hersh D, Kranzler HR, Meyer RE. Persistent delirium following cessation of heavy alcohol consumption: diagnostic and treatment implications. Am J Psychiatry. 1997;154(6):846–51.
34. Landefeld CS, Palmer RM, Kresevic DM, Fortinsky RH, Kowal J. A randomized trial of care in a hospital medical unit especially

designed to improve the functional outcomes of acutely ill older patients. N Engl J Med. 1995;332(20):1338–44.
35. Kang J, Lee M, Ko H, Kim S, Yun S, Jeong Y, et al. Effect of non-pharmacological interventions for the prevention of delirium in the intensive care unit: a systematic review and meta-analysis. J Crit Care. 2018;48:372–84.
36. Girard TD, Exline MC, Carson SS, Hough CL, Rock P, Gong MN, et al. Haloperidol and ziprasidone for treatment of Delirium in critical illness. N Engl J Med. 2018;379(26):2506–16.
37. Schneider LS, Dagerman KS, Insel P. Risk of death with atypical antipsychotic drug treatment for dementia: meta-analysis of randomized placebo-controlled trials. JAMA. 2005;294(15):1934–43.
38. Lonergan E, Britton AM, Luxenberg J, Wyller T. Antipsychotics for delirium. Cochrane Database Syst Rev. 2007;(2):CD005594.
39. Breitbart W, Marotta R, Platt MM, Weisman H, Derevenco M, Grau C, et al. A double-blind trial of haloperidol, chlorpromazine, and lorazepam in the treatment of delirium in hospitalized AIDS patients. Am J Psychiatry. 1996;153(2):231–7.
40. Shehabi Y, Riker RR, Bokesch PM, Wisemandle W, Shintani A, Ely EW, et al. Delirium duration and mortality in lightly sedated, mechanically ventilated intensive care patients. Crit Care Med. 2010;38(12):2311–8.
41. Lat I, McMillian W, Taylor S, Janzen JM, Papadopoulos S, Korth L, et al. The impact of delirium on clinical outcomes in mechanically ventilated surgical and trauma patients. Crit Care Med. 2009;37(6):1898–905.
42. Sakuramoto H, Subrina J, Unoki T, Mizutani T, Komatsu H. Severity of delirium in the ICU is associated with short term cognitive impairment. A prospective cohort study. Intensive Crit Care Nurs. 2015;31(4):250–7.
43. Pandharipande PP, Girard TD, Jackson JC, Morandi A, Thompson JL, Pun BT, et al. Long-term cognitive impairment after critical illness. N Engl J Med. 2013;369(14):1306–16.
44. Ely EW, Shintani A, Truman B, Speroff T, Gordon SM, Harrell FE Jr, et al. Delirium as a predictor of mortality in mechanically ventilated patients in the intensive care unit. JAMA. 2004;291(14):1753–62.
45. Pisani MA, Kong SY, Kasl SV, Murphy TE, Araujo KL, Van Ness PH. Days of delirium are associated with 1-year mortality in an older intensive care unit population. Am J Respir Crit Care Med. 2009;180(11):1092–7.

46. Meagher DJ, Leonard M, Donnelly S, Conroy M, Adamis D, Trzepacz PT. A longitudinal study of motor subtypes in delirium: frequency and stability during episodes. J Psychosom Res. 2012;72(3):236–41.
47. McCusker J, Cole M, Dendukuri N, Han L, Belzile E. The course of delirium in older medical inpatients: a prospective study. J Gen Intern Med. 2003;18(9):696–704.

Index

A
Absent brainstem reflexes, 623
Absent corneal reflex, 624
Acute ischemic stroke, 256, 257
Acute kidney injury (AKI), 651
Acute kidney injury network (AKIN) criteria, 651
Adenosine triphosphate (ATP), 550
Adult respiratory distress syndrome, 653
Airway access
  bronchoscopy
    airway evaluation, 92–94
    airway preparation, 91
    anatomy, 87–89
    basic and standard pre-procedure steps, 90, 91
    flexible bronchoscope, 87, 88
    history, 86
    indications, 89, 90
    patient sedation, 91
    pitfalls, 95, 96
    post-procedural care, 95
  infraglottic devices
    anatomy, 58, 59
    direct laryngoscopy, 60–67
    ETT, 57
    indications and contraindications, 57, 58
    insertion, 59
    video laryngoscopy, 67–71
  larynx, 44, 45
  mouth, 44
  nose, 44
  PDT
    advantage, 79
    bleeding, 85
    inadequate site, 86
    mobile trachea, 86
    pliable trachea, 86
    puncturing, 85
    technique, 79–85
  supraglottic device
    LMA, 50–57
    OPA and NPA, 46, 47, 49, 50
  surgical airway
    cricothyroidotomy, 73–76
    indications, 72, 73
    indications and contraindications, 72
    pitfalls and troubleshooting, 78, 79
    tracheostomy, 76–78
  trachea, 45
Airway pressure release ventilation (APRV), 419

Alcohol withdrawal syndrome (AWS)
  benzodiazepine-based protocol, 544
  management of, 536
  pharmacotherapy, 536–537
  primary literature, 538–543
  symptom-guided lorazepam, 537
Alpha-to-delta power ratio (ADR), 517
American Academy of Neurology (AAN), 618
American association for the study of liver diseases (AASLD), 138
American Epilepsy Society (AES), 384
American Society for Apheresis (ASFA), 579
Analgosdation, 284
Analgo-sedation, 277
Ancillary testing, 630–636
Angioplasty, 515
Anticoagulation, 589–590, 662, 663
Antipsychotics, 686
Apheresis, 579, 580
Apnea testing, 625–628
Arterial catheters
  indications, 39, 40
  pitfalls and troubleshooting, 41, 42
  technique/methods, 40
  types of kits, 40–42
Arteriovenous (AV), 661
aSAH-induced vasospasm, 511
Ascending cholangitis, 350
Ascitic fluid leakage, 149
Asymmetrical fascial thickening, 353
Atelectatic lung, 212
Atrioventricular fistula (AVF), 20, 588
Autoimmune diseases, 601
Aztreonam, 341

B
Baclofen, 159
Bacterial meningitis, 324, 328–335
Bag-mask ventilation (BMV), 47
Basilar artery vasospasm, 513
Basilic vein, 34
Bat sign, 483
Becker drain, 176
Bedside lung ultrasound in emergencies (BLUE) protocol, 212, 213, 485, 486
Behavioral pain scale (BPS), 282
Benzodiazepines, 279, 370
Bilevel positive pressure ventilation (BIPAP), 419
Bowel perforation, 149
Brain death
  ancillary testing, 618
  current evidence and guidelines, 636–640
  definition of, 617
  ECMO, 641, 642
  flow diagram for determination of, 638
  procedure for declaration of death
    absence of brain-stem reflexes, 617
    ancillary testing, 630–636
    apnea testing, 625–628
    certification and medical record documentation, 636
    clinical examination, 622–624
    diagnosis of, 619
    establishing irreversibility, 619, 620
    modified apnea test, 628, 629
    pre-apnea test recruitment maneuver, 630

pre-requisites and
exclusions, 620, 621
therapeutic hypothermia, 640,
641
Brain oxygenation monitoring,
184–186
Brain stem death, 258, 259

C
Candida auris, 328
Candida krusei, 328
Candida lusitaniae, 328
Candida tropicalis, 328
Cardiac arrhythmias, 522
Cardiac output (CO), 226, 447,
455
Cardiac tamponade, 125, 126
Cardiac ultrasound
right ventricular function and
pulmonary embolism,
231, 232
transthoracic views, 213, 214
apical four-chamber view,
216–218
inferior vena cava
longitudinal view, 218,
219
parasternal long-axis view,
215, 216
parasternal short-axis
view, 215–217
subcostal long-axis view,
217, 219
utility of
fluid responsiveness,
222–227
left ventricular systolic
function, 220–222
tamponade, 227–230
Cardiogenic shock, 28, 30,
456
Carotid artery, 16
Catecholamines, 552
Catheter-associated UTI
(CAUTI), 351

Cefepime, 342
Ceftaroline, 353
Central and lateral transtentorial
herniation, 299–300
Central fever, 319
Central venous catheters
(CVCs), 587, 588
canalization sites, 13
history, 13
non-tunneled CVCs
femoral approach, 16, 17
IJV, 16
indications, 13, 14
subclavian approach, 16
pitfalls, 18, 19
tunneled CVCs, 14
Central venous pressure (CVP),
458
Cerebral autoregulation curve,
293
Cerebral blood flow (CBF),
469–470, 631–633
Cerebral blood flow velocity
(CBFV), 512
Cerebral blood volume (CBV),
470
Cerebral microdialysis (CMD),
526
Cerebral perfusion pressure
(CPP), 245, 292, 502
Cerebral vasospasm, 511
Cerebrospinal fluid (CSF), 157,
175
Cervical traction
case presentation, 272, 273
definition, 265
Garner-Wells tongs
patient positioning, 268
pin placement, 270
pre-medication, 266
preparation, 267–269
traction/reduction, 271
indications, contraindications,
and caveats, 265,
266
post-procedural care, 271

Chest tube thoracostomy
  equipment preparation, 115, 118
  indications, 114
  patient preparation, 115
  pitfalls/troubleshooting, 123, 124
  pleural cavity, 113
  procedure, 118–123
Chlorhexidine, 166
Cholecystitis, 350
Cholinesterase inhibitors, 686
Chronic inflammatory demyelinating polyneuropathy (CIDP), 581, 606, 607
Cilostazol, 520, 523
Circle of Willis, 247
Cirrhosis, 139, 140, 149
Cisatracurium, 310
Cisternal irrigation, 521
Clazosentan, 520
ClearSight, 461
Clostridium difficile induced diarrhea (CDI), 350
Cold crystalloid infusion, 397
Colonization, 338
Coma, 622
Community-acquired meningitis (CAM), 321
Confirmatory tests, 630
Contaminated sample, 338
Continuous glucose monitoring systems (CGMS), 557
Continuous hemodynamic monitoring, 40
Continuous positive airway pressure (CPAP), 628
Continuous positive pressure ventilation (CPAP), 419
Continuous renal replacement therapy (CRRT), 585
  advantages of, 660
  anticoagulation, 662, 663
  diagnosing AKI, 651
  dosing, 661
  modes of, 658, 659
  neurocritical care patients, 666–669
  principles of, 657–658
  protocol decision for, 667
  regional anticoagulation, 663–664
  RIFLE/AKIN/KDIGO criteria, 652
  risk factors for renal injury, 650
  systemic anticoagulation, 664–665
Convulsive status epilepticus (CSE), 366
Cortical spreading depolarizations (CSD), 517
COVID-19 pandemic, 642
Critical Care Pain Observation Tool (CPOT), 283
CT angiography (CTA), 514
Cuffless tubes, 431
Cytarabine, 159

D

Dantrolene, 519
Decannulation, 436–441
Deep venous thrombosis (DVT)
  screening and diagnosis, 201, 202
  two-point DVT screen, 202–204
Delirium
  cause of, 685
  clinical presentation, 682–685
  epidemiology, 679–680
  identifying, 682
  management, 686–688
  neuroimaging and biomarkers, 684
  outcomes, 688, 689
  prevention, 685–686
  rating scales, 683, 684
  risk factors for, 680, 681
  role of EEG, 684
Dexamethasone, 552

Dexmedetomidine, 686
Diabetic ketoacidosis (DKA), 558
Dialysis, 581
Diastolic volume-pressure curve, 448–450
Diffusion-weighted and perfusion-weighted imaging (DWI/PWI), 516
Digital subtraction angiography (DSA), 515
Diltiazem, 519
Direct laryngoscopy (DL), 60–67
Distributive shock, 456
Disuse atrophy, 415
Diverticular abscess, 350
Drainage system, 175
Duke's criteria, 348
Dynamic CT perfusion scan, 516

E

Electroconvulsive therapy, 383
Electroencephalographic (EEG) patterns, 367
Electroencephalography (EEG), 517, 620
Electrolyte derangements, 565
Electrolyte management
  calcium management, 566–567
  electrolyte reference ranges, 566
  hyperkalemia management, 571
  hypophosphatemia, 568
  laboratory testing, 572
  magnesium management, 567–568
  phosphorus homeostasis, 568
  potassium management, 570–572
  sodium management, 572–576
Electrophysiological function, 634–635
Elevated ICP, 292
ELISA test, 350

Empyema, 114
End diastolic velocities (EDV), 243
Endotracheal intubation (ETI)
  advantages and adverse effects, 500–501
  anatomy, 502, 503
  confirming proper placement, 506
  indications and contraindications, 497–498
  induction, suggested dose, 500–501
  medications, 498–499
  neurocritical patient, 499–502
  preparation, 503–505
  protocol for, 507–508
  technique, 505–506
Endotracheal intubation protocol, 507
Endotracheal tube (ETT), 57, 58, 60, 64
Endovascular cooling, 398–399
Epidural hematoma, 166
Epilepsia partialis continua (EPC), 367
Esophageal cooling devices, 399
Ethanol, 535
European association for the study of the liver (EASL), 138
Extended length (XLT) tracheostomy tube, 430
External ventricular drain (EVD), 175–177, 180–182, 185, 187–189, 338
  advantages and disadvantages, 181, 182
  catheter passing, 180
  completion, 181
  Heiss self-retaining retractor, 179
  patient positioning, 177, 178
  patient preparation, 177–179
  securing catheter, 180, 181

Extracorporeal membrane oxygenation (ECMO), 641, 642
Extravascular lung water (EVLW), 471, 472

F
Fasudil, 519
Femoral approach, 16, 17
Femoral vein, 32, 33
Fever in Intensive Care Unit (ICU), 318
Fiberoptic intracranial pressure monitor, 182–184
Fidaxomycin, 350
Flotrac, 460, 488
Fluid overload, 469
Fluid responsiveness
  dynamic parameters, 224–227
  static parameters, 223, 224
Foam cuffed tracheostomy tubes, 431
Focused assessment sonography in trauma (FAST), 232–234
Folstein Mini-Mental State Examination (MMSE), 682
Fractional shortening (FS), 221
Frank-Starling curve, 447–448
Fresh frozen plasma (FFP), 590
Fundoscopy, 302
Fungal meningitis, 325–327

G
Gabapentin, 686
Gamma-aminobutyric acid (GABA), 535
Gauge system, 3
Glasgow Coma Scores (GCS), 510
Global end diastolic volume (GEDV), 472
Glucose homeostasis, 550–552
Glucose transporters (GLUT), 550
Glutamate dehydrogenase (GDH), 350
Gram-negative rod NVM, 342
Guillain-Barré syndrome (GBS), 580, 581, 605

H
Haemophilus influenzae (Hib), 332
Hagen-Poiseuille equation, 6
Haloperidol, 687
Haptoglobin, 525
Hemodialysis (HD), 588, 657
Hemodialysis catheters, 20, 22
Hemodynamic monitoring
  application, 487–488
  Bat sign, 483
  BLUE protocol, 486
  cardiogenic and non-cardiogenic pulmonary edema, 478
  determination of volume status, 488
  diagnostic threshold, 467
  dynamic air bronchograms, 480, 481
  fluid resuscitation
    arterial system, 446
    diastolic volume-pressure curve, 448–450
    Frank-Starling curve, 447–448
    isovolumetric contraction, 450
    mean systemic filling pressure, 451–452
    venous return, 452–454
  hemodynamic profiles of shock
    cardiogenic shock, 456
    distributive shock, 456

Index 701

    methods of assessment, 458–468
    septic shock, 455
  hyperechoic lines, 477
  intravascular volume status assessment, 445
  pulmonary edema, 477
  role of ultrasound artifacts, 475–482
    extravascular lung water, 471, 472
    fluid overload, 469
    image acquisition, 473, 474
    Neuro-Science Intensive Care Unit, 484–487
    real images, 482–487
  seashore sign, 476
  shock states characterization, 457
  stratosphere sign, 476
  technical application of, 462–466
  tools, 457
  ultrasonographic based techniques, 446
  venous return and cardiac output, 453
  venous return curve and diminished cardiac output, 454, 455
Hemofiltration (HF), 657
Hemothorax, 114
Heparin, 520
Herniation syndromes, 296–298
Hydrophilic guidewires, 42
Hypercalcemia, 566
Hyperglycemia and hypoglycemia
  glucose homeostasis, 550–552
  management of, 554–561
  NCCU, 552–554
Hyperkalemia, 415, 570
Hypermagnesemia, 568
Hypernatremia, 573
Hyperphosphatemia, 570
Hypertonic saline (HTS), 308, 309
Hypocalcemia, 566
Hypokalemia, 570
Hypomagnesemia, 567
Hyponatremia, 572
Hypophosphatemia, 568
Hypotension, 149, 470
Hypothermia, 382, 395

I
Iatrogenic vasospasm, 509
Immune system regulation, 603
Immune-related protein substitution, 603
Induced normothermia or hypothermia, 396
Induction agents, 416
Infective endocarditis (IE), 348
Inferior vena cava (IVC), 458
Infraglottic devices
  anatomy, 58, 59
  direct laryngoscopy, 60–67
  ETT, 57
  indications and contraindications, 57, 58
  insertion, 59
  video laryngoscopy, 67–71
InnerCool RTx® Endovascular cooling system, 398
Intermittent hemodialysis (IHD), 655
Internal jugular vein (IJV), 16, 32, 33
International League against Epilepsy (ILAE), 366
International normalized ratio (INR), 141
Intracardiac shunting, 31
Intracerebral hemorrhage (ICH), 412, 620
Intracisternal thrombolysis, 521

Intracranial access
  archaeological evidence, 173
  cerebrospinal fluid, 175
  ICP, 173, 174
    brain oxygenation
      monitoring, 184–186
    external ventricular drain
      placement, 177–182
    fiberoptic intracranial
      pressure monitor,
      182–184
    indications, 175–177
  neurocritical care, 174
  SDH
    indications, 186
    SEPS, 190, 191
    subdural drain, 187–189,
      191
Intracranial hypertension
  causes of, 294
  CBF monitoring, 293
  clinical features, 294, 295, 298
  definitive measures for
    management, 306
  elevated ICP, 293
  external lumbar drain, 311
  fundoscopic examination, 302
  general measures for
    management, 303–305
  herniation syndromes,
    296–298
  HTS, 308, 309
  indications for ICP
    monitoring devices, 298
  management of, 303, 305
  mannitol, 307, 308
  medications with doses, 309
  non-invasive modalities,
    301–302
  pathophysiology of, 290–293
  sedation, 310
  surgery, 305–306
  symptoms and signs in, 295
  therapeutic hypothermia, 311
Intracranial pressure (ICP), 173,
  174, 292, 295, 412
  brain oxygenation
    monitoring, 184–186
  external ventricular drain
    placement
    advantages and
      disadvantages, 181, 182
    catheter passing, 180
    completion, 181
    Heiss self-retaining
      retractor, 179
    patient positioning, 177,
      178
    patient preparation,
      177–179
    securing catheter, 180, 181
  fiberoptic intracranial
    pressure monitor,
    182–184
  indications, 175–177
Intracranial vasospasm, 509, 510
Intrathecal lidocaine, 166
Intravascular/implantable access
  devices (IVADs), 587
Intravenous immunoglobulin
  (IVIG), 602, 605
  adverse effect and
    management, 608–613
  clinical manifestations of,
    609–612
  CIDP, 606, 607
  composition, 602
  MAC formation, 602
  mechanism of action, 603, 604
  multifocal motor neuropathy,
    607, 608
  neurological diseases, 605
  neutralizes pathogenic
    cytokines, 602
  protocol for, 612
Intraventricular hemorrhage
  (IVH), 620
Introducer sheaths, 20, 22
Intubation, 416
Invasive transducer monitoring
  system, 298
Iopropyl alcohol, 167

Isovolumetric contraction, 450
IVC distensibility index, 224

J
Jackson sizing, 429

K
Ketamine, 279
Ketogenic diet, 382
Klebsiella, 342

L
Laryngeal mask airway (LMA)
  anatomy, 50, 51
  history, 50
  indications and contraindications, 51, 52
  pitfalls/troubleshooting, 56, 57
  techniques and methods, 52–55
  types of, 55, 56
Left ventricular ejection fraction (LVEF), 220
Left ventricular end-diastolic diameter (LVEDD), 221
Left ventricular end-diastolic pressure (LVEDP), 28
Left ventricular end-systolic diameter (LVESD), 221
Left ventricular systolic function, 220–222
Lemierre's syndrome, 346, 348
Licox, 182, 184
Ligamentum flavum, 159
Light's criteria, 347
Lindegaard index (LI), 513
Linear air bronchogram, 481
Listeria, 334
Logistic organ dysfunction system (LODS), 318
Lorazepam-based alcohol withdrawal protocol, 544
Low-molecular heparin (LMWH), 664
Lumbar drainage of CSF, 521
Lumbar puncture (LP), 333
  anatomy, 159, 160
  complications
    epidural hematoma, 166
    infection, 166, 167
    intrathecal lidocaine, 166
    needle deformation, 168
    post lumbar puncture headache, 167, 168
  contraindications, 159
  CT guidance, 165, 166
  fluoroscopy guidance, 162, 163, 165
  history, 157
  indications, 158, 159
  lumbar puncture kit, 160, 161
  needle gauge, 162
  position techniques, 160
  spine level location, 160
  Tuffier's line, 158
  types of needles, 161, 162
  ultrasound guidance, 162
Lung sliding, 475
Lung ultrasound
  abnormal patterns
    B-lines, 208–210
    BLUE protocol, 212, 213
    consolidation, 211, 212
    pleural effusions, 210, 211
    pneumothorax, 207, 208
  acoustic impedance, 204
  normal patterns
    A-lines, 206, 207
    lung sliding, 205, 206
    pleural line, 205

M
MACOCHA score, 414
Magnesium, 382

Mallampati classification, 414, 503
Mannitol, 307, 308
Mean arterial pressure (MAP), 292, 447
Mean flow velocity (MFV), 252, 254, 256
Mean systemic filling pressure, 451–452
Mechanical ventilation
  airway assessment, 412–413
  difficult mask ventilation, 414
  indications for intubation, 412
  intubation assessment, 414
  MACHOCHA variables, 415
  modes of ventilation
    APRV, 419
    considerations for, 415
    controlled vs assisted breaths, 418
    in neurologically injured patients, 418
    NIPPV, 419, 422
    PRVC, 419
    weaning protocol, 422–424
  predictors of difficult intubation, 413–415
  predictors of difficult ventilation, 413
Melatonin, 686
Membrane filtration, 585
Membrane plasma separation (MPS), 585
Meningitis, 321
Meningococcus (MCM), 328
Methotrexate, 159
Micro-RNA (mRNA), 526
Midazolam, 310, 387
Middle cerebral artery (MCA) vasospasm, 512
Milrinone, 522, 523
Mitral annular plane systolic excursion (MAPSE), 222
Modified Duke's criteria, 349
Multifocal motor neuropathy (MMN), 607, 608
Multimodality monitoring, 311
Multi-organ failure (MOF), 653

N
Nasopharyngeal airway (NPA)
  BMV, 46
  contraindication, 47, 48
  indication, 47, 48
  sizing, 47–49
  techniques and methods, 49, 50
Necrotizing fasciitis (NF), 353
Negative predictive value (NPV), 511
Neurocritical care society (NCS), 384
Neuro-critical care unit (NCCU), 289, 411, 552–554, 650
  AMP-C groups of microbes, 344
  antibiotics and CSF penetration, 335–337
  bacterial meningitis, 324, 328, 332–335
  blood-brain barrier, 317
  CAM, 321, 324
  CAM (bacterial) in adults, 322–323
  catheter related bloodstream infections, 352
  CAUTI, 351
  CDI, 350
  CSF findings, 333
  fever in ICU, 320
  fungal meningitis, 325
  infectious causes of fever, 321–328
  infective endocarditis, 348
  measurement of body temperature, 320
  musculoskeletal infections, 352
  non-infectious causes of fever, 354–355
  NVM, 338
  organisms causing NVM, 339

oro-pharyngeal infections, 348
protocol for fever management, 355–356
sino-pulmonary infections, 346, 347
skin and soft tissue infection, 353
toxic shock syndromes, 353
traumatic brain injury related meningitis, 345
UTI, 351
viral meningitis, 324
Neurogenic fever (NF), 319
Neuro-intensivist, 317
Neurological illness, 650
Neuromuscular blocking agents, 417
Neuromuscular disease, 415
Neuro-science intensive care unit, 484–487
Nicardipine, 519
Nifedipine, 519
Nimodipine, 518
Nitric oxide (NO), 520
N-methyl-D-aspartate (NMDA) receptors, 537
Nonaneurysmal PSAH (NPSAH), 510
Non-convulsive status epilepticus (NCSE), 367, 383
Non-invasive monitoring systems, 298
Noninvasive positive pressure ventilation (NIPPV), 419, 422
Non-steroidal anti-inflammatory drugs (NSAIDs), 671
Normal ICP waveform, 291
Normocapnia, 402
Normoglycemia, 402
Normokalemia, 402
Normomagnesemia, 402
Normoxia, 402
Nosocomial ventricular meningitis (NVM), 338, 341–343
NxStage, 585

O

Oropharyngeal airway (OPA)
BMV, 46
contraindication, 47, 48
indication, 47, 48
sizing, 47–49
techniques and methods, 49, 50
Oxyhaemoglobin, 509

P

Papaverine, 520
Paracentesis
anesthetizing, 144
ascitic fluid, 138
cessation of flow of ascitic fluid, 153
complications
acute kidney injury, 149
ascitic fluid leakage, 149
bleeding, 148, 149
bowel perforation, 149
hypotension, 149
infection, 149
contraindications, 140, 141
equipment selection, 143
fluid pocket localization, 151
indications, 138–140
lack of aspiration of fluid, 152
local anesthetic injection, 152
locations for needle entry, 143, 144
needle insertion, 145–147
patient positioning, 141, 142
patient preparation, 141
peritoneal cavity, 137
peritoneal fluid, 147, 148
post-procedural ascitic fluid leak, 153, 154
site of needle puncture, 141, 142
skin preparation, 142
types of kits, 150–152
Parasternal approach, 130
Passive leg raise (PLR), 226
Passy-Muir speaking valve, 437

Peak systolic velocity (PSV), 243
Penicillin (PNC), 334, 341
Pentobarbital, 310
Percutaneous coronary intervention (PCI), 31
Percutaneous cricothyroidotomy, 75
Percutaneous dilatation tracheostomy (PDT)
  advantage, 79
  bleeding, 85
  inadequate site, 86
  mobile trachea, 86
  pliable trachea, 86
  puncturing, 85
  technique, 79–85
Perforated viscus, 350
Pericardiocentesis
  apical approach, 129, 130
  cardiac tamponade, 125, 126
  complications, 132–136
  diagnostic pericardial fluid sampling, 126
  equipment, 127, 128
  management, 131, 132
  parasternal approach, 128, 130
  subxiphoid approach, 128, 129
Peripheral antecubital veins, 587
Peripheral intravenous catheter (PIVC)
  advantages, 9
  disadvantages, 9
  indications, 6, 8
  method of insertion, 8
  midline catheters, 9, 10
Peripheral vascular catheters
  French system, 4
  Hagen-Poiseuille equation, 6
  incidence, 3
  midline catheters, 9, 10
  PICC, 10–12
  PIVC
    advantages, 9
    disadvantages, 9
    indications, 6, 8
    method of insertion, 8
Peripherally inserted central catheter (PICC), 10–12
Phenobarbital-based alcohol withdrawal protocol, 545
Phosphorus homeostasis, 568
Plasma filtration, 581
Plasmapheresis, 580
Pleural effusions, 210, 211, 484
Pneumothorax, 114, 207, 208
Point-of-care ultrasound (POCUS)
  cardiac ultrasound (*see* Cardiac ultrasound)
  definition, 195
  echogenicity, 196
  FAST, 232–234
  lung ultrasound (*see* Lung ultrasound)
  positioning and probe control, 198
  probe selection, 196, 197
  vascular ultrasound
    access, 199–201
    DVT screening and diagnosis, 201–204
Polyvinyl chloride (PVC), 431
Popliteal vein (PV), 203
Port-CVCs, 589
Positive end expiratory pressure (PEEP), 628
Positive predictive value (PPV), 511
Positron emission tomography scan (PET Scan), 514
Post lumbar puncture headache, 167, 168
Posterior cerebral artery (PCA), 516
Post-traumatic vasospasm, 511
Pressure regulated volume control (PRVC), 418
Primary ventriculitis, 343
Prismaflex, 585

Prophylactic transluminal balloon angioplasty, 521
Propofol, 310, 499
Protocolized tracheostomy care, 435
Pulmonary artery catheters, 21
  history, 27
  indications
    cardiogenic shock, 28, 30
    intracardiac shunting, 31
    PCI, 31
    pulmonary hypertension, 30
    severe heart failure, 28
    shock, 28, 29
  pitfalls and troubleshooting, 36–38
  technique/methods, 31–35
  types of kits, 35, 36
Pulmonary artery occlusion pressure (PAOP), 458
Pulmonary artery pressure, 455
Pulmonary capillary wedge pressure (PCWP), 28, 455
Pulmonary embolism (PE), 201, 231, 232
Pulmonary hypertension, 30
Pulmonary infections, 346
Pulmonary vascular resistance (PVR), 30
Pulsatality index (PI), 245
Pulse contour cardiac output monitors (PiCCO), 459
Pulse pressure variation (PPV), 458
Pyridoxine, 382

Q

Quick Sequential Organ Failure Assessment (qSOFA), 319
Quincke needle, 161
Quinolones, 342

R

Radiological vasospasm, 510
Randomized controlled trials (RCTs), 606
Rapid 4-step technique, 76
Rapid sequence intubation, 499
Refractory status epilepticus (RSE), 367
Regional anticoagulation, 663–664
Regional citrate anticoagulation (RCA), 664
Regional heparin anticoagulation (RHA), 664
Relative alpha power variability (RAV), 517
Renal replacement therapy (RRT)
  comparison of modalities for, 656
  CRRT, 657–659, 661
  IHD, 655
  indications of, 651–653
  timing of, 653–655
Resistive index, 243
Reversal agent, 417
Rho-kinase inhibitor, 523
Richmond Agitation and Sedation Scale (RASS), 282, 544
Richmond Agitation and Sedation Score, 282
Right ventricular function, 231, 232
Riker Sedation-Agitation Scale (SAS), 282

S

Seashore sign, 476
Sedation and analgesia management
  drug selection, 279
  indications for, 278
  pharmacological agents for, 279–282
  sedation vacations, 283–284
  tools for objective measuring, 282–283

Seldinger technique, 75
Sepsis, 318
Septic shock, 455
Sequential organ failure assessment (SOFA), 318
Severe heart failure, 28
Shivering, 405, 406
Shock, 28, 29
Sickle cell disease (SCD), 259, 260
Simplified lung edema scoring system (SLESS), 485
Single-photon emission computed tomography (SPECT), 515
Sinusitis, 346
Skin and soft tissue infections (SSTI), 353
Skin counter warming, 401
Specialty catheters
  hemodialysis, 20, 22
  introducer sheaths, 20, 22
Spinraza, 159
Spontaneous bacterial peritonitis (SBP), 139
Spontaneous breathing trials (SBT), 423
Static methods, 458
Statins, 520
Status epilepticus (SE)
  acute symptomatic etiologies, 366
  alcohol abuse, 366
  autoimmune disease, 366
  benzodiazepines, 366
  convulsive status epilepticus
    anti-epileptic drugs, 370, 373–375
    clinical and electrographic seizures, 368
    current evidence, 384–387
    fourth therapy phase, 377, 381, 382
    initial therapy phase, 369–371
  NCSE, 383
  refractory and super refractory status epilepticus, 378–380
  second-therapy phase, 371, 372
  stabilization phase, 368, 369
  status epilepticus treatment protocol, 385
  third therapy phase, 372, 376, 377
  treatment of status epilepticus, 384
  drug toxicity/withdrawal, 366
  symptomatic and cryptogenic, 365
Stenosis, 256, 257
Stenotrophomonas, 341, 342
Stratosphere sign, 476
Streptococcus pneumoniae, 332
Stroke Outcomes and Neuroimaging of Intracranial Atherosclerosis (SONIA) trial, 256
Stroke volume (SV), 225
Subarachnoid hemorrhage (SAH), 241, 242, 255, 256, 412, 619
Subclavian approach, 16
Subclavian vein, 32, 33
Subcutaneous immunoglobulin (SCIg), 604
Subcutaneous insulin, 559
Subdural evacuating port system (SEPS) placement, 190, 191
Subdural hematomas (SDH)
  indications, 186
  SEPS, 190, 191
  subdural drain, 187–189, 191
Super refractory status epilepticus (SRSE), 367
Supraglottic device
  LMA, 50–57

OPA and NPA, 46, 47, 49, 50
Surface cooling (SFC), 397–398
Surgical airway access
   contraindications, 72, 73
   cricothyroidotomy, 73–76
   indications and
      contraindications, 72
   pitfalls and troubleshooting,
      78, 79
   tracheostomy, 76–78
Swan-Ganz catheter, 35, 36
Sympathetic storming, 319
Systemic anticoagulation,
   664–665
Systemic inflammatory response
   syndrome (SIRS), 318
Systemic vascular resistance
   (SVR), 447, 455
Systolic blood pressure (SBP),
   40, 621

T

Tamponade, 227–230
Targeted temperature
   management (TTM)
   conventional methods, 397
   endovascular cooling,
      398–399
   EVC, 399
   indications and
      contraindications, 396
   induction phase, 400, 401
   normothermia, 402
   oxidative stress, 395
   procedures, 399
   protocol, 400–405
   SFC, 398
   shivering, 405, 406
   techniques for, 397
   therapeutic hypothermia, 402
Therapeutic apheresis, 580
Therapeutic cytapheresis
   (hemapheresis), 581
Therapeutic hypothermia, 311,
   640, 641
Therapeutic plasma exchange
   (TPE), 581
   anticoagulation, 589–590
   AV fistula, 588
   centrifugation techniques, 586
   complications and
      monitoring, 594–595
   contraindications, 596
   CVC, 588
   definition, 579
   estimate plasma volume, 591
   immunoadsorption, 586
   indications of, 581–584
   mechanisms of action,
      583–584
   membrane filtration, 585, 586
   peripheral antecubital veins,
      587
   port-CVCs, 589
   principles, 583
   replacement fluids, 590–591
   therapeutic plasma exchange,
      592–593
   vascular access, 587
Thermodilution, 458
Thin-walled atraumatic needles,
   168
Thoracentesis
   definition, 103
   equipment and yourself
      preparation, 106, 107
   indications, 103, 104
   patient preparation, 104, 105
   pitfalls/troubleshooting, 110,
      111
   procedure, 107–109
3-Dimensional (3D) angiography,
   515
Thrombocytopenic purpura
   (TTP), 590
Time- averaged mean maximum
   velocity (TAMM), 247
Time of flight-MR angiography
   (TOF-MRA), 514
Toxic shock syndromes (TSS),
   353

Tracheostomy care
    characteristics and features of, 428–429
    chronic tubes, 427
    decannulation, 436–441
    guidelines, 441
    long-term care, 440, 441
    post-placement care, 433–436
Tracheostomy tubes, 430, 431
Transcranial Color Doppler (TCD) ultrasound, 247, 248, 511–513
    acute ischemic stroke, 256, 257
    brain death evaluation, 258, 259
    doppler shift equation, 243
    equipment, 246–248
    insonation angles, 244, 245
    intracranial vessels, 241
    low-resistance spectral waveforms, 243, 244
    pulsatality index, 245
    SCD, 259, 260
    spectral Doppler waveform, 243
    stenosis, 256, 257
    TBI, 258
    technique, 249–252
    transducer, 242
    vasospasm, 242, 252–256
Traumatic brain injury (TBI), 258, 412
Traumatic Brain injury related Meningitis, 345
Tricuspid annular plane systolic excursion (TAPSE), 232

U
Uniform Determination of Death Act (UDDA), 618
Urinary tract infection (UTI), 351

V
Vagal nerve stimulation, 383
Vascular access, 587
Vascular ultrasound
    access, 199–201
    DVT screening and diagnosis, 201–204
Vasospasm, 252–256
    cerebral vasospasm, 511
    diagnostic modalities
        cilostazol, 520
        cisternal irrigation, 521
        clazosentan, 520
        CTA, 514
        dantrolene, 519
        DSA, 515
        DWI/PWI, 516
        dynamic CT perfusion scan, 516
        EEG, 517
        estrogens and erythropoietin, 520
        fasudil, 519
        heparin, 520
        intracisternal thrombolysis, 521
        lumbar drainage of CSF, 521
        nitric oxide, 520
        papaverine, 520
        PET-scan images, 514
        prevention of, 518–521
        prophylactic transluminal balloon angioplasty, 521
        SPECT, 515
        statins, 520
        TCD, 511–513
        TOF-MRA, 514
        xenon (Xe)-133 clearance, 516
        xenon enhanced computed tomography, 516
    endovascular therapy, 523–524

pharmacological treatment, 522–523
protocol for, 525
treatment of, 521, 522
Venous return, 452–454
Venovenous (VV), 661
Ventilator-associated pneumonia (VAP), 346
Verapamil, 519
Viral meningitis, 324

W

Weaning protocol, 422–424

Whittacre needle, 161
Windkessel effect, 447

X

Xenon (Xe)-133 clearance, 516
Xenon enhanced computed tomography, 516

Z

Z-track technique, 145, 146

GPSR Compliance

The European Union's (EU) General Product Safety Regulation (GPSR) is a set of rules that requires consumer products to be safe and our obligations to ensure this.

If you have any concerns about our products, you can contact us on ProductSafety@springernature.com

In case Publisher is established outside the EU, the EU authorized representative is:

Springer Nature Customer Service Center GmbH
Europaplatz 3
69115 Heidelberg, Germany

Batch number: 08823220

Printed by Printforce, the Netherlands

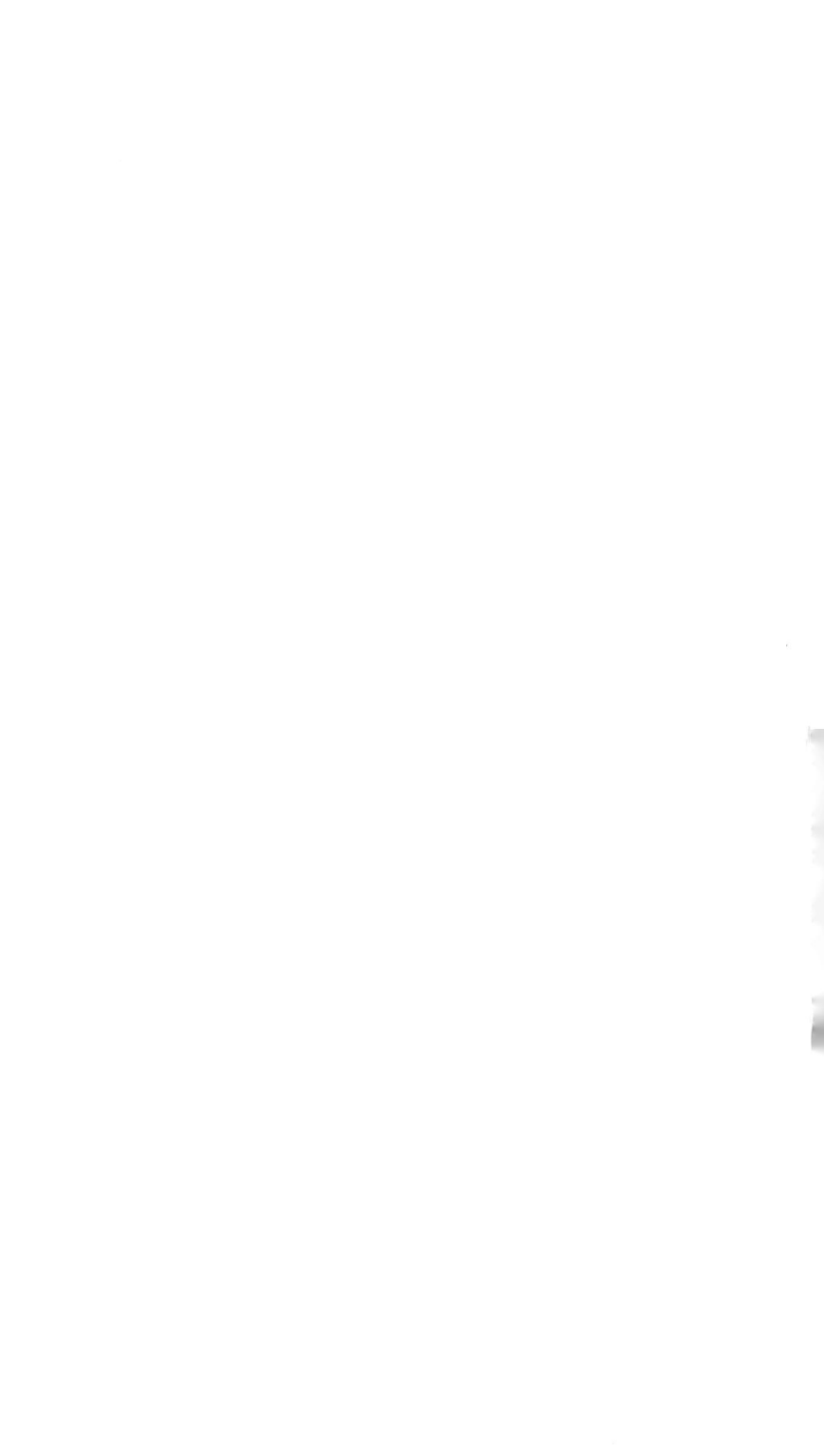